Neuropeptides

Cellular and Molecular Neuroscience
Charles F. Stevens, editor

Gary Banker and Kimberly Goslin, editors,
Culturing Nerve Cells, 1991

Gary Banker and Kimberly Goslin, editors,
Culturing Nerve Cells, second edition, 1998

Fleur L. Strand,
Neuropeptides: Regulators of Physiological Processes, 1999

Neuropeptides

Regulators of Physiological Processes

Fleur L. Strand

A Bradford Book
The MIT Press
Cambridge, Massachusetts
London, England

This book was set in Bembo on the Monotype "Prism Plus" PostScript Imagesetter by Asco Trade Typesetting Ltd., Hong Kong and was printed and bound in the United States of America.

Library of Congress Cataloging-in-Publication Data

Strand, Fleur L.
Neuropeptides : regulators of physiological processes / Fleur L. Strand.
p. cm. — (Cellular and molecular neuroscience series)
"A Bradford book."
Includes bibliographical references and index.
ISBN 0-262-19407-4 (hc : alk. paper)
1. Neuropeptides. I. Title. II. Series.
[DNLM: 1. Neuropeptides—physiology. WL 104 S897n 1998]
QP552.N39S73 1998
573.8′465–dc21
DNLM/DLC
for Library of Congress

97-52765
CIP

Contents

Foreword

Charles F. Stevens

It has been claimed that at least three of the seven deadly sins are mediated by neuropeptides. This book explains what the neuropeptides are, where they come from, and how they work.

Classical neuroscience focused on rapid synaptic transmission, but the slower neuromodulatory processes have been coming under increasingly intense study in the past several decades as the field has moved into the modern era. The time is at hand, then, to bring together what we have learned about the hormones of the brain, and this is the goal of Professor Strand in this book. The growth of the neuropeptide field has largely depended on new techniques that have made routine what could not even be imagined just a short while ago. Each methodological advance in our ability to manipulate peptides, from the protein sequencing methods half a century ago to the dazzling gene manipulation techniques of recent years, has fueled the exponential growth in our understanding of neuropeptides. Professor Strand has beautifully organized this information, from peptide biosynthesis and processing through targeting and secretion to the incredibly diverse peptide actions.

This work not only tells us where we are and places the neuropeptides in a larger neurobiological and evolutionary context, but it points out the directions the field will take in the future.

Preface

As an active researcher in the field of neuropeptides and as a teacher of a graduate course on neuropeptides, I have been inspired by the excitement of this robust area of neuroscience. The widespread occurrence of neuropeptides through evolution, their presence in the brain and in almost all peripheral tissues, their ability to act as hormones, neuromodulators, and neurotransmitters, forcefully indicate their importance as regulators of physiological processes.

My colleagues, my students, and I have all felt the need for a book that would comprehensively discuss the basic principles of neuropeptide action, such as their biosynthesis, processing, transport, and distribution. The powerful techniques of molecular cloning of genes and receptors, transgenic procedures, gene knockouts, and single-gene mutations contribute new insights into the mechanisms involved in neuropeptide action. These topics, as well as the intimate interaction between the neuropeptides, stress, and the immune system, are all discussed in the first part of the book, which provides insight into the common properties of the vast number of neuropeptides presently identified.

In the second part of the book, the regulatory functions of the families of neuropeptides are considered in sufficient detail to provide both the advanced student and senior investigators a thorough understanding of the most important neuropeptides. This is achieved by consideration of the actions of individual neuropeptides on several levels of regulation: evolution, molecular biology, distribution, receptors, second messengers, physiological and behavioral actions, and clinical implications. An attempt has been made to discuss the most significant facts and controversies based on experimental evidence wherever possible. A comprehensive summary at the end of each chapter focuses on the main concepts for easy review. For those readers who wish to delve deeper into the material, extensive up-to-date references are listed in the form of books, reviews of the literature, and original articles.

Additional neuropeptides are being discovered and new functions for "old" neuropeptides are reported constantly in almost every issue of scientific journals. The common thread throughout this book is an integrative, regulatory role for neuropeptides as they coordinate, integrate, and regulate physiological processes in all organisms. Neuropeptides have been shown to regulate physiological and behavioral processes during development, puberty, reproduction, regeneration, and senescence. It is anticipated that many fascinating questions will inspire new investigations: Is there is a window of time and a tissue-sensitivity that limits neuropeptide actions? Can one neuropeptide economically replace another in this vast family, or is there a fail-safe mechanism or sheer redundancy that governs their actions? How do the complex receptor subtypes function to regulate the reactions of the cell bombarded by the immense number of information-bearing molecules? We still have so much to learn but I hope this book will provide the fundamental information necessary to begin that quest.

Acknowledgments

It is a pleasure to acknowledge my gratitude and indebtedness to my colleagues who have critically reviewed this book, generously corrected errors or omissions, and made helpful suggestions. There will undoubtedly be further corrections needed as new information is forthcoming, but that lends excitement and vitality to this rapidly developing field. My editor, Michael Rutter of The MIT Press, has been an unending source of support through constant communication and encouragement in all aspects of this book, from the overall concept down to the complications of getting permissions for the cover art. I would also like to thank the many authors and publishers who generously permitted me to reprint their original material. Bill Boland, Editor of the *Annals of the New York Academy of Sciences*, deserves my special thanks for his patience with my many requests. Most of the library research was done in New York University libraries, and I am most indebted for the help I received from their librarians.

As part of my support system throughout my career, I am particularly grateful to David de Wied and Abba Kastin, leaders in neuropeptide research for many years, for their invaluable help, friendship, and advice.

There can be no adequate acknowledgment of the loving encouragement I have received from my husband and daughter while writing this book, despite the long hours taken from family life. The splendid meals prepared by Curt, his patience with my long hours at the computer and at the library, his loving reassurance and support when it all seemed too much to manage, have made my task much easier.

General Characteristics of Neuropeptides

I

The Neuropeptide Concept and the Evolution of Neuropeptides

1

1.1 The Neuropeptide Concept

Since the late 1960s and early 1970s when it was shown that the hypothalamic regulatory factors, stimulating and inhibitory, are peptides, that the endorphins and enkephalins are peptides, and that the gut peptides, such as cholecystokinin (CCK), vasoactive intestinal polypeptide (VIP), and somatostatin, are also produced in the brain, the intensity of research on peptides has increased enormously. What makes a peptide a neuropeptide? Several groups of scientists, working independently and sometimes together, showed that there was a dissociation between the classical endocrine effects of the peptide adrenocorticotropic hormone (ACTH) acting on the adrenal cortex, and ACTH effects on complex behavioral processes such as learning and memory. Furthermore, it was a clear indication that a peptide had a direct effect on the nervous system, a concept that has been fortified by the demonstration that synthetic fragments of ACTH, devoid of adrenocorticotropic action, were potent neuroactive molecules, both in the central and peripheral nervous systems. The demonstration that brain peptides have a direct effect on neurons, via specific peptidergic receptors, and that the peptides have highly specific physiological properties, led to the formulation of the neuropeptide concept, to which De Wied and his Utrecht group (De Wied, 1969) and Kastin and his colleagues in New Orleans (Kastin et al., 1979) have been the main contributors.

This concept, that peptides produced in the brain and gut have direct effects on neurons, took many years to gain the acceptance that it presently enjoys. Neuroactive peptides are the *neuropeptides* to be discussed in this book, but today the description of a neuropeptide is even more encompassing. Neuropeptides affect non-neural tissues and organs as well as neurons, and it has become increasingly clear that one of the most important functions of neuropeptides is the integration of the functions of the brain and the systems of the body. The long list of functions with which neuropeptides are involved include regulation of reproduction; growth; water and salt metabolism; temperature control; food and water intake; cardiovascular, gastrointestinal, and respiratory control; behavior; memory; and affective states. Neuropeptides are involved in many autonomic responses. They affect nerve development and regeneration. Neuropeptides may act as neurohormones, neuromodulators, or neurotransmitters and are often co-localized with the classical neurotransmitters such as acetylcholine (ACh) and the monoamines. Many peptides with neurogenic activities have been isolated from sources as disparate as frog skin, shark mouth, the invertebrates, and even plants; they affect mammalian tissues as well as their host tissues.

Neuropeptides may be divided into families with similar or identical genes that express large precursor molecules which may give rise to several family members. Often there is a strong evolutionary link between members of a neuropeptide family. Multiple neuropeptides may regulate a specific physiological or behavioral function such as food ingestion, sexual behavior, or reproduction. Consequently, in vitro models must be extrapolated with care into the whole organism as we try to unravel the complex coordination of the many neuropeptides involved in the regulation of physiological processes. The question to be considered seriously, therefore, is the specificity of all these neuropeptides and the possibility that they may constitute an evolutionary fail-safe series of redundant controls. These issues are being resolved today with the help of highly advanced molecular biology techniques, transgenic and genetic knockout animals, immunocytochemistry, high-performance liquid chromatography, and mass spectrometry. Of great importance has been the ability to clone peptide receptors, and the development of selective agonists and antagonists. The answers will probably be as revolutionary for our present ideas of physiology as the neuropeptide concept was for the classical field of endocrinology, but the rewards will be not only in basic science but also in applications to clinical therapies for many pathological conditions.

1.2 The Neuroendocrine System

Complex organisms require complex integrating systems for efficient function. Earlier concepts of integration of organ systems through the nervous and endocrine systems fused into the perception that, in many cases, these two regulating systems themselves were integrated into a neuroendocrine system. The concept of a neuroendocrine system in which neurons secreted hormones into the circulation was introduced by Ernst and Bertha Scharrer in 1937 and later expanded (1963). In the late 1940s intensive research demonstrated hypothalamic neurons to be rich in secretory material which could be localized not only in their soma but also in their axon terminals projecting to the pituitary gland. Our understanding of the neuroendocrine system has developed from the initial discovery of hypothalamic control over the secretions of the anterior pituitary gland, and consequently of its target endocrine organs, to the realization that endocrine secretions, in turn, influence neuronal function. Because several target endocrine organs, such as the gonads and the adrenal cortex produce steroid hormones, most of the earlier research concentrated on the relationship between these peripherally produced steroids and the central, regulating neurosecretory cells in the hypothalamus and pituitary gland. Demonstration of feedback control, chiefly negative, by the circulating steroids on the hypothalamus and pituitary reflected this intimate relationship.

In the last three decades, however, our understanding of the role of the hypothalamic and pituitary hormones, all of which are peptides, has been expanded greatly. The classic endocrine effects of these hormones have been shown to be only part of their repertoires. For example, the pituitary neuropeptide ACTH not only stimulates the adrenal cortex to produce corticosteroids but has profound effects on central and peripheral neuronal functions. These include cognitive abilities, such as memory, learning, and attention, as well as effects on the development and regeneration of peripheral neurons. To complicate matters further, ACTH is produced in many tissues and cells besides the hypothalamus and pituitary gland; it is produced in other brain areas, in the gastrointestinal tract, and by lymphocytes. A close interrelationship between ACTH and the immune system has been discovered and may help to elucidate the association between stress and disease. This diversity of site of production and of extraendocrine functions holds true for many, if not all, of the hypothalamic and pituitary peptides.

1.3 Nonendocrine Neuropeptides

ACTH is not the only neuropeptide present in nonendocrine cells, for a vast array of neuropeptides exists outside the neuroendocrine system. They are found in the brain, spinal cord, and almost all peripheral organs where they may act locally as autocrine, paracrine, or endocrine factors. The small-diameter sensory neurons of the spinal ganglia contain substance P, somatostatin, VIP, and CCK, among other peptides. The coexistence of neuropeptides with the classical neurotransmitters such as ACh, norepinephrine, or γ-aminobutyric acid (GABA) extends the dispersion of many neuropeptides to central, autonomic, and peripheral nerve terminals. This, together with the widespread distribution of the enkephalins, opiate peptides that mediate analgesia, and the rich reservoir of neuropeptides existing in the gut, indicates a regulatory role for neuropeptides that complements and greatly extends their endocrine functions.

1.4 Plasticity of Neuropeptides

The expression of genes for neuropeptides and their receptors is highly variable during ontogeny and later development. Some neuropeptides are expressed early in development, then suppressed as the organism matures, to be expressed once more if there is a marked change in metabolism or severe injury, such as nerve section (Hökfelt et al., 1994). Similarly, tissue responsiveness to a specific neuropeptide changes with maturation so that there is a "window of opportunity" for a given neuropeptide during which it may powerfully regulate physiological processes; once the window is shut, the neuropeptide is ineffective (Strand et al., 1991). Depending on the tissue substrate, the stage of development, the metabolic state, the presence or absence of other hormones, growth factors, or even neurotransmitters, neuropeptide action may be highly specific, merely permissive, or perhaps even redundant. Neuropeptides may play a fail-safe role so that in the absence of other regulatory factors, neuropeptides provide the necessary critical control.

1.5 Evolution of Neuropeptides

1.5.1 The Evolutionary Clock

The presence of neuropeptides in unicellular organisms and plants, as well as in invertebrates and vertebrates ranging from the lamprey to humans, indicates their basic importance as chemical messengers (table 1.1). Proteins appear to evolve at a constant rate (Zuckerkandl and Pauling, 1962). If mutations occur at a relatively constant rate one can use the amino acid sequence homology to determine the evolutionary time at which two related proteins diverged. This

Table 1.1
Some "vertebrate" neuropeptides found in unicellular organisms, plants, and invertebrates

Protozoa	Bacteria	Fungi	Plants	Invertebrates
ACTH	ACTH		TRH	ACTH/MSH
β-Endorphin	β-Endorphin		β-Endorphin	β-Endorphin
Insulin	Insulin	Insulin		Insulin
Gonadotropin	Gonadotropin			Glucagon
CCK				Gastrin
Calcitonin				GnRH
Somatostatin				Bombesin
				CCK
Glucagon				Angiotensin I
Vasotocin				ANH
				Pancreatic peptide
				Vasopressin
				VIP

ACTH, adrenocorticotropic hormone; ANH, atrionatriuretic hormone; CCK, cholecystokinin; GnRH, gonadotropin-releasing hormone; MSH, melanocyte-stimulating hormone; TRH, thyrotropin-releasing hormone; VIP, vasoactive intestinal polypeptide.

has been quantified into a system known as the unit evolutionary period, which is the length of time, in millions of years, needed for 1% of the amino acids to change in two related proteins. This permits the calculation of the time at which evolutionary divergence of various species occurred. As an interesting example consider the calculation of the evolutionary divergence of prolactin (PRL) and growth hormone (GH), two closely related neuropeptides. When the alignments of bovine, rat, and human GH and PRL sequences are compared using this method (figure 1.1), the separation of GH and PRL genes appears to have been established more than 350 million years ago (Miller et al., 1983).

1.5.2 Rules for Neuropeptide Evolution

Niall (1982) suggested, half-humorously, that there are four basic rules for peptide evolution:

1. Conserve the biologically important part of the molecule—you can play around with the rest.
2. Never make a new peptide if you can use an old one.
3. Everything is made everywhere.
4. Gene duplication is the name of the game.

1.5.2.1 Conservation of Structure

The structure of neuropeptides has been strongly conserved throughout evolution, indicating that mechanisms must exist to perpetuate these signal molecules. It has been suggested by Stefano (1989) that the evolutionary force may be the stereoselective nature of the neuropeptides, together with the other components of the signaling system, including receptors, processing enzymes, and inactivation. Logically this must require the simultaneous evolution of these components through the corresponding genes.

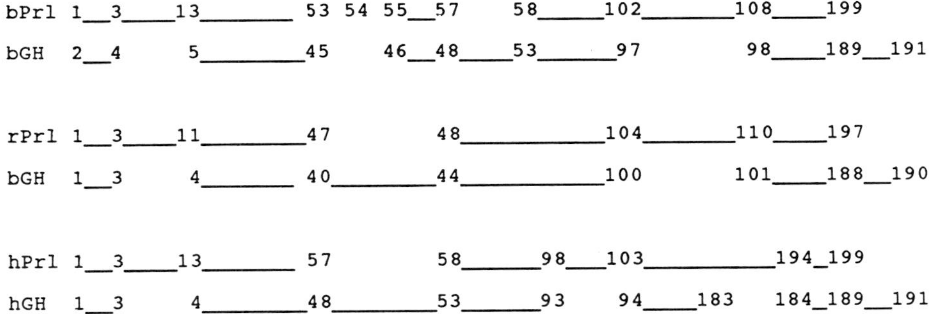

Figure 1.1
Alignment of prolactin (Prl) and growth hormone (GH) sequences from bovine (top), rat (middle), and human (bottom). (From Miller et al., 1983.)

Once this ancient integrated system had evolved in simple organisms it would probably remain intact in more complex animals, retaining or conserving the biologically active part of the molecule. For example, the mammalian insulins are very highly conserved with only one or two sequence differences between porcine, bovine, and human insulin, suggesting that almost all of the insulin structure is essential to its functions, which include not only binding to its receptor but probably also the regulation of the stereoselective processing of the biosynthetic precursor to insulin and the storage of insulin granules. On the other hand, porcine and rat relaxin, a peptide hormone produced during pregnancy, show little homology, with about half the amino acids differing in their sequences, indicating considerable divergence between these two species.

1.5.2.2 Never Make a New Peptide if You Can Use an Old One

Conservation of structure does not prevent the primitive system from gaining new functions. The economy of evolutionary development has resulted in the retention of the chemical structure of many neuropeptides even as their functions and receptors have changed. Prolactin, one of the oldest peptide hormones, has changed its function radically throughout evolution. In all species, from fish to humans, PRL is concerned with water and salt metabolism; in birds it is vital for the production of crop milk; in mammalian females it is responsible for lactation; and in mammalian males, including humans, PRL is involved in spermatogenesis, testosterone synthesis, and male libido.

The common ancestry of many neuropeptides is further suggested by the ability of peptides derived from plants, amphibians, fish, and lower mammals to activate physiological processes in humans. Morphine, an alkaloid of opium culled from a species of poppy, will produce the same effects in humans as the endorphins, a term imaginatively coined in 1975 by Eric Simon (Simon and Hiller, 1978) from "endogenous morphine." Thyrotropin-releasing hormone (TRH), a hypothalamic hormone, is also found in spinach. While the effects of these compounds in humans are well known, we have no idea as to their function in the plant. Neuropeptides from species as different as bacteria and humans often have similar effects on cells: human neuropeptides affect bacteria; human endorphins inhibit feeding behavior of bacteria; vasopressin from fish causes water retention in mammals.

1.5.2.3 Everything is Made Everywhere: Classification of Neuropeptides

One of the first attempts at classifying neuropeptides was based on their source, either as hypothalamic or pituitary peptides, as this was the first well-documented interrelated neuroendocrine system. The hormones of neurosecretory hypothalamic cells either stimulated or inhibited the release of the hormones of the anterior pituitary gland, forming a well-regulated neuroendocrine system. Furthermore, the hypothalamic hormones vasopressin and oxytocin were stored in the posterior pituitary gland, available for release into the circulation on appropriate stimulation. The subsequent discovery of these hypothalamic and pituitary peptides in several other discrete brain regions gave rise to the concept of the "endocrine brain," described so well by Dorothy Krieger (1979, 1981). The endocrine brain refers to a diffuse system of neurons, widely distributed throughout the central nervous system (CNS), that produce neuropeptides. These may reach their sites of action through axons, blood vessels, or the cerebrospinal fluid (CSF). The mechanisms that regulate the synthesis and release of brain neuropeptides differ from those controlling pituitary and hypothalamic neuropeptides, topics that are discussed in detail in later chapters.

The diversity of this system became more apparent when peptides considered to be "gut peptides," like CCK, were also found in the brain, and hypothalamic and pituitary peptides were found in the viscera or gut. Table 1.2 shows the wide dispersal of neuropeptides as it is presently known. A more functional classification is based on the similarity of neuropeptide structure, or amino acid sequence, permitting the division of neuropeptides into families, often with similar or overlapping roles (table 1.3).

1.5.2.4 Gene Duplication and Neuropeptide Families

Neuropeptides are formed from large precursor preprohormones and prohormones, which are progressively split by specific proteolytic enzymes. Several modulator sites exist in addition to the active site so that the chain can be considered a result of a multiple evolution. The amino acid sequence will influence the conformation of the active peptide chain, regulating its flexibility or rigidity. Our understanding of the evolutionary relationships of peptide hormones is incomplete, but the existence of families of neuropeptides indicates that they were generated through successive events of gene duplication within a common ancestral peptide. This process temporarily frees one part of the genome from selective pressure and permits a small error rate of mutation. Such duplication is a fundamental mechanism for increasing both the size and number of peptide chains. Similarly, new receptors and processing enzymes probably evolved from existing receptors through gene duplication and show familial relationships as befits their neuropeptide ligands and substrates, respectively.

This process has been described by Acher and Chauvet (1995) as the molecular model of neuroendocrine control of organismal functions—a neuroendocrine regulatory cascade which is dependent upon the conformational recognition of two molecules at each step. Each interaction causes a conformational change in the recognized protein, which in turn becomes a recognizer for the following molecule. The initial step involves the processing of the precursor polypeptide, followed by its passage into storage vesicles and ultimate secretion into the blood. The circulating hormone must recognize membrane receptors on its target cells. The receptors, in turn, transduce the message to the biochemical effector within the cell, leading to the specific physiological function. The cascade presumes that each step along the way relies upon specific molecular recognition and that the molecular components must have evolved synchronously. The complexity of the cascade in higher animals is due to subsequent differential processing of the precursor, the emergence of several types of receptors for each hormone, and the variety of effects triggered by second messengers while retaining the common fundamental structure.

Families such as the growth hormone family (which includes PRL), the insulin-like family, the enkephalins, the gut hormones, and the tachykinins have extensive amino acid sequence homology. For example, the tachykinins (substance P, neurokinin A, neurokinin B, eledoisin, and physalaemin) all share the amino acid sequence 7–11 of substance P. Another example is found in the three major branches of the opiate family: the large precursor molecule, pro-opiomelanocortin (POMC), contains three similar amino acid sequences of α-, β-, and γ-melanocyte-stimulating hormone (MSH). POMC also contains ACTH and β-endorphin. Similarly, the pro-enkephalin molecule contains six copies of met-enkephalin and one leu-enkephalin sequence, while the third branch of this family, pro-dynorphin, contains three leu-enkephalin sequences (figure 1.2). These multiple copies of related molecules are best explained by the concept of gene duplication, and the existence of distinct receptors for the peptide fragments lends credence to coordinated evolution mentioned above. The evolutionary success of this peptide system of communication requires the synthesis and processing of the neuropeptide; its storage, secretion, transport, and binding to receptor; and finally its metabolism. In most cases, a feedback system controlling the synthesis of the neuropeptide is involved. Such a complex system requires coordinated evolution.

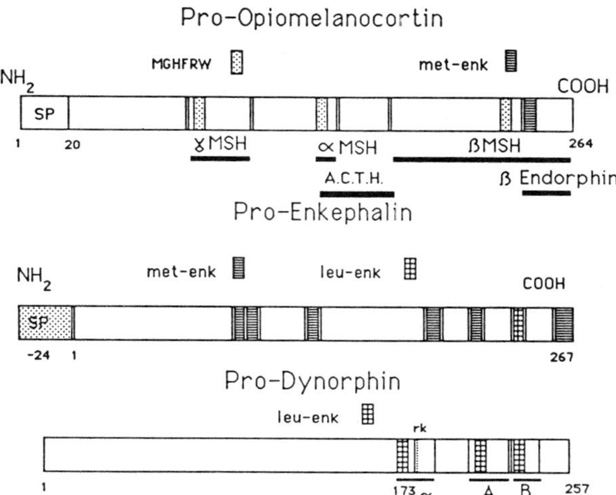

Figure 1.2
Structural relationships among the prohormone, precursor forms of the three major branches of the opiate peptides, depicted as bar diagrams. The length in amino acid residues is indicated by the number at the corresponding C-terminus. Basic amino acid sequences that are cleavage sites for processing are indicated by single or double vertical lines within the bars. SP, substance P; MSH, melanocyte-stimulating hormone; A.C.T.H., adrenocorticotropic hormone. (From Cooper et al., 1986.)

a. Gene duplication in the neurohypophyseal family

The neurohypophyseal hormones OT and VP have been examined in all classes of vertebrates and each species has two neurohypophyseal nonapeptides: the OT-like peptides, which are involved in reproduction, milk ejection, and uterine contractility; and the VP-like peptides, which have antidiuretic and pressor functions. The VP family of peptides have in common a basic amino acid residue at position 8, whereas

Table 1.2
Mammalian neuropeptides classified according to principal source (other sources in parentheses)

Hypothalamic Peptides
β-endorphin (pituitary)
Corticotropin-releasing hormone (pituitary, median eminence, brain, spinal cord)
Galanin (locus ceruleus)
Gonadotropin-releasing hormone (placenta, gonads?)
Growth hormone–releasing hormone (placenta)
Oxytocin[a] (posterior pituitary, brain, spinal cord)
Pituitary adenylate cyclase–activating polypeptide (hypothalamus, posterior pituitary, testis, pancreas)
Pro-opiomelanocortin (pituitary)
Somatostatin (brain, spinal cord, gut, salivary glands, excretory system)
Thyrotropin-releasing hormone (brain, spinal cord, gut, pancreas)
Tyr-MIF-1 (hypothalamus, cerebral cortex)
Vasopressin[a] (posterior pituitary, brain, spinal cord, peripheral nerves)

Anterior Pituitary Peptides
Adrenocorticotropin (median eminence, brain, spinal cord, placenta, gut, lymphocytes)
β-Endorphin (median eminence, placenta, gut)
Follicle-stimulating hormone (median eminence, placenta)
Growth hormone (median eminence, placenta)
Luteinizing hormone (median eminence, placenta)
Melanocyte-stimulating hormone (median eminence, brain, spinal cord, peripheral nerves)
Prolactin (median eminence, brain, spinal cord, placenta)
Secretoneurin (brain, pituitary, adrenal medulla, retina)
Thyroid-stimulating hormone (median eminence, placenta)

Brain and Spinal Cord Peptides
Delta sleep–inducing peptide (hypothalamus, pituitary, adrenal medulla, milk)
Dynorphin
Endorphins (pituitary)
Met- and leu-enkephalin (myenteric neurons, peripheral nerves)
Neurotensin (cardiovascular system, gastrointestinal tract)

Gut and Pancreatic Peptides
Amylin
Calcitonin gene–related peptide (sensory systems, hypothalamus, thyroid, motor neurons)
Cholecystokinin (brain, pituitary, adrenal medulla, peripheral nerves)
Galanin (brain, spinal cord, almost all peripheral systems and organs)
Gastrin (pituitary, spermatozoa)
Gastric inhibitory peptide
Gastrin-releasing peptide[b] (spinal sensory ganglia, spinal cord, brain)
Glucagon (brain, median eminence)

Table 1.2 (continued)

Glucagon-like peptide-1
Insulin (neonatal brain, fetal liver)
Motilin (brain? peripheral nerves?)
Neuromedin B (spinal cord)
Neuropeptide Y (brain, peripheral nerves, adrenal medulla, vascular endothelium)
Opiates (brain, spinal cord, peripheral nerves)
Pancreatic polypeptide
Peptide histidine isoleucine (cerebral cortex, hypothalamus)
Neurotensin (median eminence, hypothalamus, pituitary, entire central nervous system)
Peptide YY (brain stem)
Secretin (brainstem, hypothalamus, cerebral cortex)
Somatostatin (hypothalamus, brain, spinal cord, thyroid, excretory system)
Substance P (brain, spinal cord, peripheral nerves)
Vasoactive intestinal polypeptide (salivary glands, cerebral cortex, hypothalamus, peripheral nerves)
Placental Peptides
Chorionic gonadotropin
Corticotropin-releasing hormone (pituitary)
Follicle-stimulating hormone (ovary)
Growth hormone (pituitary)
Growth hormone–releasing hormone (pituitary)
Inhibin (gonads)
Prolactin (pituitary)
Pro-opiomelanocortin (hypothalamus, pituitary)
Somatostatin (brain, spinal cord, gut, salivary glands, excretory system)
Thyrotropin-releasing hormone (brain, spinal cord, gut, pancreas)
Adrenal Medullary Peptide
Adrenomedullin (vasculature, pituitary, central nervous system)
Cardiac Peptide
Atrionatriuretic hormone (hypothalamus)
Blood Peptide
Angiotensin II (brain, pituitary, hypothalamus, pons)
Thyroid and Parathyroid Peptides
Calcitonin (lungs, adrenals, thymus, brain, neuromuscular junctions)
Parathyroid hormone (brain, hypothalamus)
Parathyroid-related protein (brain, vascular smooth muscle, milk, placenta, tumors)

[a] Produced in the hypothalamus but stored in the neurohypophysis and called neurohypophyseal peptides.
[b] Bombesin-like peptide.

Table 1.3
Families of neuropeptides based on structural similarities

Family	Abbreviation	Precursor
ACTH, MSH, and Opiates		
Adrenocorticotropin	ACTH	Pro-opiomelanocortin for all
Melanocyte-stimulating hormone	MSH	
β-Lipotropin		
β-Endorphin		
Bombesin-like Peptides		
Bombesin		Probombesin
Gastrin-releasing peptide	GRP	Pro-GRP
Neuromedin B	NMB	Pro-NMN
Rantensin		Proranatensin RT
Calcitonin Gene–Related Peptides		
Calcitonin		Procalcitonin
Calcitonin gene–related peptide	CGRP	Pro-CGRP
Cholecystokinin		
Cholecystokinin	CCK	Pro-CCK
Gastrin		Progastrin
Enkephalins		
Met-enkephalin		Proenkephalin A
		Proenkephalin B
Leu-enkephalin		Proenkephalin A
		Proenkephalin B
Dynorphin		Proenkephalin B
Glucagon, Secretin		
Glucagon		Proglucagon
Secretin		Prosecretin
Vasoactive intestinal polypeptide	VIP	Pro-VIP/pro-PHI
Peptide histidine isoleucine	PHI	Pro-VIP/pro-PHI
Pituitary adenylate cyclase–activating peptide	PACAP	Pro-VIP/pro-PHI
Gastric-inhibitory peptide	GIP	Pro-GIP
Growth hormone–releasing hormone	GHRH	Pro-GHRH
Glycoprotein Hormones		
Thyroid-stimulating hormone	TSH	Pro-TSH
Follicle-stimulating hormone	FSH	Pro-LH/pro-FSH
Luteinizing hormone	LH	Pro-LH/pro-FSH
Chorionic gonadotropin	CG	Pro-CG

Table 1.3 (continued)

Family	Abbreviation	Precursor
Insulin-like Growth Factors		
Insulin		Proinsulin
Insulin-like growth factors I and II		Pro-IGF-I and -II
Relaxin		Prorelaxin
Neurotensin		
Neurotensin	NT	Proneurotensin/proneuromedin
Neuromedin		Proneurotensin/proneuromedin
Angiotensin II	AT-II	Proangiotensin
Oxytocin, Vasopressin		
Oxytocin	OT	Pro-OT/proneurophysin I
Vasopressin (antidiuretic hormone)	VP (ADH)	Pro-VP/proneurophysin II
Vasotocin		Provasotocin
Pancreatic Polypeptides		
Pancreatic polypeptide	PP	Pro-PP
Neuropeptide Y	NPY	Pro-NPY
Peptide YY	PYY	Pro-PYY
Somatotropins		
Growth hormone	GH	Pro-GH
Prolactin	PRL	Pro-PRL
Placental lactogen (choriomammotropin)	PL	Pro-PL
Tachykinins		
Substance P	SP	α-, β-, or γ-Protachykinins for these tachykinins
Neurokinin A	NKA	
Neurokinin B	NKB	
Tyr-MIF-1		
MIF-1		
Tyr-MIF-1		
Tyr-W-MIF-1		
Tyr-K-MIF-1		

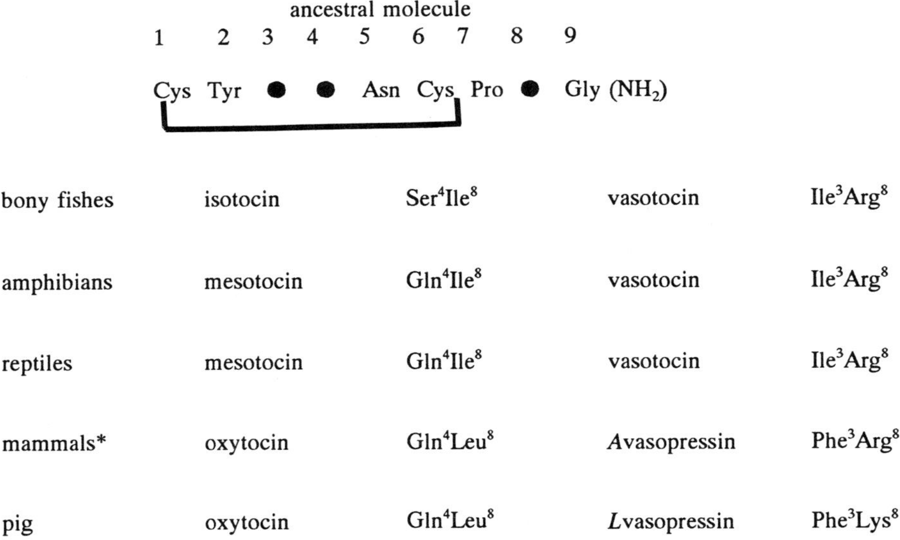

Figure 1.3
Hypothetical scheme of evolution of neurohypophyseal hormones. One gene duplication and a series of subsequent single substitutions in positions 3,4, or 8 produce two molecular lines. The substituted amino acids and their positions in a hormone are listed to the right of each hormone. All oxytocin-like peptides in column 2 have Il^3. *A*, arginine; *L*, lysine; *, except pig. (From Acher, 1980.)

the OT-related peptides have a neutral amino acid in this position. Duplication of the gene followed by mutation of residue 8 in one of the genes, resulted in the dual evolution of the two lines of peptides and their separate receptors (figure 1.3). The neurohypophyseal hormones are discussed in more detail in chapter 11. Gene duplication occurred before the appearance of elasmobranchs (cartilaginous fish) and teleosts (bony fish). Mammalian VP is probably derived from vasotocin, whereas the OT precursor was probably the mesotocin of amphibians. On the basis of calculations of the evolutionary distances and structural organization of precursors, Urano et al. (1992) suggest that this divergence occurred about 230 million years ago. Indeed, this may have occurred much earlier as invertebrates, such as the mollusc *Lymnaea*, appear to contain only a VP-like peptide which has the structural characteristics of VP and the functional attributes of OT (Van Kesteren et al., 1995). Precursor genes for these hormones antedate the appearance of the neurohypophysis in vertebrates and existed in the animal kingdom before the divergence of vertebrates and invertebrates, perhaps 700 million years ago. The invertebrate precursors are processed in exactly the same way as vertebrate precursors, suggesting that the processing machinery also predates divergence (Acher, 1995).

b. Gene duplication in the neuropeptide Y family: brain-gut peptides

Another excellent example of neuropeptide evolution may be seen in the neuropeptide Y (NPY) family. NPY, so named because it begins and ends in tyrosine (single-letter anino acid code Y; see appendix C), is a member of the pancreatic polypeptide (PP) family, which also includes the gut endocrine peptide YY (PYY) and pancreatic polypeptide (PP in tetrapods; PY in fish). Each of these peptides consists of 36 amino acids and a C-terminal amide. NPY has been extremely well conserved during vertebrate evolution and can be found in cartilaginous fish such as the shark and ray and also in the brain of cyclostomes (lampreys) which diverged from the main vertebrate line about 450 million years ago (Pieribone et al., 1992). There is an extraordinarily high sequence identity (92%) between the ray *Torpedo marmorata* and mammals, an evolutionary time distance of more than 400 million years (Blomqvist et al., 1992). There is perfect sequence identity in mammalian NPY except for the three artiodactyls, cow, sheep, and pig. Chicken NPY differs from human NPY by only one amino acid.

While there is some overlap, in general NPY is found in abundance in the central and peripheral nervous systems, PYY in the intestine and PP only in the pancreas, an organ found uniquely in vertebrates. Throughout evolution the pancreas has developed gradually into the anatomically discrete organ that contains four types of islet of Langerhans cells capable of producing four distinct hormones: insulin, glucagon, somatostatin, and PP. In animals lower than the sharks and rays, the islet cells produce two or three of these hormones, but not PP, which is only produced by the gut mucosa. Sharks and rays and the higher vertebrates all have the distinct four-hormone islet cell model. PYY is also produced by the gut endocrine cells so it has been suggested that since both PP and PYY are derived from gut mucosa, the PP gene arose from duplication of the PYY gene (Larhammar et al., 1993a), as depicted in figure 1.4. Figure 1.5 shows the alignment of all known NPY sequences. Conserved sequences are believed to represent functionally active portions of the molecule. Blomqvist et al. (1992) suggest that the strong sequence conservation of NPY implies that it has important physiological functions, acting either directly or through other molecules. Some of the functions influenced by NPY include blood pressure, food intake, circadian rhythms, and sexual behavior.

It is assumed that the common precursor molecule for NPY and its subgroups was expressed in neuronal cells as NPY and in gut endocrine and pancreatic endocrine cells as PYY, PY, and PP (see figure 1.4). Since PP acts on receptors distinct from the NPY and PYY receptors, the gene duplication of the NPY or PYY gene that gave rise to the PP gene was presumably paralleled or followed by a gene encoding an NPY or PYY receptor (Larhammar et al., 1993b).

c. *Significance of gene duplication*

The duplicated amino acid sequences can be enzymatically cleaved from the precursor molecule and can then exist as separate moieties or they can be colocalized in secretory granules. Even greater variation on this theme is acccomplished by differences in enzymatic cleavage and subsequent processing of the fragments in different tissues. Repetitive gene duplication could involve initial fusion of amino acid chains but eliminate fusion in the last steps, to result in several lines of homologous proteins, each with internal homology. Duplication may be the most efficient way to increase the size of the genome and then, through mutations, increase the number and functions of proteins. As a gene is duplicated a redundant copy is formed, permitting the original hormone to continue its function while the duplicate gene is free to mutate and interact with a structurally different set of receptors, which in turn have probably evolved

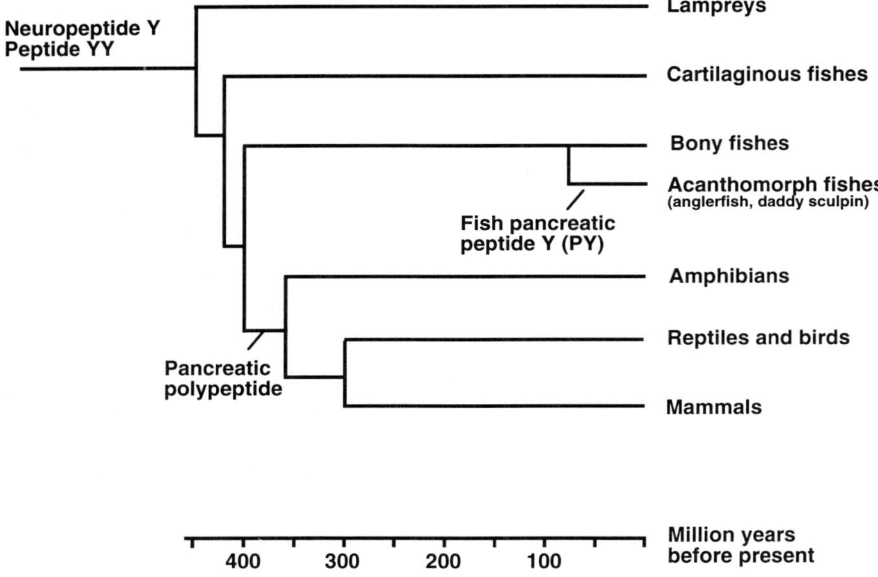

Figure 1.4
Probable gene duplication events in the neuropeptide Y (NPY) family shown in a schematic vertebrate evolutionary tree. Both NPY and peptide YY (PYY) were present in the ancestral vertebrate. Pancreatic peptide (PP) probably arose early in tetrapod evolution by duplication of the PYY gene. Fish pancreatic peptide (PY) may be an independent duplication of the PYY gene in acanthomorph fishes. Alternatively, acanthomorph PY may be a rapidly diverged form of the true PYY gene. (From Larhammar et al., 1993a.)

from existing receptors by their own process of gene duplication. Not all duplicate genes are functional but it makes evolutionary sense for a new hormone, slightly different from the original hormone, to establish a new hormone–new receptor complex, including the entire process of processing, secretion, transport, and binding rather than evolving an entirely new gene.

1.6 Summary

Early ideas of neuroendocrine control related to hypothalamic neuropeptides controlling pituitary secretion of tropic hormones, which in turn stimulated target endocrine organs. The neuropeptide concept, developed since the 1960s, widened this to include peptides produced by nerve cells and that have widespread extraendocrine functions. As many non-neural tissues have been found to produce the same peptides as neural tissues, it has become clear that neuropeptides serve to integrate the brain and organ systems, acting as neurohormones, neurotransmitters, and neuromodulators to maintain physiological homeostasis and influence important behavioral patterns. Neuropeptides are highly plastic in their actions, which vary according to age, tissue, metabolism, and the presence of other hormones or neurotransmitters.

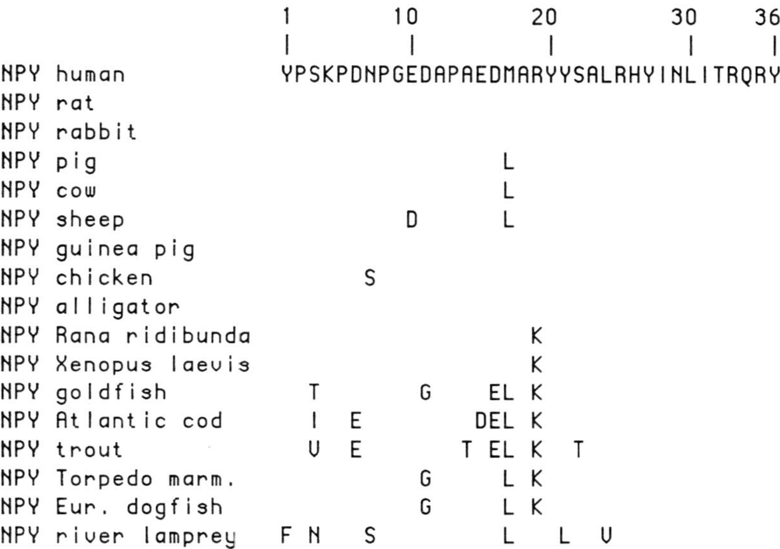

Figure 1.5
Alignment of neuropeptide Y (NPY) sequences. Only positions that differ from the top sequence are shown. Amino acids are shown according to their single letter codes (see appendix C) (From Larhammar et al., 1993a.)

The structure of many neuropeptides has been maintained throughout evolution, with the most important biologically active sequences conserved even though their function may have changed. Neuropeptides can be classified into families on the basis of the similarity of their amino acid sequences. Gene duplication is believed to be a fundamental process for neuropeptide evolution, accompanied by a neuroendocrine regulatory cascade that results in the coevolution of suitable receptors and regulatory molecules. The neurohypophyseal hormones OT and VP are excellent examples of gene duplication, as are the members of the NPY family.

Chapter 2 considers some of the many methods and techniques used to study the localization of neuropeptides and their enormously diverse functions.

Methods of Studying Neuropeptides

2

There are many ways to study neuropeptides and only an introduction to the concepts of the most frequently used techniques can be attempted here. Detailed descriptions of the exact methodologies of these and many more techniques may be found in the references for this chapter.

2.1 Bioassays

Classically, the bioassay is the technique used for the functional identification of a hormone based on the effect of administration of that hormone, usually to an animal from which the endogenous source of that hormone has been removed. Removal of the thyroid gland will result in several severe metabolic disturbances which can be returned to normal through the administration of the hormone thyroxine (T_4). These disturbances can be measured in the whole animal (metabolic rate, body temperature) or in the tissue slices, dissociated cells, or cell fragments from the organs that are the target for T_4. As most hormones have many effects, different assays are needed to investigate a specific effect, for example, the effect of T_4

on cell respiration (oxygen consumption, adenosine triphosphate (ATP) utilization) or induction of tadpole metamorphosis (tail resorption); the effect of ACTH on adrenocortical secretion (cortisol determinations at specific times of a 24-hour period); or hormonal effects on nerve regeneration (return of sensory and motor function).

In vivo bioassays also quantify the concentration of a hormone in tissue, plasma, or urine. However, most in vivo bioassays are not sensitive enough to measure normal or below-normal levels of the hormone. In vitro bioassays using complete organs, organ sections, or perfused organs permit more accurate and sensitive assays of hormonal effects on the target organ. The cytochemical bioassay developed by Chayen and Bitensky (1983) is an extremely sensitive technique. It is based on the development of a colored precipitate formed as a result of a hormone-dependent intracellular reaction. The precipitate is analyzed by microspectometry and microdensitometry and therefore requires highly specialized equipment.

2.2 Radioimmunoassays

The *radioimmunoassay (RIA)* was developed by Stanley Berson and Rosalyn Yalow in 1960. Yalow was awarded half the Nobel prize in 1977, with Roger Guillemin and Andrew Schally sharing the other half, for her work in endocrinology and the development of the RIA technique. (Stanley Berson had died before that date; the Nobel prize is not given posthumously.) The RIA is less sensitive and less demanding than the cytochemical assay but it is far more sensitive than the classical bioassay techniques, permitting the determination of physiological and subphysiological concentrations of hormones in the range of femtomoles (10^{-15} mol) of neuropeptide. The RIA has been the technique of choice of endocrinologists since the 1960s but has been considerably modified and refined since those early days.

For the RIA, neuropeptides, which are usually less than 50 amino acids long, must first be conjugated to a carrier protein to generate high-affinity and high-titer antibodies against these peptides. The conjugated peptide must then be labeled, usually with ^{125}I. Using monoclonal antibodies permits the production of almost unlimited amounts of high-affinity and high-specificity antibody. Monoclonal antibodies are single idiotype antibodies produced by immortal, monoclonal, hybridoma cell lines that are formed by the fusion of antibody-secreting spleen or plasma cells, and myeloma cell lines. A basic problem with RIAs is that the RIA results do not always conform to the physiological status of the organism since the number of antigenic sites in a sample is not always the same as the number of active hormone molecules (Chayen and Bitensky, 1983). This may be due to several factors: antibodies may react with only a small portion of a natural ligand, which may not be the biologically active portion; inactive metabolic products of the hormone may still retain immunoreactivity if the antibodies bind to the degraded portion of the hormone; or antibodies may bind to inactive precursors of the hormone. Consequently, RIA results are frequently considerably higher than those determined by bioassay. Despite these drawbacks, RIA remains the most convenient and accurate method of neuropeptide determinations and has been pivotal in characterizing the rhythms of the release of many of the hypothalamic and pituitary hormones.

It is now possible to produce designer antibodies by molecular biology techniques. Using the genome for a constant portion of the antibody, customized genes can be inserted for different regions and thus produce ultraspecific, high-affinity antibodies against almost any ligand (Bissette and Ritchie, 1992).

The *radioreceptor assay (RRA)* is more specific than the RIA for it quantifies the binding of a hormone to its biological receptor. However, it cannot distinguish between different forms of a hormone that may have different physiological effects, nor can it depict the cumulative binding that would be more characteristic of the physiological state (Bangham, 1983). An additional problem with RRAs is that they bind antagonists as well as agonists.

2.3 Immunocytochemical Techniques

2.3.1 Anatomical Localization of Neuropeptides

Immunocytochemistry permits the anatomical localization of specific peptides through their immunoreactivity as detected by specific antisera. Reactivity can be visualized at the light microscopic level using immunohistofluorescence, a technique first introduced by Falck et al. (1962) and used extensively to demonstrate the presence of monoamines and their pathways in the CNS (Dahlstrom and Fuxe, 1965; reviewed by Fuxe et al., 1985). More detailed structural analysis at both the light and electron microscope levels can be obtained through the use of immunoperoxidase methods. Reliable immunocytochemistry depends upon the raising of polyclonal and monoclonal antibodies to specific neuropeptides and is subject to the same constraints as discussed under RIAs, that is, the antibodies recognize biologically inactive parts of the peptide. Consequently, careful investigators usually refer to the reactivity as "-like," as in gonadotropin-like immunoreactivity.

Immunocytochemistry has clarified many neuroendocrine functions in the CNS, demonstrating the synaptic connections between transmitter systems and neuroendocrine cells, sites of neuropeptide synthesis and release, products of peptide processing, and the coexistence of transmitters and neuropeptides in secretory granules. Changes in peptidergic systems after manipulation of transmitter systems can be followed visually by immunocytochemical techniques and correlated with functional alterations resulting from these manipulations. Immunocytochemistry has been the basic technique leading to the concept of colocalization of peptides and transmitters (figure 2.1). It combines a high degree of specificity with the resolution of the light and electron microscope and the amount of immunoreactivity often can be quantified.

Combination of immunocytochemistry with other techniques is now used extensively to determine peptidergic neuronal pathways and synapsing transmission systems. Immunochemistry may be combined with *intracellular filling of neurons* with horseradish peroxidase or biocytin after electrophysiological characterization of the neurons to correlate anatomical and physiological characteristics. Immunocytochemical techniques together with *anterograde labeling* (e.g., from afferent fibers to postsynaptic neurons) and *retrograde labeling* (e.g., from terminals of motor neurons to connected premotor neurons) are used to characterize projection neurons. Biocytin and biotinylated dextrans are valuable anterograde tracers. The lipophilic fluorescent tracer 1,1-dioctadecyl-3-3-3′-3′-tetramethylcarbocyanine (DiI) can be used in vivo for either anterograde or retrograde tracing of axons. To follow chains of neurons across their synapses and even to follow peripheral nerves to their connections in the brain, live neuronal viruses are frequently used as transneuronal tracers. The viruses are replicated in the recipient neurons after anterograde or retrograde transport. Because the virus replicates so vigorously in the recipient cell, strong labeling can be detected with

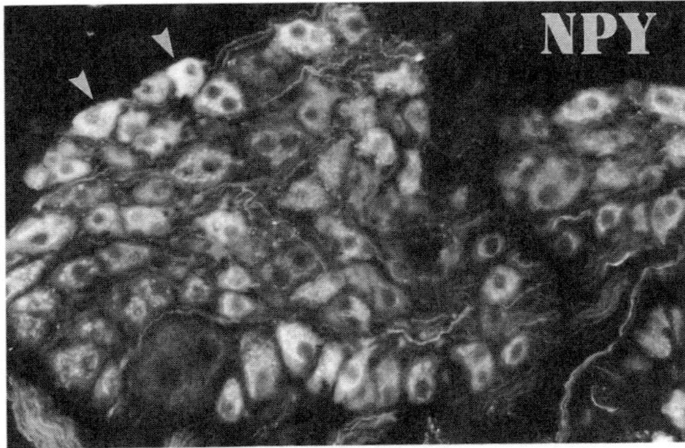

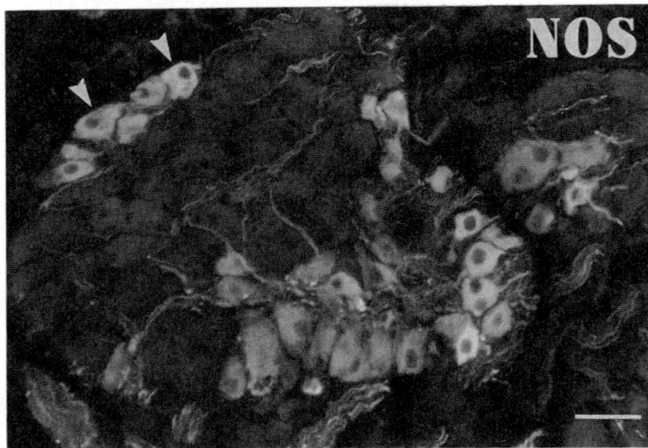

Figure 2.1
Immunofluorescence micrographs of section of the guina pig pelvic ganglion after double-staining for neuropeptide Y (NPY) and nitric oxide synthase (NOS). Almost all neurons contain NPY, which coexists with NOS in a subpopulation of cell bodies (arrowheads). Bar: 50 μm. (Courtesy of K. Holmberg, L. Elvin, and T. Hökfelt.)

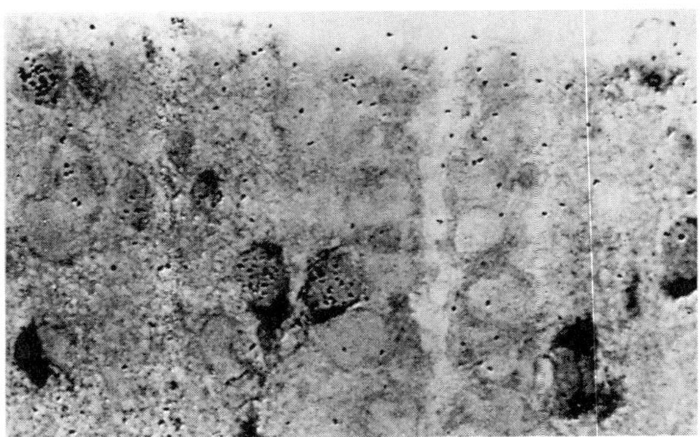

Figure 2.2
Thaw-mount autoradiogram of anterior hypothalamus prepared 1 hour after [^{3}H]estradiol injection into an ovariectomized colchicine-treated rat and stained by the immunoperoxidase method with somatostatin antibodies. Note the nuclear concentration of [^{3}H]estradiol in somatostatin neurons. (From Sar and Stumpf, 1989.)

immunocytochemical techniques. The live viruses used may be one of two herpesviruses or one of two rhabdoviruses (Kuypers and Ugolini, 1990). This valuable blend of methods elucidates neuronal circuits better than most other techniques.

Simultaneous localization of steroid hormones and neuropeptides in the same tissue preparation ingeniously shows the morphological relationships, and inferentially, the functional interdependence, of different hormones. This method combines *autoradiography* and *immunocytochemistry* (Sar and Stumpf, 1989). Steroid hormones regulate certain neuropeptide-producing cells by activating their genomes, and the visualization of their anatomical relationships can provide invaluable information about sites of action and sites of target cell response. An example of [^{3}H]estradiol simultaneously localized with somatostatin antibodies in the rat hypothalamus is shown in figure 2.2.

2.3.2 Localization by Cellular Activity: Immediate Early Genes

Immediate early genes are genes that are expressed early (within an hour) in response to a stimulus. They are themselves transcription factors, the products of which can evoke the transcription of the later expression of target genes. The transcription of immediate early genes is activated within minutes after the addition of a growth factor; the induction of these genes is transient and the levels of transcription return to normal, undetectable levels by 30 minutes after activation. Immediate early genes are rapidly and transiently expressed in active neurons, or in nondividing cells that are stimulated by growth factors, cytokines, or neuropeptides. Cellular activity can be marked through neuroanatomical techniques that locate immediate early genes within cells.

The best-studied immediate early genes are *c-fos* and *c-jun*. Fos, the protein of the *c-fos* gene, binds to Jun, the product of the *c-jun* gene, to form a heterodimer that regulates gene transcription. Figure 2.3 illustrates the induction of *c-fos* in spinal cord neurons after a brief, 30-minute treatment with α-MSH, a potent stimulus for neurite outgrowth. Fos immunocytochemistry requires a dramatic increase in neuronal activity to be a useful technique, but by

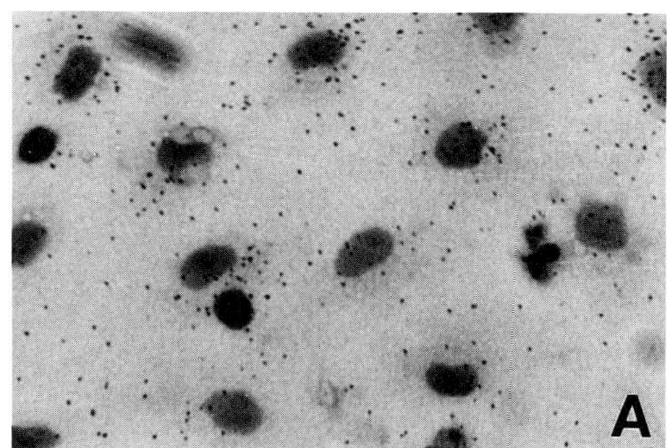

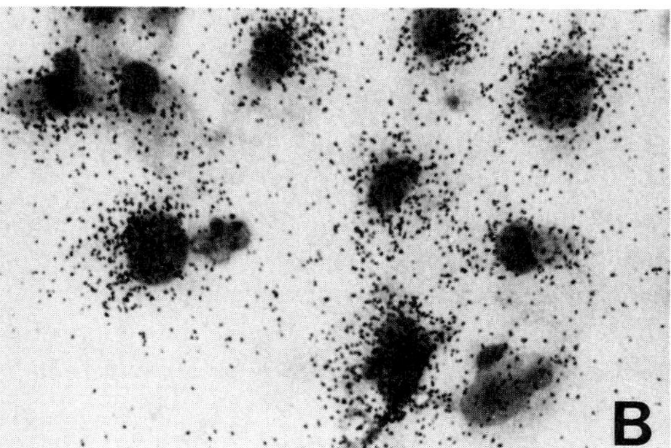

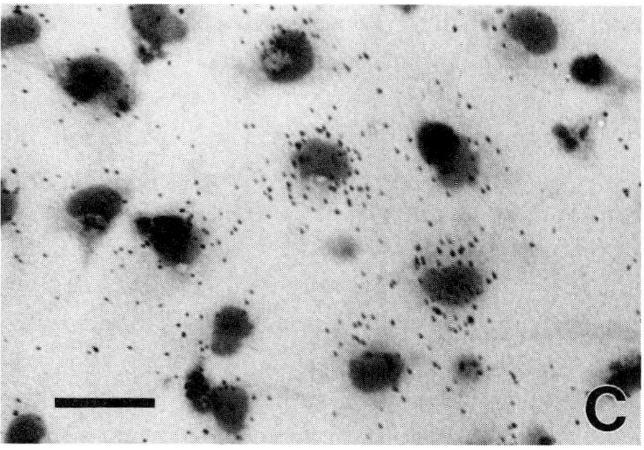

Figure 2.3
The expression of the immediate early gene *c-fos* upon a 30-minute treatment of spinal cord neurons with 10 μM α-MSH (melanocyte-stimulating hormone). Before treatment, the cells were deprived of growth factors. (A) Under control conditions, almost no *c-fos* mRNA is detectable. (B) *C-fos* expression is strongly induced after treatment with α-MSH. (C) The presence of the calcium chelator ethyleneglycoltetraacetic acid (EGTA) during treatment with α-MSH almost completely abolishes the induction of *c-fos*. Bar: 8.5 μm. (From Hol et al., 1994).

combining it with neuropeptide immunocytochemistry or with pathway tracing methods, it provides a powerful tool for defining activated neuropeptide and neurotransmitter pathways (Sagar and Sharp, 1992).

2.3.3 *Administration of Labeled Neuropeptides*

Important information can be derived from the localization of the target tissue or cell to which a peptide hormone binds. Visualization of the binding site generally relies on the direct radioactive labeling of the peptide and subsequent incubation of tissue slices or cell cultures with the labeled hormone, which is then identified through *autoradiography*. Labeling, or other techniques to identify the peptide, is necessary as the small size of the peptide makes most of the amino acids inaccessible to antibodies once the peptide is bound to the membrane receptor. Several other methods can be used to label the peptide, such as rhodamine labeling with subsequent *fluorescent microscopy*, or conjugation of the peptide with biotin followed by several steps which ultimately permit its visualization. Peptides can be conjugated with larger molecules such as ferritin or horseradish peroxidase, which are then more easily identified under the microscope. Another excellent technique involves labeling with colloidal gold which is especially well suited for *electron microscope studies* because it is electron-dense and can be obtained in a wide range of sizes (Jennes et al., 1989; Varndell and Polak, 1984). It must, however, be stated that in many cases there is a poor correspondence between the anatomical distribution of peptide-containing nerve fibers and terminals and the distribution of the expected binding sites. This discrepancy may be due to problems with lack of specificity of the ligands or the techniques used may label only the high-affinity receptors when perhaps only low-affinity receptors correspond to the release sites of the peptides.

2.4 Neuropeptide Receptors

Receptors for endogenous substances such as neuropeptides or for exogenous compounds like drugs have a dual function: to recognize the ligand with high specificity and affinity and to transduce the information from this messenger into cellular function. *Microscopic receptor mapping* is a procedure whereby receptors are selectively labeled and visualized microscopically on autoradiograms. This provides far greater anatomical resolution and sensitivity than biochemical binding methods. Receptors may be labeled in vivo or in vitro.

2.4.1 *In Vivo Labeling*

In vivo receptor labeling requires the systemic administration of the radioactive ligand, which, if it has a high affinity for the receptor, will bind in sufficient amounts to be detectable on the autoradiogram. Unbound drug will be excreted. This technique requires the removal of tissues for autoradiography and consequently the sacrifice of the animal. Many of the difficulties involved in in vivo labeling are eliminated in noninvasive procedures which use *positron emission tomography (PET)* (Kuhar, 1987): the selected ligand emits positrons that can be detected in the living organism. However, PET scans do not have very high resolution and require extremely expensive equipment and highly trained technicians. Another drawback is that the material being detected must be sufficiently metabolically stable to persist long enough to be measured. The comparable advantages and disadvantages of these techniques and their comparisons with biochemical receptor binding methods are clearly described by Grigoriadis and De Souza (1992).

2.4.2 In Vitro Labeling

In vitro visualization of receptors is amplified through image-intensified fluorescence microscopy and fluorophores, the most commonly used being fluorescein and rhodamine derivatives. This method is sensitive enough to detect a small number of receptors per cell or the limited number of reactive groups free for coupling of the fluorophore with small neuropeptides such as enkephalin, a 5–amino acid molecule (Blanchard et al., 1989).

Receptors can also be localized using the high-affinity *avidin-biotin complex*. Biotinylated peptide hormones, which retain their high binding affinity and biological activity, can be synthesized and target tissues exposed to the labeled hormone. The tissues can then be processed for immunocytochemistry using biotin-tagged antibodies to localize the sites of the neuropeptide hormone. However, since the advent of receptor cloning, in situ hybridization techniques have become the method of choice of most investigators to visualize the receptor messenger RNAs (mRNAs) and thus the cells that synthesize the receptors. The cloning of genes that code for many neuropeptides and their receptors has greatly facilitated the study of their structure, function, and regulation.

2.5 Measurement of Neuropeptide Release

2.5.1 In Vivo

2.5.1.1 Radioimmunoassay and Immunocytochemical Methods

These techniques can demonstrate the presence or absence of neuropeptides in discrete brain areas, but they are limited in their sensitivity and especially in their inability to detect dynamic changes. Measurement of the steady-state content of specific neuropeptides gives no information concerning the balance between their synthesis and utilization. However, an indirect method of measuring the in vivo dynamics of the synthesis and utilization of neuropeptide stores has been described by Mocchetti and Costa (1987). An evaluation of the gene expression of the neuropeptide precursor can be achieved using *complementary deoxyribonucleic acid (cDNA) hybridization analysis*, a technique that measures the accumulation or depletion of mRNA coding for specific neuropeptide precursors. The precursor content is then determined, as is the content of the biologically active peptide fragments processed from the precursor. A commonly used assay method for RNA-cDNA hybridization is the Northern gel blot on nitrocellulose which allows quantification of specific species of mRNA.

2.5.1.2 In Situ Hybridization Histochemistry (ISHH)

This is a powerful tool for studying the regulation of selected mRNA species in single neurons, a distinction that cDNA hybridization does not permit. This technique is based on the ability of radiolabeled DNA that is complementary to a specific mRNA to bind to specific mRNA in tissue sections. Either an oligonucleotide or an RNA probe is usually selected for ISHH. Oligonucleotide probes are single-stranded, short, and easily labeled. RNA probes are chosen when there are no nucleic acid sequence data for the genes encoding the mRNAs. The autoradiographic signal generated by either the oligonucleotide or RNA probe is detected by film and emulsion autoradiography, and the data analyzed using an image-analysis system recording optical density or grain count. The sections can then be counterstained (figure 2.4). The label is usually in the perikarya of

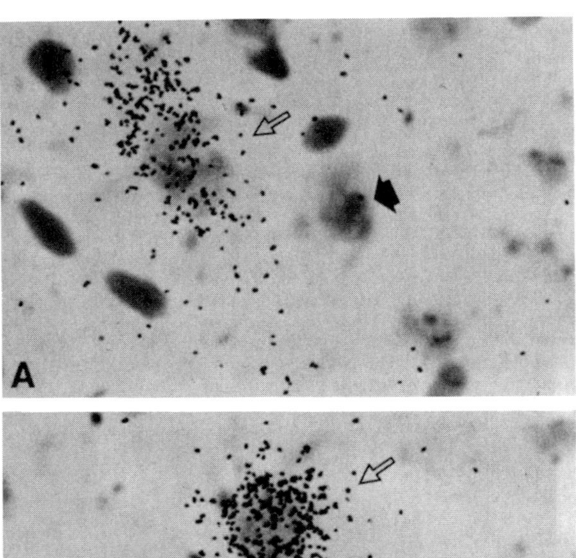

Figure 2.4
In situ hybridization with RNA probes. Sections of mouse brain were incubated with a sulfur 35–labeled RNA probe complementary to the mRNA coding for glutamic acid carboxylase. The open arrows point to labeled cells in the substantia nigra reticulata (A) and the cerebral cortex (B), Note the counterstained nuclei and the dense accumulations of silver grains over the unstained cytoplasm of the labeled cells, contrasting with the low background and the presence of unlabeled cells (solid arrows). (From Baldino et al., 1989.)

the cell because mRNA is confined mainly to the cell body. If one wants to localize both the hybridization signal and an immunohistochemical label within the same cell, immunohistochemistry is usually performed before in situ hybridization (Baldino et al., 1989).

2.5.1.3 In Vivo Sampling and Microdialysis

Pulsatility of neuropeptide release is an important feature of the mammalian neuroendocrine system and has been shown to be more effective than a continuous release of hormones into the circulation. Techniques have been developed which permit both sampling and administration of pulses of hormones in unanesthetized, freely moving rodents.

a. Sampling

To monitor peripheral hormone pulsatility, indwelling atrial cathers are used and the recommended sampling frequency is at least three times the maximal endogenous pulse frequency. Care must be taken to protect the animals from excessive loss of body fluids and concomitant stress; thus the duration of the experiments is usually limited to less than 5 hours.

b. Microdialysis

In microdialysis the duration of the experiments is almost unlimited as fluid is not directly withdrawn from the animal. The microdialysates are usually collected continuously and the longer the duration, the greater the absolute recovery rate of the neuropeptide. This technique is based on the concept that exchange of solutes will occur across a semipermeable membrane which separates a stationary fluid pool from a moving fluid pool. The direction and magnitude of the exchange depends on the concentration gradient. This technique and the sampling technique are described in detail by Levine et al. (1994). For the measurement of neuropeptide hormones in small structures such as

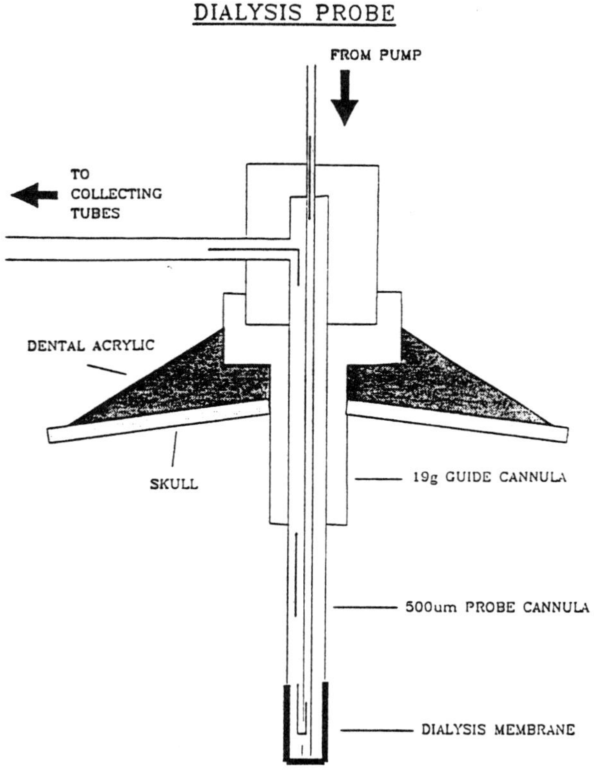

Figure 2.5
Diagram of a dialysis probe used for chronic implantation to monitor pulsatile release of neuropeptide hormones from the hypothalamus or pituitary gland of conscious, freely moving rats. (From Levine et al., 1991.)

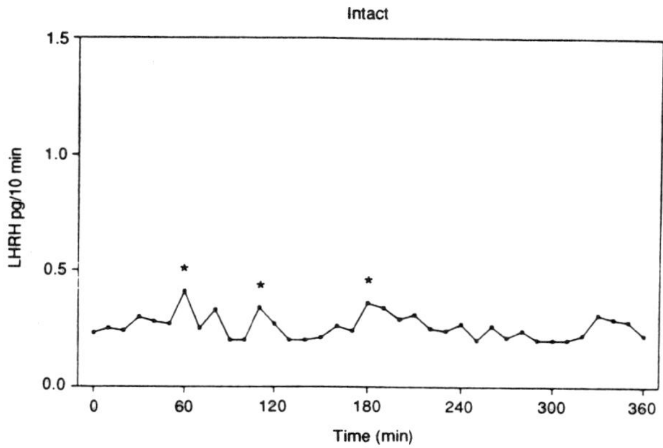

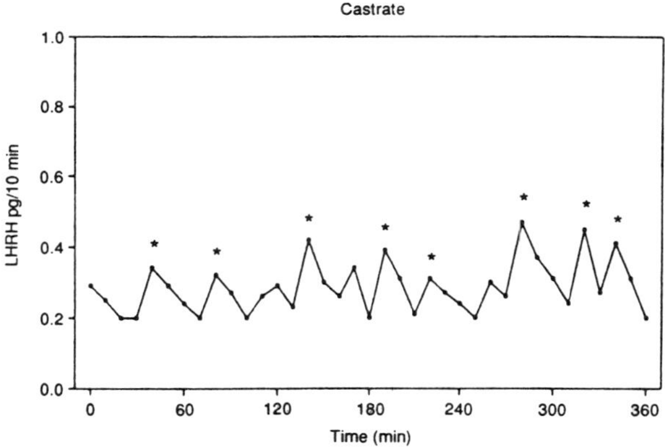

Figure 2.6
Pulsatile luteinizing hormone–releasing hormone (LHRH) patterns in intrahypophyseal microdialysates obtained from an intact and a castrated male rat. Pulse frequency was analyzed by ULTRA analysis and is clearly increased in rats deprived of testosterone. (From Levine et al., 1994.)

the hypothalamus or pituitary gland, stereotaxic coordinates are used to guide the placement of the microdialysis probes (figure 2.5). Figure 2.6 illustrates the marked increase in the frequency of pulsatile release of luteinizing hormone–releasing hormone (LHRH) that occurs in male rats after castration, due to removal of negative inhibition of testosterone on LHRH secretion. The disadvantage of microdialysis is that it recovers only very small amounts of neuropeptides.

2.5.1.4 Antibody Microprobes

The probes are coated with antibodies specific for a particular peptide and implanted into CNS tissue. The endogenous peptide in the extracellular fluid binds to the antibodies on the surface of the probe. The probe is then incubated in specific tracer in vitro, and after exposure to x-ray film the site of the endogenous peptide can be seen. This is not a quantitative method for neuropeptide release but qualitative comparisons under different experimental conditions can give a fair indication of relative release (Waterfall et al., 1994).

2.5.2 In Vitro

2.5.2.1 Perfusion Methods

Release of neuropeptides can be measured through the perfusion of synaptosomes, tissue slices, and small organs such as the posterior pituitary gland. These perfusion systems are all based on controlled infusion and withdrawal of the artificial, physiological perfusing fluid that bathes the organelles, tissues, or organs. The basal release is taken as a control value with which changes induced by the addition of stimulants or inhibitors of the system can be compared. Basal values may provide important information about the spontaneous release of neuropeptides, which is often of an oscillating, pulsatile nature.

2.5.2.2 Reversed-Phase High-Performance Liquid Chromatography (HPLC)

This method permits the evaluation of the synthesis, processing, and secretion of neuropeptides. Reversed-phase HPLC is a high-resolution analytical tool well suited for the separation and characterization of neuropeptides that are biologically active at the picogram to nanogram level. Figure 2.7 demonstrates the use of reversed-phase HPLC to study the metabolism of the proenkephalin A peptide, peptide E, which contains one copy of Met-enkephalin, one copy of Leu-enkephalin, and several other peptides. After enzymatic cleavage the separate fragments can be analyzed by reversed-phase HPLC, a method that is ideally suited for the separation of peptides that differ in structure by as little as the configuration of one asymmetrical carbon (Smith and Hanly, 1997). This technique is often combined with *micropunch dissection* of frozen sections, which enables the quantitative mapping of neurotransmitters and neuropeptides in specific, anatomically minute sections of the brain. Small pieces of tissue are punched out of brain slices, solubilized, and the amount of peptide measured by a specific RIA (Palkowits, 1973). When HPLC is combined with electrochemical detection and applied to micropunched tissue, much higher specificity and sensitivity are achieved (Kilts, 1992).

2.5.2.3 Cell Blot Assay

This is an in vitro method that measures hormone secretion by individual cells and thus can demostrate the functional heterogeneity of a tissue, such as cells of the anterior pituitary gland. Cells are incubated, then bound to a transfer membrane onto which the secreted hormones are bound. The membrane is then processed for the Western blot method as a result of which the released hormone becomes visible as a zone immediately surrounding the cell. The different secretion zones can be analyzed and quantified to differentiate between the secretions of the various anterior pituitary cells (Kendall and Hymer, 1989).

2.5.2.4 Reverse Hemolytic Plaque Assay

This technique permits the detection of hormone-secreting cells among a heterogeneous population of dispersed endocrine cells. A hemolytic plaque forms around the actively secreting cells when the cells are incubated as a monolayer with staphylococcal protein

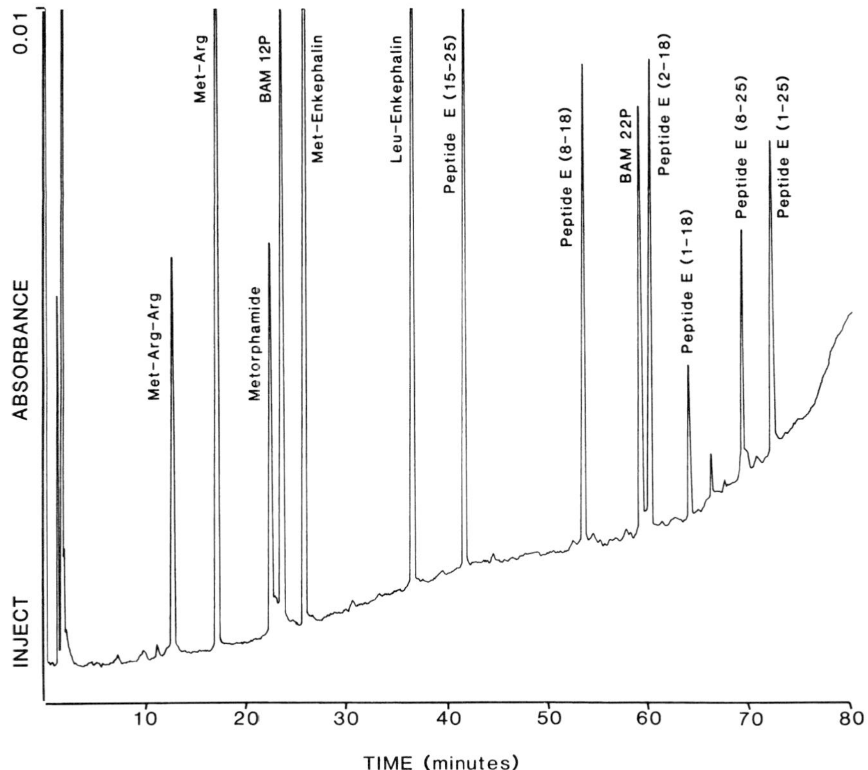

Figure 2.7
Reversed-phase high-performance liquid chromatography (HPLC) of peptide E (1–25) and 12 related fragments. Each peak represents 300 ng of peptide on the separation column. All HPLC peaks were confirmed by amino acid analysis of hydrolyzed samples. BAM, bovine adrenal medullary peptides. (From Davis, 1991.)

A–linked ovine erythrocytes in the presence of hormone antiserum and complement (Neill and Frawley, 1983). Electron microscopy can then define the ultrastructural features of the plaque formers to show the distribution of the neuropeptide in the subcellular compartments of the cell. Modifications of this technique make it possible to measure hormone release from individual cells in vitro (Castano et al., 1994).

2.6 Isolation and Characterization of Peptides

Many methods have been used for the isolation and characterization of peptides, including biological and chemical assays, peptide purification, peptide and nucleotide sequence determination, and molecular biotechnology. Peptides isolated on the basis of one biological function have usually been found to have many other functions. Peptides isolated on the basis of their chemical characteristics frequently have no known biological function, often because the biological activity depends on important post-translational modifications. On the other hand, many synthetic peptides, manufactured on the basis of their amino acid sequence in the precursor hormone, have potent biological effects, yet cannot be demonstrated convincingly to exist in physiological systems. The ACTH 1–39 neurotrophic fragment ACTH 4–10 has potent effects on behavior, nerve development, and regeneration, yet has not been shown to be processed endogenously from the parent molecule. However, the search for more potent peptides has produced some excellent analogs with more specific and longer-lasting effects than the endogenous peptide, a result that has both clinical and basic research benefits.

Some of the more frequently used methods of neuropeptide isolation and structure analysis are listed below:

2.6.1 Fast Atom Bombardment Mass Spectrometry

This is a new ionization technique which uses a particle beam consisting of the neutral atoms of xenon or argon. The gas atoms are first ionized and accelerated in the fast atom bombardment gun and then neutralized on the counterelectrode. The sample on the probe tip is ionized by the beam and sputters charged particles that are then accelerated in the ion source and analyzed (Silberring, 1997a).

2.6.2 Size-Exclusion HPLC Linked to Electrospray Ionization Mass Spectrometry

Electrospray ionization mass spectrometry has several advantages over other mass spectrometric techniques. It serves as a sensitive and structure-specific on-line detector for the analysis of complex peptide mixtures (figure 2.8). When combined with size-exclusion liquid chromatography, peptides in the range of 0.5 to 7.0 kD can be separated (Silberring, 1997b).

2.6.3 Matrix-Assisted Laser Desorption Ionization Time of Flight Mass Spectrometry

This method determines the mass of a peptide by mixing peptides with an ultraviolet-absorbing matrix and using matrix-assisted laser desorption ionization time of flight mass spectrometry. This is a rapid and sensitive method for mass determination of biomolecules over a very large range of molecular weights (up to 55 kD), whereas the mass spectrometry techniques described above are usually limited to a mass range of less than 25 kD. This technique is described in detail by Critchley and Worster, 1997.

2.7 Neuropeptide Antagonists

The development of peptide antagonists, which selectively block the action of the peptide, presumably by binding to the neuropeptide receptors, has been of spectacular help in elucidating the function of those peptides for which antagonists have been developed. Antagonists are usually the substance of preference for use in binding studies of agonists, since they bind better and are less likely to be displaced by ions.

The opiate antagonist naloxone is a specific narcotic antagonist and has been used extensively in studies to determine the specificity of opiate action. Naloxone and naltrexone, morphine antagonists that are devoid of analgesic and addicting agonist properties, are sometimes used in the treatment of addicts. Many nonpeptidergic agonists and antagonists have been synthesized for use both in basic research and

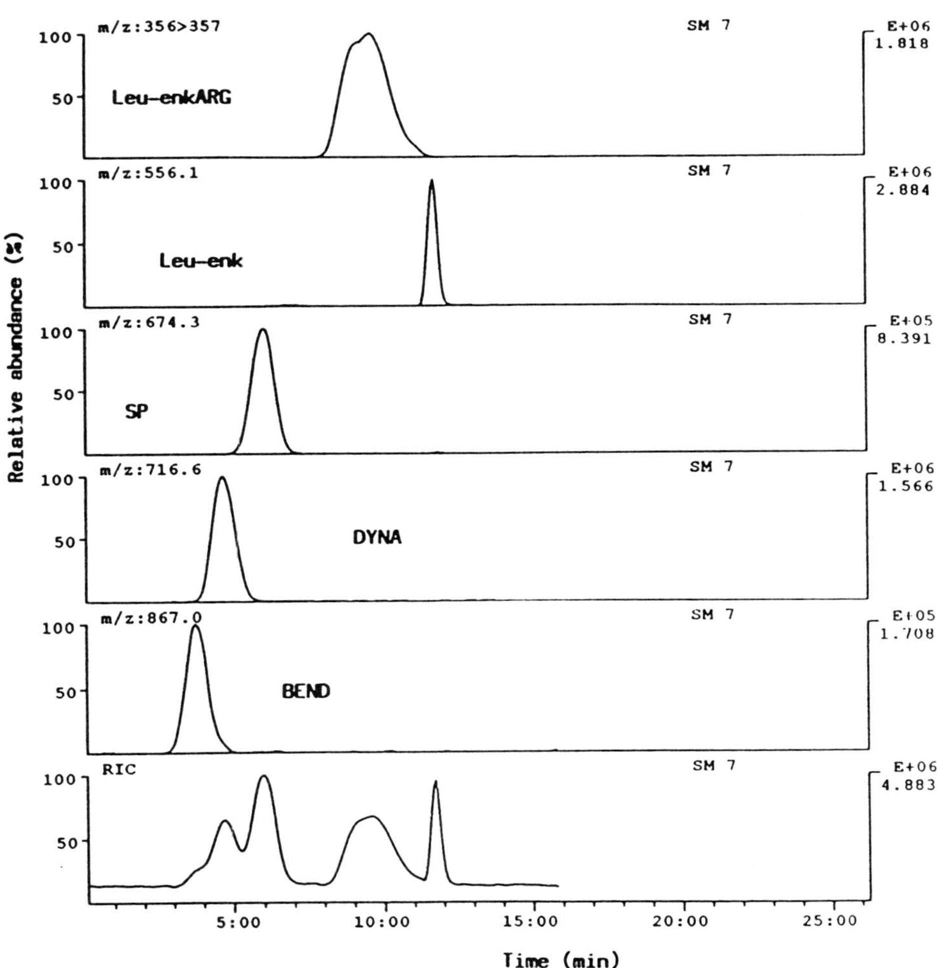

Figure 2.8
Electrospray ionization mass chromatogram of a peptide mixture, separated by size-exclusion chromatography. The selected ion current profiles represent the particular peptides (labeled with names) at various charge states. BEND, β-endorphin; DYNA, dynorphin; SP, substance P; Leu-enkARg, leu-enkephalin-Arg^6; Leu-enk, leu-enkephalin. Sample load: 5 μg of each peptide (2 μg of Leu-enkephalin). (From Silberring, 1997b.)

in the clinic. Synthetic antagonists to substance P and other members of the tachykinin family have permitted the identification of several receptor subtypes (Maggi et al., 1991).

2.8 Electrophysiological Techniques

Anatomical identification of neuropeptide-containing cells ultimately only gains relevance if there is a functional correlation. Neuropeptides can modulate the excitability of neurons by changing the ion permeability of the neuronal membrane. The primary effector system linked to peptide receptors in the mammalian brain is a potassium channel (I_K), either alone or together with a nonselective cation channel ($I_{Na,K}$) (Boden, 1995). Many neuropeptides act as neurotransmitters or neuromodulators, or both, and these functions can best be investigated by electrophysiological methods. Stimulated neuropeptide secretion can be linked with increased electrical activity of the peptidergic cell. In the periphery, changes in electromechanical responses of denervated skeletal muscle after neuropeptide adminstration provide convincing evidence for a neurotrophic action of the melanocortins, short fragments of ACTH.

2.8.1 In the Central Nervous System

2.8.1.1 In Vivo

The macroelectrophysiological techniques used for the study of drugs on the brain in vivo are well adapted for investigating neuropeptide effects in the intact organism, whether animal or human. These techniques include the electroencephalogram (EEG), the electrocorticogram, evoked potentials, and multiple unit activity. These techniques, as well as microelectrophysiological techniques as affected by neuropeptides, are discussed in detail by Urban (1986). Microelectrophysiological techniques involve the stereotaxic placement of recording electrodes in brain regions that contain peptidergic neurons, to record the electrical activity of these neurons under various conditions, from spontaneous rhythmic firing to bursts of potentials elicited by electrical or physiological stimulation. Using chronically implanted microelectrodes, it is possible to obtain single-cell recordings from conscious animals. It is necessary to confirm the accuracy of the placement of the electrodes by subsequent histological sections that illustrate the electrode tracks. The accuracy of the localization of the electrodes is increased if a direct current is passed through the electrode tip after the experimental recordings are completed. The current produces a small lesion at the electrode tip which identifies the site of the recordings (figure 2.9). Alternatively,

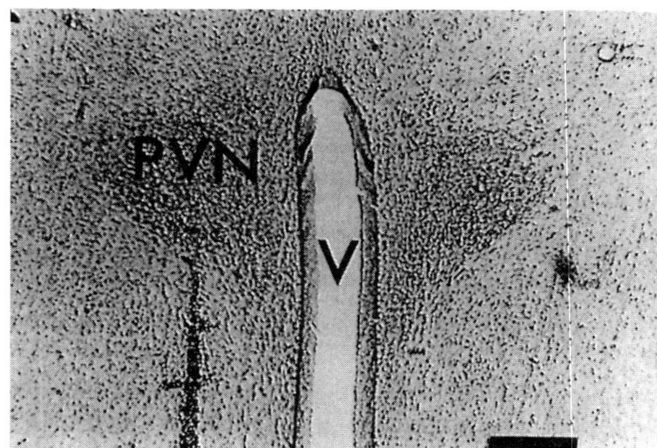

Figure 2.9
Photomicrograph of a 100-μm cresyl violet–stained coronal section through the medial hypothalamus of a rat. Below left is a blood-filled micropipette trajectory to the paraventricular nucleus (PVN) inserted from the ventral hypothalamus. V, portion of the third ventricle. Calibration bar: 100 μm. (From Ferguson and Renaud, 1987.)

a dye marker such as lucifer yellow or cresyl violet can be ejected through the electrode tip by current application.

Figure 2.10 shows that neurons synthesizing the neurohypophyseal hormones VP or OT can be distinguished on the basis of the pattern of their firing. VP neurons may fire in either a phasic or continuous mode and respond, through baroreceptor afferents stimulated via an increase in mean arterial blood pressure, by a reduction in firing. On the other hand, OT neurons fire continuously and do not respond to changes in baroreceptor stimulation.

Neuropeptides may be administered directly onto individual cells by *microiontophoresis or pressure ejection* and the response, or lack of response, of the target cell recorded. Microiontophoresis expels charged molecules from within the micropipette when an electric field is applied to that pipette; pressure ejection relies on pressure rather than charge to eject the peptide. The advantages and disadvantages of these two techniques are discussed by Ferguson and Renaud (1987). These methods have proved valuable in distinguishing the action of the applied neuropeptide as a neurotransmitter, neuromodulator, or neurohormone, depending on the change in membrane potential of the responding cell.

2.8.1.2 In the Peripheral Nervous System

Electrical stimulation of denervated muscle through its regenerating nerve serves as a reliable measure of the rate and quality of nerve regeneration and pre-

PUTATIVE VP NEURONS :

• Phasic.

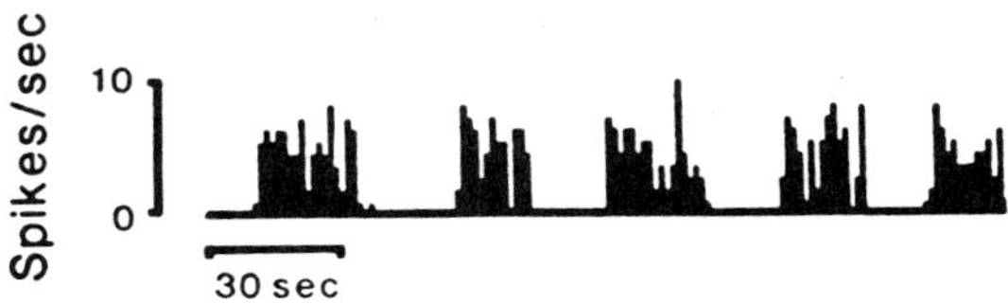

• Continuous, BP-sensitive.

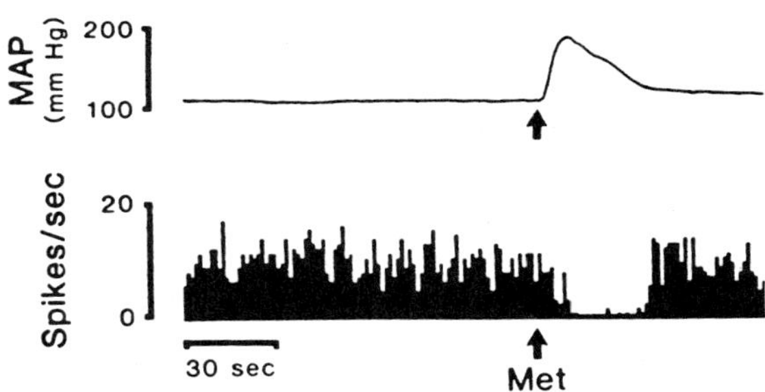

PUTATIVE OXY NEURONS :

• Continuous, BP-insensitive.

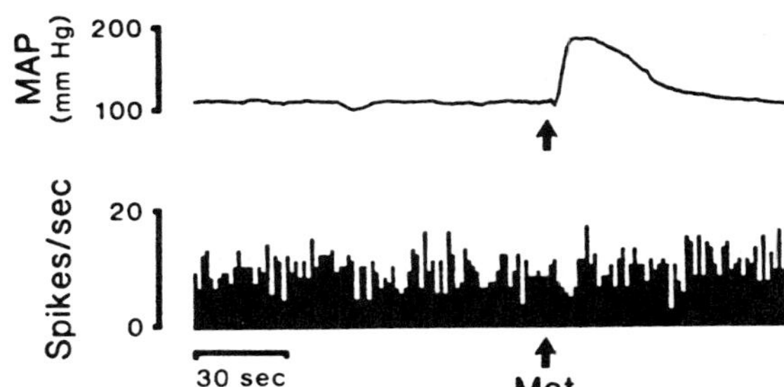

Figure 2.10
Ratemeter records and corresponding mean arterial blood pressure (MAP) illustrate recordings that distinguish between vasopressin (VP)- and oxytocin (OT)-synthesizing neurons in the hypothalamus BP, blood pressure. See text. (From Renaud et al., 1985.)

vention of muscle atrophy. This in situ preparation serves as a model to test the neurotrophic effects of neuropeptides, especially the melanocortins, ACTH or MSH 1–13 and its smaller fragments, none of which are corticotropic. Immediately after a controlled crush of the sciatic or peroneal nerve, intraperitoneal administration of the neuropeptide commences, with the optimal pattern of administration being 40 μg/kg 48 h. Electromechanical testing commences at 7 days, just before reinnervation of the extensor digitorum longus (EDL) muscle by the peroneal nerve, and subgroups of animals are tested at various intervals to monitor the course of reinnervation. [The values of the muscle twitch and tetanus, fatigue curves, motor unit recruitment, and conduction velocity, contribute to the evaluation of the effectiveness of the peptide.] Morphological studies of nerve terminal branching within the endplate, the size of the endplate itself, and the number, size, and myelination of the regenerating axons supply additional information. In addition, behavioral responses such as recovery of motor function and withdrawal of the injured limb from a noxious stimulus permit an integrated evaluation of the competence of the neuropeptide in studies of regeneration (Saint-Come and Strand, 1985; Strand et al., 1993). Figure 2.11 illustrates the change in tetanic amplitude and the fatigue curve of EDL muscle after peroneal nerve crush and adminstration of ACTH 4–10 or its analog BIM 22015.

2.9 Perfusion and Tissue Culture Studies

2.9.1 *Perfusion*

Many different in vitro perfusion preparations are available, ranging from autonomic and sensory ganglia, to the isolated pituitary gland or one of its three lobes, to chunks of tissue such as hypothalamic-neurohypophyseal explants or slices of spinal cord. With these larger tissue explants it is possible to maintain more of the neural and vascular connections. The tissue is then perfused with an artificial medium through the attached arteries, which maintains it in good condition for subsequent electrophysiological and pharmacological studies.

The mechanisms and routes of *transport of neuropeptides across the blood-brain barrier (BBB)* have been extensively studied. Several separate and distinct transport systems have been identified. Saturable uptake mechanisms for peptides have a high affinity and a low capacity so that brain perfusion methods, which permit extended exposure of the peptide to the brain endothelium, are required. Autoradiographic studies have demonstrated the presence of receptors for a number of peptides on the circumventricular organs, indicating a more permissive general entry for some neuropeptides into brain extracellular fluid, although some of the ependymal cells surrounding these areas are joined by tight junctions and rates of diffusion are slow (see chapter 5).

The *brain uptake index* is a measurement of the uptake of substances that enter slowly into the brain after intravenous (i.v.) injection: the brain-to-blood ratio of the substance relative to a reference substance is calculated. To take into consideration the many physiological variables in such a system, a multiple-time regression analysis method is utilized. The details of these techniques are clearly discussed in Jaspan et al., (1994). Brain-to-blood efflux systems can be measured either by ventriculocisternal perfusion or by measuring the neuropeptide in the blood after intracerebroventricular (i.c.v.) injection (Banks and Kastin, 1994). Although this technique is not sensitive enough to measure the passage of low amounts of neuropeptides, it has provided good results for sugars,

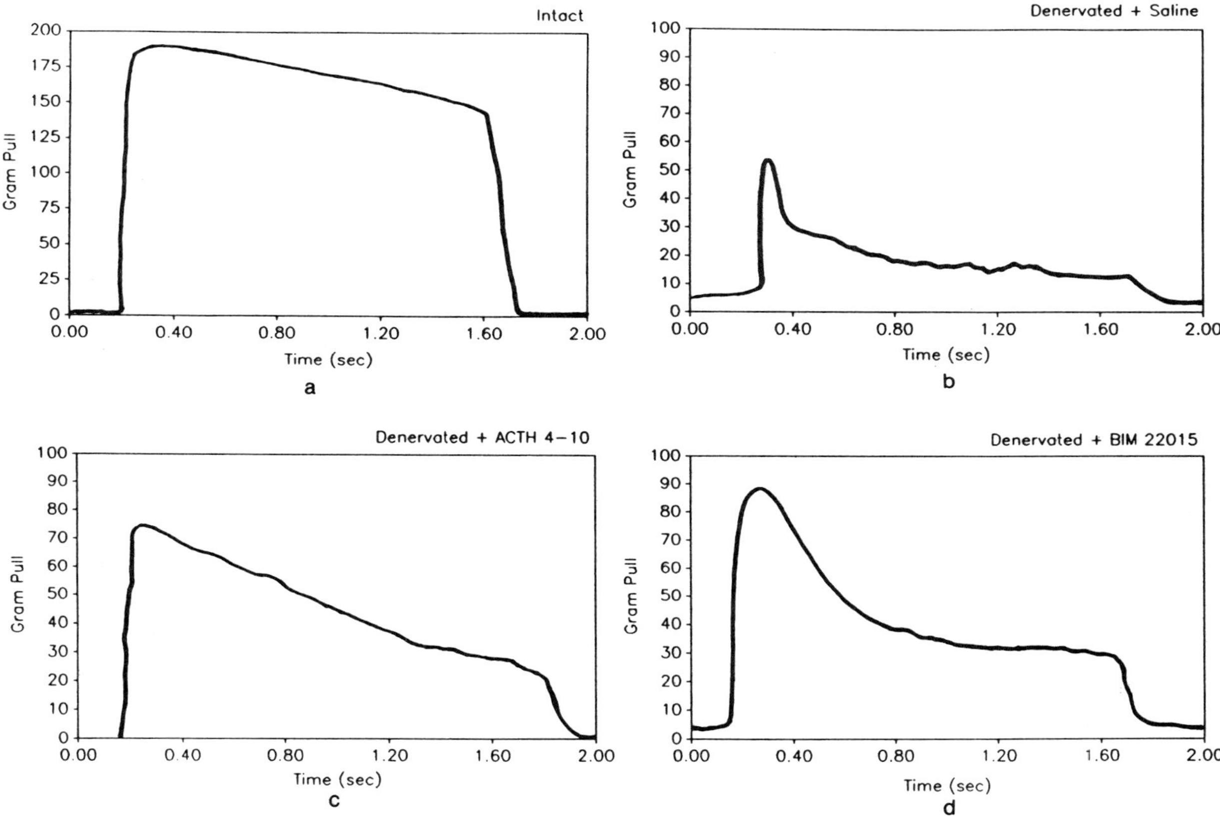

Figure 2.11
Representative traces showing peak tetanic contraction amplitude and decline from peak (fatigue) of extensor digitorum longus muscle during peroneal nerve stimulation 11 days after peroneal nerve crush. Treatment with adrenocorticotropic hormone (ACTH) 4–10 or the ACTH 4–10 analog BIM 22015 or saline commenced immediately after nerve crush. Peptide dosage was 40 μg/kg/48 hours intraperitoneally. Both peptides partially restore the ability of denervated muscle to maintain tetanic tension. Note the difference in scale of grams pull (contraction amplitude) for intact muscle. (From Strand et al., 1993.)

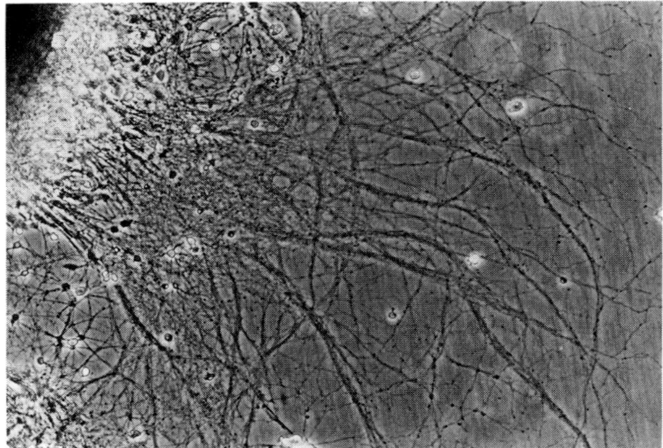

Figure 2.12
Outgrowth of fetal spinal cord slices in a liquid culture medium to which 0.1 nM α–melanocyte-stimulating hormone had been added. (From Van der Neut et al. 1988.)

amino acids, and similar molecules present in higher concentrations.

2.9.2 Tissue Culture

Fetal spinal cord slices or dissociated spinal and sensory neurons can be propagated in a liquid culture medium (figure 2.12) or in a semisolid agar culture medium and the effects of neuropeptides on neurite growth determined (Van der Neut et al., 1988; Mandys et al., 1991). A novel modification of this technique, which allows for more accurate measurement of neurite outgrowth, incorporates the *three-chambered tissue culture system* (Campenot, 1977). Collagen-coated culture dishes receive scratches 200 μm apart made on the surface of the collagen and a drop of growth medium containing methylcellulose is placed on the center of the scratched medium. Teflon dividers divide the culture dish into three compartments. Dissociated cells (spinal cord, dorsal root ganglia) are plated in the center compartment which contains the growth medium. The two side compartments contain the experimental solutions of neuropeptides. As the neurites grow out into the side compartments parallel to the surface scratches, their length can be accurately measured (figure 2.13). This technique clearly differentiates between the neurotrophic potencies of nerve growth factor (NGF) and ACTH 4–10 and its analog, BIM 22015 (figure 2.14).

2.10 Behavioral Techniques

The pioneering studies by De Wied's group (De Wied, 1964) and Kastin and his colleagues (Kastin et al., 1976) clearly demonstrated that ACTH and its related noncorticotropic peptide fragments have profound effects on adaptive behavior in rats. Behavioral deficits induced by removal of the anterior pituitary gland can be corrected by administration of these peptides. The array of behavioral tests includes extinction of shuttle-box and pole-jumping avoidance behavior, maze performance, passive avoidance behavior, food- or sex-motivated behavior, conditioned taste aversion, and amnesia produced by carbon dioxide inhalation or electroconvulsive shock, all of which are improved by peptide administration. Other important behavioral techniques used to study neuropeptides involve analysis of learning and memory, attention, locomotion, food intake, open field behavior, spatial orientation, and excessive grooming. Social behaviors are especially interesting and include aggression, and maternal and sexual behavior. Rewarded behavior, such as self-administration of heroin and electrical self-stimulation into the ventral tegmental area (an area associated with opiate reward) is also modulated by neuropeptides, When ACTH peptides are administered i.c.v., a stretching and yawning

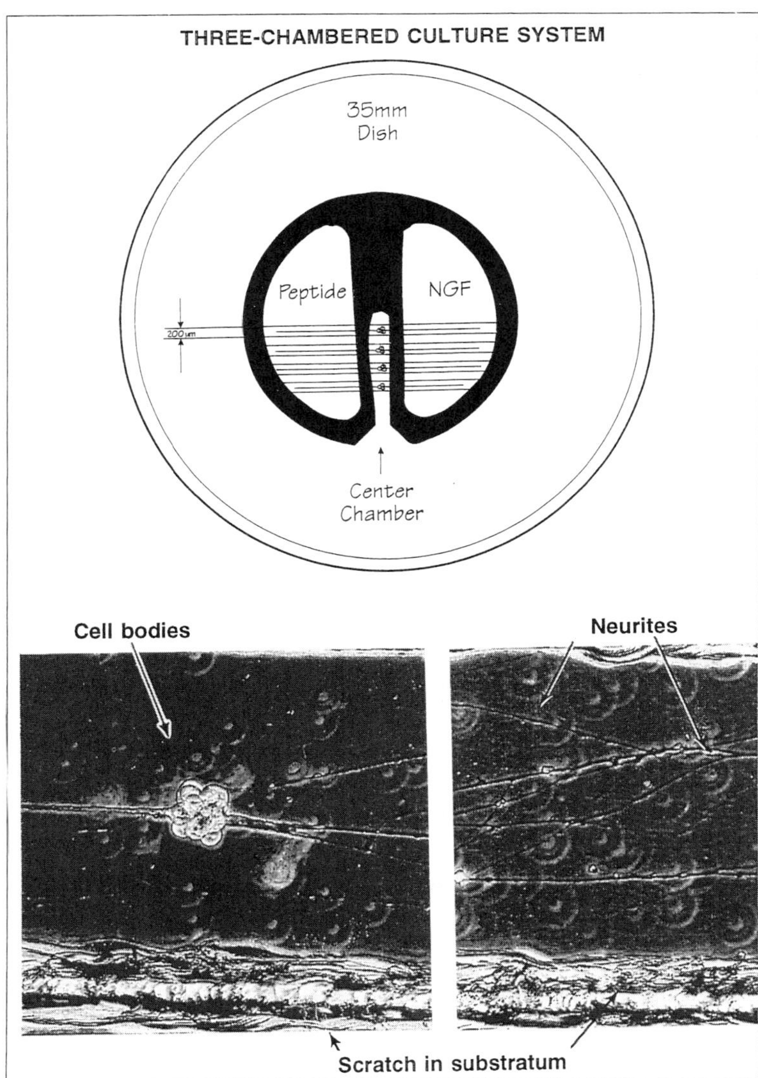

Figure 2.13
Three-chambered tissue culture system. Neurons of either dorsal root ganglia or spinal cord cells are plated in the center chamber. Neurite outgrowth extending from the center to either side is measured at 14 days in vitro. Below is an enlargement of a single track containing cell bodies and their neurites. (From Lee, 1995.)

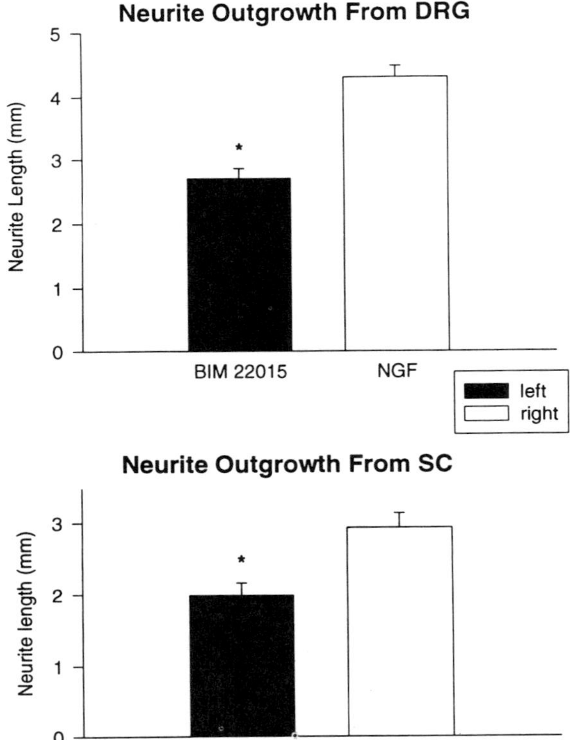

Figure 2.14
Neurite outgrowth from dorsal root ganglion (DRG) and spinal cord (SC) cells into side chambers containing either nerve growth factor (NGF) or the ACTH 4–10 analog BIM 22015 (100 ng/mL), 14 days in vitro. It is unusual to have neurite outgrowth in a medium lacking NGF. $^*P < .05$. (From Lee, 1995.)

syndrome can be induced in dogs, and excessive grooming and penile erection in rodents.

Not only the ACTH peptides of the anterior pituitary but the neurohypophyseal neuropeptides VP and OT, and an analog of VP, [des-Gly^9-Lys^8] VP, which has virtually no pressor activity, can also rectify many behavioral deficits. A number of opiate peptides, such as β-lipotropin, which share the precursor molecule POMC with the ACTH peptides, have similar effects on behavior. Behavioral tests are reviewed in detail by Bohus (1986), De Wied (1990) and De Wied et al. (1993). These tests are sensitive enough for structure-activity studies which have successfully located the active moieties of the various neuropeptides (Coy and Kastin, 1986; Gispen and Isaacson, 1986; van Nispen and Greven,1986). It must be emphasized, however, that it takes practice, patience, and skill to achieve reliable results with behavioral tests.

Behavioral tests in humans include tests of visual detection and discrimination, attention, and memory in normal subjects, in elderly patients, and in mentally retarded persons. In general, it appears that attentional and processing abilities may be enhanced by the ACTH or MSH fragments (Kastin et al., 1986; Sandman and O'Halloran, 1986). There is some correlation between changes in brain peptides and schizophrenia, aging, and Alzheimer's disease, as determined from brain sections analyzed by RIA and immunocytohemistry (Crow et al., 1982; Chan Palay, 1987) and reviewed by Spruijt et al. (1990).

2.11 Transgenic Models and Gene Targeting

2.11.1 Transgenic Models

The creation of transgenic mice has opened new potentials to trace the role of individual neuropeptides in the developing and mature animal. A *transgenic animal* is defined as one in which copies of an artificial gene sequence are stably integrated into the genome of every cell of that animal.

2.11.1.1 Techniques Used to Produce Transgenic Animals

There are essentially three ways of producing transgenic animals. One is the retroviral integration of the new gene into an early embryo, another the injection of intact or altered gene sequences into the pronuclei of fertilized oocytes, and a third, the transfection of embryonic stem cells, in culture, by electroporation or facilitated uptake. These techniques have been used most successfully in mice and are described in detail by Evans et al.(1994). The generation of transgenic mice has become a powerful device for focusing on the mechanisms of gene regulation, gene promoter characteristics, enhancer sequences, transcription factor site interactions, mutations, and tissue-specific expression. A large number of neuropeptide genes have been tested for their ability to target expression to the hypothalamus and pituitary in transgenic mice, which has resulted in the ablation or immortalization of specific cell types and analysis of transcription regulatory sequences (Waschek, 1995).

2.11.1.2 Physiological Consequences Seen in Transgenic Animals

The oocytes or embryonic cells containing the altered gene are implanted into the uterus of a hormonally prepared female and allowed to develop. The insertion of the new gene, by homologous recombination, results in a mouse that has the gene in the right place, under the control of the normal regulatory elements, and in the normal genetic environment, in all of its cells. The overall physiological consequences of a specific, artificial mutation can now be investigated in the whole animal. This is an incredibly valuable technique for neurophysiologists interested in the effects of overproduction or underproduction of a specific neuropeptide. In a mouse model that expresses a transgene that causes an overproduction of corticotropin-releasing hormone (CRH), the animals exhibit endocrine abnormalities involving the hypothalamo-pituitary-adrenal (HPA) axis and serve as a genetic model for chronic stress. The CRH transgene is expressed in regions where CRH is normally expressed and transgenic animals have markedly elevated signals for CRH mRNA in almost all tissues in which CRH is found in normal mice. The transgenic mice show all the behavioral effects of chronic stress, such as decreased food consumption, enhanced fear responses, and decreased sexual activity. These animals also display features characteristic of Cushing's syndrome (Stenzel-Poore et al., 1996). In addition, the immune system is markedly suppressed, another indication of the physiological effects of hypersecretion of CRH (see chapter 8).

2.11.2 Gene Targeting

An important and ingenious research tool is gene targeting, a procedure in which a single gene is selected and inactivated, or "knocked out." The inactivated (null) gene is then injected into early mouse embryos and by homologous recombination, the introduced inactive gene replaces the normal gene in the mouse chromosome (figure 2.15). Subsequent generations of deficient mice have an inheritable, complete loss of function in all tissues, at all stages of development. The specific role of the knocked-out gene can then be determined by observing the physiological and structural changes that result from the absence of the normal gene. Gene knockout technology, for example, can produce a CRH-deficient

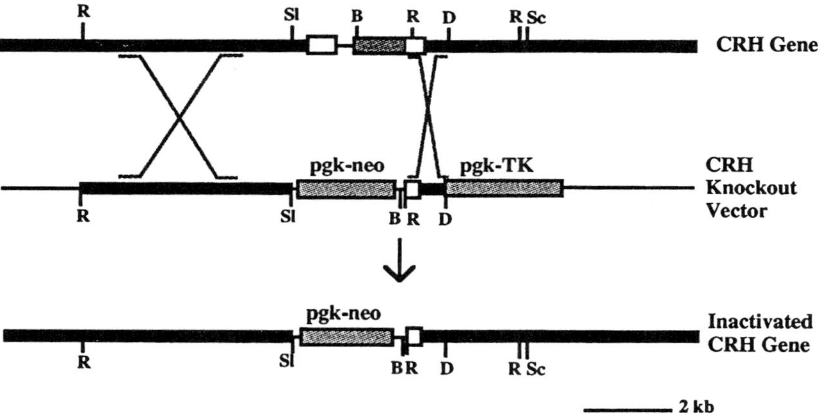

Figure 2.15
Corticotropin-releasing hormone (CRH)–deficient mice produced by targeted disruption in embryonic stem cells. The strategy is to inactivate the CRH gene by homologous recombination. After electroporation of the CRH targeting vector into 3-day-old embryonic stem cells, successful homologous recombination (shown by stippled lines) should occur between the endogenous CRH gene and the targeting vector to create an inactive CRH allele. Thick black line, CRH gene-flanking regions; open boxes, CRH noncoding exons; upper stippled box, prepro-CRH–coding region; stippled boxed, pgk-neo and pgk-TK genes. Restriction sites: R, EcoRI; Sl, SalI; B, BamHI; D,DraI; and Sc, SacI. (From Muglia et al., 1994.)

mouse by targeted mutation in embryonic stem cells and with consequent deficiencies in stress responses, diurnal rhythms, and feeding behavior. Some of the methods and problems involved in producing the null CRH gene are discussed by Muglia et al. (1996).

2.11.3 Site-Directed Mutagenesis

With the ability to create almost any desired mutation in a given DNA sequence, site-directed mutagenesis permits the introduction of a selected mutation into specific locations. It is a powerful technique by which specific changes in a target DNA molecule can be generated for structure-function studies (Viville, 1994). It is an invaluable approach to the study of neuropeptides, their precursors, and the precise sequence(s) responsible for such processes as receptor binding. Details of this revolutionary technique are given by Yang et al. (1994).

2.12 Integrated Physiological Techniques

Measurements of food and water intake are used to investigate the integrated physiological responses to neuropeptides. Lesions in the CNS can isolate the level at which the integration occurs. Figure 2.16 shows that both control and decerebrate rats decrease sucrose intake after peripheral injection of bombesin, indicating that caudal brainstem regions isolated from the cerebral cortex are sufficient to integrate the afferent signals from bombesin and taste receptors to depress ingestive behavior (Flynn, 1994). Neuropeptide Y and galanin are two hypothalamic neuropeptides that affect a variety of physiological actions specifically

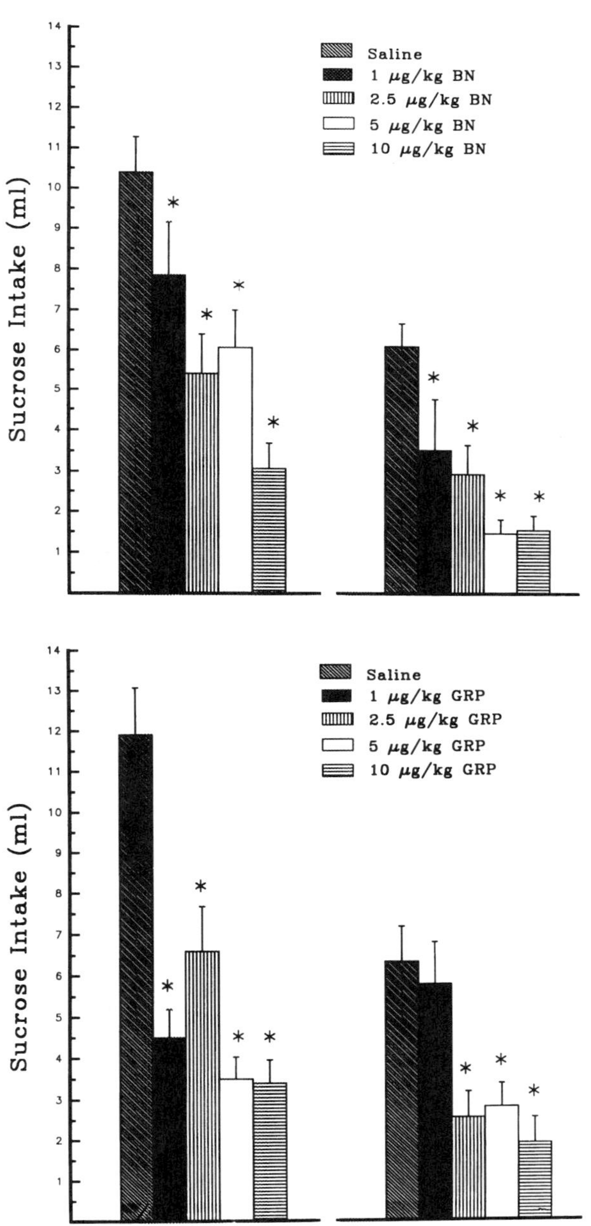

related to nutrient and energy homeostasis; to study these interactions, endocrine, metabolic, behavioral, and neural techniques are required (Leibowitz, 1994). Similarly, the complex physiological responses to the administration of stress-evoked neuropeptide hormones (CRH, ACTH, VP, OT, endorphins and enkephalins, and prolactin) are interpreted through measurements of cardiac and pressor changes, alterations in reproductive endocrinology and behavior, analgesia and locomotor activity, and alterations in the immune system.

The actions of neuropeptides are widespread and demonstrable at all biological levels—molecular, cellular, tissue, organ, and integrated systems—and through the ingenuity of the scientist coupled with the startling developments of modern technology, we are accumulating more information than can readily be absorbed. The challenge is to bring order and understanding into the mass of data and discover the pattern by which neuropeptides regulate vital physiological processes.

2.13 Summary

Methods of studying neuropeptides can be organized into those that determine the following:

1. The amount of neuropeptide in a cell, tissue, organ, or in body fluids, such as plasma or CSF. These include bioassays and radioassays.

Figure 2.16
Intraoral sucrose intake after peripheral injections of saline or bombesin (BN) in control and chronic decerebrate (CD) rats. GRP, gastrin-releasing peptide. Asterisk indicates a reliable reduction in intake compared to saline injections. (From Flynn, 1994.)

2. The anatomical site of neuropeptides. These include immunocytochemistry, together with neuronal labeling, to characterize projection neurons; and administration of labeled neuropeptides followed by autoradiography or electron microscope studies, depending on the size and type of label.

3. The localization of receptors using receptor labeling and visualization microscopically or on autoradiograms, in vivo or in vitro.

4. The amount of neuropeptide released using RNA-cDNA hybridization, in situ hybridization histochemistry, in vivo sampling, and microdialysis. In vitro techniques include perfusion, HPLC, and the cell blot assay.

5. The structure of neuropeptides through isolation and chemical and physical techniques, peptide and nucleotide sequencing, and molecular biotechnology.

6. Structure-function relationships of closely related peptides through a wide variety of behavioral tests.

7. The function of neuropeptides, particularly through the use of peptide antagonists and agonists, electrophysiological techniques, and integrated physiological studies. The introduction of a mutated gene (animals); the elimination of a gene (gene knockout technology); change in a specific sequence of a precursor neuropeptide molecule (site-directed mutagenesis) provide excitingly exact information about neuropeptide function.

In chapter 3 the synthesis of neuropeptides from large, inactive precursor molecules is followed through their processing to smaller, biologically active peptides. The POMC gene is discussed as an example of the organization of a precursor gene. Examination of neuropeptide secretion and inactivation completes the sequence of events that began with precursor synthesis.

Biosynthesis, Processing, Secretion, and Inactivation of Neuropeptides

3

3.1 Neuropeptides as Physiological Regulators

Neuropeptides ranging in size from 3 to 40 amino acid residues constitute a major group of intercellular agents for cell-to-cell communication, either as messenger hormones or as neurotransmitters and neuromodulators. The regulatory function of neuropeptides may be regarded as a long cascade of molecular interactions, affecting all physiological functions and being in turn regulated by feedback mechanisms at all levels, from the molecular to the organismal. This cascade commences within the neurosecretory cell, with the expression of the promessenger gene, precursor processing, storage of the neuropeptide in vesicles, and finally the secretion of the neuropeptide (Acher and Chavet, 1995). The response of the target cell depends on neuropeptide recognition of specific membrane receptors and the consequent transduction of the message through a second intracellular cascade to result in activation of the effector. Consequently, information concerning neuropeptide synthesis and processing is essential to a fundamental understanding of how these regulators are regulated.

Like all polypeptides and proteins, neuropeptides are produced by cleavages from large precursor molecules synthesized on ribosomes and subsequently subjected to enzymatic proteolysis to yield neuropeptides with varying characteristics and potencies. The first prohormone, proinsulin, was discovered some 20 years ago and since then many prohormones have been discovered and sequenced. The precursors may contain one or more sequences for closely related peptides, as well as for unrelated peptides. Depending on the enzymatic complement of the cell and the precise vesicles in which the enzymes may be sequestered, the excision of specific neuropeptides may vary.

This method greatly increases the diversity of neuropeptides available for chemical signaling between cells and brings some logic to the cellular process of synthesizing large inactive precursors, which then must be cleaved to attain biological activity. The nascent precursors are closely associated with the intracellular membranes of the cell, through which they are translocated, chemically processed, packaged, and prepared for secretion.

3.2 Biosynthesis and Processing of Neuropeptides

3.2.1 Preprohormones and the Signal Peptide Sequence

The initial precursor polypeptide chain containing the amino acid sequence of the neuropeptide, plus the signal sequence at its N-terminus that guides it through the ribosome and into the lumen of the rough endoplasmic reticulum (RER), is known as the *preprohormone*. The prefix "pre-" indicates that there is an N-terminal presequence of about 15 to 30 amino acid residues, the *signal peptide*, a sequence found on precursors of hormones that are designed to be secreted. The large preprohormones common to most neuropeptides range in size from approximately 10 to 35 kD. Some preprohormones are schematically illustrated in figure 3.1.

Synthesis of the preprohormone starts in the cytosol with the formation of a complex between the ribosome, mRNA, and a group of protein factors. Synthesis proceeds until the amino acid chain is about 60 to 70 amino acids in length, at which time the nascent signal peptide binds to a signal recognition particle which inhibits further extension of the polypeptide chain. Led by the signal peptide, the preprohormone is inserted and translocated through the RER membrane, in an ATP-mediated process (figure 3.2). This is in sharp contrast to the biosynthesis of conventional small molecule transmitters and hormones, such as ACh and the catecholamines. These small molecules or their immediate precursors can be synthesized and transported directly into mature secretory granules (Mains et al., 1987).

The *signal sequence* that directs the preprohormone through the RER has a region of about 10 hydrophobic amino acids a fixed distance from the cleavage site, which is dominated by a region with small, neutral amino acids, for example, alanine, cysteine, serine, and glycine. The insertion of the preprohormone into the lipid of the RER membrane is facilitated by the hydrophobicity of the signal peptide. Once inside the membrane, the signal sequence is rapidly removed by a signal endopeptidase during the process of translation. Therefore the structure of the primary translation product of a neuropeptide gene can only be deduced from the cDNA and not through biochemical analysis of the proteins the cell synthesizes. Consequently, techniques that permit the analysis of cDNA sequences have been invaluable in predicting the primary structure of a precursor protein and in determining the derivation of multiple peptides from a single precursor (Alberts et al., 1983)

The signal peptide sequence has a hydrophilic N-terminus and is followed by a peptide separated from the next peptide in the parent molecule by some combination of two basic amino acids, usually Lys-Arg. Depending on the specific preprohormone, other active or inactive peptide sequences within the parent molecule are usually separated by combinations of Lys-Arg, Arg-Arg, or Lys-Lys from the C-terminal region, although some separation may occur at a single basic amino acid (see figure 3.1). The signal peptide that has emerged from the big subunit of the

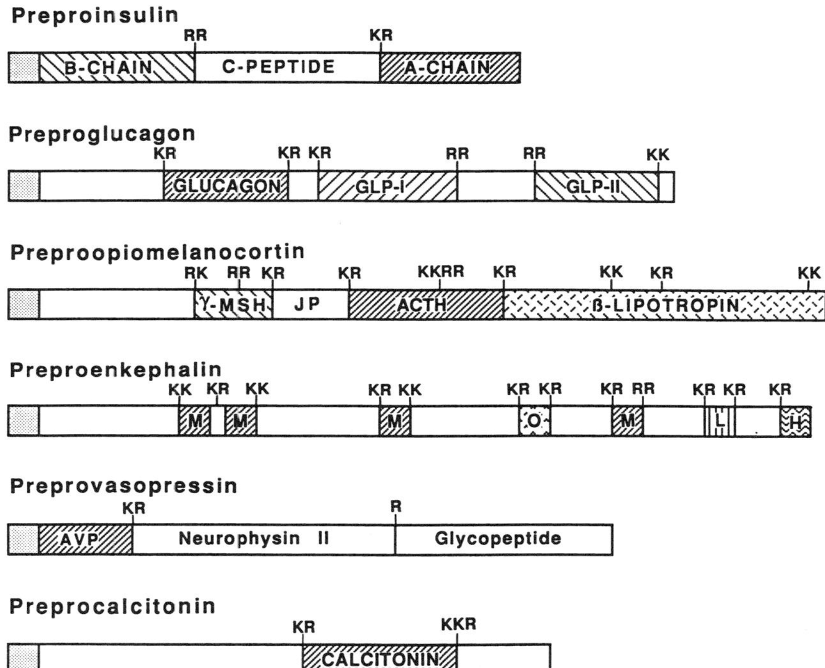

Figure 3.1
Preprohormone structures. The precursor structures for several peptide hormones are schematically illustrated. All pre-prohormones contain an N-terminal signal sequence. Peptide hormone domains within the precursor are indicated as shaded areas. The signal sequence is represented by the dotted box at the N-terminus of each preprohormone. GLP, glucagon-like peptide; MSH, melanocyte-stimulating hormone; JP, joining peptide; ACTH, adrenocorticotropic hormone; M, met-enkephalin; O, met-enkephalin-Arg^6-Gly^7-Leu^8; L, leu-enkephalin; H, met-enkephalin-Arg^6-Phe^7; AVP, arginine vasopressin; K and R represent single-letter codes for lysine and arginine, respectively. (From Hook et al., 1994.)

ribosome promotes the formation of a junction between the 60S subunit of the ribosome and the membranes of the RER. Blobel and Dobberstein (1975) suggest that the interaction between the signal protein and the membrane recruits membrane receptors (transmembrane glycoproteins), causing them to associate through ionic bonds to form a tunnel, which is further stabilized by the binding of the big ribosomal subunit to the membrane. The tunnel facilitates the translocation of the peptide chain through the RER membrane at which time the leading signal peptide is cleaved from the nascent peptide chain by signalase, an endopeptidase (see figure 3.2). The cleavage mechanism is highly conserved: microsomal membranes from sources as diverse as bacterial cells, amphibians, and mammals can cleave signal sequences from the proproteins from equally diverse sources (Boileau et al., 1981).

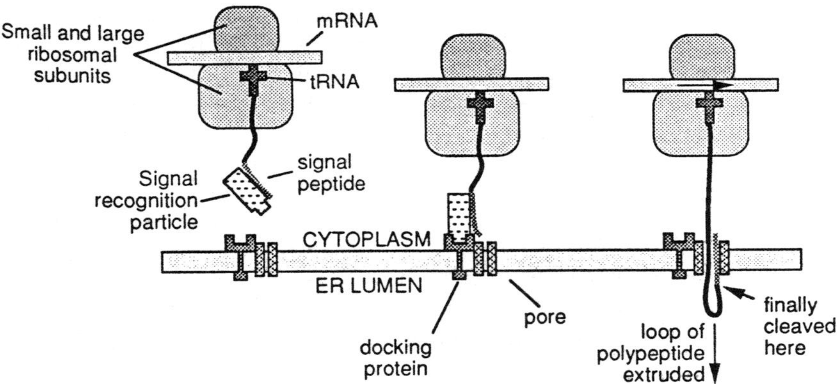

Figure 3.2
The signal peptide targets a secreted protein to the endoplasmic reticulum (ER). See text for details. mRNA, messenger RNA; tRNA, transfer RNA. (From Hardie, 1991.)

3.2.2 Prohormones and Precursor Processing

The peptide chain with the signal peptide removed is the *biologically inert prohormone* containing one or multiple copies of the final active neuropeptides, and this chain must be proteolytically processed into smaller active peptides (figure 3.3). Protein folding occurs in the cisterna of endoplasmic reticulum (ER) cisterna. The prohormones and proneuropeptides, released from the signal peptide, are immediately shuttled to the *cis*-face of the Golgi apparatus, then targeted to the *trans*-Golgi network.

Packaging of the precursors into secretory granules occurs in the *trans*-Golgi network, where they are actively sorted away from other proteins into the granules of the regulated secretory pathway. Sections of the Golgi network filled with the prohormone bud off to form prohormone-filled granules or vesicles (figure 3.4). Proteolysis, except for the removal of the signal peptide, begins at the *trans*-Golgi network and continues in the granules.

3.2.2.1 The Role of Prohormones

The role of prohormones is varied; proinsulin ensures the correct folding and disulfide formation between the A and B chains of the insulin molecule. The neurophysins may serve a similar purpose for OT and VP. Protein folding occurs in the ER cisterna and in some cases the propeptides also undergo N-linked glycosylation or disulfide bond formation within this cellular compartment, structural modifications essential to the secondary structure of the neuropeptides (Loh et al., 1993). Prohormones vary considerably in size, as do their respective preprohormones, with the median size being about 15 kD, but the size of the prohormone has little relationship to the size of the final neuropeptide. The enkephalins are very small, only 5 amino acids, but are derived from a large prohormone, proenkephalin (see figure 1.3). Some prohormones are simple linear chains of amino acids, giving rise to as few as two products for example, OT and OT-neurophysin. Growth hormone (GH) is syn-

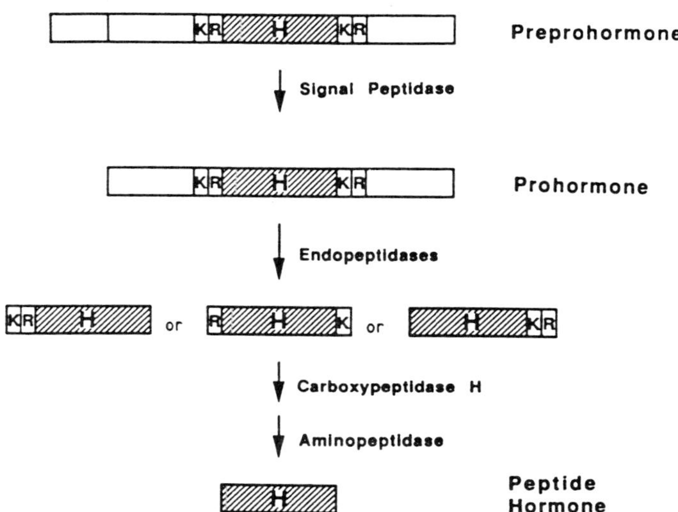

Figure 3.3
Preprohormone processing. A model preprohormone is illustrated, with the active hormone (H) indicated by the shaded area. The N-terminal signal peptide is removed by signal peptidase. The Lys-Arg (K-R) paired basic cleavage sites in many prohormones may be Arg-Arg, Lys-Lys, or Arg-Lys. The prohormone is cleaved by endopeptidases at the N-terminus between two basic residues, or at the C-terminus of the paired basic residues. Basic residue extensions are removed by carboxypeptidase H and aminopeptidase to yield the active hormone. (From Hook et al., 1994.)

thesized as a prohormone, that is, the hormone is secreted intact after removal of the signal sequence. Other prohormones are very complex, giving rise to many products, both biologically active neuropeptides and sequences which apparently have no function. POMC is a good example of a very complex prohormone that contains multiple peptides which become active once the prohormone has been processed, as well as some apparently biologically inert fragments (see figure 1.3 and section 3.2.5 below).

3.2.2.2 Secretory Granule Function

Within the granules, and sometimes before packaging in the Golgi network, *post-translational precursor processing* occurs: the excision of peptide sequences from the prohormone by endoproteases to generate a diversity of biologically active peptides. The granules contain a series of co-packaged processing enzymes which sequentially attack the prohormone as the granules move from the cell body down to the nerve terminals (figure 3.5). The active peptide sequences to be excised are usually, but not always, flanked by dibasic amino acids, where cleavage occurs, first by endopeptidases, followed by exoproteolyis by amino- and carboxypeptidases, and in some cases by special amidating enzymes to free the active neuropeptide. During their transit through the Golgi network, precursors may be subjected to many of the enzymatic modifications illustrated in figure 3.4: initial endoproteolytic processing, glycosylation, phosphorylation,

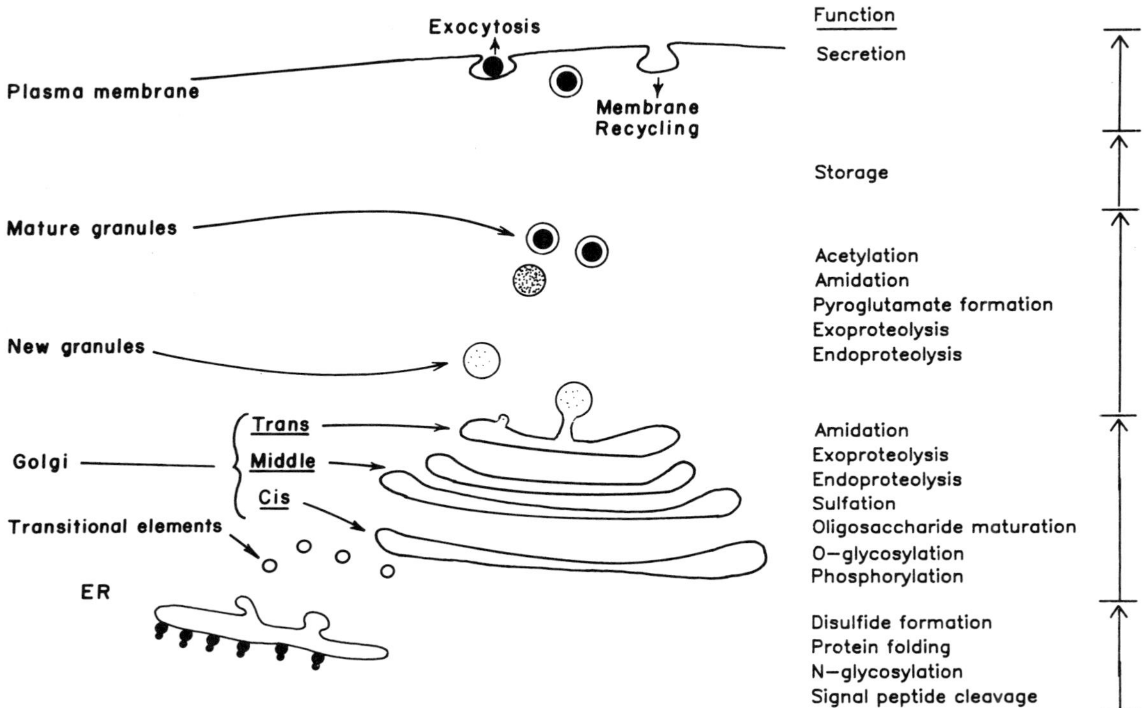

Figure 3.4
The major steps involved in the conversion of preprohormones into their final products are listed next to their primary site of occurrence ER, endoplasmic reticulum. (From Mains et al., 1990.)

sulfation of tyrosyl residues or oligosaccharides, and hydroxylation of lysine residues (Mains et al., 1987).

Figure 3.4 also shows that the final stages of shortening and clipping the large prohormone occur in the secretory granules. As peptides containing C-terminal basic residues are not found, the exoproteolytic removal of these residues probably occurs soon after endoproteolytic cleavage (Fricker, 1992). Thus the synthesis of the bioactive neuropeptides is first through the endopeptidases, followed by the exoproteolytic trimming of the ends of the resulting peptide fragments, and finally the modifications of the N- or C-terminal amino acids by α-*N*-acetylation, *O*-acetylation, formation of pyroglutamic residues, and α-amidation. The processing events in secretory granules require a few to several hours, but because neuroendocrine cells secrete hormones very slowly, it is not surprising that the turnover time for peptides stores is greatest in the granules; some studies indicate that it would take a week to replace corticotropic peptides stored in the anterior pituitary cells (May and Eipper, 1986).

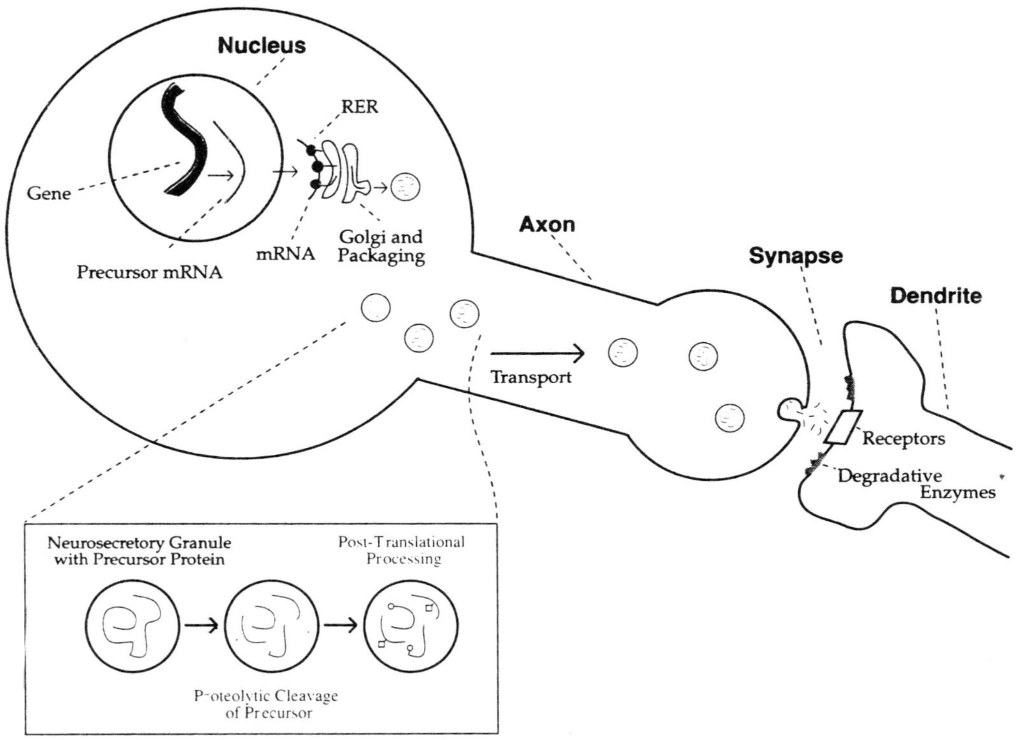

Figure 3.5
The biosynthesis, processing, transport, and secretion of neuropeptides from a model neuron. This scheme illustrates the progressive stages of neuropeptide expression in neuropeptide neurons. The inset represents the three stages of neuropeptide post-translational processing occurring during neurosecretory granule axonal transport: packaging, proteolytic cleavage, and modification (e.g., amidation, glycosylation, phosphorylation, etc.) mRNA, messenger RNA; RER, rough endoplasmic reticulum. (From Sherman et al., 1989.)

3.2.2.3 Regulatory and Constitutive Secretory Pathways

Peptide hormones and neuropeptides synthesized in neuroendocrine cells are secreted by a *regulatory secretory pathway*, in which peptides are stored in secretory granules (figure 3.6) and secreted in response to secretagogues—an "on demand" mechanism (Loh, 1987). This is in contrast to many other secretory proteins, such as growth and trophic hormones, plasma proteins, and membrane-associated receptors, which are transported to plasma membranes by a *constitutive secretory pathway* (a continuous mechanism) from their precursors in a Golgi network–related compartment, a pathway that apparently does not involve storage or regulation. The Golgi apparatus is responsible for sorting the secretory proteins between these two pathways.

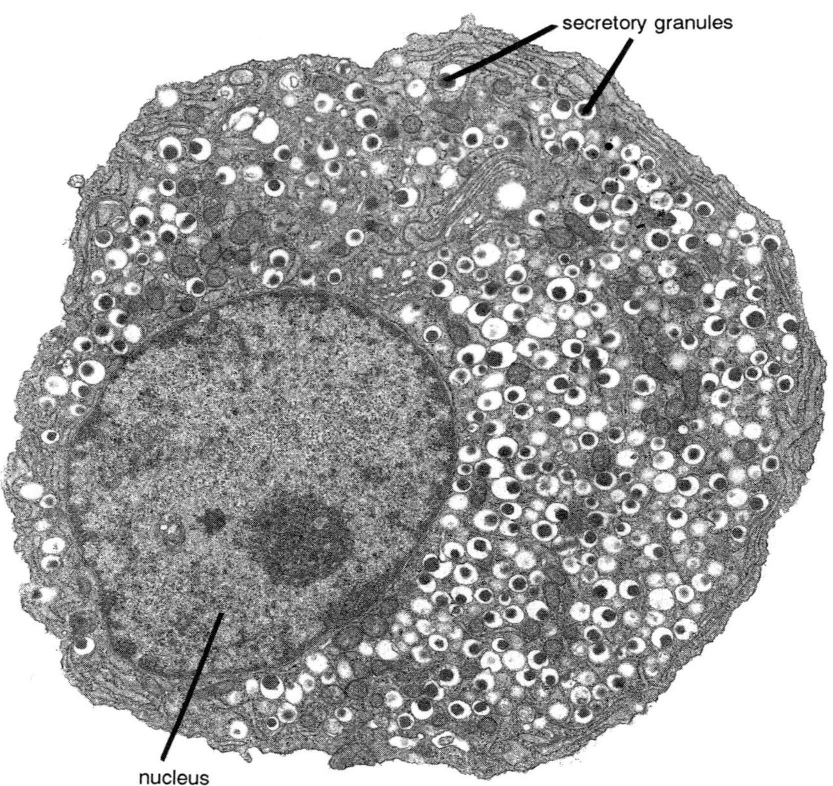

Figure 3.6
Electron micrograph of a pancreatic beta-cell from the islets of Langerhans showing insulin stored within the membrane-bound secretory granules. The dense granule core is irregular in shape and separated from the limiting membrane by a wide halo. Magnification X12,000 (From Orci and Perrelet, 1975.)

Several mechanisms have been proposed for this sorting procedure. One is that during passage of the prohormone through the Golgi stacks, the different transport vesicles are covered with distinctive protein coats, such as clathrin, and the coat selects the cargo protein that the vesicle will carry (Rothman and Orci, 1996). This intracellular trafficking of neuropeptides is cell type–specific (Castro and Morrison, 1997). There may also be prohormone binding proteins, called *sortases*, present in the Golgi apparatus, which could be vital to the regulation of the route taken by the prohormone.

Another mechanism for the sorting of the proteins has been suggested. Recent work has shown that there is a *sorting signal motif* in POMC that determines how the molecules destined for storage in secretory granules are sorted and sent with apparent accuracy to their final destinations. The sorting signal is present in the form of a heart-shaped 13-amino acid amphipathic loop in the N-terminal region of POMC, the stability of which depends on the integrity of a disulfide bridge within the loop. Using site-directed mutagenesis (see chapter 2), Loh and her colleagues demonstrated for the first time that only this 13–amino acid loop is necessary to direct POMC to the regulated secretory pathway and that there are no other essential sorting signals in the rest of the POMC molecule (Cool et al., 1995). If this heart-shaped loop is absent, the mutant POMC is sent along the constitutive (default) secretory pathway.

A sorting signal alone is not sufficient to cause sorting to the regulated secretory pathway. A sorting receptor, *carboxypeptidase E*, has been identified which specifically binds regulated secretory pathway proteins, including prohormones. Carboxypeptidase E does not bind constitutively secreted proteins. In a mutant mouse lacking this receptor the pituitary prohormone POMC is missorted to the constitutive pathway and secreted in an unregulated manner. This sorting confusion results in multiple endocrine disorders (Cool et al., 1997). However, additional mechanisms may regulate the differential distribution of peptides or proteins into these secretory pathways; for instance, isoforms of an important endoproteolytic enzyme, prohormone convertase PC5-A and PC5-B, are differentially sorted depending on the unique C-terminal 38 amino acids of PC5-A (de Bie et al., 1996). These enzymes are discussed in detail in section 3.2.3.1 (Prohormone Convertases).

3.2.3 Post-Translational Processing

3.2.3.1 Endoproteolysis

Peptide bond hydrolysis of the prohormone usually occurs through a trypsin-like endopeptidase at precursor sites represented by pairs of basic amino acids, aranged in doublets adjacent to the bioactive peptide sequences. The most common pair is Lys-Arg, although Lys-Lys and Arg-Arg are also sites of cleavage. Most of the dibasic sites which are cleaved in vivo are in exposed regions of the precursor structure, the special features of which are essential for recognition by the dibasic-specific endoproteases (Brakch et al., 1989). Figure 3.1 shows the cleavage sites of several proproteins within the preprohormone illustrating that there is no consistent pattern for the positioning of the active fragments inside the prohormone. In proinsulin the active chains (B and A) are at the ends of the prohormone; glucagon and calcitonin are more central; there are several copies of met-enkephalin as well as one leu-enkephalin in proenkephalin; and POMC contains several different biologically active neuropeptides.

Paired basic cleavage enzymes have stringent substrate specificity: if one of the amino acids is mutated, cleavage is totally blocked. Not all basic residue pairs serve as sites of cleavage nor do all proteolytic cleavages occur at basic pairs of amino acids. Cleavage at single arginine residues occurs in the biosynthesis of atriopeptin, somatostatin 28, CCK, dynorphin, pancreatic polypeptide, and growth hormone–releasing hormone (GHRH). Prosomatostatin contains both dibasic and monobasic cleavage sites (figure 3.7). The dibasic site probably is involved in the production of somatostatin 14, whereas cleavage of the monobasic site is involved in the production of somatostatin 28 (Beinfeld et al., 1989). However, there are several constraints over single arginine cleavages, one of which is the requirement of another basic residue within about two residues of the cleavage site.

a. Prohormone Convertases

Identification of these precursor processing endopeptidases as *prohormone convertases* (*PCs*) is an impor-

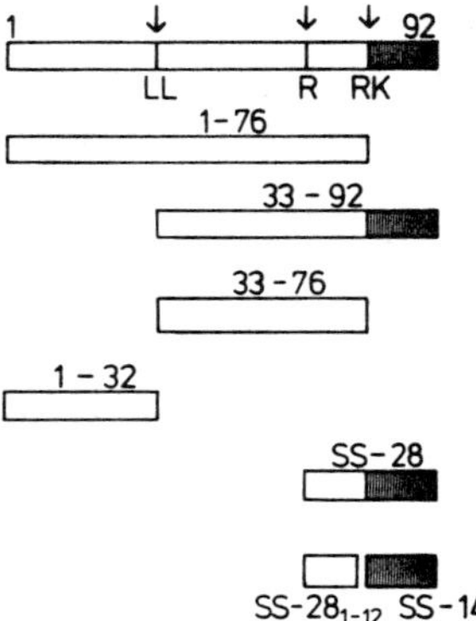

Figure 3.7
Schematic representation of the pathway of processing of mammalian prosomatostatin. The arrows show sites of proteolytic cleavage at a Leu-Leu (LL) bond, at a single arginine (R) monobasic processing site, and at a Arg-Lys (RK) dibasic processing site. (From Conlon, 1989.)

tant recent advance. Convertases are protease enzymes that clip off the active segments from the prohormone at single, specific basic residues or pairs of basic residues. The convertases form a family of seven mammalian proteases that resemble a bacterial protease called *subtilisin*, with extensive homologies in their N-terminal portions, indicating strong evolutionary conservation of these residues. The PCs identified are PC1 (also known as PC3), furin, PC4, PACE4, PC5, PC6, and PC7. Each enzyme has its unique structural characteristics as well as characteristics common to the members of this family such as membrane association, calcium ion dependency, and substrate specificity toward paired basic residues (Mizuno and Matsuo, 1994; Seidah, 1995). All the PCs contain a signal peptide, a prosegment, a catalytic segment, and a P-domain. The P-domain is critical to the intracellular folding of the convertases within the ER. Furin has a somewhat different requirement for cleavage: it requires a motif of 4 amino acids (Arg-X-Lys–Arg-Arg) rather than the simpler dibasic site targeted by PC1/PC3 and PC2.

The active site triad of Asp, His, and Ser residues, and the catalytically important Asn, along the polypeptide chain is characteristic of subtilisin-like serine proteases and has been identified in bacteria, yeast, molluscs, insects, nematodes, and coelenterates, as well as in amphibians and mammals. The yeast functional homolog of the mammalian endoprotease kexin (KEX2) is able to cleave neuropeptides such as proinsulin or POMC at distinct dibasic sites. It is important to note that only PC2 contains an Asp rather than an Asn in the catalytic site, a substitution which provides it with unique binding properties.

PC1/3, PC2, and KEX2 share common structural features including an N-terminal signal peptide followed by a propeptide of 80 to 90 residues terminating in a cleavage motif, Arg-X-Lys–Arg-Arg, a catalytic domain related to subtilisin that contains the characteristic triad, Asp, His, and Ser residues. They also share a well-conserved domain of about 150 residues that is essential for activity (Rouille et al., 1995). In addition to their selectivity for the specific base pairs they cleave, the prohormone convertases also require certain secondary and tertiary structures of the precursor for their enzymatic activity (Plevrakis et al., 1989). Processing proteases possess clear preferences for prohormone substrates: for example, in chromaffin granules of the adrenal medulla, proenkephalin and POMC are cleaved by the 70-kD aspartic protease but not by PC1/3 or PC2, whereas pro-NPY is cleaved by another protease, *prohormone thiol protease*, which also cleaves proenkephalin and POMC (Hook et al., 1994). Consequently, the specificity of the PCs and other proteases determines the cell type and the time at which the biologically active peptides are derived from the inactive precursor and thereby vitally affects cellular development and activity (Seidah and Chrétien, 1997).

b. Distribution of prohormone convertases

Furin and PC7 are widely expressed in all mammalian cells, and gene knockout experiments of furin in mice are embryonically lethal. Similarly, PC5 and PACE4 are found throughout the embryo but in the adult PC5 is limited to the gut, endothelial and Sertoli cells, and the adrenal cortex. The isoforms PC5A and PC5B are differentially sorted, the former being sent to dense-core secretory granules, whereas PC5-B is found chiefly in the *trans*-Golgi network (de Bie et al., 1996). PC4 is only expressed in the germ cells of the testis.

PC1/3 and PC2 are primarily expressed in endocrine and neural cells and, like PC5-A, are mostly localized within dense-core secretory granules in regulated cells. Several genes have now been found that code for convertases, and the genes for PC1/PC3 and PC2 have been cloned. These genes are active in cells where prohormone cleavage occurs and there is an especially high expression of these genes in neuropeptide-secreting cells, such as in the paraventricular nucleus (PVN), supraoptic nucleus (SON), pituitary, hypothalamus, and the insulin-secreting cells of the pancreas. These PCs are therefore believed to be the processing enzymes for the precursors of neuropeptides in the regulated secretory pathway. Furin is probably responsible for the maturation of many secretory and membrane-bound proteins within the constitutive secretory pathway.

Other modifications of the prohormone may be post-transcriptional but pretranslational: calcitonin and calcitonin gene–related peptide (CGRP) seem to be derived from a single gene after alternate splicing at the mRNA level. Here the primary product is tissue-specific since thyroid cells produce mRNA for calcitonin, whereas hypothalamic cells produce mRNA for CGRP (figure 3.8).

3.2.3.2 Exoproteolysis and Neuropeptide Segregation

Exoproteolysis follows the cleavage of the peptide precursor by endoproteolysis. After endoproteolytic cleavage the newly exposed C-terminal basic residues are removed by *carboxypeptidase E*, a carboxypeptidase B–like exopeptidase that has a high specificity for basic residues. This enzyme is also referred to as enkephalin convertase and carboxypeptidase H (see figure 3.3). After removal of C-terminal basic residues, peptides having an exposed C-terminal glycine residue often undergo conversion of this residue to an amide.

Most of the proteolytic processing of neuropeptides, at least as far as studies of POMC and proinsulin indicate, occurs within the secretory granules after they have been formed in the *trans*-Golgi network. Usually the products of proteolytic cleavage are stored and secreted in equimolar amounts. Depending on the sequential processing of the prohormone, the specific neuropeptide content of the vesicles will vary; if the prohormone undergoes endoproteolysis before being packaged in a vesicle, the vesicle may contain only one of the active sequences of the prohormone. On the other hand, if endoproteolysis occurs within the vesicle, that vesicle may enclose several different biologically active neuropeptides. This segregation of neuropeptides within different vesicles, or their coexistence within the same vesicle, is of utmost significance in determining the pattern of release of these regulatory agents after stimulation.

3.2.3.3 Post-Translational Enzymatic Modifications

Neuropeptides in the secretory granules may undergo glycosylation, removal of the C-terminal basic

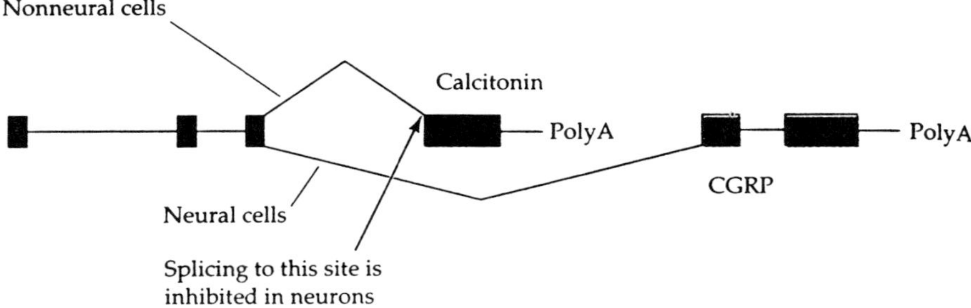

Figure 3.8
Neural-specific splicing. The calcitonin gene–related peptide (CGRP) gene is alternately spliced to produce calcitonin in nonneural cells and CGRP in neural cells. This regulation is brought about by neural-specific inhibition of splicing to exon 4, which encodes calcitonin. (From Lemke, 1992.)

residues by carboxypeptidase B–like exopeptidases, amidation, acetylation, phosphorylation, and sulfation, alterations that in most cases are crucial to the biological activity of the neuropeptide (see figure 3.4). The enzymes essential to the processing of the prohormones are in the dense-core vesicles of the regulated secretory pathway. It is important to emphasize that these modifications are, in many cases, remarkably species- or tissue-specific.

a. *Glycosylation*

Glycosylation of proteins is a complex process and depends on certain structural cues within the amino acid sequence of the protein (Bennett et al., 1993). The anterior pituitary hormones thyroid-stimulating hormone (TSH), luteinizing hormone (LH), follicle-stimulating hormone (FSH), and the closely related chorionic gonadotropin, are *N*-glycosylated, a process that permits the formation of the necessary dimer structure of these hormones and is essential to their biological activity. Human chorionic gonadotropin (HCG) undergoes glycosylation in which a core of high-mannose oligosaccharide is attached to the asparagine residues of the nascent polypeptide chain by an *N*-glycosidic linkage. The N-terminus of POMC is *O*-glycosylated and begins in the RER as core sugars are attached to the prohormone. The process is completed in the Golgi apparatus with several modifications to the carbohydrate side chain. However, blocking of glycosylation does not appear to affect the biosynthesis or release of the mature peptide (Vaudry et al., 1986).

b. *C-terminal amidation*

For many neuropeptides, C-terminal α-amidation is essential to biological activity. The enzyme responsible is peptidylglycine α-amidating monoxygenase (PAM), which converts, by two distinct catalytic steps, peptides that terminate in glycine to the corresponding des-Gly peptide amide; the C-terminal glycine is mandatory. This requires prior endoproteolytic cleavage and/or removal of C-terminal basic amino acids. High concentrations of PAM are found in the heart, anterior and intermediate pituitary, salivary glands, and hypothalamus, with lesser amounts found in almost all other tissues. Amidation often improves the binding of neuroendocrine peptides to their receptors and may protect them from degradation in vivo. As the ability to α-amidate peptides is uniquely associated with secretory granules, it is probably specific to the post-translational processing of neuropeptides.

c. *Acetylation*

Acetylation may determine the biological potency of many peptides but the degree to which a peptide is acetylated is remarkably tissue-specific. Acetylation not only affects the biological activity of neuropeptides either positively or negatively but may increase the longevity of the peptide in the circulation. It is also a mechanism by which the biological activities of different neuropeptides derived from the same precursor may be selectively potentiated or diminished, thus offering an additional means for the regulation of hormone activity. The acetyl group for the enzymatic reaction is derived from acetyl–coenzyme A. Acetylation of α-MSH and β-endorphin occurs in secretory granules of the intermediate lobe of the pituitary and markedly potentiates the activity of α-MSH but abolishes the opiate activity of β-endorphin. Acetylation does not occur within the anterior lobe as the secretory granules of this tissue do not contain peptide acetyltransferase.

Other examples include the post-translational acetylation of 5% of the histones on the N-terminus of GH in the hypothalamus, whereas 25% of the histones in leu-enkephalin in the posterior pituitary are acetylated. Dynorphin, a prohormone for leu-enkephalin, is found in both the hypothalamus and posterior pituitary, but its leu-enkephalin sequences are not acetylated. VP is inactivated by *N*-acetylation.

d. *Phosphorylation*

Phosphorylation of peptides is accomplished by cyclic adenosine monophosphate (cAMP)–dependent protein kinases. In the rat anterior pituitary 50% of ACTH molecules and 66% of corticotropin-like intermediate lobe peptide (CLIP) molecules are phosphorylated at serine 31; in the mouse the degree of phosphorylation of both these molecules is less than one third of that in the rat. In the human, phosphorylation is 33% and bovine ACTH and CLIP are not phosphorylated at all. Interestingly, phosphorylation does not seem to affect the biological activity of ACTH, which may explain the variability of this process. Many other neuropeptides are phosphorylated, although the specific sites have not all been identified: peptides derived from gastrin and proenkephalin precursors, parathormone (PTH), GH, PRL, proatrial natriuretic hormone, and HCG.

e. *Sulfation*

Tyrosine sulfation is the most common post-translational modification of Tyr residues. CCK, gastrin, and the amphibian peptide caerulein are derived from a common ancestral peptide and they have identical C-terminal pentapeptides, the active site for the sulfation of tyrosyl residues of these related neuropeptides. Sulfation dramatically affects the biological activity of certain neuropeptides, of which the CCK family is the best example. CCK undergoes successive cleavage to CCK 33, CCK 12, CCK 8, and CCK 4, of which all but CCK 4 are sulfated. Sulfation increases the effectiveness of CCK 33 260 times. Sulfation is essential to stimulating gallbladder emptying and pancreatic secretion, which explains the inactivity of CCK 4 on these processes. Many enkephalins are sulfates and sulfation may prolong the half-life of these and other neuropeptides by protecting exposed tyrosine residues from the extracellular environment.

3.2.4 *Summary of Biosynthesis and Processing*

The major steps in the conversion of preprohormones into their final products that occur during biosynthesis and their subsequent transport through the Golgi complex are illustrated in figure 3.4 and may be summarized as follows:

1. In the RER, cleavage of the signal peptide occurs and the resulting prohormone undergoes disulfide formation, folding, and perhaps *N*-glycosylation in the cysternal space of the ER.
2. These products are transferred to the Golgi complex in which a number of maturational processes may occur: the transitional products from step 1 may undergo phosphorylation, acetylation, *O*-glycosylation, oligosaccharide maturation, sulfation, endoproteolysis, exoproteolysis, amidation, or any combination of these. Proteolytic processing is significant in that it may activate or deactivate a molecule. Almost all the prohormones are biologically inactive, or active only at very high concentrations, and attain potency only after they are processed. On the other hand, further intracellular processing may inactivate the neuropeptide, for example, CCK 8 is active, CCK 4 is inactive; ACTH 1–39 is processed to several smaller molecules, one of which, CLIP, is generally inactive, although it may have some mild lipotropic effect.
3. Alternatively, the conversion of the prohormone to the hormone may occur in the early granules packaged by the Golgi complex. For example, newly formed gastrin granules containing the prohormone are fairly small and highly electron-dense. During the maturation process they become larger and electron-lucent. At this time there is a progressive change from gastrin 34 to gastrin 17, probably due to extensive proteolytic cleavage within the granule. These mature granules are then available for exocytotic secretion (Häkanson et al., 1982).

3.2.5 Tissue-Specific Processing

POMC was the first prohormone to be shown to be differentially processed in a tissue-specific manner to yield multiple active neuropeptides. In the anterior lobe of the pituitary gland, cleavage of POMC yields chiefly a large N-terminal fragment, ACTH 1–39, and β-lipotropin. These reactions are generated by PC1/3. PC1/3 is also present in the intermediate lobe where it again functions to generate ACTH and β-lipotropin, but PC2, which is present in the intermediate lobe but not the anterior lobe, further hydrolyzes them to produce the shorter neuropeptides, γ-lipotropin, β-endorphin, and α-MSH. Additional amino acid sequences, joining peptide (JP), and CLIP, of unknown biological activity, are also produced in the intermediate lobe (figure 3.9). This exemplifies tissue-specific processing of POMC due to the different expression of the two processing enzymes, PC1/3 and PC2.

In vitro studies have shown that an aspartic proteinease, purified from intermediate lobe secretory vesicles, and named *POMC-converting enzyme* (*PCE*), processes POMC between or on the carboxyl side of pairs of basic residues. PCE can generate all the major peptides found in the anterior pituitary but does not cleave ACTH 1–39 or β-endorphin (figure 3.10). As PCE is co-localized with α-MSH in intermediate lobe secretory vesicles, it is highly probable that this enzyme has a physiological role in POMC processing. Aspartic proteinases are selective in their substrate, most readily cleaving POMC but also cleaving proenkephalin, provasopressin, and pro-NPY (Hook et al., 1996).

Thus the differential processing patterns of a prohormone may depend on variations in the relative amounts of the individual convertases within a neuroendocrine cell (Rouille et al., 1995). Although POMC also contains the met-enkephalin sequence, this short sequence does not appear to be cleaved from POMC but instead is formed from a different prohormone, proenkephalin (see figure 1.3).

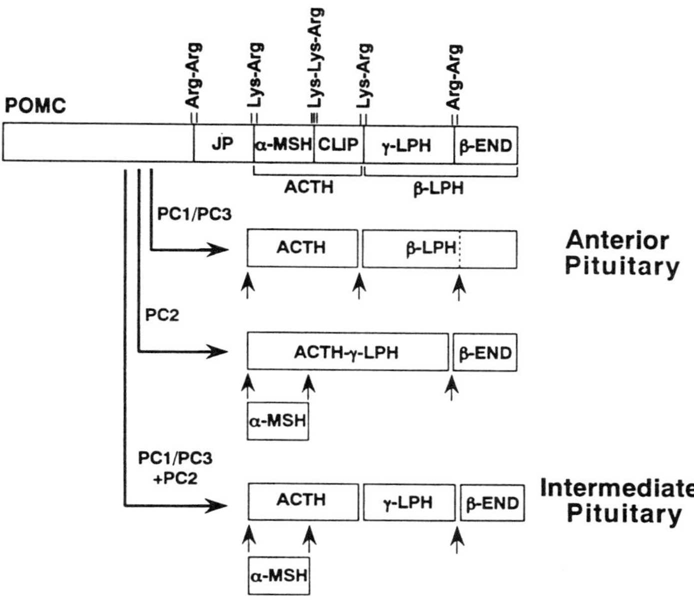

Figure 3.9
Tissue-specific processing of pro-opiomelanocortin (POMC), which is processed to ACTH and β-lipotropin (β-LPH) by proconvertase PC1/PC3 in the anterior lobe of the pituitary. In the intermediate lobe it is processed to smaller peptides such as melanocyte-stimulating hormone (α-MSH), corticotropin-like intermediate peptide (CLIP), and β-endorphin (β-END) by both PC1/3 and PC2. (From Mizuno and Matsuo, 1994.)

There is a satisfactory overlap of the expressions of PC1/PC3 and PC2 in the *early postnatal pituitary* with POMC expression and parallel changes in the POMC endoproteolytic processing pattern, indicating that the biosynthesis of these enzymes and their substrates may be regulated coordinately during ontogeny (Zheng et al.,1994).

Further support for the dependence of tissue-specific processing comes from the differential cellular distribution of the PCs in the PVN and SON, in which PC1 is colocalized with both VP and OT in intracellular secretory granules, but PC5 is colocalized only with OT mRNA. There is also selective regulation of PC1 by glucocorticoids (Dong et al., 1997). Differential processing of prohormones is an efficient method by which the tremendous functional diversity of the nervous system is achieved.

3.3 Precursor Genes

3.3.1 Localization of the Genes

Are the genes coding for neuropeptide precursors expressed in the same cells as the precursor? As described in chapter 2, gene expression in terms of mRNA levels can be measured by hybridization with the

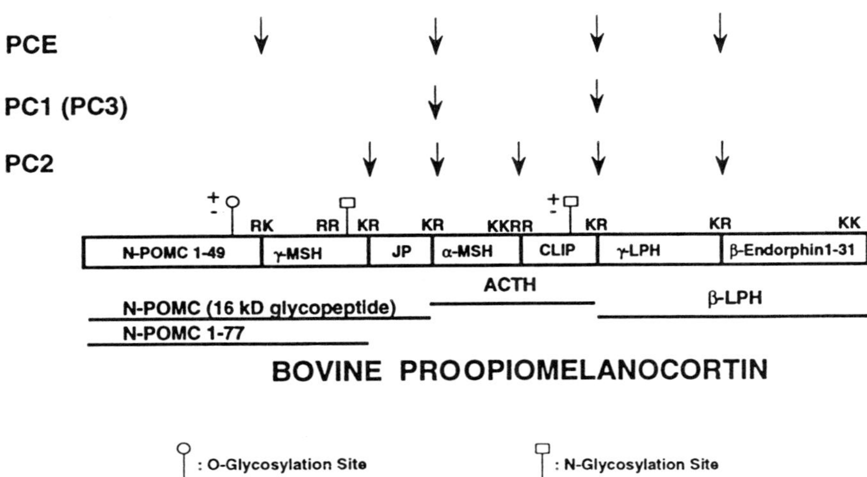

Figure 3.10
Diagrammatic representation of pro-opiomelanocortin (POMC). The cleavage sites are denoted by single-letter codes (R, arginine; K, lysine) and the processed products indicated. The arrows represent the sites cleaved by the three processing enzyme candidates: PCE, PC2, and PC1/3 (see text). LPH, lipotropin; MSH, melanocyte-stimulating hormone; ACTH, adrenocorticotropin; JP, joining peptide; CLIP, corticotropin-like intermediate peptide. (From Loh et al., 1993.)

appropriately labeled oligonucleotide probes prepared from the known nucleotide sequence of the cDNA or mRNA coding for the neuropeptide precursor. Northern blot analysis is used to measure the size of the message. In situ hybridization enables the specific mRNA to be localized in the cell and thus to identify the gene coding for the precursor. This technique permits the differentiation between cells that synthesize the neuropeptide and those that may only store the neuropeptide once it has been transported from some other site, a very important functional distinction.

3.3.2 Organization of a Precursor Gene: The Pro-opiomelanocortin Gene

The isolation and characterization of POMC mRNA and the organization of the POMC gene have been extensively studied and serve as a model for most neuropeptides. The mRNA coding for POMC and its translation products makes up almost one-third of the total translation products in the bovine pituitary intermediate lobe. The first POMC gene fragment described was that in the human and subsequently the whole POMC gene was determined in the cow (Nakanishi et al., 1979, 1981). The basic structure of the POMC gene has been highly conserved. The most conserved regions of nucleotide sequence are centered around each of the MSH units. The POMC gene contains three exons and two introns. In all cases studied, the large 3′ exon contains the nucleotides coding for all the biologically active neuropeptides (ACTH and α-MSH, β-lipotropin, β-MSH, and β-endorphin, and γ-MSH) and most of the N-terminal part of the precursor (figure 3.11). Exon 1 includes

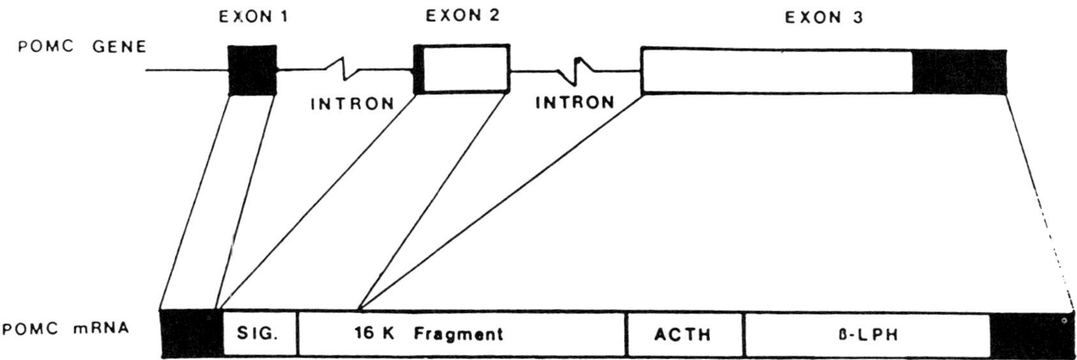

Figure 3.11
Schematic representation of the pro-opiomelanocortin (POMC) gene in mammals. The shaded regions on the POMC gene correspond to untranslated regions on the POMC mRNA. SIG, signal peptide; ACTH, adrenocorticotropic hormone; β-LPH, β-lipotropin. (From Dores, 1988.)

the nucleotide sequence complementary to the 5′ sequence of POMC mRNA and is a noncoding exon. Exon 2 codes for the signal peptide and the first 18 amino acids of POMC. There is a repetition of the melanotropin core heptasequence Met-Glu-His-Phe-Arg-Tryp-Gly in ACTH, α-MSH, β-MSH, and γ-MSH. The differential processing of these neuropeptides is discussed in chapter 12. The POMC gene has been localized to chromosome 2 in the human and to chromosome 19 in the mouse (Uhler et al., 1983).

3.3.3 *Regulation of Gene Expression*

Neuropeptide gene expression is usually regulated by a complex series of negative and positive controls. In the anterior pituitary lobe, the secretion of POMC peptides is stimulated by CRH and VP, and inhibited by glucocorticoids from the adrenal cortex. In the intermediate lobe, the release of POMC peptides is inhibited by the neurotransmitters dopamine and GABA. These secretory changes are preceded by the appropriate increase or suppression of POMC mRNA activity in the pituitary. Hypothalamic POMC mRNA levels also are controlled by gonadal steroids, especially estrogen, which markedly reduces POMC mRNA in ovariectomized rats (Wilcox and Roberts, 1985).

3.4 Excitation-Secretion Coupling

3.4.1 *Electrical Stimulation*

Neuroendocrine cells use their excitability to respond to physiological stimuli. The plasma membrane of neuroendocrine cells contains voltage-gated sodium, calcium, and potassium channels that mediate the all-or-nothing potentials associated with the rise in $[Ca^{2+}]_i$. Four major types of Ca^{2+} channels have been identified, three of which remain open long enough to cause a large transient increase in $[Ca^{2+}]_i$ with a time to peak of less than 1 second and a slower decay phase (2 to 4 seconds) (Schlegel and Mollard, 1995). These changes are illustrated in figure 3.12). After

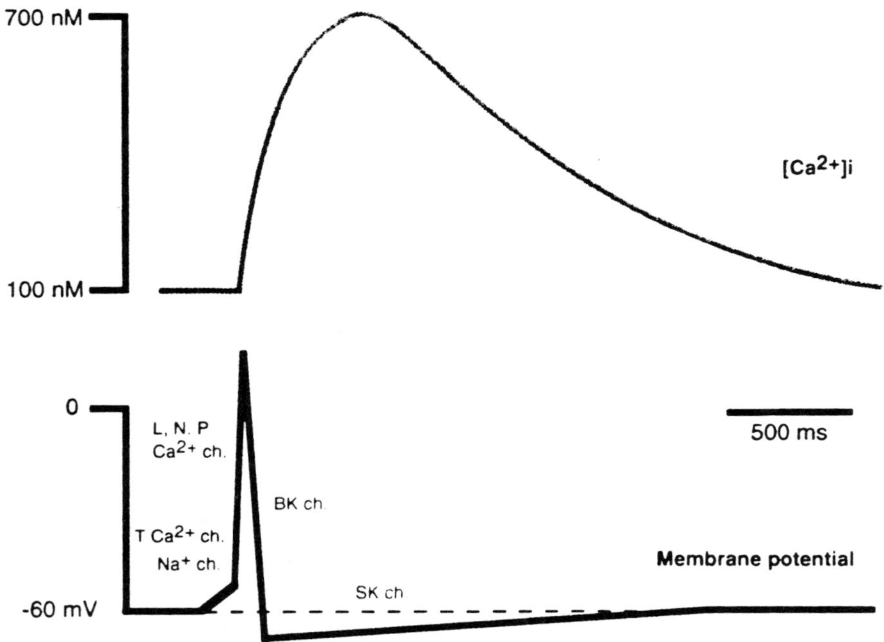

Figure 3.12
Relationship between ionic channels and membrane potential. Lower trace diagrams an action potential and the ionic channels involved. The upper trace illustrates the ensuing $[Ca^{2+}]_i$ change. Four calcium channels (ch.) are shown: T, transient, activated, and inactivated at low voltage; L, long-lasting; P, originally found in Purkinje cells; N, neither L nor T type. L, P, and N are activated at high voltage and inactivate slowly. (From Schlegel and Mollard, 1995.)

a rise in cytosolic free Ca^{2+}, neuroendocrine cells demonstrate a wide repertoire of electrical responses to secretatagogues (figure 3.13). Some cell types generate one or two patterns, for example, the beta cells of the endocrine pancreas respond to glucose with patterns c and g (see figure 3.13), whereas TRH–stimulated lactotrophs display almost all these patterns (Schlegel and Mollard, 1995).

3.4.2 Hormonal Stimulation

Hormones as well as action potentials induce secretion in neuroendocrine cells via the release of intracellular Ca^{2+} stores in response to the second-messenger inositol 1, 4, 5-triphosphate (IP_3), and IP_3 receptors are present in secretory vesicles of neuroendocrine cells (Blondel et al., 1995). However, it has not yet been conclusively shown that physiological hormone levels evoke an increase in cellular IP_3 (Petersen, 1996).

3.5 Exocytosis: A Calcium-Dependent Cell Function

Exocytosis entails the formation of fusion pores between membrane-bound vesicles and the presynaptic

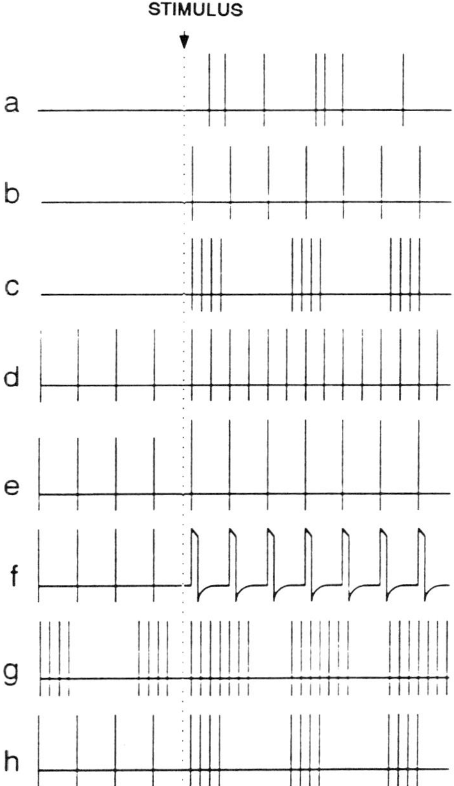

Figure 3.13
Patterns of electrical response of neuroendocrine cells to secretagogues grouped according to their prestimulation excitability: *In silent cells*, action potentials (APs) triggered by agonist application can appear (a) randomly (random mode); (b) as single spikes firing at near constant frequency (pacemaker mode); (c) as bursts of spikes separated by silent intervals (bursting mode). *In cells that are active prior to stimulation*, the stimulatory modulation can be observed as (d) an increse in spike frequency; (e) an increase in amplitude; (f) an increased duration of spikes; (g) a decrease in the silent interval between bursts or spikes; (h) a shift from one mode to another, for example, pacemaking to bursting. (From Schlegel and Mollard, 1995.)

membrane and the subsequent release of the contents of the vesicle into the extracellular space. The process involves multiple Ca^{2+} binding proteins with different affinities and a Ca^{2+} sensor for the final fusion with the plasma membrane. In neuroendocrine cells, two pathways of exocytosis exist:

1. In *constituted exocytosis* the vesicle membrane fuses with the presynaptic membrane as soon as the vesicle migrates from the *trans*-Golgi network and approaches the cell surface, so that the molecules stored in the vesicles are readily released into the extracellular milieu. This is the nonregulated process used by proteins that are continuously secreted.
2. *Regulated exocytosis of the classical neurotransmitters*, which are stored in *small electron-lucid synaptic vesicles (SSVs)* involves the orderly storage of the vesicles at active sites on the presynaptic membrane. Triggered by Ca^{2+} entry, fusion of the SSVs with the plasma membrane occurs within less than 1 ms, followed by the retrieval and refilling of the vesicles from nerve terminal stores. The delay between excitation and secretion is about 200 μs for fast synapses.

Regulated exocytosis of neuropeptides, which are are contained within *large (>70 nm) dense-core vesicles (LDCVs)*, is in many ways is more like the secretion of hormones from endocrine cells than the release of transmitters from the SSVs, with the delay between excitation and secretion being about 3 to 50 ms. A few vesicles may be waiting at the inner face of the plasma membrane until a cytosolic messenger triggers the *fusion event*, the initial phase of secretion. In many neuroendocrine cells, where both pathways for exocytosis exist, the rise in cytosolic Ca^{2+} due to the voltage-gated Ca^{2+} influx through the plasma membrane is sufficient to trigger exocytosis. Measurements at the single-cell level have shown that action potentials, or simulated spikes, effectively induce release of the vesicular contents (Zhou and Misler, 1995).

The first phase of secretion, the fusion event, is followed by a Ca^{2+}-dependent recruitment of vesicles or secretory granules that are further away from the plasma membrane. This migration involves a Ca^{2+}-dependent dissociation of the intracellular actin web of filaments by actin-severing proteins. This frees the vesicles to move toward the plasma membrane, where they may then be docked in place by synaptotagmin, a transmembrane protein, also Ca^{2+}-dependent. It is believed that synaptotagmin may position the secretory vesicle precisely at the site of entry of Ca^{2+} (i.e., voltage-dependent Ca^{2+} channels) and thereby facilitate excitation-secretion coupling (Littleton and Bellen, 1995). Figure 3.14 is a model of exocytosis in pancreatic beta cells, showing the various pools in which the secretory granules are believed to exist.

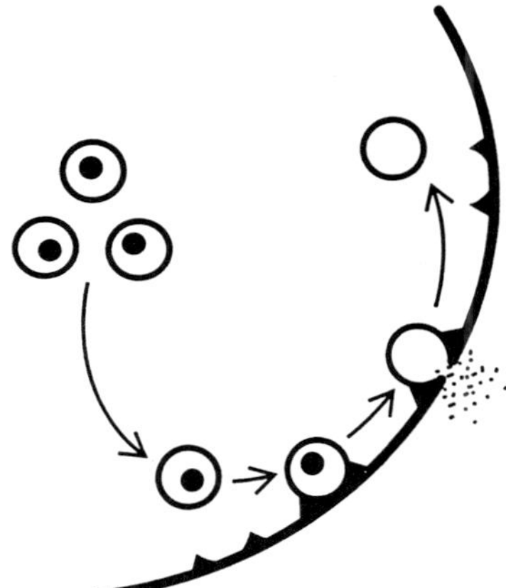

Figure 3.14
Model of exocytosis in pancreatic beta cells. The secretory granules are believed to exist in several pools, one of which is readily releasable (5% to 10%) and already docked with the plasma membrane. The docking sites are indicated by the hatched triangles on the plasma membrane. In addition, there is a much larger pool of granules not immediately available for release and which must be translocated or chemically modified to become releasable. Elevation of Ca^{2+} triggers the fusion of the secretory granules with the plasma membrane and subsequent release of the granule contents. Following exocytosis, empty secretory granules may be retrieved by endocytosis. (From Aschcroft and Rorsman, 1995.)

Characteristics of LDCV exocytosis in neuroendocrine cells include the following (Nicholls, 1994; Burgoyne and Morgan, 1995):

1. LDCVs are not usually docked before stimulation on the plasma membrane, as are SSVs, but may be released at regions other than the synaptic cleft and may not be directly targeted to postsynaptic receptors.
2. LDCVs are not neatly recycled at the terminals but must be refilled through the axonal transport of neuropeptides newly synthesized in the cell body. The components of the vesicle membrane are selectively recycled through an endocytotic pathway within the nerve terminal to generate new vesicles.
3. LDCVs lack many of the membrane and membrane-associated proteins that coat the SSVs, such as clathrin and the synapsins. They do possess three essential proteins, synaptobrevin, syntaxin, and synaptosome-associated protein 25 (SNAP 25), proteins also essential to neuronal exocytosis.
4. Both LDCVs and SSVs coexist in most neuroendocrine cells and may be differentially released. The LDCVs containing neuropeptides are released after a bulk increase in Ca^{2+} rather than a local coupling between Ca^{2+} channels and exocytosis, whereas stronger and more frequent stimulation will preferentially release SSVs, with their content of classical neurotransmitters (see chapter 4, section II. A).
5. Exocytosis in neuroendocrine cells is regulated by a Ca^{2+} binding protein with a Ca^{2+} affinity an order of magnitude higher than that in neuronal cells.

The fundamental differences in biosynthetic pathways, vesicular compartmentalization, and uptake and metabolism of catecholamines and neuropeptides have been concisely demonstrated using cultured neurons of the superior cervical ganglion which express high levels of both catecholamines and NPY. A clearly independent regulation of NPY and catecholamine content and release was shown (May et al., 1995).

Of considerable significance is the extracellular conversion of some neuropeptides after release into neuropeptides which may have effects that are similar, different from, or even the inverse of the parent neuropeptide, thus extending and increasing the selectivity of the role of the parent neuropeptides to influence a wide range of physiological processes. The several biologically active derivatives of the POMC molecule are a fine example of such diversification (De Wied, 1987).

3.6 Inactivation of Neuropeptides

In general, there is remarkably little *intracellular degradation* of neuropeptides, in contrast to their rapid inactivation in plasma. Some of the products of proteolytic cleavage are biologically inactive and many of the enzymatic modifications of the precursor may yield inactive metabolites. Degradation of neuropeptides to their inactive fragments or metabolites occurs in the RER or in the Golgi complex within about 30 minutes of precursor synthesis, whereas later cleavages occur in the secretory granules in which the products may then be stored for days. Thus the necessary enzymes must be present in the RER, Golgi complex, and the secretory granules (see figure 3.5).

Extracellular inactivation through enzymatic degradation occurs rapidly in plasma and by other cells, including glia, due to the widespread presence of peptidases. Neuropeptides are quickly inactivated in the gastrointestinal tract and therefore are ineffective if administered orally. It should be noted, however, that the effects of peripherally administered neuropeptides extend far longer than their biological half-life (about 15 to 20 minutes); this is due to their tenacious binding to cell membranes which apparently protects them from proteolysis and permits them to perpetuate the cascade of receptor-mediated second-messenger effects for several hours

3.7 Summary

Neuropeptides designed to be secreted are synthesized first as large preprohormones, polypeptide chains that include a signal sequence, which is removed by an endopeptidase during translation. The remaining peptide chain, the prohormone, is inactive and must be processed proteolytically into smaller fragments, both biologically active and inactive peptides. The prohormone is transported through the *cis*-face of the Golgi network to the *trans*-Golgi network where it is packaged into secretory granules, in which proteolytic processing by endoproteases (prohormone convertases), followed by exoproteases, continues, excising biologically active (and some inactive) sequences. Cleavage usually occurs at dibasic amino acid sites. Proteolysis begins at the *trans*-Golgi network and continues in the granules. During the transit through the Golgi network, the precursors may be subjected to enzymatic modifications such as glycosylation, phosphorylation, sulfation, or hydroxylation. Prohormones may be differentially processed in different tissues, yielding different amounts of the active peptides. Neuropeptide gene expression is regulated by a complex series of negative and positive controls by other neuropeptides and neurotransmitters.

Neuropeptides are secreted by a regulatory secretory pathway in which peptides are stored in secretory granules and released in response to secretagogues. Specific amino acid sequences in the prohormone form a sorting signal in the Golgi network that separates the molecules destined for secretory granules from the constitutive (default) secretory pathway.

Regulated exocytosis of neuropeptides, which are contained in LDCVs, is Ca^{2+}-dependent. They may be released together with small, clear synaptic vesicles containing classical transmitters, but the stimuli for release of neuropeptides are of higher frequency and longer duration. Unlike the classical transmitters, neuropeptides are not recycled at the nerve terminals but have to be refilled by newly synthesized neuropeptides delivered from the cell body. Again, unlike the relatively specific inactivating mechanisms for the classical neurotransmitters, there is little intracellular neuropeptide inactivation, apart from degradation to inactive metabolites in the RER or in the Golgi complex. Inactivation by peptidases occurs rapidly in plasma and in other cells.

Chapter 4 considers where neuropeptides are found in the central and peripheral nervous systems, their co-localization with other neuropeptides and neurotransmitters, and the implications this has for their role as neuromodulators, neurotransmitters, and integrators of physiological functions.

Distribution and Localization of Neuropeptides

4

4.1 Distribution in the Central and Peripheral Nervous Systems

4.1.1 Hypothalamus, Preoptic area, Pituitary Gland, and Spinal Cord

The richest sources of neuropeptides in the CNS are several hypothalamic nuclei, the preoptic area, and the pituitary gland. However, many of the neurosecretory hypothalamic neurons have projection axons long enough to reach fairly distant areas of the CNS so that these neuropeptides are found in high concentrations in nerve terminals in many regions of the brain and spinal cord.

4.1.2 The Endocrine Brain

Other brain areas also contain neuropeptides, as indicated in tables 4.1 and 4.2. In addition to their concentration in hypothalamic nuclei and the pituitary gland, several neuropeptides such as somatostatin, TRH, neurotensin, substance P (SP), insulin, CCK, VIP, and the enkephalins are found in perikarya generously distributed in certain areas of the CNS, areas that are rich in both peptide-immunoreactive cell bodies and terminals. These include the dorsal horn of the spinal cord, the dorsal vagal complex, the nucleus accumbens, the stria terminalis bed nuclei, the amygdala, and the periaqueductal central gray. This extensive distribution of neuropeptides in the brain has led to the concept of the brain as an endocrine organ. The "endocrine brain," as defined by Palkowits (1980), is a system of CNS neurons that produce neuropeptides. However, unlike the extensive peptidergic pathways of the hypothalamic neurosecretory neurons, the pathways of neurons in extrahypothalamic brain areas are obscure and it is likely that they act chiefly on neighboring neurons in a paracrine manner. These brain neuropeptides are not susceptible to the tight regulation by target organ secretions that control the secretion of the hypothalamic and pituitary neuropeptides, as considered in detail in chapters 12 and 13.

Table 4.1
Coexistence of neurotransmitters and neuropeptides

Transmitter	Neuropeptide	Tissue
Dopamine	Neurotensin	Mesencephalon
	CCK	Mesencephalon
	Neurotensin, galanin, GnRH	Median eminence
	Calcitonin	Chick ultimobranchial
Norepinephrine	Enkephalin	Locus ceruleus
		Superior cervical ganglion
	Neuropeptide Y	Locus ceruleus
		Medulla oblongata
	Pancreatic polypeptide	Hindbrain, pancreas
		Sympathetic nerves
	Somatostatin	Sympathetic ganglia
Epinephrine	Neurotensin	Medulla oblongata
	Neuropeptide Y	Medulla oblongata
	Substance P	Medulla oblongata
	TRH	Medulla oblongata
	Enkephalin	Medulla oblongata
		Pons, adrenal medulla
Acetylcholine	VIP	Cerebral cortex
		Autonomic ganglia
		Submandibular gland
	Enkephalin	Cochlear nerves
	Substance P	Pons
GABA	Somatostatin	Thalamus
	Motilin	Cerebellum
Serotonin	Somatostatin	Thyroid
	Calcitonin	Thyroid
	Substance P	Medulla oblongata
		Raphe
	TRH	Medulla
	Insulin	Pancreas
Substance P[a]	CCK	Dorsal horn

CCK, cholecystokinin; GnRH, gonadotropin-releasing hormone; TRH, thyrotropin-releasing hormone; VIP, vasoactive intestinal polypeptide; GABA, γ-aminobutyric acid.
[a] May be classified here as a neurotransmitter.

Table 4.2
Coexistence of neuropeptides in the same neuron

Neuropeptide	Site of Neurons
ACTH, α-MSH, β-endorphin[a]	Arcuate nucleus, pituitary
Enkephalin, dynorphin	Arcuate nucleus
Neurotensin, galanin	Arcuate nucleus
Neurotensin, galanin, GnRH (LHRH)	Median eminence
Dynorphin, vasopressin	Supraoptic nucleus
Gastrin, cholecystokinin	Supraoptic nucleus
Cholecystokinin, oxytocin	Paraventricular nucleus
α-Neoendorphin, dynorphin	Magnocellular hypothalamus
Somatostatin, pancreatic polypeptide	Telencephalon
Enkephalin, somatostatin	Adrenal gland
ACTH, α-MSH, gastrin	Antropyloric gastrin cells
Met- and leu-enkephalin[a]	Stomach wall, myenteric plexus
TRH, substance P	Medulla oblongata
Substance P, leu-enkephalin	Avian ciliary ganglion

ACTH, adrenocorticotropin; MSH, melanocyte stimulating hormone; GnRH, gonadotropin-releasing hormone; TRH, thyrotropin-releasing hormone; LHRH, luteinizing hormone releasing hormone.
[a] Common precursor: located in same dense-core vesicles.

4.1.3 The Periphery

Table 1.2 shows that whereas some neuropeptides appear to be restricted to the CNS, others are more widely distributed in various regions of the body, especially mucosal cells in the gastrointestinal tract, the pancreas, adrenal medulla, gonads, the placenta, and peripheral nerves.

4.2 Localization of Neuropeptides

The presence of a neuropeptide in a tissue, as determined by immunocytochemical methods, is not proof that it was synthesized in that tissue since it may have been transported there by the hypothalamic-hypophyseal portal system, the vascular system, through the CSF, via axonal transport, or by accidental contamination. However, modern techniques, such as mRNA determination of the biosynthetic precursor, provide more accurate information as to the site of neuropeptide synthesis. The concentration of brain peptides (10^{-12} to 10^{-15} moles/mg protein) is infinitely less than that of the classical neurotransmitters such as ACh and norepinephrine (NE) (10^{-9} to 10^{-10}) and they are physiologically effective at nerve terminals at these extremely low concentrations. However, pituitary and gut peptides, which are diluted through the circulation before they reach their targets, are present at their sites of synthesis in concentrations considerably higher than those of the brain peptides. Similarly, administration of neuropeptides into the ventricles of the brain (intracerebroventricular, i.c.v.) requires far less peptide than intravenous (i.v.) administration to evoke a physiological response. Intravenous administration, of course, involves not only dilution of the neuropeptide in the circulation but involves problems of breaching the blood-brain barrier (BBB).

4.2.1 Coexistence of Neurotransmitters and Neuropeptides

4.2.1.1 Dale's Principle

The discovery that more than one neurotransmitter may be liberated from a neuron is often considered to violate Dale's principle. However, what Dale noted in 1935 was that if the sensory peripheral terminals of a neuron secreted ACh, then it was likely that the central terminals of this neuron would secrete the same chemical. This concept was extended by Eccles (1957) into what he termed Dale's principle, stating that "any one class of nerve cells operates at all its synapses by the same chemical transmission mechanism." At that time, there was little evidence that more than one transmitter could be synthesized by a neuron, but whereas we now know that several transmitters, including neuropeptides, can be produced and secreted by a neuron, the assumption is still that all branches of the neuron contain the same selection of neurotransmitters, supporting Dale's principle of the metabolic and functional unity of the neuron. It has been suggested that since the smaller neurotransmitter molecules are stored in small vesicles and the larger neuropeptide molecules are stored in dense-core vesicles, that there could be some selectivity of one axonal branch for the larger or smaller package (Whittaker, 1984). There is considerable evidence that there is selective release of large and small vesicles depending on the frequency and duration of nerve stimulation, but these modifications do not negate Dale's principle. In general, peptide release requires bursts of high-frequency stimulation (figure 4.1), but in some cases it is the continuous repetitive stimulation rather than the bursting pattern that regulates peptide release (Peng and Horn, 1991). The neuropeptide is frequently responsible for a slow and long-lasting response in contrast to the rapid and short-lasting effects of classic transmitters, such as ACh and NE (see figure 4.1).

4.2.1.2 Evidence for Coexistence of Neuropeptides and Neurotransmitters

Hökfelt et al. (1984, 1986), in a series of classic papers, have clearly demonstrated the coexistence of neuro-

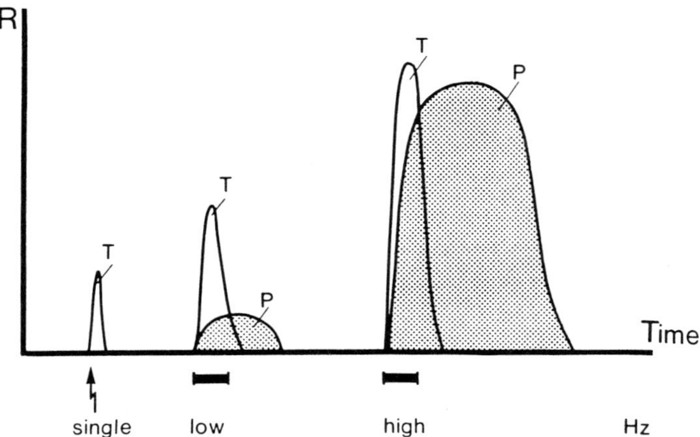

Figure 4.1
Contribution of the classical transmitter (T) and coexisting peptide (P) to the functional response (R) of neuronal activation induced by increasing frequency of electrical stimulation. A single nerve impulse preferentially induces a response due to the classical transmitter. With higher frequencies, the slower, graded, and longer-lasting peptide effect is evoked. (From Lundberg and Hökfelt, 1985.)

transmitters and neuropeptides within the same neuron, sometimes even within the same vesicle, in both central and peripheral neurons. Table 4.1 lists some of the combinations that have been demonstrated; many others probably exist. Interestingly, there is little evidence for the coexistence of two or more classical neurotransmitters, such as ACh and NE, or dopamine (DA) and serotonin (5-HT), in one neuron, although GABA has been shown to be colocalized with DA or 5-HT (Belin et al., 1983). In some neurons, two or more neuropeptides may be present in the same or separate secretory granules depending on the processing of the prohormone (see table 4.2). These variations lend immense flexibility to the regulation and modification of synaptic events. The coexistence of neurotransmitters and neuropeptides and their simultaneous or sequential release require multiple forms of receptors on both postsynaptic and presynaptic membranes, resulting in diverse, receptor-mediated effects on the excitability of the target cell. Figure 4.2 diagrams the possible vesicular combinations of a classical neurotransmitter 5-HT with the neuropeptides SP, TRH, and neurokinin A (NKA) in spinal autonomic systems.

Lundberg and Hökfelt (1985) have suggested possible variations in regulatory control that arise from the coexistence of a classic transmitter and a neuropeptide in nerve terminals synapsing on a postsynaptic cell (figure 4.3):

1. One transmitter acts on one postsynaptic receptor (R).
2. The transmitter acts on multiple types of postsynaptic receptors (R′α, R′, R′β).
3. The transmitter acts in addition on a presynaptic receptor (Rp1) to affect its own release
4. The enlarged nerve terminal shows that multiple compounds peptide (M1–3), possibly differentially

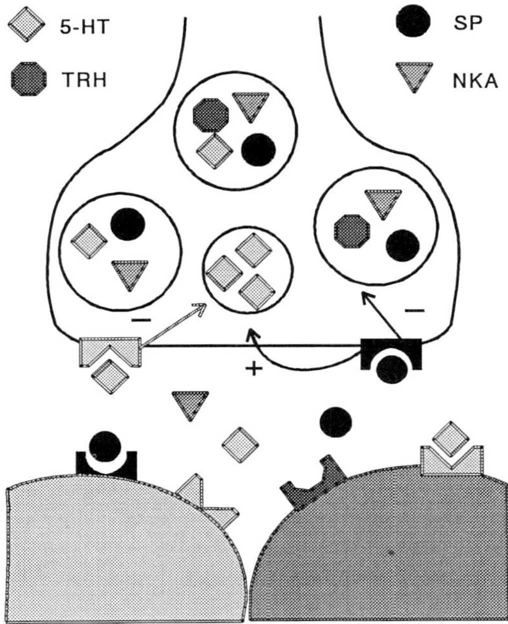

Figure 4.2
Schematic of a nerve terminal in the interomediolateral cell column of the thoracic spinal cord showing the coexistence of serotonin (5-HT), subtance P (SP), neurokinin A (NKA), and thyrotropin-releasing hormone (TRH), potential vesicular storage sites, and presynaptic receptor–mediated release of 5-HT and SP. The inhibitory effects of the presynaptic 5-HT_{1B} and the NK_1 receptors are on the evoked release of 5-HT and SP, respectively. The facilitory effect of the NK_1 receptor activation is on the basal release of 5-HT. (From Helke and Yang, 1996.)

stored in small vesicles (classical transmitters) and in large, dense-core vesicles (classical transmitter plus peptide) are released from the same nerve ending. The main possible interactions are:

a. inhibition of the release of the second messenger (peptide M2) by the classical transmitter (M1) via presynaptic action (Rp′1);

b. interaction at the postsynaptic receptor (R′β) level between M1 and M2;

c. facilitation or inhibition of release of the classical transmitter by the peptide (M3) via action on a presynaptic receptor (Rp″);

d. activation by the peptide (M3) of electrical activity in the postsynaptic neuron via a postsynaptic receptor (R‴).

4.3 Neurohormone, Neurotransmitter, or Neuromodulator?

4.3.1 Neurohormone or Neurotransmitter?

When neurons secrete their hormones into a vascular system to be transported to relatively distant target organs, they fulfill the classical definition of a hormone, or in this case a neurohormone. However, many of the axon terminals of a neurosecretory cell may also secrete their products at synapses to directly affect a postsynaptic cell, thus acting as neurotransmitters. Consequently, the classification of a neurohormone is often blurred and a neuropeptide may justly be considered a neurohormone at one terminal and a neurotransmitter at another.

4.3.2 Neurotransmitter or Neuromodulator?

Traditionally, a neurotransmitter is secreted from nerve endings in response to Ca^{2+} influx and causes a change in the membrane potential of the postsynaptic cell, to either depolarize or hyperpolarize it, changes that result in either stimulation or inhibition of the postsynaptic cell. A neuromodulator, such as a neuropeptide, is also secreted in response to Ca^{2+} influx and is capable of altering the postsynaptic potential but not sufficiently to evoke either an excitatory (EPSP) or

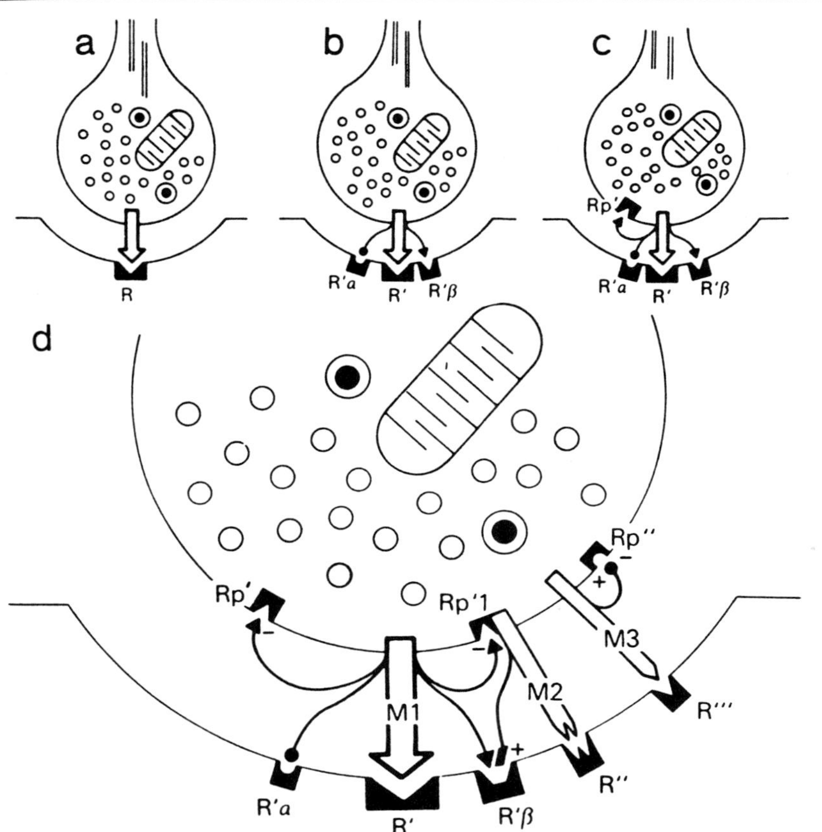

Figure 4.3
Schematic representation of possible regulatory actions of multiple transmitters at a synapse. See text. (From Lundberg and Hökfelt, 1985.)

inhibitory (IPSP) postsynaptic potential. The neuromodulator may facilitate an EPSP and exacerbate an IPSP evoked by the neurotransmitter. The neuromodulator may affect the intensity and the duration of the response after the short, intense response evoked by the neurotransmitter. Figure 4.4 illustrates an example in which the action of the neuropeptide prolongs that of the transmitter. In sympathetic nerves terminating in the salivary gland, the transmitter noradrenaline (NA) (also known as norepinephrine) induces secretion by a salivary acinus as well as vasoconstriction of the supplying blood vessels, the latter effect being prolonged by the colocalized NPY. In parasympathetic nerves to this gland, ACh causes salivary secretion and vasodilation, increasing blood flow through the gland, the latter effect being prolonged by the colocalized VIP, or perhaps due to VIP.

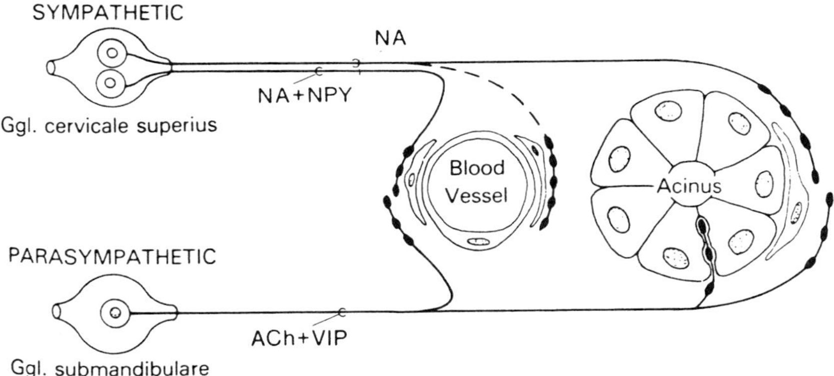

Figure 4.4
Innervation of the cat submandibular gland by autonomic neurons containing multiple neurotransmitters with different effects upon the target organs. Noradrenaline (NA) induces salivary secretion and vasoconstriction which is blocked by α- and β-adrenoreceptor antagonists. Neuropeptide Y (NPY), co-localized with NA, has no effect on secretion but causes prolonged vasoconstriction. Acetylcholine (ACh) increases secretion and causes vasodilation which is blocked by atropine. Vasoactive intestinal polypeptide (VIP), co-localized with ACh, has no effect on secretion but causes prolonged vasodilation. (From Lundberg and Hökfelt, 1985.)

In the complexity of the CNS, a neuropeptide may act as a neurotransmitter at some synapses and a neuromodulator at others. This topic is considered in detail in chapter 7. It is therefore simpler to refer to these neurosecretions in general as neuropeptides and consign their definition as hormone, neurotransmitter, or neuromodulator to a specific neuropeptide at a specific site.

4.3.3 Volume Transmission

Fuxe and Agnati (1991) have emphasized the importance of neuropeptides as volume transmission signals, a concept that envisions extrasynaptically co-released transmitters, each matched to its selective, high-affinity receptor. Volume transmission is characterized by three-dimensional conduction of the signal within the extracellular fluid. Figures 4.5 and 4.6 illustrate the different types of intercellular communication and how they may be involved in volume transmission. These include autocrine and paracrine transmission for short distances, neuroendocrine-like transmission though the CSF for longer distances, and even the use of nerve bundles as preferential diffusion pathways for longer distances. Thus, for this type of communication, it is essential that nerve terminals contain multiple classical transmitters and high-affinity receptors, selective for each of these chemical signals.

4.4 Pathway-Specific Neuropeptide Content

As has just been discussed, some neurons may contain several neuropeptides in addition to a nonpeptide neurotransmitter such as 5-HT, ACh, or NE. In some cases the coexisting neuropeptides appear to have synergistic or at least similar postjunctional effects, yet

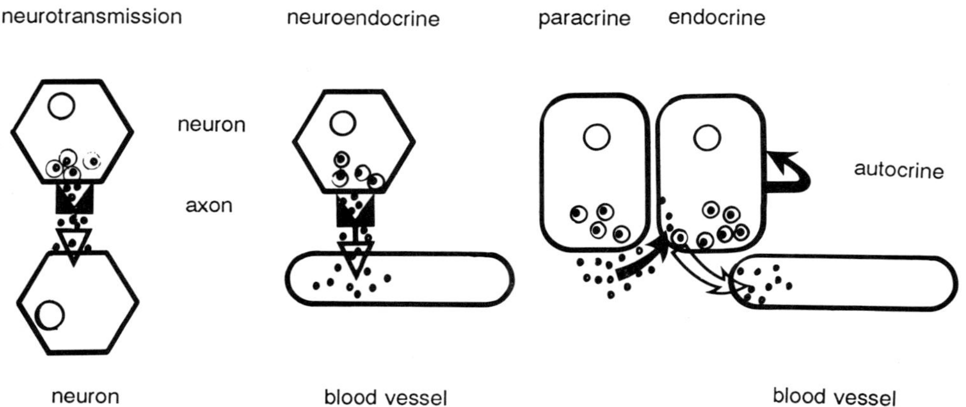

Figure 4.5
Chemical communication between cells. Transmitter release from one neuron to an adjacent neuron, neurotransmission; secretion by a neuroendocrine cell into the circulation, neurohormonal; secretion by one cell to affect an adjacent cell, paracrine; secretion by a cell to affect itself, autocrine; secretion from an endocrine cell into the circulation, hormonal.

there are examples of opposing postjunctional actions. If neuropeptides are indeed regulators of physiological functions, how are they in turn regulated? It appears that anatomical distribution may be some indication of their ultimate function.

4.4.1 Correlation Between Neuropeptide Content and Target Tissue

There does seem to be some pattern to the coexistence of neuropeptides according to the neuronal pathways in which they are found. There is a high degree of correlation between the combination of peptides in a neuron and the peripheral tissue to which that neuron projects (Gibbins, 1989). This is well documented for autonomic and sensory neurons. Dorsal root ganglia (DRG) contain several populations of neurons, each of which has a distinct combination of neuropeptides and a specific projection to its target organ. Table 4.3 shows that some DRG neurons possess SP, CGRP, CCK, and dynorphin, and that these neurons project to the skin, forming free sensory endings around small dermal blood vessels. Other DRG neurons contain SP, CGRP, and CCK, but not dynorphin, and these neurons project to small blood vessels in skeletal muscles. Yet another group of DRG neurons contains SP, CGRP, and dynorphin, but not CCK, and innervate the pelvic viscera. Similar pathway-specific neuropeptide combinations occur in sympathetic ganglia.

On the other hand, all the neurons in some peripheral ganglia appear to have the same neuropeptide combination and all project to the same tissue, for example, all the cholinergic ciliary ganglion cells contain SP as well as ACh and they all innervate the muscles of the iris of the eye. This is complicated by the fact that each population of neurons contains additional unique combinations of other neuropeptides: SP is also found in the sensory neurons innervating the iris, but in this neuronal population SP is combined

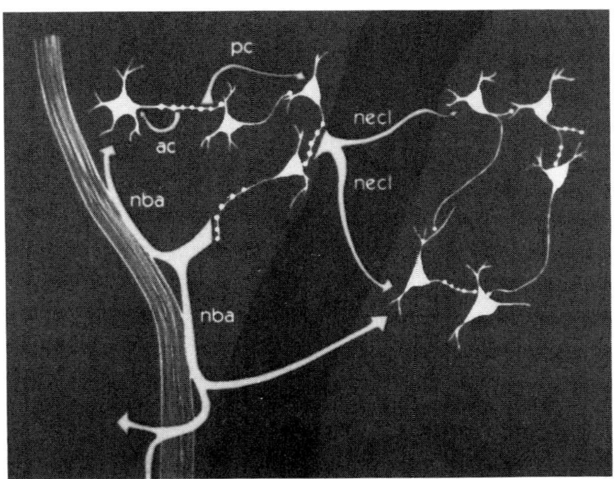

Figure 4.6
Schematic representation of the different types of intercellular communications involved in volume transmission in the CNS. Autocrine (ac) and paracrine (pc) transmission take place over short distances (short arrows). Nerve bundle–associated (nba) transmission is the preferential diffusion route for long-distance volume transmission (long arrows), while neuroendocrine-like (necl) transmission involves the cerebrospinal fluid as a route. (From Fuxe et al., 1994.)

Table 4.3
Peptide content and peripheral projections of unmyelinated dorsal root ganglion neurons of guinea pigs

Peptide combination	Main peripheral targets
CGRP, SP	Heart, most blood vessels, abdominal viscera
CGRP, SP, CCK	Blood vessels in skeletal muscles
CGRP, SP, dynorphin	Pelvic viscera, airways
CGRP, SP, CCK, dynorphin	Skin, iris
CCK	Viscera

From Gibbins, 1989.
CGRP, calcitonin gene–related protein; SP, substance P; CCK, cholecystokinin.

with CGRP, dynorphin, and CCK. Similarly, NPY is found in both sympathetic and parasympathetic neurons, and dynorphin occurs in both sympathetic and sensory neurons (figure 4.7).

4.4.1.1 Significance of Pathway-Specific Distribution

Some of the implications of the distribution of neuropeptides according to their anatomical origin are summarized by Gibbins (1989) as follows:

1. A tissue may be innervated by different classes of neurons containing the same peptide, as illustrated in figures 4.4 and 4.7.
2. Functionally similar neurons may contain different neuropeptides. There are marked differences in the peptide-containing neurons that result in vasodilation: those innervating the cranial blood vessels contain VIP, those innervating the pelvic blood vessels contain VIP, NPY, dynorphin, and somatostatin.
3. Neurons may contain families of gene-related peptides. Neuropeptides that are produced from the same precursor are often present in the same neuron. The products of POMC (ACTH, α-MSH, β-endorphin) coexist, as do the products of preprotachykinin (SP, NKA, or substance K). However, owing to differential processing of some neuropeptide precursors, not all the products of the same gene necessarily coexist in the same cell.

4.4.1.2 Integrative Role for Coexisting Neuropeptides

The widespread coexistence of neuropeptides and neurotransmitters in all types of neurons, except myelinated sensory neurons and most myelinated motor nerves, may have a functional significance that extends beyond their roles as transmitters of slow events or as neuromodulators. The parvocellular neurons of

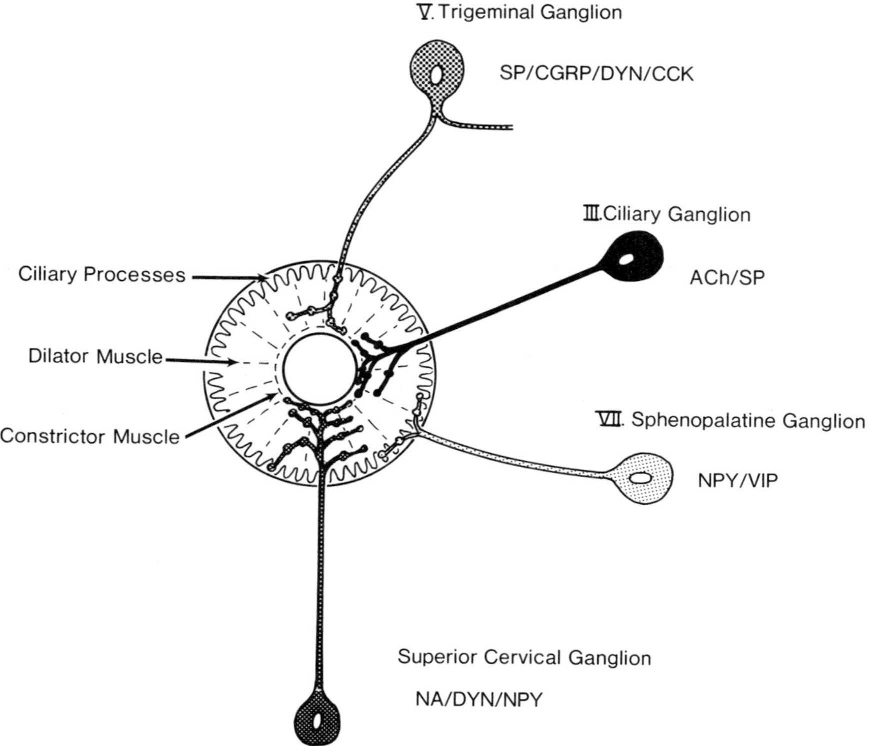

Figure 4.7
Diagram summarizing the innervation of the albino guinea pig iris by peptide-containing autonomic and sensory neurons. Substance P (SP), neuropeptide Y (NPY), and dynorphin (DYN) each occur in two functionally and anatomically different populations of neurons. However, the combination of peptides in any particular neuronal population is unique. CCK, cholecsytokinin; VIP, vasoactive intestinal polypeptide; NA, noradrenaline, ACh, acetylcholine. Roman numerals refer to the cranial nerve pathway in which the ganglia lie. (From Gibbins, 1989.)

the hypothalamus that are best known for their production of CRF can synthesize at least seven neuropeptides: the hypothalamic magnocellular neurons that secrete OT and/or VP are capable of secreting several other neuroactive compounds, expressed at much lower concentrations than OT and VP (Sawchenko at al., 1992). These observations indicate differential regulation of coexisting molecules within the same neuron, a very delicate type of "fine control."

Unmyelinated sensory neurons not only have central processes that transmit information to the CNS but their peripheral axons release a cocktail of neuropeptides (SP, NKA, and CGRP) that synergistically act to reduce neurogenic inflammation. SP may further enhance wound healing through increasing the rate of fibroblast cell division. Since CRGP inhibits SP breakdown, both centrally and peripherally, and CCK and dynorphin regulate these effects, the intricacies of neuropeptide interaction permit subtleties of regulation that we are only beginning to comprehend.

4.4.1.3 Neuropeptides: Fail-Safe, Redundant, or Special?

At the beginning of the neuropeptide decade, we believed that each neuropeptide had a specific and identifiable action upon a certain tissue. This concept has not stood the test of time and it is unlikely that there is a "one peptide, one response" phenomenon in a living, intact physiological system. Could it be that if one peptide is not readily available, another may readily take its place?

Many cellular functions have overlapping controls, indicating a remarkable degree of redundancy or fail-safe precautions. These precautionary measures range from the redundancy of respiratory control mechanisms within the CNS to the plethora of communications conveyed by second-messenger molecules. An excellent example of apparent overlap may be seen in the number of agents that appear to have beneficial effects on nerve regeneration. Cells particiating in nerve repair in vivo condition the local milieu through the release of factors that stimulate Schwann cell adhesion, migration, and proliferation. Exogenously administered gangliosides, guide tubes, sex steroids, the growth-associated protein B50, calcium antagonists, melanocortins, growth hormone, TSH, and ciliary neurotrophic factor, all enhance peripheral nerve regeneration to about the same extent. This suggests that the role of neuropeptides is complex, that they are probably multifunctional, and that very often one one neuropeptide can replace another. Their effects and effectiveness may vary according to their metabolic milieu, their interaction with other growth factors, including steroid hormones, the genetic sex of the organism, the stage of development of the target organ, and possible guidance messages from the target organ. In addition, physical factors such as surface molecules, piezoelectrical effects, and magnetic fields all alter nerve growth. Some specific examples may be found in Strand et al. (1990). The neuropeptides are functioning in a complex jungle of competing and coordinating agents and it will be our task to sort out which actions are undeniably specific from those that are merely redundant, so that we may eventually assess to what extent a physiological fail-safe system exists.

4.5 Summary

Not only are the hypothalamus and pituitary gland rich in neuropeptides but many brain regions produce neuropeptides, which act in a paracrine or autocrine manner. Many neuropeptides are found in peripheral organs. A neuron can synthesize several neuropeptides and neurotransmitters, but in general, the smaller transmitters are stored in small, clear vesicles, whereas the larger neuropeptides are stored in bigger, dense-core vesicles. The pattern, duration, and frequency of stimulation will determine the simultaneous or selective release of neuropeptide or transmitter. The existence of many different receptors, pre- and postsynaptic, permits many variations in regulatory control at the synapse. Neuropeptides may sometimes act as neurotransmitters, neuromodulators, or neurohormones, depending on the synapse or tissue. Extrasynaptically coreleased neuropeptides may act as volume transmission signals within the extracellular fluid, but require selective, high-affinity receptors.

In some cases, there is a pattern to the coexistence of neuropeptides according to the neuronal pathway in which they are found and the peripheral tissue to which those neurons project. Examples are found in DRG neurons that project to the skin and in peripheral ganglionic neurons projecting to the iris of the eye. Functionally similar neurons may contain different neuropeptides. Neurons may contain families of gene-related peptides, as they are produced from the same precursor. The several different neuropeptides that are released at the nerve endings of unmyelinated sensory nerves may act synergistically to reduce inflammation. As many neuropeptides seem to have overlapping functions, the question arises as to whether they are redundant, fail-safe, or special.

In chapter 5 the organization of the neuroendocrine system is described and the transport systems that carry neuropeptides through this system are considered. The important topic of how neuropeptides enter the CNS is discussed in terms of the structure and function of the blood-brain barrier.

The Neuroendocrine System and the Transport of Neuropeptides

5

5.1 The Neuroendocrine System

5.1.1 Neuropeptide Pathways

As discussed in chapter 4, neuropeptides are present in almost all tissues, but they are especially concentrated in the CNS. The hypothalamus, especially its preoptic area; the median eminence (ME); and the pituitary gland contain the highest concentrations of neuropeptides, which, except for the anterior pituitary gland, are less concentrated in the cell bodies and axons than in nerve terminals. Special neural and vascular pathways provide the routes by which these brain and neuroendocrine secretions reach their targets. These pathways are the *hypothalamic-median eminence-anterior pituitary neuropeptide system* and the *hypothalamic–posterior pituitary pathway*. In addition, many neurosecretory neurons send axon collaterals directly to CNS neurons.

Neuropeptides synthesized in peripheral tissues, such as the pancreas and gut, reach their local target cells via paracrine and autocrine mechanisms, but also have endocrine effects (see figure 4.1) as they travel through the systemic circulation to reach the brain and spinal cord. This communication between central and peripheral actions in many cases requires passage of neuropeptides through the BBB.

5.1.2 Anatomical Structure of the Neuroendocrine System

5.1.2.1 Hypothalamic-Median Eminence-Anterior Pituitary System

a. The hypothalamus

The hypothalamus forms the base of the diencephalon and has reciprocal neural connections with much of the cerebral hemispheres and brainstem, essential to its role in the maintenance of homeostasis and integration of behavioral patterns. In addition to its purely neural connections, many of the hypothalamic areas contain neurosecretory cells which release their secretions either through a vascular route to the anterior pituitary gland, to regulate the release of the pituitary tropic hormones, or through a neural route to the posterior pituitary (figures 5.1, 5.2, and 5.3). This forms the *neuroendocrine system*, which has two main components, which are illustrated in figures 5.2 and 5.4 and described below.

The first component was described in the early days of neuroendocrine research by Berta and Ernst Scharrer in 1937. This is the *magnocellular neuroendocrine system*, consisting of large cells in the paraventricular nucleus (PVN) and the supraoptic nucleus (SON). Axons from these cells pass through the stalk or infundibulum to terminate in the posterior pituitary gland, where they release their secretions, oxytocin (OT) and vasopressin (VP), into the venous circulation.

The second component, the *parvocellular neurosecretory system*, is formed by cells in the hypothalamic region, including the preoptic area, and the ventromedial, dorsomedial, posterior hypothalamic, premammillary, and suprachiasmatic nuclei, the axons of which liberate their releasing or release-inhibiting secretions into a vascular system in the ME. Table 5.1 summarizes the anatomical source of most of the hypothalamic regulatory neuropeptides.

b. The median eminence

The fibers from these hypothalamic regions run in three bundles to terminate in the ME. CRH, gonadotropin-releasing hormone (GnRH), and TRH fibers and terminals run mainly in the medial part, with GnRH and DA fibers in the two lateral parts (Halász, 1994). Some axons from the magnocellular nuclei of the hypothalamus, the paraventricular and supraoptic nuclei, also terminate in the ME but most of these axons pass directly to the posterior pituitary, as described below. Neuropeptides synthesized in other brain areas are also conveyed to the ME. All the known hypothalamic neuropeptides can be found in the ME, making it a particularly rich source of these hormones. The most important pathways are formed by the axons of the cells of the parvocellular nuclei (Palkowits, 1980). Fibers from the preoptic area and the forebrain may contain LHRH, TRH, or somatostatin. Other axons terminating in the ME, especially from the arcuate and anterior periventricular nuclei, contain neurotransmitters, such as DA.

c. The pituitary gland and the hypothalamic-hypophyseal portal system

The pituitary gland (hypophysis) is an unpaired organ recessed in the sella turcica of the sphenoid bone of the skull. It is divided into the *adenohypophysis*, which consists of the large anterior lobe; the *pars tuberalis* and the thin layer of the *intermediate lobe*, a structure that is fused with the anterior lobe in humans; and the *neurohypophysis*, which is comprised of the ME, posterior pituitary, and the stalk or infundibulum, which connects the posterior pituitary to the hypothalamus. The anterior pituitary is derived from oral ectoderm, whereas the posterior pituitary is derived from neural

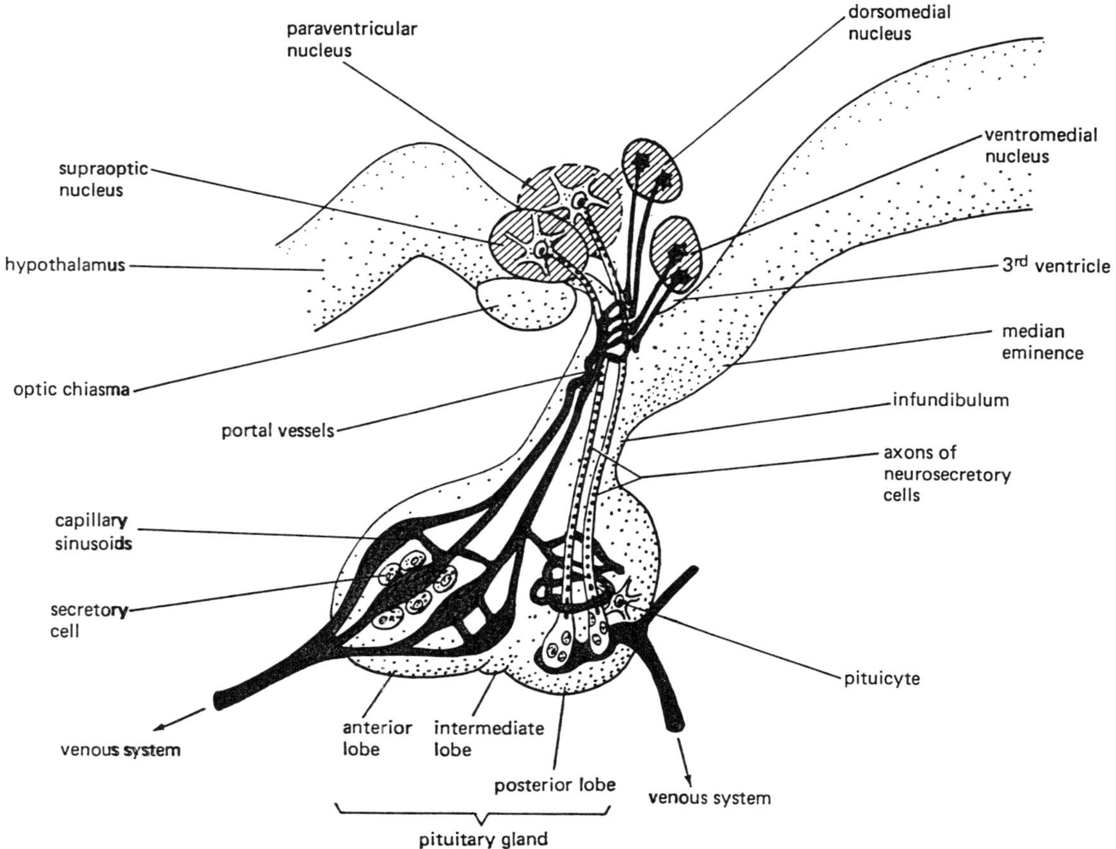

Figure 5.1
The pituitary gland and its neural and circulatory connections to the hypothalamus. Four hypothalamic nuclei are shown. Cells of the dorsomedial and ventromedial nuclei form part of the parvicellular neurosecretory system and deposit their hypothalamic secretions in the region of the median eminence, where they enter the portal system that leads to the anterior pituitary. The magnocellular neurosecretory system is composed of large cells within the paraventricular and supraoptic nuclei, the axons of which extend through the infundibulum to the posterior pituitary. Not shown are the parvicellular elements of these nuclei which send branches into the region of the median eminence. (From Strand, 1983.)

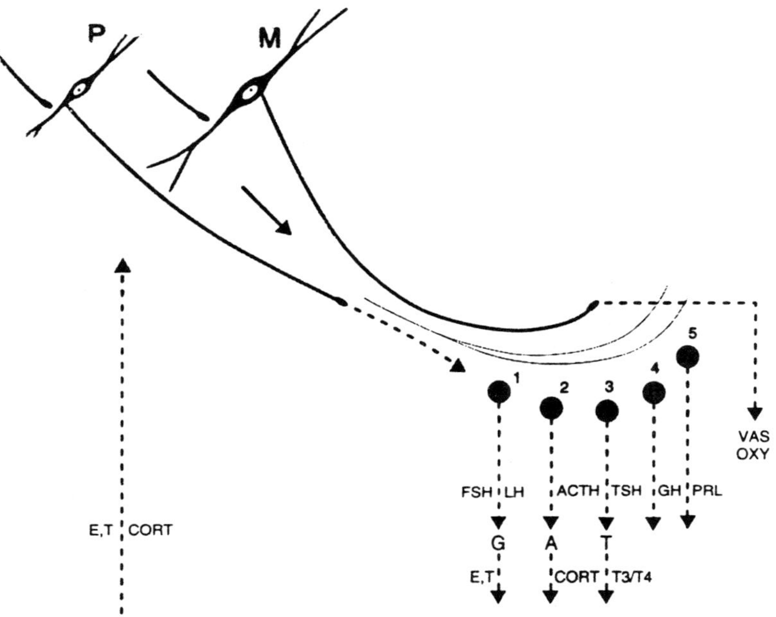

Figure 5.2
The neuroendocrine system consists of parvicellular (P) and magnocellular (M) neurons in the hypothalamus that send their axons to the stalk of the pituitary gland. Magnocellular axons end in the posterior lobe, where they release vasopressin (VAS) and oxytocin (OXY) into the systemic circulation. Parvocellular neurons release stimulating or inhibiting factors from the hypothalamus into the portal system in the median eminence for delivery to the anterior pituitary gland, where they regulate the release of hormones from the five classical endocrine cell types: 1, gonadotrophes release FSH and LH which act on the gonad (G) to release estrogen (E), progesterone (not shown), or testosterone (T); 2, corticotrophes secrete ACTH to stimulate the adrenal cortex to release corticosterone (CORT) and related glucocorticoids; 3, thyrotrophes stimulate the release of thyroid hormones (T3/T4) from the thyroid gland; 4, somatotrophes secrete growth hormone (GH); 5, lactotrophs release prolactin (PRL). As shown on the left, gonadal and adrenal hormones exert a negative feedback control on the hypothalamus. (From Swanson, 1993.)

ectoderm. The anterior lobe has a double arterial circulation, receiving blood from the superior hypophyseal artery, which supplies the base of the hypothalamus and the ME with arterial blood to form the primary capillary network. The anterior lobe also receives blood from the inferior hypophyseal artery, a branch of the internal carotid artery, to create the secondary capillary network of large sinusoids. The primary and secondary capillary beds are connected by the relatively long straight portal vessels, forming the hypothalamic-hypophyseal portal system, first described in detail by Popa and Fielding (1930) and Wislocki and King (1936) and shown in figures 5.1 and 5.3, providing an anatomical route for control of the pituitary by the hypothalamus. These vessels bring neuropeptide-rich, venous blood from the hypothalamus to regulate the secretory activity of the anterior pituitary gland.

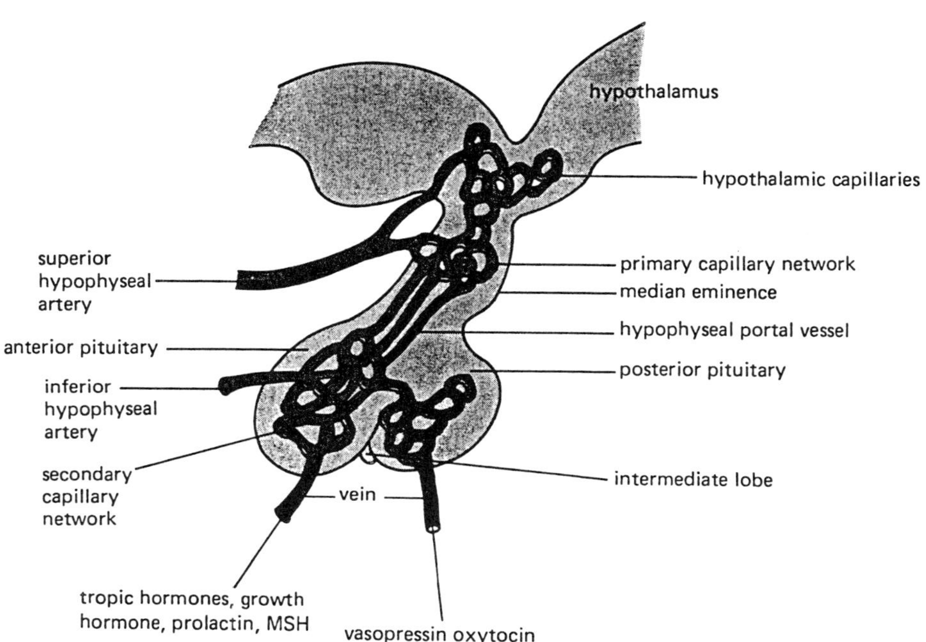

Figure 5.3
The double arterial system of the anterior pituitary gland. The capillaries formed in the median eminence by the superior hypophyseal artery are connected by the relatively straight hypophyseal portal vessels to blood sinuses in the anterior lobe. These sinuses, and those of the posterior lobe, are formed by the inferior hypophyseal artery. MSH, melanocyte-stimulating hormone. (From Strand, 1983.)

The functional importance of the hypothalamic-hypophyseal portal system was first realized by the English physiologist Geoffrey Harris (Green and Harris, 1947). Harris (1955) demonstrated that severance of these portal vessels prevents ovulation in the rabbit, for the gonadotropic-stimulating hormones from the hypothalamus are unable to reach the anterior pituitary and consequently FSH and LH, pituitary hormones essential to ovulation, are not secreted. All the hypothalamic neuropeptides that stimulate or inhibit the secretion and release of the anterior pituitary peptides are deposited in the region of the ME. The many thousands of axons that terminate in the ME lack the synaptic specializations characteristic of CNS synapses and the neuropeptides are released into the pericapillary space that surrounds the fenestrated capillaries of the primary portal plexus. This specialized structure permits the rapid entrance of the relatively large neuropeptides into the portal vessels and thence into the sinusoids of the anterior pituitary. In addition to these long portal vessels, there are short portal vessels that pass through the intermediate lobe to connect the neural posterior lobe to the anterior lobe. The tropic neuropeptides secreted by the anterior pituitary in response to hypothalamic (and other) stimuli are released into the venous system.

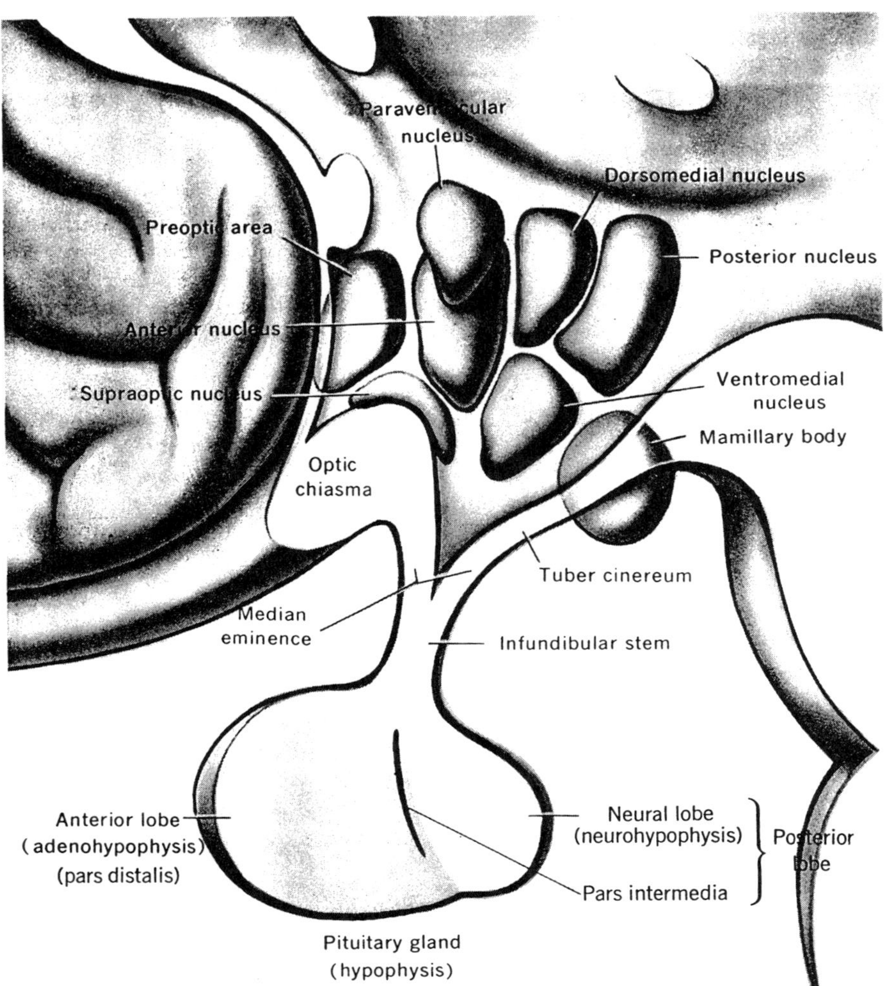

Figure 5.4
The pituitary gland and some hypothalamic nuclei. The hypothalamus is composed of four nuclear areas: (1) the preoptic area (telencephalic region); (2) the supraoptic or anterior area, including the paraventricular nucleus, anterior nucleus, and supraoptic nucleus; (3) the tuberal or middle area, including the dorsomedial and ventromedial nuclei; and (4) the mamillary or posterior area, including the posterior nucleus and the mamillary body. (From Noback and Demarest, 1975.)

Table 5.1
Anatomical source of hypothalamic regulatory neuropeptides

Region	Neuropeptide Hormone
Septal, preoptic, suprachiasmatic, infundibular, and premammillary nuclei	Gonadotropin-releasing hormone
Paraventricular nucleus (parvocellular portion)	Corticotropin-releasing hormone
Arcuate nucleus and lateral hypothalamus (medial perifornical)	Growth hormone–releasing hormone
Paraventricular nucleus (parvocellular portion), preoptic nucleus, dorsomedial nucleus, laterobasal hypothalamus	Thyrotropin-releasing hormone
Periventricular area, anterior hypothalamic nuclei, lateral hypothalamus, preoptic area	Somatotropin-release inhibiting factor (somatostatin)
Arcuate nucleus and ventral anterior periventricular nucleus (tuberoinfundibular dopamine neurons)	Prolactin-inhibiting factor, dopamine

d. *Modifications of the portal system*

Subsequently, it has been shown that the circulation between the hypothalamus and pituitary is much more complex, consisting not only of the anterograde flow just described but also, a system of vascular switches in the posterior pituitary, through which blood may be shunted in a retrograde manner to the anterior pituitary, hypothalamus, and other brain areas to directly modify brain function. In addition, hypothalamic and pituitary neuropeptides may reach distant parts of the brain through the CSF flowing through the ventricles and the subarachnoid spaces (Dogtorom et al., 1977).

An additional transport system is formed by *tanycytes*, specialized cells in the floor of the third ventricle and also in the ME. Tanycyte processes have end-feet that support the portal blood vessels and block nerve endings containing hypothalamic factors from reaching the pericapillary spaces in the ME. In turn, the tanycytes are regulated by DA released by DA-containing nerve endings; when DA inhibition is removed, the tanycytes contract, permitting the neuropeptide-containing nerve terminals access to the portal blood vessels. Processes from these cells, together with neurosecretory terminals, end near the portal capillaries (figure 5.5). These various systems provide a selection of routes by which neuropeptides may reach the brain and affect phenomena as diverse as sleep, pain, orgasm, and headache (Bergland and Page, 1979).

5.1.2.2 Hypothalamo–Posterior Pituitary Pathway

The posterior lobe arises from an outgrowth from the floor of the third ventricle and is connected by a stalk to the hypothalamus. The magnocellular neurons of the SON and PVN secrete the neuropeptides VP and OT, which, together with their carrier neurophysin molecules, travel down the axons through the stalk to be stored in nerve terminals in the posterior lobe. The neuropeptide-rich terminals in the neurohypophysis are surrounded by small pituicytes and by a rich capillary circulation (see figures 5.1 and 5.3). Some axons from the PVN appear to terminate in the ME and many neuropeptide-containing axons from the SON and PVN project to the medulla oblongata, especially the nucleus of the tractus solitarius and the spinal cord, thus integrating the neuroendocrine and autonomic systems.

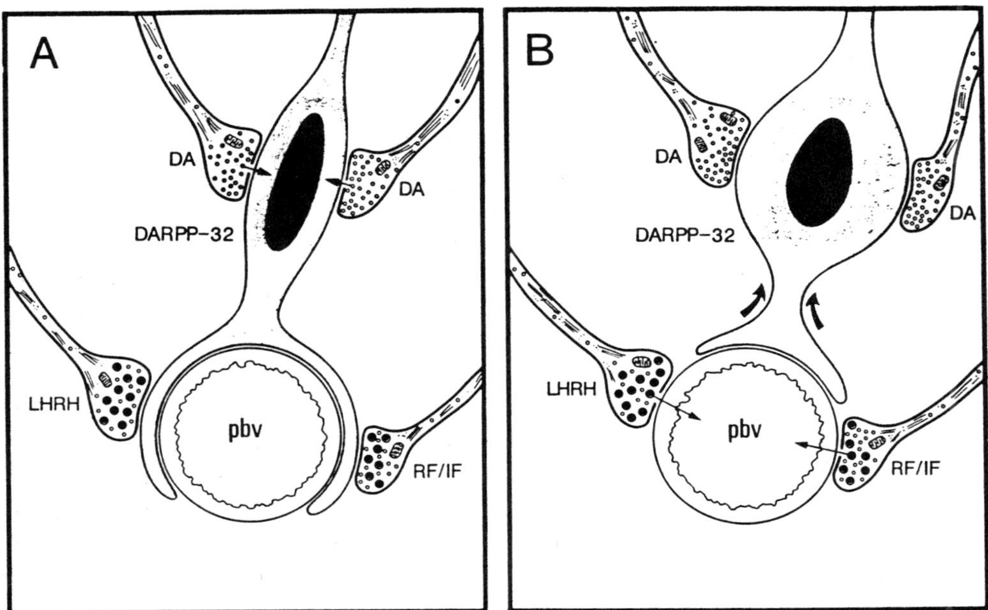

Figure 5.5
Schematic drawing illustrating the hypothetical role of tanycytes in the median eminence. (A) Tanycytes containing dopamine (DA) have end-feet that surround the portal blood vessels (pbv). Dopaminergic nerve endings control the dynamic state of the tanycyte by releasing DA. Tanycyte processes prevent nerve endings containing luteinizing hormone–releasing hormone (LHRH) or some other releasing factor (RF) or inhibiting factor (IF) from having free access to the pericapillary space. (B) When DA inhibition is reduced, the tanycyte contracts and permits the neuropeptide-containing terminals access to the portal blood vessels. DARPP-32, a cAMP-regulated phosphoprotein. (Modified from Everitt et al., 1994.)

5.1.3 Neurotransmitter Regulation of the Neuroendocrine System

The hypothalamus and ME are also rich in nerve terminals containing important monoaminergic neurotransmitters, such as NE, DA, and 5-HT, which are closely involved in neuroendocrine control mechanisms, especially those controlling ACTH secretion. Many of the neurons contain complex mixtures of neuropeptides and neurotransmitters, coexisting in the same cell. The detailed anatomical organization of the monoaminergic neurons in the hypothalamus is described by Everitt et al. (1992).

Not only the catecholamines but also ACh, GABA, and histamine are involved to varying extents in the regulation of neuroendocrine secretion. Both ACh and histamine appear to activate the hypothalamic-hypophyseal-adrenal axis, whereas GABA probably exerts an inhibitory action. Experimental results are often difficult to interpret as the effects differ according to the species and the type of neurotransmitter manipulation, for example, administration of the neurotransmitter, its agonist or antagonist, synthesis inhibitors, reuptake blockers, and so on (Müller and Nisticò, 1989). Specific neurotransmitter control mechanisms for individual hypothalamic, pituitary, and adrenocortical hormones are discussed in later chapters.

5.2 The Blood-Brain Barrier

The existence of a barrier between the blood and the brain was first demonstrated by Paul Ehrlich at the beginning of this century in his search for chemotherapeutic agents, a search which led to the discovery of the sulfonamides. He observed that many dyes, injected IV, stained the whole body but not the brain. Goldmann (1909) provided the decisive experiment, using a vital dye, trypan blue. Intravenous injection of trypan blue left the brain unstained and no dye was found in the CSF, although the choroid plexus and meninges were stained. However, if the dye were injected into the CSF, the entire brain was stained, but none was found in the blood, indicating that the impediment existed regardless of the direction from which the dye approached the barrier.

Today we consider that the BBB is not merely a passive protective barrier maintaining the nutritive environment and the general homeostasis of the brain but that it acts as a dynamic interface regulating the flow of information, in terms of nutrients and regulatory substances such as neuropeptides, between the CNS and the periphery (Jaspan et al., 1994).

5.2.1 Morphology of the Blood-Brain Barrier

5.2.1.1 Cerebrospinal Fluid

CSF is mainly formed by the choroid plexuses, highly vascularized modifications of the pia mater that extend into the roofs of the third and fourth ventricles and the walls of the lateral ventricles. The choroid plexus is lined by modified ependyma to form the high-secretory choroid epithelial cells. Drainage of CSF is mainly through the openings of the subarachnoid spaces into the large venous sinuses of the dura mater. Separation of the blood in the CNS capillaries from the extracellular fluid (ECF) of the brain parenchyma and separation of the blood in the choroid plexus and circumventricular organs are the function of the BBB.

5.2.1.2 Structure of the Blood-Brain Barrier

The BBB exists in two forms: the endothelial barrier and the ependymal barrier. The endothelial barrier consists of tight junctions between cerebral capillary endothelial cells. The ependymal barrier exists at the choroid plexus and the circumventricular organs. It is more usual to apply the term *blood-brain barrier* to the barrier formed by the tight junctions of the fused endothelial cells of the brain capillaries (figure 5.6). The capillaries may be seen as an endothelial tube some 3 μm in diameter, formed by a single layer of endothelial cells some 100 to 150 nm thick. The cytoplasm of these cells is dense and, unlike the endothelium of peripheral tissue capillaries, contains few pinocytotic vesicles. The brain microvessels are almost completely covered by the foot processes of astrocytes, which at one time were believed to be the physical component of the BBB. However, tracer studies by Brightman (1977) clearly showed that it is the unfenestrated, continuous endothelial cells with their tight junctions that construct the BBB. A detailed description of the morphology of the BBB may be found in Davson and Segal (1995).

An enzymatic barrier is also a component of the BBB as the BBB contains highly active degradative peptidases that rapidly cleave peptides. However,

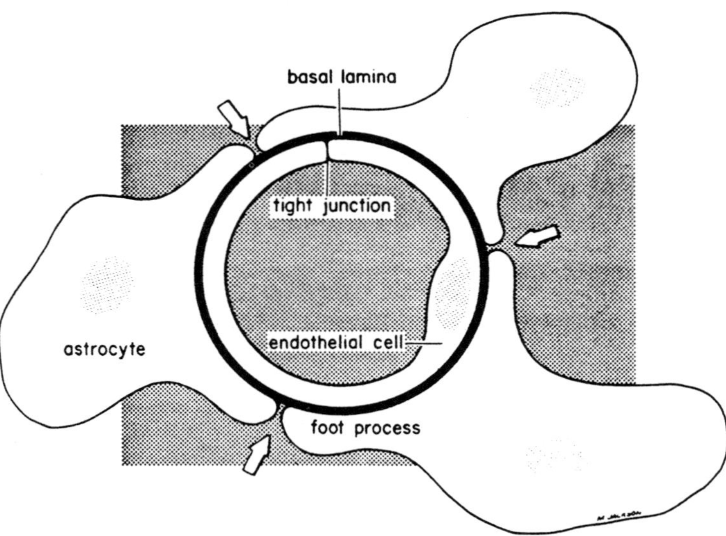

Figure 5.6
Diagram illustrating the close association of endothelial cells in brain capillaries with foot processes extending from astrocytes. The blood-brain barrier is produced by the tight endothelium. The astrocytes encircle the microvessels, but are not sealed together, and interstitial fluid has access (arrows) to the basement membrane and abluminal surface of the endothelial cell. (From Goldstein, 1988.)

many neuropeptides and their analogs cross the BBB intact in both directions (Begley, 1994). It has also been suggested that the cerebral endothelium may act as an endocrine organ by secreting potent growth factors at crucial times in the development and maintenance of the nervous system (Joó, 1987).

5.2.2 Functions of the Blood-Brain Barrier

5.2.2.1 Neuronal and Non-Neuronal Communication

The BBB is both a structural and functional barrier, selectively preventing the passage of certain substances and facilitating the passage of others between the blood and the ECF of the brain. This results in a stable and protected milieu intérieur for the brain, an internal environment that differs considerably from that of the other tissues of the body. Cserr and Bundgaard (1984) suggest that the phylogenetic development of a BBB provides a unique milieu for neuronal and non-neuronal communication. Short-term variations in the composition of intracellular fluid (ICF) that result from neuronal activity may act as signals to affect the electrical activity of neighboring neurons and glia. In this way, the BBB isolates the interstitium from the capillary plasma and thus permits this additional information to be retained over the short term. In the long term, the BBB maintains the homeostasis of the neuronal microenvironment. These two important functions, neuronal and non-neuronal com-

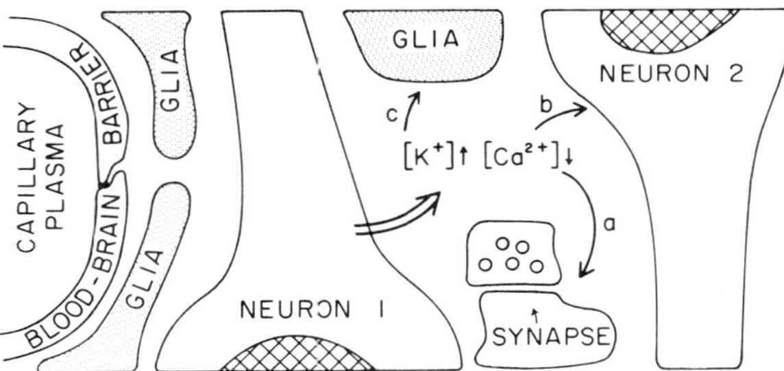

Figure 5.7
Schematic drawing illustrating that impulses in neurons lead to changes in brain interstitial fluid composition, which may in turn represent meaningful signals to neighboring neurons and glial cells, thus increasing the brain's integrative capacity. In the absence of the blood-brain barrier (BBB, left) these signals would be attenuated due to free diffusional exchange with plasma. Activation of neuron 1 causes increase in interstitial fluid Ca^{2+}, changes that influence synaptic transmission, threshold of neuron 2, and glial metabolism (arrows a, b, and c respectively). Responses are nonlinear. By providing a stable base level of concentration (homeostasis) the BBB ensures that responses to a given change in ionic concentration will be independent of ionic changes in plasma. (From Cserr and Bungaard, 1984.)

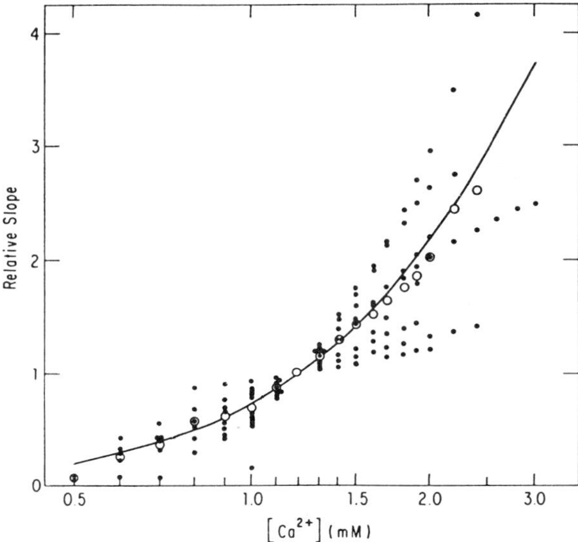

Figure 5.8
Excitatory synaptic transmission (expressed as relative slope) in rat hippocampal slices is nonlinearly dependent on $[Ca^{2+}]_o$. (From Dingeldine and Somjen, 1981.)

munication, are illustrated in figures 5.7 and 5.8. The bidirectional transport from brain to blood as well as from blood to brain assures integration of central neural functions with peripheral physiological systems.

5.2.2.2 Selected Restrictive Passage Results in Differences Between CSF and Plasma

Tight junctions prevent the passage of substances between the cells and thus exclude a direct aqueous connection between the plasma and brain ECF, in contrast to the relatively free movement of fluid and small solutes across the capillary bed of peripheral tissues (figure 5.9). In general, larger molecules penetrate more poorly, hydrophilic substances penetrate less well, and lipid-soluble substances such as alcohol and steroids penetrate extremely rapidly. Owing to the absence of pathways between brain endothelial cells, a high electrical resistance of 1500 to 2000 ohms/cm^2 is established across the cerebral endothelium, resulting in an effective barrier to hydrophilic molecules. Thus, as is characteristic of peripheral capillary membranes, uncharged or negatively charged particles penetrate the BBB more readily than positively charged particles or ions. However, a number of polar metabolic substances cross the cerebral endothelium via highly stereospecific, self-saturable, and inhibitable transport systems (Davson et al., 1987). Peptides have difficulty crossing the BBB by permeation as they are highly polar and some may lack a specific carrier-mediated transport system.

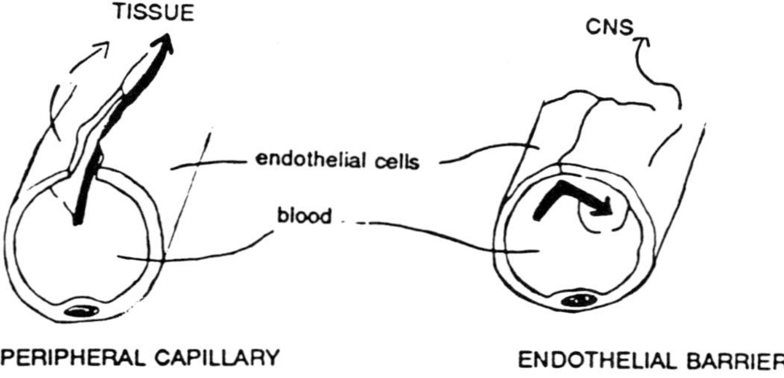

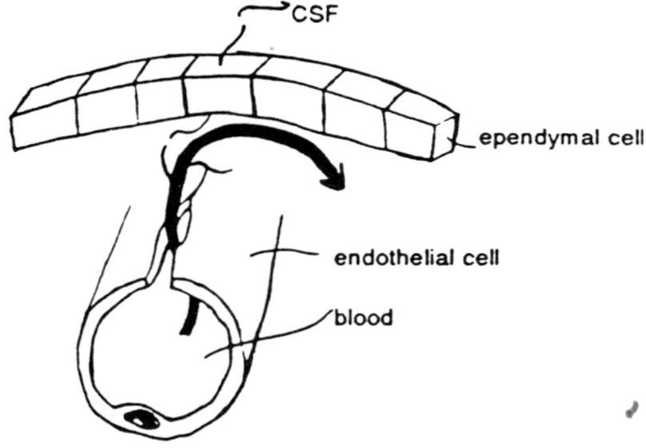

Figure 5.9
Capillary and barrier mechanisms. In peripheral capillaries, intercellular clefts between the individual endothelial cells that make up the capillary wall allow the movement of fluid and solutes (solid line) across the capillary bed. The endothelial barrier in CNS capillaries is due to the fusion of opposing membranes of the endothelial cells, virtually eliminating the intercellular clefts. Transmembrane diffusion and carrier-mediated transport (broken line) become the dominant mechanisms determining movement across the CNS capillary bed. In a few areas of the brain (circumventricular organs and choroid plexus) the tight junctions and the resulting barrier occur at the level of interfacing ependymal cells. (From Banks and Kastin, 1988.)

Table 5.2
Composition of plasma and cerebrospinal fluid (CSF) (mEQ/L)

Substance	Plasma	CSF
Protein (mg/100 g)	6500	25
Glucose	6.2	4.0
Lactate	0.9	2.0
Urea	11.1	6.5
Amino acids	2.5	0.9
Na^+	163	158
K^+	4.8	2.7
Ca^{2+}	5.3	3.1
Mg^{2+}	1.4	1.8
Cl^-	132	144
HCO_3^-	25.5	24.1

As a result of these selective characteristics of the BBB, the plasma-CSF ratio of many ions, such as Na^+ and K^+, differs considerably from their plasma–interstitial fluid ratio. In addition, the ratios of important organic molecules such as protein, glucose, amino acids, and urea diverge remarkably in plasma and CSF: in almost all species the concentrations of these substances is lower in CSF than in plasma. CSF contains very little protein, is almost isotonic to plasma, is slightly alkaline, and almost cell-free. The concentration of Na^+ in the CSF does not differ much from that of plasma, but the K^+ concentration is considerably lower in CSF (table 5.2). Whereas the exact concentrations vary somewhat in different species, the ratios are very similar. An almost perfect CSF K^+ concentration is maintained through bidirectional carrier-mediated transport. When plasma K^+ is high, influx is limited by carrier saturation. When K^+ levels are low, transport is facilitated, thus achieving a steady CSF concentration regardless of fluctuations in plasma concentrations. Efflux becomes operational only when K^+ becomes high. Brain capillaries not only slow the exchange of solutes but play an active role in the passage of small neuropeptides by secretion.

5.2.3 The Circumventricular Organs and the "Weak" Blood-Brain Barrier

The BBB is often referred to as "weak" in certain areas, which are known as the *circumventricular organs (CVOs)*. The CVOs, as their name implies, lie close to the ventricles of the brain and consist of the choroid plexus, the ME, the neurohypophysis, the pineal gland, the organ vasculosum terminalis, the subfornical organ, the subcommissural organ, and the area postrema (figure 5.10). The choroid plexus is the largest of the CVOs and the ependyma of this organ is in direct contact with the CSF and may permit easier transport for some solutes.

These structures have fenestrated capillary endothelium in contrast to the tight junctions characteristic of the capillaries of the rest of the brain (Bouldin and Krigman 1975) (figure 5.11). However, whereas there is no endothelial barrier at the CVO, the ependymal cells surrounding these areas are joined by tight junctions to form the second type of BBB. Experiments with horseradish peroxidase have demonstrated open junctions between ependymal cells of the choroid plexus that permit direct exchange between ME capillaries and the CSF of the third ventricle. Whereas these organs are often credited for the passage of large hydrophilic molecules across the BBB, their sum total surface area is small, 0.02 cm^2/g tissue as compared with the 100 to 150 cm^2/g of high-resistance BBB vessels (Begley, 1994). In addition, transport of peptides from blood to brain has been demonstrated in areas in which there are no CVOs, such as in the cerebral cortex and cerebellum (Kastin et al., 1996).

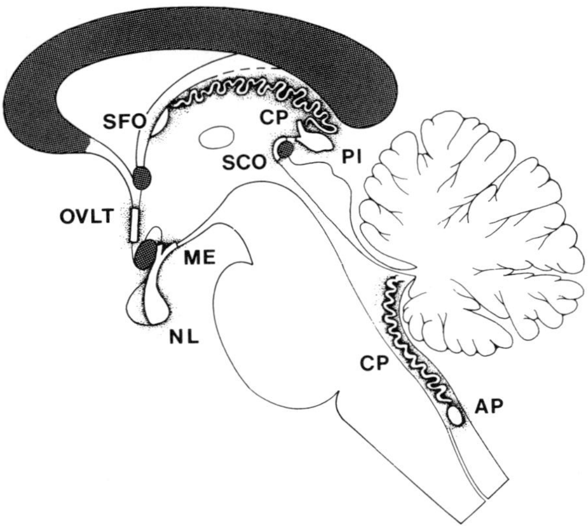

Figure 5.10
Drawing of the median sagittal aspect of the human brain showing the seven circumventricular organs and the choroid plexus (CP). AP, area postrema; ME, median eminence; NL, pituitary neural lobe; OVLT, organum vasculosum of the lamina terminalis; PI, pineal gland; SCO, subcommissural organ; SFO, subfornical organ. (From Gross and Weindl, 1987.)

5.3 Passage of Neuropeptides Across the Blood-Brain Barrier

How circulating peptides exert their central effects has been the topic of considerable debate over the last two decades. The BBB forms an effective structural barrier to the passage of large neuropeptides, yet there is convincing evidence that systemically administered peptides have potent effects on the CNS (De Wied 1969; De Wied et al., 1975; Kastin et al., 1984; Banks and Kastin 1995b). It can also be shown that the selectivity of the BBB differentiates between those neuropeptides that are synthesized and released centrally from those that are synthesized and released from peripheral tissues. In general, there are three mechanisms by which circulating neuropeptides may cross the BBB and exert central effects:

5.3.1 Penetration via Pores and Pinocytosis

Whereas this method is common for penetration of particles through capillaries in other tissues, it is mostly precluded in the brain by the lack of fenestrations, few pinocytotic vesicles, and tight junctions between the endothelial cells of brain capillaries. However, the structural components that form the BBB are not completely leakproof as it can be shown that a small amount of albumin enters the CNS resulting in a concentration of albumin in the CSF that is only about 0.5% of the concentration of albumin in the serum.

5.3.2 Transmembrane Diffusion

Diffusion through the endothelial membrane is highly dependent on the physicochemical properties of the substance, especially its lipid solubility. However, other characteristics of compounds also affect permeability. These include ionization, molecular weight, and the ability to form electroneutral complexes. Recently, hydrogen bonding has been proposed as the best predictor of membrane (BBB) penetration. Passage by transmembrane diffusion is nonsaturable and increases linearly with increase in peptide concentration. Several peptides, for example, [^{125}I]N-Tyr-delta sleep–inducing peptide, the tripeptide TRH, and α-MSH, cross the BBB by this route (Banks and Kastin, 1984; 1995a; 1995b; Banks et al., 1987b Jaspan et al., 1994). Insulin also crosses the BBB by

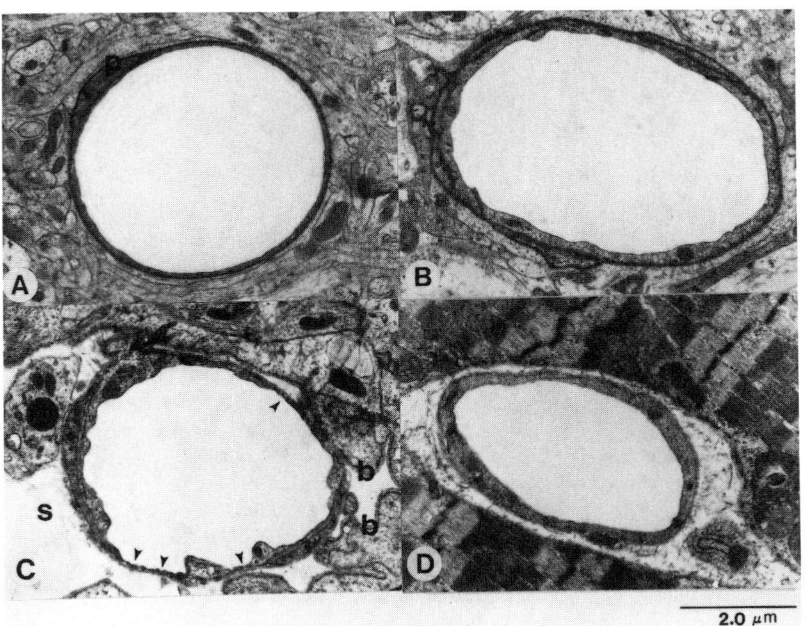

Figure 5.11
Comparison of the ultrastructure of microvessels in various tissues of the mouse. (A) Cerebral cortex. (B) Anterior area postrema. (C) Posterior area postrema. (D) Skeletal muscle. The vascular endothelium of A, B, and D lack fenestrations or "pores." C lacks a blood-brain barrier and is characterized by extensive regions of fenestrated endothelial cells (arrowheads) which contain vesicles. Note the large perivascular space (s) and the double basal lamina (b). (From Coomber and Stewart, 1985.)

transmembrane diffusion, but the major mechanism for its transport appears to be a saturable transport system (Baura et al., 1993).

5.3.3 Specific Carrier-Mediated Mechanisms

Water-soluble molecules, such as glucose and amino acids, are transported almost exclusively by specific carrier-mediated transport systems. Most neuropeptides are water-soluble, and those that lack a carrier transport system are excluded from the brain. Neuropeptide transport systems share the characteristics of similar systems in other tissues, that is, saturability, a high degree of specificity, and some stereospecificity. Despite their low lipophilicity, relatively large size, and susceptibility to enzymatic degradation, one way by which neuropeptides might cross the cerebral capillary endothelium of the BBB is, arguably, by specific *receptor-mediated* mechanisms. This involves three steps:

1. Binding of the neuropeptide to specific receptors on the capillary endothelium;

Table 5.3
Peptide receptors demonstrated within circumventricular organs[a]

Angiotensin II	Neuropeptide Y
Arginine vasopressin	Oxytocin
Atrial natriuretic hormone	Pancreatic polypeptide
Bradykinin	Prolactin
Brain natriuretic peptide	Somatostatin
Endothelin	Substance P
Insulin-like growth factors	Vasoactive intestinal polypeptide
Insulin	

Adapted from Ermisch et al. (1993) by Begley (1994).
[a] Receptors were localized using autoradiographic methods.

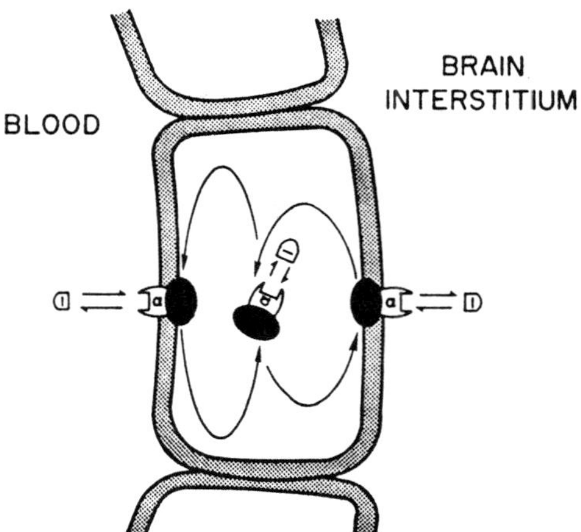

Figure 5.12
Transcytosis of insulin (I) through the blood-brain barrier (BBB) is viewed as three sequential steps: (1) receptor-mediated endocytosis of the peptide at the blood side of the BBB; (2) diffusion of the peptide or peptide receptor complex through the endothelial cytoplasm; and (3) receptor-mediated exocytosis of the peptide at the brain side of the BBB. a, receptor. (From Pardridge, 1986.)

2. internalization of the peptide-receptor complex and migration through endosomes in the endothelial cytoplasm; and
3. release of the peptide by exocytosis on the other side of the barrier.

The resulting receptor-mediated synaptic signal is relayed to other central neurons. This controversial hypothesis is supported by the localization of many different neuropeptide receptors within the CVOs (table 5.3). Receptor-mediated endocytosis may provide for the bidirectional transport of some large peptides (Pardridge 1990), including insulin (Frank and Pardridge, 1987; Pardridge 1988, 1990), although the main mechanism for insulin uptake appears to be through nonsaturable transmembrane diffusion. When receptor-mediated endocytosis is combined with exocytosis of the neuropeptide, the transport system is referred to as *transcytosis* (figure 5.12). The classical transport systems of glucose, electrolytes, amino acids, and so on do not use this mechanism.

5.3.3.1 Neuropeptide Transport Systems

Different neuropeptides probably use different routes and mechanisms for penetration, and neuropeptides and their analogs cross the BBB to varying degrees. Neuropeptide transport systems can be saturable and highly stereospecific and do not transport amino acids but may be regulated by them (Banks et al., 1987a). Most transport systems that have been located are in the choroid plexus or the capillary bed of the CNS. The specificity of these transport systems is shown by the more than tenfold variation in penetration for gastrin, delta sleep–inducing peptide, VIP, calcitonin, and neurotensin. Some of these systems transport peptides into the brain, some transport peptides out of

Table 5.4
Some peptides transported across the blood-brain barrier by saturable systems[a]

Direction of Saturable Transport		
Influx	Efflux	Influx and Efflux
MIF-1	Met-enkephalin[b]	Arginine vasopressin
Peptide T analog	Tyr-MIF-1	Leu-enkephalin
Delta sleep–inducing peptide[c,d]	Oxytocin[b]	GnRH
Dynorphin analog[c]	PACAP 27	PACAP 38
ACTH 4–10 analog[c]	Somatostain analog	
Leu–enkephalin	Tyr-W-MIF-1[b]	
Glutathione[c]		
Insulin[c]		
Pancreatic polypeptide		

Adapted from Banks and Kastin (1995b).
MIF, melanocyte-stimulating hormone inhibiting factor; PACAP, pituitary adenylate cyclase–activating polypeptide; GnRH, gonadotropin-releasing hormone.
[a] Regulatory peptides omitted.
[b] Influx not tested.
[c] Efflux not tested.
[d] In guinea pig but not in rat.

the brain, and some transport peptides bidirectionally (table 5.4).

a. Separate transport systems for different neuropeptides

There are at least two separate systems for the brain-to-blood transport of neuropeptides. One system, the *peptide transport system-1 (PTS-1)* transports small peptides with an N-terminal tyrosine such as the tetrapeptides Tyr-MIF-I (Tyr-Pro-Leu-Gly-NH_2) and Tyr-W-MIF-1 (Tyr-Pro-Trp-Gly-NH_2), which have antiopiate and antidepressant properties, and the analgesic peptides Met-enkephalin, Leu-enkephalin, and dynorphin 1–8. PTS-1 transports only in the direction of brain-to-blood, apparently not having a blood-to-brain, or influx, component. These small peptides appear to share the same carrier: Tyr-MIF-I and Met-enkephalin clear at the same rate after icv injection. Leu-enkephalin, which is transported in both directions, probably uses another transport system for influx (Banks and Kastin, 1984, 1985, 1995). In addition, a β-glycoprotein transporter exists for some peptides like cyclosporine.

A second system transports VP-like peptides, which appear to have saturable, bidirectional transport systems at the BBB. Arginine vasopressin (AVP) crosses the BBB intact, in both directions, from blood to brain and from brain to blood, and AVP receptors may be responsible for the cellular uptake or binding, or both, of the neuropeptide.

b. Demonstration of neuropeptide transport systems

Specific saturable uptake of neuropeptides has been demonstrated through several very careful methodologies. The brain uptake index (BUI) measures the uptake of substances into the brain after IV injection by calculating the brain-to-blood ratio of the substance relative to a reference substance, water. Figure 5.13 shows the BUI for heroin, glucose, morphine, and enkephalin in comparison with water, which penetrates very readily. It can be seen that both morphine and enkephalin have low rates of penetration. A more sensitive method for the detection of passage of substances for which the uptake is too low to be detected by the BUI has been developed based on a multiple time regression analysis method (Patlak et al. 1983).

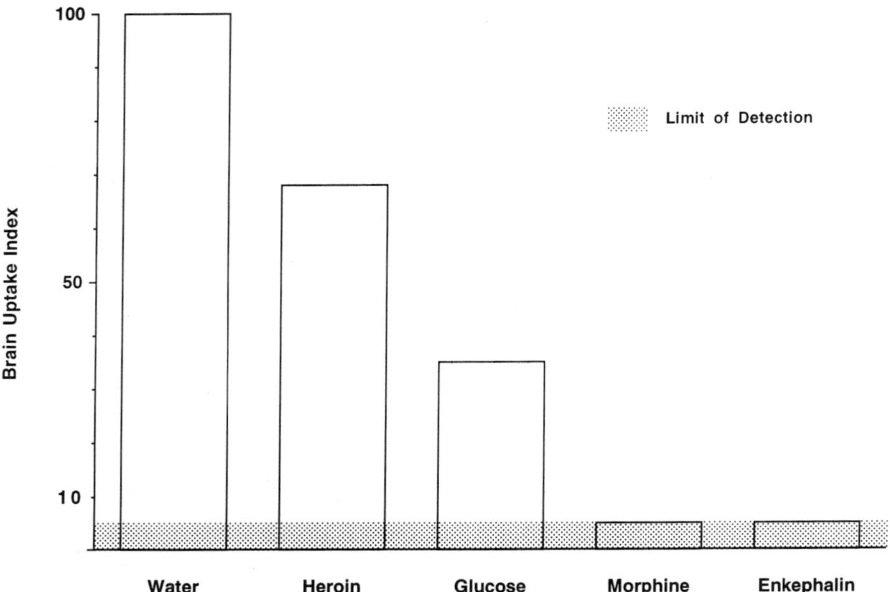

Figure 5.13
Brain uptake index for the reference standard, water, compared with compounds shown. (From Jaspen et al. 1994.)

5.4 Modification and Disruption of the Blood-Brain Barrier

5.4.1 Circumvention of the Blood-Brain Barrier via Retrograde Axonal Transport

Blood-borne molecules such as neurotoxins and neurotropic viruses may travel via a retrograde axonal route from peripheral synaptic clefts through the axoplasm to the lysosomes in the neuronal soma of cranial nerves, neurosecretory neurons, autonomic preganglionic fibers, and lower motor nerves, thus circumventing the BBB. Figure 5.14 illustrates retrograde transport from the axon terminal to the dendritic branches of a neuron.

5.4.2 Neuropeptide Regulation of the Blood-Brain Barrier

Neuropeptides themselves may alter the permeability of the BBB to other substances by affecting not only the functions of the tight junctions but also the rate of transport by saturable systems, and even through changes in the composition of the endothelial membrane. Neuropeptides may produce hemodynamic effects in the periphery and thus alter cerebral blood flow and consequently the blood-to-brain passage of substances that are flow-dependent. AVP regulates the entry of several amino acids, including leucine, whereas leucine, enkephalin, bradykinin, angiotensin, and cytokines increase the permeability of the BBB to other peptides, the transfer of K^+, and the penetration

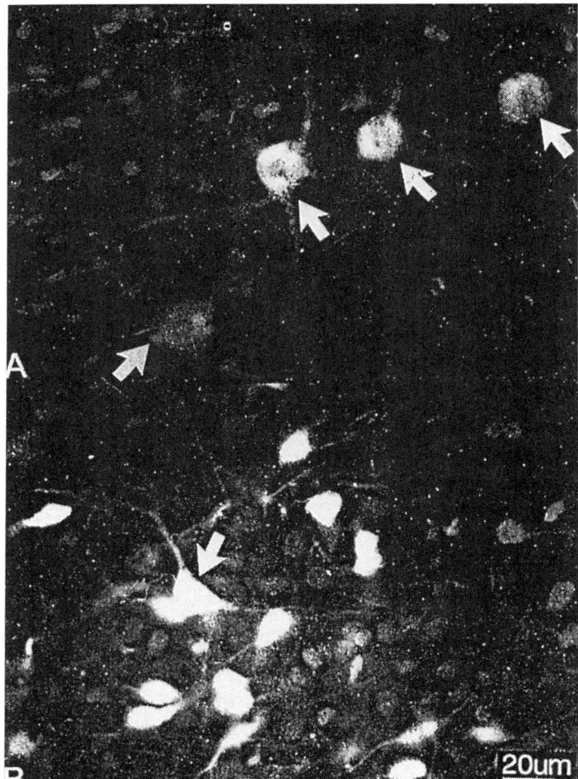

Figure 5.14
High magnification of β-endorphin–positive neurons, lacking endogeneous β-endorphin, after injection of β-endorphin into the lateral ventricle. An intense cytoplasmic staining of accumulated β-endorphin is seen all the way from the nerve cell soma out into the dendritic branches after postulated retrograde transport from the axon terminal. The nerve cells, indicated by arrows, show the morphological appearance of neuropeptide Y neurons. Bar: 10 μm. (From Fuxe et al., 1994.)

of water. The melanocortins appear capable of altering the permeability of the BBB through several of these methods (Banks and Kastin, 1995a) These complex regulatory mechanisms are discussed in detail by Ermisch et al. (1993).

5.4.3 Pharmacological Techniques and Clinical Implications

5.4.3.1 Physicochemical Alterations

The physicochemical characteristics of the neuropeptide may be changed or stable analogs may be synthesized, changes which may increase its ability to penetrate the BBB (Banks and Kastin, 1985). Elbiratide, an ACTH 4–9 analog, crosses the BBB 10 to 100 times more rapidly than other melanocortins because of a saturable transport system. The diversity of actions of many neuropeptide fragments, such as those of the melanocortin family, may derive from differences in transport rates that depend on small structural changes. *Absorptive-mediated endocytosis* is another way by which the transport of modified neuropeptides may be increased. The charge of the protein can be changed by cationization via the linkage of primary ammonium groups; uptake is based on an electrostatic interaction between the positively charged protein and negative charges on the surface of the brain capillary endothelium.

A novel technique has been developed by Simpkins et al. (1994) based on the concept of molecular packaging and in vivo sequential metabolism. Both the C- and the N-termini are modified to increase the lipid solubility of the peptide and to prevent cleavage by BBB aminopeptidases. Other alterations of a substance may enhance its penetration through the BBB. Lipid solubility, glycosylation and cationization, liposome entrapment, and coupling to carriers are possible mechanisms.

5.4.3.2 Peptidase Inhibitors

Many endogenous blood-borne neuropeptides are metabolized before they can enter the CNS intact which complicates the treatment of CNS diseases with peptide-based drugs. Specific *peptidase inhibitors* that protect neuropeptides from enzymatic inactivation prolong or enhance their biological activity and ease their passage across the BBB. For example, the passage of enkephalins across the BBB can be enhanced by peptidase inhibitors (Brownson et al., 1994). However, the great variability in neuropeptide access to carrier systems and their differential lipid solubility requires the development of many neuropeptide-specific analogs or peptidase inhibitors.

5.4.3.3 Physiological and Pathological Factors

Passage of neuropeptides across the BBB is affected by many physiological factors, including age, stress, light, diurnal rhythms, and amino acids such as leucine. In addition, drugs, neurotoxins, radiation, and structural disruption of the BBB are associated with CNS disorders such as hypertension and seizures. It has been suggested that there is a faulty BBB in Alzheimer's disease, epilepsy, and paranoid psychosis. Membrane permeability to lipophilic substances, including neuropeptides, is increased by aluminum, permitting the inference that aluminum may lead to dementia by altering BBB permeability (Banks and Kastin, 1985). A failure to metabolize leucine, resulting in the hyperleucinemia characteristic of maple syrup urine disease, is associated with an inhibition of enkephalin transport out of the CNS, and the consequent increase in CSF enkephalins may be responsible for the severe CNS symptoms of this disease.

Experimentally, the BBB can be opened by increased intravascular pressure, hyperosmolar solutions, or substances that alter the endothelial surface charge, but these alterations may have serious side effects. Therapeutically, it may be possible to increase the permeability of the BBB to chemotherapeutic agents, but the use of neuropeptides for this purpose is still in its infancy.

5.5 Summary

Neuropeptides from the hypothalamus reach the pituitary gland via one of two routes: the vascular hypothalamic-ME-anterior pituitary route, or the neural pathway from the hypothalamus to the posterior pituitary. Peripherally produced neuropeptides reach the CNS through the systemic circulation but also have paracrine and autocrine effects in the tissues that produce them. The two main components of the neuroendocrine system are formed by the magnocellular nuclei, the PVN and SON, which contain the large neurons that send their peptide-filled axons via the neural route to the posterior pituitary; and the parvocellular system, which consists of several hypothalamic nuclei which liberate the regulatory peptides into a vascular system in the ME. Fibers from other brain regions, containing neuropeptides and neurotransmitters, also terminate in the ME.

The anterior pituitary is well supplied with arterial blood and, in addition, receives venous blood through the hypothalamic-hypophyseal portal system that delivers regulatory neuropeptides from the hypothalamus. Blood may also be shunted in the reverse direction. Tanycytes form an additional transport system so that neuropeptides from the pituitary and ME may reach the brain via several routes, bypassing the systemic circulation. The neurons of the PVN and SON secrete OT and VP, which, together with their carrier neurophysin molecules, are axonally transported through the stalk to the posterior lobe for storage in the nerve terminals. There is a vascular link between the posterior and anterior lobes which passes through the intermediate lobe. Many neurotransmitters regulate hypothalamic and pituitary secretion, acting either as activators or inhibitors.

To reach the CNS from the systemic circulation neuropeptides must pass through the BBB which consists of an endothelial and ependymal barrier, the latter existing at the choroid plexus, and the CVOs. The endothelial barrier is formed by the tight junctions of the fused endothelial cells of the brain capillaries. The BBB is both a structural and functional barrier to the passage of substances between the blood and the brain. Tight junctions restrict the passage of many substances: in general, large molecules penetrate poorly, hydrophilic substances scarcely penetrate at all, and lipid-soluble substances penetrate very rapidly. Uncharged or negatively charged particles penetrate more readily than positively charged ions. Consequently, the composition of CSF varies considerably from that of plasma. The CVOs have fenestrated endothelium, but the ependymal cells surrounding these areas are joined by tight junctions to form the second type of BBB, with some open junctions. This is the "weak" BBB through which neuropeptides may more easily penetrate, but the total surface area is small.

Systemically adminstered neuropeptides have potent effects on the CNS and there are three ways by which they may cross the BBB: to a very small degree via pores and pinocytosis; by transmembrane diffusion, a nonsaturable process, highly dependent on the physicochemical properties of the substance; and by specific carrier-mediated mechanisms. Neuropeptide transport systems are saturable and stereospecific, some transporting peptides into the brain, others transporting peptides out of the brain, and some transporting bidirectionally. There are separate transport systems for different peptides. The BBB may be modified by neurotoxins, neurotropic viruses, and several neuropeptides, as well as age, stress, light, and diurnal rhythms. Facilitation of neuropeptide penetration of the BBB may be achieved by altering the physicochemical properties of synthetic neuropeptides, and their biological activity may be prolonged by peptidase inhibitors.

Chapter 6 examines the mechanisms by which neuropeptides activate their target cells by binding to cell surface receptors and exciting second-messenger systems, many of which are interconnected, resulting in a wide variety of physiological responses.

Neuropeptide Receptors as Regulators of Cellular Functions

6

6.1 Cellular Messenger Systems

Neuropeptides form an exceedingly complex system for coordinating the intercellular information needed for the intricate, specialized physiological systems essential to life. This coordination is critical during the organization, differentiation, maturation, and aging of the organism. The neuropeptide information system shares many of the characteristics of the faster-acting neurotransmitters, a topic which is discussed in detail in chapter 7, and there is mounting evidence for synchrony of function with neuropeptides influencing neurotransmitter release and function, and vice versa.

The *first messengers* are the neuropeptides and neurotransmitters, which signal the target cell to modify its properties. For the target cell to respond, the message must be received by an acceptor molecule, the *receptor*, a macromolecule such as a protein or glycoprotein. Neuropeptides, due to their insolubility in the plasma membrane, cannot cross this membrane barrier and therefore must exert their effects by interacting with receptors on the cell surface. This interaction between the neuropeptide ligand and the surface receptor usually results in a change in the three-dimensional structure of the receptor, a conformational change that triggers a cascade of biochemical events in the cell, eventually leading to modification of the cell properties (figure 6.1).

An interesting facet of some neuropeptides is their promiscuity—they may not be not highly selective and may interact with a variety of receptor types and subtypes, with varying degrees of activity, including

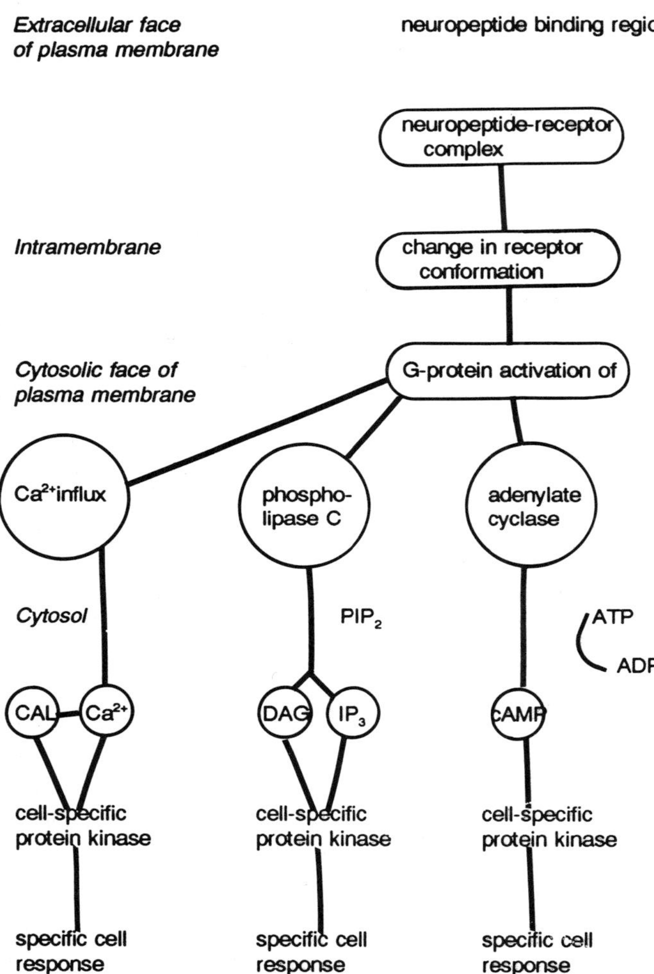

Figure 6.1
Interaction between a neuropeptide, the first messenger, with the surface receptor, and the subsequent conformational change in the receptor that activates a membrane-bound intermediary, a G protein. The G protein activates membrane-bound enzymes that catalyze the production of cytosolic second messengers to regulate a wide variety of cell functions. In many cases, there is signal transduction crosstalk between the different second-messenger systems. PIP_2, phosphatidylinositol 4,5-biphosphate; ATP, adenosine triphosphate; ADP, adenosine diphosphate; CAL, calmodulin; DAG, diacylglycerol; IP_3, inositol triphosphate; cAMP, cyclic adenosine monophosphate.

nonspecific binding, as depicted in table 6.1. Neuropeptides may also interact indirectly with other related or unrelated receptors, including neurotransmitter receptors, by affecting the number of binding sites or their affinity for another ligand. The interaction can lead to coupling of the receptors with various membrane-bound ion channels, typically used by neurotransmitters, or the neuropeptide-receptor interaction can influence dynamic intracellular trafficking events, such as endocytosis, by which the receptor-ligand complex is internalized into the cell.

Second messengers convey the information provided by the first messengers to a complex, intercommunicating cascade of second messengers within the cell. The second-messenger system most extensively used by neuropeptide hormones occurs through the interaction of the receptor with *membrane-bound G proteins*, proteins that bind guanosine triphosphate (GTP). G proteins, in turn, activate other components of the membrane-bound portion of the cascade, such as adenylate cyclase and phospholipase C, compounds that generate intracellular second messengers to regulate cell functions via specific intracellular cascades (see figure 6.1). Although this is a highly favored route for neuropeptide receptors, a remarkably diverse number of other biologically active substances utilize G proteins, including neurotransmitters, drugs, and even sensory stimuli such as light and odorants. Much of the information we have regarding G protein–coupled receptor systems comes from the β_2-adrenergic receptor for catecholamines, but this information is generally applicable to the other members of this large family.

Other second messenger systems that do *not* use the G-protein route are the guanylate cyclase receptors, tyrosine kinase receptors, the cytokine receptors (see sections 6.4, 6.5, and 6.6) and a relatively recently described second messenger/neurotransmitter, the freely diffusible gas, *nitric oxide (NO)*, which may act as a neurotransmitter and/or a second messenger, as discussed in section 6.7.

The *time element* in ligand-receptor response is also crucial; some responses are elicited in milliseconds to minutes when ion channels are involved, whereas other ligand-receptor interactions may require hours, such as those involving protein synthesis. Obviously, the diversity and lack of specificity make interpretation of neuropeptide function in the intact organism extremely difficult. To unravel this puzzle, the tools of molecular biology have been most helpful; the cloning of many receptors and their subtypes permits detailed study of these interactions, requirements, and affinities under controlled in vitro conditions. The challenge is to apply these observations to the intact, living organism.

6.2 General Characteristics of Neuropeptide Receptors

6.2.1 Affinity, Reversibility, Specificity, Number, and Saturability

Hormones, including neuropeptides, exert their effects by binding with selected receptors on the target cell membrane. Hormone concentrations in vivo are normally very low, requiring that the receptor have a high affinity for that ligand. Receptor affinity can be decreased by phosphorylation, an effective regulatory mechanism discussed further in section 6.2.2. Allosteric changes in the receptor also decrease its affinity, for example, the insulin receptor can exist either as an α_2,β_2-tetramer or the α,β-dimer: the tetramer has a higher affinity for insulin than the dimer. Hormone-receptor binding is reversible, resulting in the decay of the evoked effect after hormone removal or inactivation.

Table 6.1
Neuropeptides coupled to different G proteins

	Receptor Subtype
Peptide Receptors Using G_s and Adenylate Cyclase	
Pituitary glycoproteins (LH/HCG, FSH)	
Pituitary melanocortins (ACTH/MSH)	MC1–5
Pituitary adenylyl cyclase–activating peptide (PACAP)	1, 2, 3
Hypothalamic releasing hormones (CRH, LHRH, GHRH)	
Hypothalamic magnocellular hormones (VP in kidney)	VP_2
Small peptide family[a]	
Calcitonin	$C1_a$, $C1_b$
CGRP	$CGRP_1$, $CGRP_2$
Glucagon	
Glucagon-like peptide 1	
Parathormone (PTH), PTH-like peptide	
Secretin	1, 2
VIP	VIP_1, VIP_2
Peptide Receptors Using G_i and Adenylate Cyclase[a]	
Galanin	3 subtypes, not named
GnRH	
Neurotensin	
NPY	Y_1, Y_2, Y_3
Opiates	δ, μ, κ
Somatostatin	1a, 1b, 2a, 2b
Peptide Receptors Using G_q and Phosphatidylinositol[b]	
Angiotensin II	AT_{1a}, AT_{1b}, AT_{1c}, AT_2, AT_3
ANH	
Bombesin, gastrin releasing peptide	2, 3
Bombesin, neuromedin B	1
Bradykinin	2
CCK, gastrin	CCK_A, CCK_{B1}, CCK_{B2}
Endothelin	ET_A, ET_B, ET_C
GnRH	
Neurokinin A	NK_2
Neurokinin B	NK_3
Substance P	NK_{1A}, NK_{1B}
TRH	
VP, oxytocin	VP_{1a}, VP_2, OT

GRP, gastrin-releasing hormone; CG4, receptors preferring a C-terminal peptide common to CCK and gastrin. For other abbreviations, see appendix A.

There are probably many additional subclasses being discovered as this table is printed. G_s activates adenylate cyclase, G_i inhibits adenylate cyclase, G_q mediates the response of the receptor to phosphatidylinositol (PI).

[a] Some peptides in this group may also use G_q and PI.

[b] Some peptides in this group may also use G_i and adenylate cyclase.

A *high specificity* ensures that closely related neuropeptides, though capable of binding to closely related receptors, nevertheless bind preferentially to their own receptors and remain functionally distinct. Some closely related hormones, such as OT and VP may cross-bind, but relative specificity is determined by the concentration of the hormone and the affinity of its receptor; that is, at low concentrations VP will bind to its receptor and evoke pressor and antidiuretic effects; at high concentrations it can evoke the classic oxytocic effects of uterine contractions and milk ejection.

Receptor number is finite so that receptors are *saturable*; this characteristic distinguishes the specific binding of a hormone from nonspecific binding. However, receptor number can be increased (*upregulation*) or decreased (*downregulation*), depending on the concentration of the hormone to which the cell is exposed. Insulin lowers the number of insulin receptor numbers by decreasing receptor half-life. Receptor number is also profoundly affected by the opposing actions of receptor *synthesis* and receptor *degradation*, processes that can also be enhanced or curtailed by hormones. Receptors are subject to *competition* by closely related compounds and are profoundly affected by specific antagonists and drugs. The measurement of receptor number and affinity and the percentage of specific binding are described in most biochemistry texts; an excellent summary is given by Bolander, 1989. Detailed examples of receptor regulation by specific neuropeptides are given in part II of this text.

6.2.2 Receptor Downregulation and Desensitization

Neuropeptides regulate the number and sensitivity of their own receptors. Desensitization is usually a decreased response to continued stimulation. Receptors modulate their sensitivity in response to the intensity and frequency of stimulation by several mechanisms of feedback regulation. These may involve the receptor itself or the downstream signaling pathway. Sequestration of receptors results in downregulation (decreased receptor number) and the loss of responsiveness to agonists may include loss of coupling to G proteins, Upon exposure to an agonist, the response peaks and then declines to some tonic level above basal but below the maximal. If the agonist is removed, desensitization generally remains, resulting in a smaller maximal response to a repeated exposure. If the agonist is absent for a prolonged period, the cell recovers from desensitization and there may be an eventual overshoot compared to the base level (upregulation) (figure 6.2).

On the other hand, decreased receptor activity in desensitization often involves phosphorylation of a receptor by a protein kinase, altering its conformation

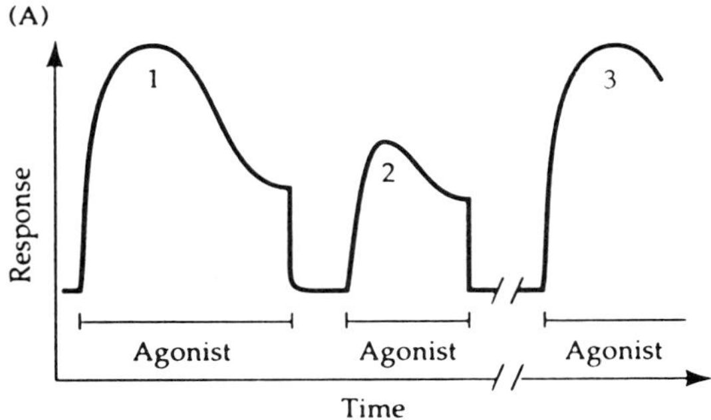

Figure 6.2
Desensitization in response to a neurotransmitter or neuropeptide (agonist). (1) Upon exposure to the agonist, the response peaks and then declines to some level above basal. (2) A repeat exposure to the agonist, after an interval, elicits a smaller response indicating remaining desensitization. (3) If the agonist is removed for an extended time, recovery from desensitization is seen. (From Ross, 1992.)

and changing its affinity for its ligand, which in some cases may enhance the binding of an inhibitory protein. Receptor phosphorylation is reversible by phosphatases. Desensitization that is confined to one receptor is called *homologous desensitization*. A more common form of desensitization is *heterologous desensitization*, which involves all the receptors that use a signaling pathway and is usually initiated by the second messenger of that pathway, for example, desensitization of the adenylate cyclase systems is initiated by cAMP acting upon cAMP-dependent protein kinase, resulting in phosphorylation of the receptor.

6.2.3 Receptor Upregulation and Sensitization

In contrast to the response to agonists, chronic exposure to antagonists can lead to an increase in the number of receptors, often accompanied by an increased sensitivity to agonists. In the case of GnRH autoregulation of its own receptors, upregulation is dependent on the secondary mobilization of extracellular Ca^{2+} caused by the continuous administration of the agonist (GnRH) (figure 6.3).

Several drugs, such as lithium and antidepressant drugs, not only affect the uptake of neurotransmitters in presynaptic nerve terminals but also alter the sensitivity of pre- and postsynaptic receptors, probably through increased transmitter release.

6.2.4 Receptor Metabolism and Recycling

Desensitization may also occur through endocytosis of the hormone-receptor complex after binding, the kinetics of which are important (see section 6.9). This ends the first-messenger signal and is an important part of desensitization. Once the endosome is safely within the cytoplasm, it becomes acidified by an ATP-dependent mechanism and the hormone be-

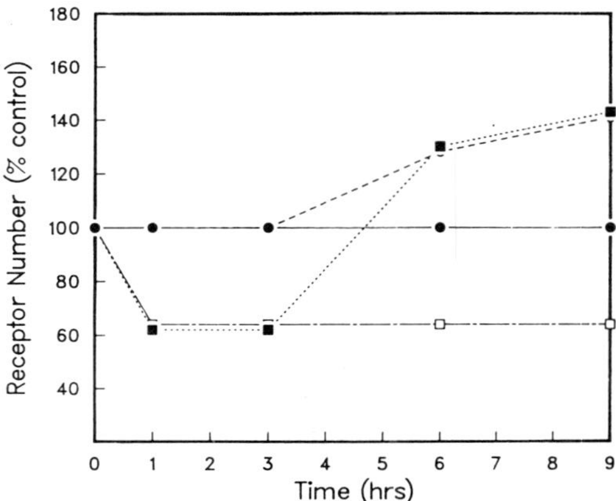

Figure 6.3
Regulation of the gonadotropin-releasing hormone (GnRH) receptor. Culture of pituitary cells with 1 nM GnRH (black squares) causes an initial decrease in receptor number, followed by an increase. The increase can be prevented by chelation of extracellular Ca^{2+} with ethyleneglycoltetraacetic acid (open squares), or provoked directly by addition of 100 nM Ca^{2+} ionophore A23187. (From Jinnah and Conn, 1988.)

comes dissociated from its receptor. The liberated receptors then return to the Golgi apparatus, where they are sorted, some being recycled to the plasma membrane while others are degraded.

An interesting hypothesis has been propounded by Elde et al. (1995). From their studies of opiate receptors, they suggest that these receptors undergo axonal transport and then are stored in presynaptic terminals awaiting incoporation into the presynaptic membrane following neuronal stimulation. Thus the release of receptors into accessible positions in the membrane may be regulated by depolarization and subsequent presynaptic terminal events (figure 6.4), a mechanism reminiscent of the release of neurotransmitters and neuropeptides as a result of neuronal activation.

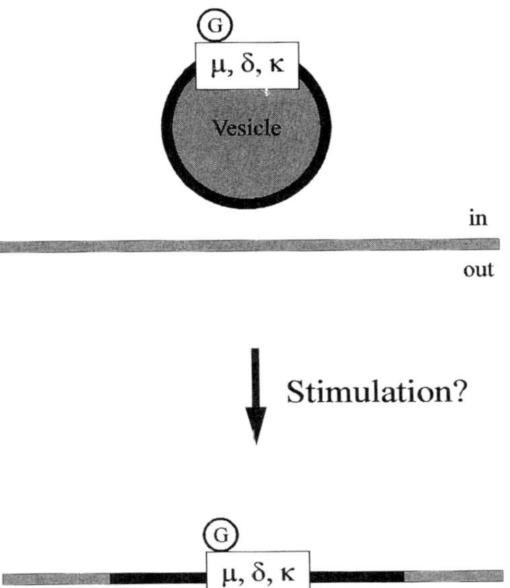

Figure 6.4
Schematic illustration of the hypothesis that presynaptic opiate receptors are inserted into the plasma membrane of the nerve terminal in an activity-dependent manner. Under normal circumstances (upper panel) a major portion of opiate receptor immunoreactivity is associated with a distinct population of vesicles. Under conditions of increased activity (lower panel) the resultant fusion of the vesicles membrane with the plasma membrane of the nerve terminal results in the externalization of the receptor. G, G proteins. μ, δ, and κ are opioid receptor subtypes. (From Elde et al., 1995.)

6.2.5 *Spare Receptors*

Because a single receptor can activate many G protein molecules (see section 6.8), maximal effectiveness often can be obtained when only a small fraction of the total receptor pool is bound by the agonist. This discrepancy is believed to be due to the presence of more receptors than are needed, that is, "spare receptors." By controlling the number of receptors on its surface, the cell can regulate its sensitivity to messengers over a wide range of concentrations.

6.2.6 *Multiple Forms of Receptors: Isoreceptors*

Isoreceptors are structurally and functionally distinct receptors for the same hormone and all bind to the same natural hormone. They are mainly classified into subtypes by specific drug agonists and antagonists, and sometimes by tissue-specific expression. The differentiation of receptor subtypes was first postulated by Dale in 1914, when he demonstrated that the actions of ACh at the neuromuscular junction could be mimicked by nicotine and blocked by curare. ACh effects in the autonomic nervous system, on the other hand, are mimicked by the plant alkaloid muscarine and blocked by atropine. Thus cholinergic receptors are differentiated into two major subtypes, nicotinic and muscarinic.

Receptor subtypes are also common to neuropeptides. Many G protein–coupled receptors have multiple isoforms that are expressed in different tissues, have different potencies, and may have quite different effects depending on the stage of development, the target cell, and interaction with other neuropeptides or neurotransmitters. The concept of multiple types of receptors explains the subtle differences in the effects of closely related neuropeptides. The structural classification of receptor subtypes is based on agonist and antagonist binding studies in vitro and in vivo, whereas behavioral studies have contributed significantly to functional classifications.

Arginine vasopressin (AVP) receptors have been divided into two broad subtypes, the V1 and V2 receptors, which are differentially distributed in tissues and use different second messengers. The $V1_a$ receptors act via phosphatidylinositol (PI) and the

Table 6.2
Distribution, second messengers, and effects of arginine vasopressin (AVP) receptors

AVP Receptor Subtype	Tissue Distribution	Second Messenger	Effect
$V1_a$	Brain and peripheral tissues, e.g., adrenals, reproductive organs, spleen, etc.	PI and Ca^{2+}	Vasopressor and CNS effects
$V1_b$	Anterior pituitary	PI and Ca^{2+}	ACTH secretion and release
V2	Kidney	Adenylate cyclase	Antidiuretic effects

PI, phosphatidylinositol.

mobilization of intracellular Ca^{2+} and mediate the vasopressor effects of AVP as well as many of its CNS effects. The $V1_a$ receptor is found in the brain and is widely distributed in many peripheral tissues, including the adrenal gland, the reproductive organs, spleen, liver, and so on. The $V1_b$ receptor is also coupled to PI turnover and Ca^{2+} mobilization, but is restricted to the anterior pituitary gland. The V2 receptor is coupled to adenylate cyclase and is located in the kidney where it mediates the antidiuretic effect of AVP (table 6.2). More information about the AVP receptors may be found in the review by Lolait et al (1995).

Another example is the family of melanocortin receptors. The five cloned receptors for the melanocortins form a multiple, pharmacologically distinct family of receptors that differ according to their tissue origin and consequently in their function. They are relatively small (297 to 360 amino acids) and have a tertiary structure different from that of other known G protein receptors (Cone et al., 1993). They are discussed in detail in chapter 12.

Through the pharmacological development of increasingly selective ligands as agonists or antagonists, it has become possible to define even more receptor types and subtypes, and perhaps even sub-subtypes for both neurotransmitters and neuropeptides. The cloning of receptors, probing of tissue-specific cDNA libraries with known receptor probes, and the use of the polymerase chain reaction (PCR) have expanded the intricacies of receptor family trees even further. However, the correlation of these various receptor subtypes with their physiological activities is not always clear and is providing molecular neurobiologists and physiologists with challenging issues for further research.

All neuropeptide receptors are proteins, most of which are glycosylated. There are three distinct structural and functional regions of the receptor that can be identified according to their location with respect to the cell membrane: an extracellular portion, a transmembrane section, and a cytoplasmic domain (figure 6.5). The specificity of the receptor depends on its distinct extracellular ligand-binding domain. There are several different classes of neuropeptide receptors, classified on the basis of their structure and the second-messenger systems which they activate.

6.3 G Protein–Coupled Receptors (GPCRs)

6.3.1 *Structure of GPCRs*

GPCRs constitute approximately 80% of neuropeptide receptors. Their extracellular portion is

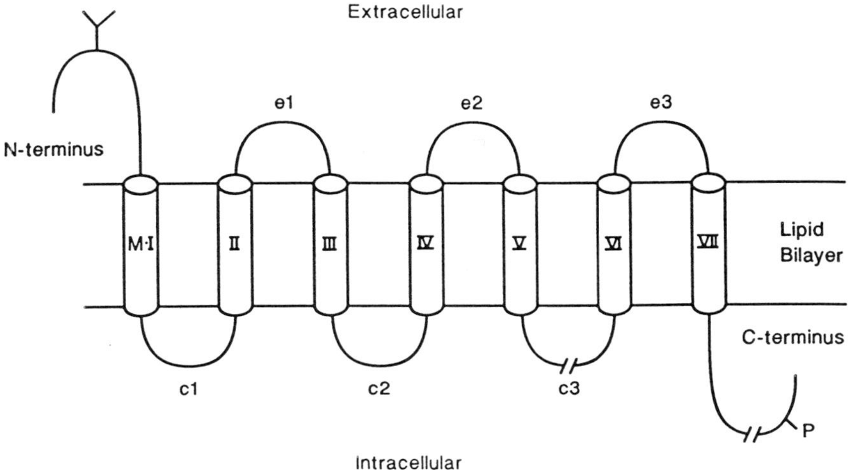

Figure 6.5
A schematic illustration of the relationship of the primary structure of a G protein–linked receptor to transmembrane topology. The domains e1, e2, and e3 are extracellular. The C1, C2, C3, and C-terminal domains are intracellular. The seven putative membrane-spanning domains are M-I to M-VII. Potential N-linked glycosylation sites (Y) are often observed on the N-terminal region and potential phosphorylation sites are usually on the C-terminal domain. (From Krause et al., 1990.)

formed by the N-terminal part of the receptor polypeptide which has potential glycosylation sites. The extracellular domain constitutes the ligand-binding domain for glycoprotein hormones. Most of these sites are the Asn-X-Ser/Thr type for N-linked oligosaccharides. Many amino acids are hydrophilic and are attracted to the extracellular milieu. Bulky neuropeptide ligands, such as LH, are bound by a large extracellular amino acid domain.

G protein–coupled receptors possess a core of seven membrane-spanning helices, the *transmembrane segments*. Seven α-helical segments, composed mostly of hydrophobic amino acid residues, are connected by alternating cytoplasmic and extracytoplasmic loops to form helical cylinders with a central pore exposed to the extracellular surface. Smaller, relatively hydrophobic peptide ligands may interact with multiple receptor domains, with several extracellular and transmembrane segments contributing to the binding. A large number of neuropeptides act through this multihelical type of receptor (see table 6.1).

The C-terminal cytoplasmic domain contains a Cys residue that represents the site for attachment to the lipid bilayer of the membrane. Both the C-terminal cytoplasmic domain and the intracellular loop contain Ser and Thr residues that are phosphorylated during receptor desensitization (see section 6.2.2).

Some examples of the structures of G protein–binding neuropeptide receptors are shown in figures 6.6 and 6.7. Figure 6.6 illustrates the receptor for substance P (SP), a member of the tachykinin family. The predominant receptor for SP has been termed the NK-1 receptor. The receptors for the other two members of this family, neurokinin A and neurokinin

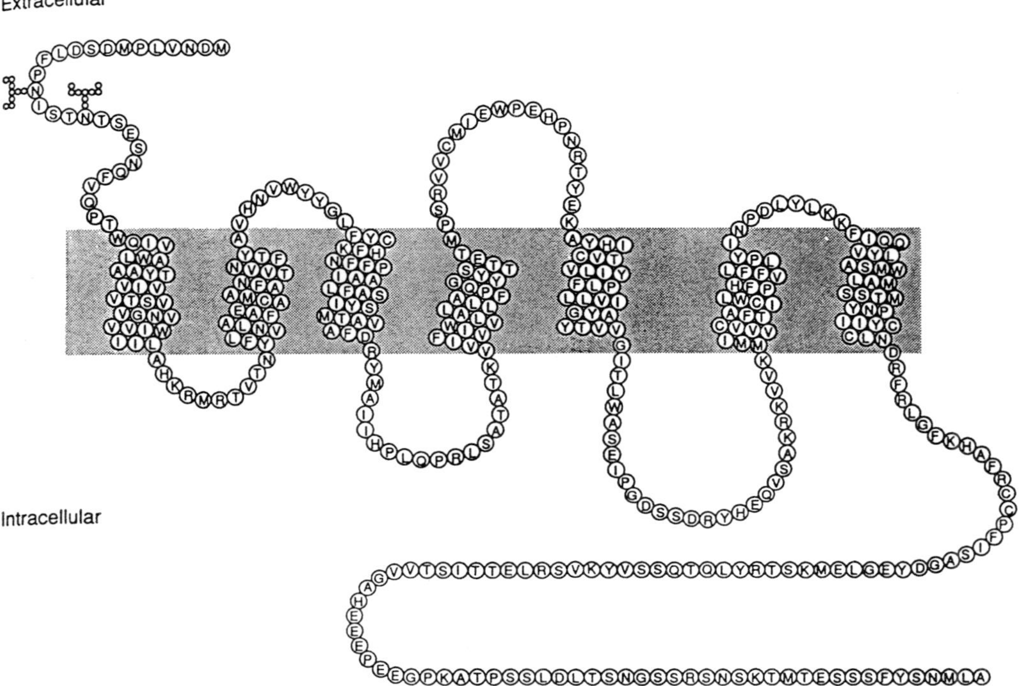

Figure 6.6
Structure of the substance P receptor. Potential glycosylation sites are indicated by branching. Codes for amino acids are given by the single letters (see appendix C). (From Poyner and Hanley, 1992.)

B, resemble the NK-1 receptor closely, but have different affinities and substrate specificities (see chapter 15). All three tachykinins use the second messengers derived from PI, diacylglycerol, and inositol 1, 4, 5-triphosphate (IP_3). However, the NK-1 receptor binds SP with an affinity that is several orders of magnitude greater than for all the other members of the tachykinin family (Boyd et al. 1995).

Figure 6.7 illustrates the structure of another subfamily of G protein–coupled receptors which includes the anterior pituitary glycoprotein hormones LH, FSH and TSH. These proteins have a common α unit but differ in their β subunits. They all act through G protein–coupled receptors to stimulate adenylate cyclase. The main characteristic of the receptors of this subfamily is the extremely long extracellular N-terminus, needed to bind these large glycoprotein ligands (Poyner and Hanley, 1992).

6.3.2 *Specific G Protein–Binding Domains*

The catalytic site in G protein–coupled receptors is composed of several cationic regions, the number that is needed to activate the G proteins varying with the

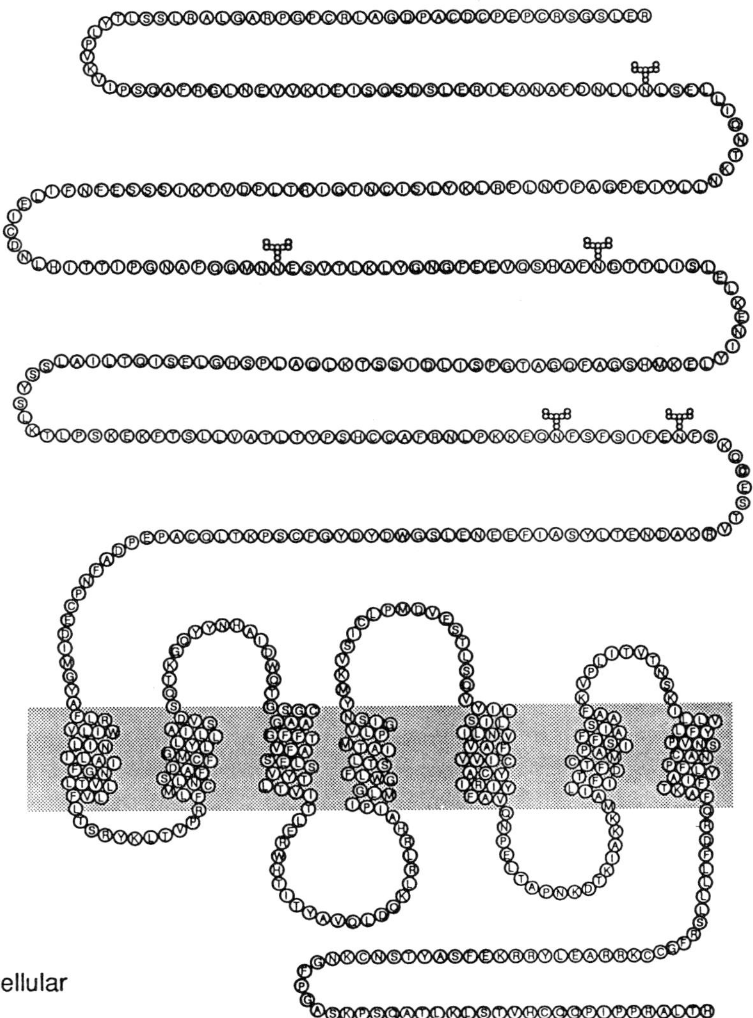

Figure 6.7
Structure of the luteinizing hormone receptor. Potential glycosylation sites are indicated by branching. Codes for amino acids are given by the single letters (see appendix C). (From Poyner and Hanley, 1992.)

specific receptor; these regions determine the receptor's selectivity among homologous G proteins:

1. the second loop that connects spans 3 and 4;
2. both stalks of the large loop that connects spans 5 and 6; and
3. cytoplasmic regions near the end of the seventh span.

In an imaginative experiment, short sequences from the second and third cytoplasmic loops of one receptor were replaced by homologous sequences from a donor receptor. These foreign sequences selectively activated only the G protein targets of the donor receptor and not those of the recipient receptor.

6.3.3 *Characteristics of G Proteins*

6.3.3.1 Structure

G proteins are membrane-bound cytoplasmic-facing proteins that bind GTP and act as intermediaries between the receptor and several second-messenger–generating enzymes, thereby controlling metabolic, neural, humoral, and developmental functions (see figure 6.1). All eukaryotic cells contain G proteins and are derived from a large gene family that encodes the subunits of the G protein. The cells may differ, however, in the subunits they express.

Each G protein is a heterotrimer consisting of a GTP-binding α subunit, and β and γ subunits. The α subunit binds GTP and can activate a variety of effector proteins in the absence of β and γ units. Subclasses of the α subunit are G_s, G_i, G_q, and G_{12}. G_s stimulates adenylate cyclase in response to a diverse group of receptors, including β-adrenergic, D_1 dopaminergic, E-type prostaglandins, VIP, and glucagon. Another group of receptors inhibits adenylate cyclase via G_i. This group includes cholinergic muscarinic M2, α_2-adrenergic, serotoninergic, somatostatin, neuropeptide Y (NPY), galanin, and enkephalinergic receptors. G_q activates phospholipase C, with G_q (and subclasses $G_{11,14-16}$) identified by insensitivity to pertussis toxin. Inactivation of G protein activity is through inherent G protein GTPase activity, which splits off inorganic phosphate from bound GTP, thereby returning to the inactive guanosine diphosphate (GDP)–bound state (figure 6.8).

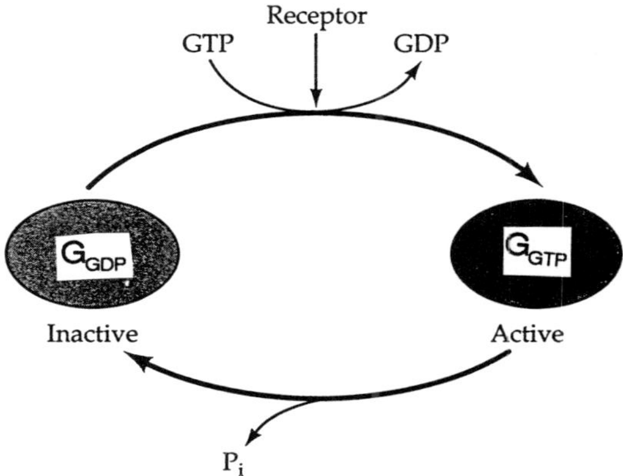

Figure 6.8
G proteins are activated by binding guanosine triphosphate (GTP). Hydrolysis of bound GTP to guanosine diphosphate (GDP) terminates activation. Receptors catalyze the release of the inactive GDP as well as the binding of GTP, and thereby increase the relative level of G protein activation. (From Ross, 1992.)

There are four different mammalian β subunit isotypes, the amino acid sequences of which are highly conserved. One of the subtypes, β_2, appears to be especially important in integrating the effects and timing of the various G protein–mediated circuits (Simon et al., 1991). There are seven different γ subunits

6.3.3.2 Trigger Action

Receptors can stimulate G proteins very rapidly and because the active state of the G proteins lasts for a relatively long time (3 to 15 seconds), each ligand-receptor can activate 10 to 20 G protein molecules. Since the G proteins also activate the next member of the signal transduction cascade, a few molecules of neurotransmitter or neuropeptide can elicit a significant cellular response. It is interesting that the classic neurotransmitters, such as ACh, epinephrine, and DA are effective in milligrams per kilogram of body weight, whereas neuropeptides are effective in the micro- to picogram range.

6.3.3.3 Regulators of G Protein Signaling

With G proteins involved in an enormous variety of biological communications systems, there should be some mechanism that would account for the specificity of the cellular response. Recent research has implicated a large family of proteins that *r*egulates the sensitivity of G protein *s*ignaling pathways, and consequently are termed the *RGS proteins*. These regulators appear to bind to the α subunit of the G protein and in this manner obstruct its normal signaling function (Siderovski et al., 1996).

6.3.4 G Protein–Activated Second Messengers

6.3.4.1 The Cyclic Nucleotide cAMP

a. Discovery of cAMP and the role of adenylate cyclase

The significance of second messengers through which hormones, the first messengers, exert their pleiotropic effects, was first demonstrated by Sutherland in 1958, for which he received the Nobel prize in 1971. Sutherland demonstrated that epinephrine increased the concentration of hepatic intracellular adenosine 3′,5′-cyclic monophosphate (cAMP), which Sutherland called the "second messenger," through the catalytic action of *adenylate cyclase* (Sutherland, 1972). Adenylate cyclase is an effector protein, a membrane-bound enzyme, which upon activation by G proteins, catalyzes the formation of cAMP from cytoplasmic ATP. cAMP is widely distributed in all organisms and is a major second messenger for neuropeptide hormones.

Both the hormone receptor and adenylate cyclase are embedded in the plasma membrane, but the stimulatory action of the hormone on adenylate cyclase is not direct. Rather it is mediated by the G proteins, also in the plasma membrane, as discussed in section 6.5. The adenylate cyclases form a heterogeneous multigene family, with several isoforms. In studies on the brain, Mons and Cooper (1995) found a selective distribution of adenylate cyclase isoforms in discrete brain regions. Selectivity even reaches ultrastructural levels in that cerebellar cells accumulate adenylate cyclase in postsynaptic densities of the dendritic spines, a characteristic that probably aids neuropeptide modulation of synaptic transmission.

b. Effects of cAMP

The main effect of cAMP is the allosteric activation of cAMP-dependent, Ca^{2+}-independent, protein kinase through binding to the regulatory subunits of the kinase, altering their conformation to their active enzymatic form. In this active form, the enzyme is able to catalyze the transfer of the γ phosphate from ATP to specific serine, threonine, or tyrosine residues on proteins, resulting in covalent modification of the proteins. This mechanism is widely utilized to regulate ion channels, enzyme activity, and the configuration of structural proteins, making cAMP a common pathway for the action of many neuropeptides and neurotransmitters.

The net concentration of intracellular cAMP is the result of the antagonistic activities of adenylate cyclase,

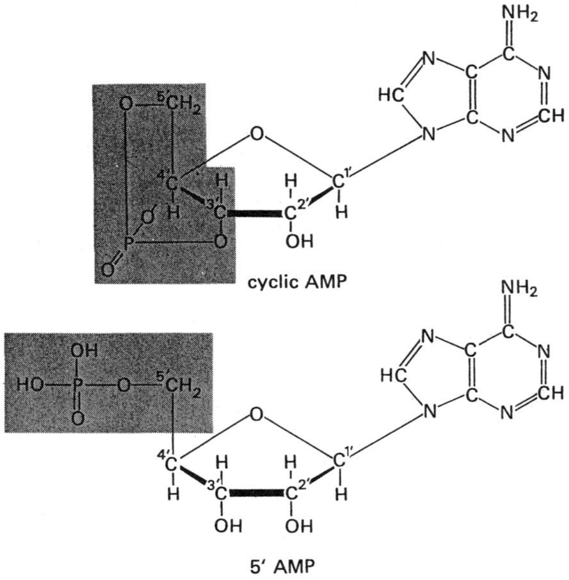

Figure 6.9
Cyclic 3′,5′-adenosine monophosphate (cAMP) has a phosphate group esterified in a cycle linking carbon atoms 3 and 5 of D-ribose. The noncyclic form, 5′-AMP, is biologically inactive.

which synthesizes it from ATP, and *phosphodiesterase*, the calcium-dependent, cytosolic enzyme that hydrolyzes cAMP to its noncyclic form, 5′-adenosine monophosphate (5′-AMP) (figure 6.9). Several hormones increase the activity of phosphodiesterase, in particular those hormones that require the rapid destruction of the second messenger in order to control metabolism on an acute basis. Examples of such hormones are ACTH, insulin, and CCK. Hormones that decrease phosphodiesterase activity regulate slower, longer-lasting processes and include the gonadotropins, the adrenal and gonadal steroids, as well as thyroxine, an iodinated amino acid derivative.

c. *Inhibition of adenylate cyclase*

The $G\alpha_i$ subfamily of G protein–coupled receptors is coupled to inhibition of adenylate cyclase. In addition, the inhibitory actions of the $G\alpha_i$ receptors include activation of K^+ channels and decreased Ca^{2+} influx through voltage-gated Ca^{2+} channels.

6.3.4.2 Phospholipase-Phosphatidylinositol–Linked Messengers

The hydrolysis of the phospholipid *phosphatidylinositol 4,5-biphosphate* (PIP_2) by membrane-bound phospholipase C produces another group of second messengers, *diacylglycerol* and IP_3 (figure 6.10). PIP_2 is a membrane lipid that projects into the cytosol and is hydrolyzed by *phospholipase C*, an enzyme which can associate with the plasma membrane and perhaps also with G proteins. In a manner reminiscent of the cyclic nucleotides, the hormones and transmitters that stimulate PIP_2 hydrolysis (e.g., TRH, VP, bombesin, and GnRH) initiate a cascade of phosphorylations. These commence with the activation of the membrane-bound Ca^{2+}-dependent, cAMP-independent protein kinase C by diacylglycerol, acting synergistically with increased physiological concentrations of Ca^{2+} released from intracellular stores by the action of IP_3 acting on its receptor in the endoplasmic reticulum.

6.4 Guanylate Cyclase Receptors

Cyclic guanosine monophosphate (cGMP) is similar in its chemical structure to cAMP, with the substitution of guanosine for adenosine as its nucleotide. However, whereas adenylate cyclase is only found tightly bound to the plasma membrane, guanylate cyclase is found in both the membrane and the cytoplasm (figure 6.11). These two forms of the enzyme apparently have different functions and are differ-

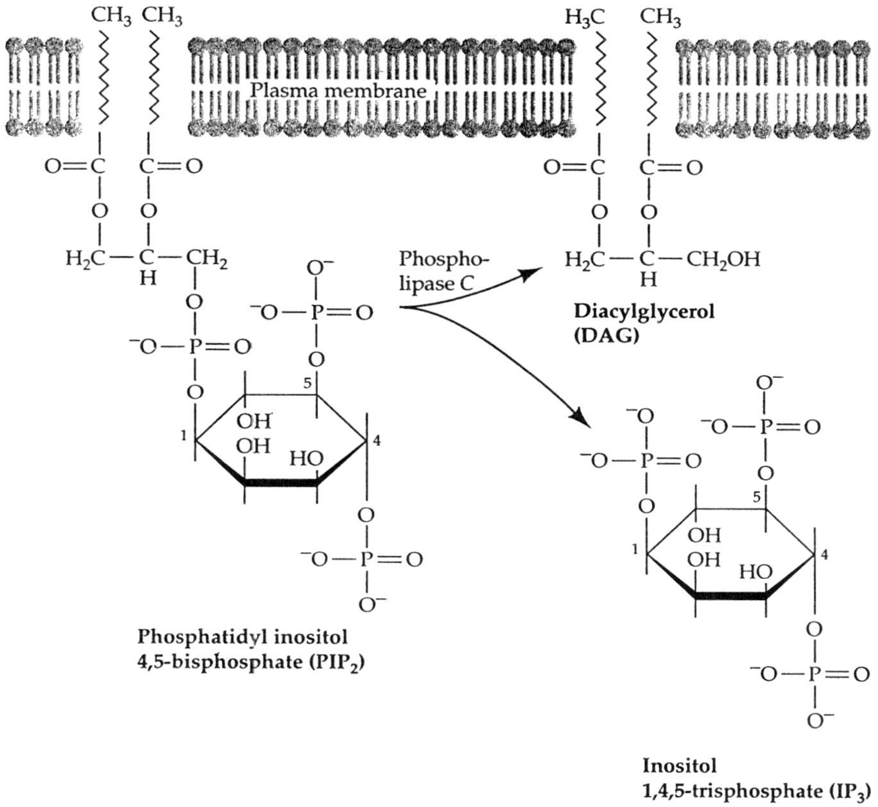

Figure 6.10
Hydrolysis products of phosphatidylinositol 4,5-biphosphate (PIP_2). PIP_2 is a phospholipid with a diglyceride backbone within the plasma membrane and a polar head oriented in the cytosol. Receptor-regulated phospholipase C catalyzes the hydrolysis of PIP_2 to produce 1,2-diacylglycerol (DAG) and inositol 1,4,5-triphosphate (IP_3). (From Kennedy, 1992.)

entially regulated. The soluble form of cGMP is activated by NO and free radicals. Membrane-bound guanylate cyclase forms part of a transmembrane receptor complex for atrial natriuretic hormone (ANH), an important neuropeptide involved in the regulation of electrolyte balance and cardiovascular homeostasis. The ANH receptor has only one membrane-spanning helix and the extracellular binding site for the neuropeptide is directly linked to the catalytic guanylate cyclase domain through this single transmembrane helix.

cGMP is not nearly as widely distributed as cAMP. It is present in highest concentration in the cerebellum and its involvement with ANH indicates it must also be in the kidney, the chief site of ANH action. cGMP activates a specific cGMP-dependent protein kinase

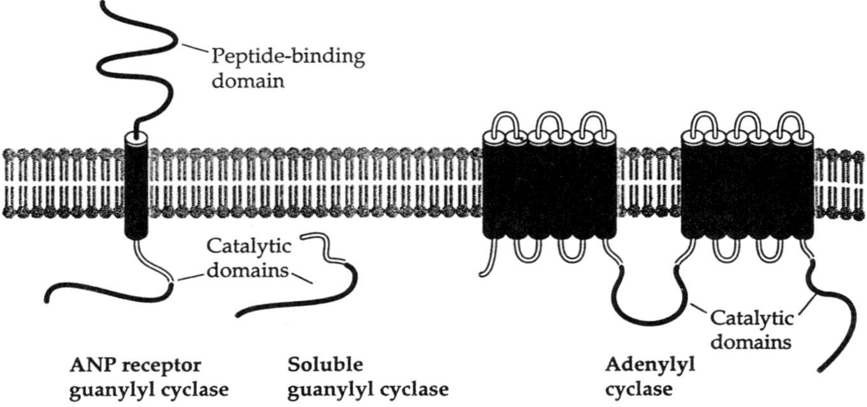

Figure 6.11
Three forms of cyclase are shown: adenylyl cyclase, membrane-bound guanylate cyclase, and soluble cytosolic guanylate cyclase. All the catalytic domains of the cyclases are similar. The membrane-bound guanalylate cyclase is a receptor for the atrial natriuretic hormone (ANP). The binding site is in the extracellular domain, whereas the catalytic site is cytoplasmic. (From Kennedy, 1992.)

which phosphorylates a 23-kD protein, named G substrate, which is expressed only in Purkinje cells of the cerebellum. A proposed role for the cGMP cascade in the cerebellum is the inhibition of phosphatases through the G substrate and thus the prolongation of the effects of phosphorylation started by other signal transduction cascades.

6.5 Tyrosine Kinase–Coupled Receptors

These receptors do not associate with G proteins and are considerably simpler in transmembrane configuration than the G protein–binding receptors, having only one membrane-spanning helix which separates the extracellular domain at the N-terminus from the cytoplasmic domain at the C-terminus. Like the more complex G protein–binding receptors, the hormone binding site is in the extracellular domain which is rich in cysteines that form stabilizing cross-linkages and, in addition, contains most of the glycosylation sites. N-linked glycosylation occurs on asparagines in the sequence Asn-X-Ser/Thr. The receptors for insulin, insulin-like growth factor, and several other growth factor receptors belong in this class (figure 6.12). The insulin receptor is glycosylated, a procedure essential to proper receptor processing.

The *cytoplasmic domain* contains a well-conserved protein kinase catalytic domain that is essential to transmembrane signaling, and several phosphorylation sites. Tyrosine kinases act by initiating a cascade of protein phosphorylations in the cytoplasm, reactions that are particularly important during development and growth. Those protein kinases that are directly regulated by second messengers phosphorylate only serine or threonine residues.

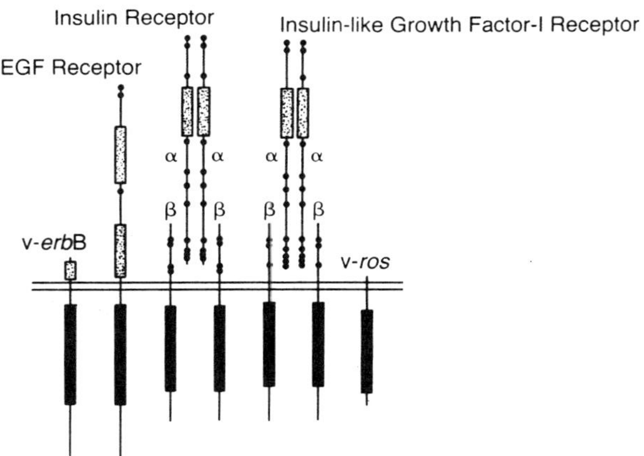

Figure 6.12
Schematic view of the insulin receptor and other tyrosine kinase receptors. Black bars in the cytoplasmic region (below the double line, representing the membrane) indicate tyrosine kinase domains. Above the line is the extracellular ligand binding domain, dominated by cysteine-rich domains (stippled) and other cysteines (black circles). The double line is the region of the single membrane-spanning helix. Both the insulin receptor and the IGF-1 receptor consist of two α and two β subunits connected by disulfide bonds to form the heterotetrameric receptor complex. Two families of receptors are shown: (1) insulin receptor, IGF-1 receptor, and related oncogene product v-*ros*; (2) epidermal growth factor (EGF) and related oncogene product v-*erb*B. (Adapted from Ullrich et al., 1986.)

6.6 Cytokine Receptors

Cytokine receptors are transmembrane glycoproteins which are classified into several families. Type I consists of the growth hormone (GH) and prolactin (PRL) receptors, which are homologous, which is not surprising considering the close homology of the two pituitary neuropeptides (see chapter 1). The GH and PRL receptors share some topological similarities with the tyrosine kinase receptors in that they have only one transmembrane region. However, they have no cysteine-rich or Ser-Thr-rich domains. They do have potential extracellular glycosylation sites. This cytokine family also includes growth factor receptors for some of the interleukins, erythropoietin, and ciliary neurotrophic factor. The other cytokine families (types II, III, and IV) do not include neuropeptides.

6.7 Nitric Oxide

The free radical gas NO may act as a neurotransmitter or a second messenger, a surprising observation first made by Garthwaite et al., 1988. NO is found exclusively in neurons and endothelial cells. This unlikely molecule is enormously versatile, an important regulator of a variety of physiological properties, including smooth muscle relaxation, vasodilation in peripheral organs and the brain, formation of cGMP in cerebellar cells, and release of transmitters. As a gas its location is difficult to pinpoint except through antibodies raised against the enzyme *nitric oxide synthase (NOS)*, an oxidative, Ca^{2+}-dependent enzyme responsible for the formation of NO from arginine. NO rapidly diffuses through cell membranes where it activates the soluble form of guanylate cyclase, thus increasing cGMP concentration. NO is not stored but is synthesized on demand; thus its formation by NOS is the only means by which it can be regulated. NOS can be inactivated by a wide variety of phosphorylating enzymes (Dawson and Snyder, 1994).

6.7.1 *Localization of NOS*

Nitric oxide synthase is found in relatively high concentrations in endothelial cells of blood vessels and in certain neurons, especially the glutaminergic granule cells of the cerebellum, the granule cells of the hippocampus, the magnocellular neurons of the PVN and

SON, and the hypothalamus. NOS is colocalized with several neurotransmitters and neuropeptides but with no apparent pattern to the selection of associated molecules. In the cerebral cortex, NOS is colocalized in neurons with ST, NPY, and the inhibitory transmitter γ-amino butyric acid (GABA). In the corpus striatum, NOS is colocalized with ST and NPY. In part of the brain stem, NOS is colocalized with choline acetyltransferase, the enzyme that synthesizes ACh.

6.7.2 *Central and Peripheral Neuronal Actions of NO*

Glutamate, an excitatory amino acid, stimulates glutamate (NMDA) receptors on cerebellar granule cells, raising the level of cGMP and probably triggering the formation of NO. NO diffuses rapidly to the adjacent Purkinje cells to activate guanylate cyclase. cGMP is selectively concentrated in Purkinje cells that receive the input of granule cells (Dawson and Snyder, 1994). Through the activation of guanylate cyclase, and perhaps by the phosphorylation of synaptic vesicle proteins, NO may influence the release of neurotransmitters. NO also may be involved in hippocampal long-term potentiation, a mechanism believed to be part of memory formation. Release of NO in the hypothalamus induces secretion of GnRH, a neuropeptide essential for ovulation and female sexual behavior (Mani et al., 1994), and the release of CRH and growth hormone (GH) (Rettori et al., 1994).

In the gut, NO causes depolarization of the myenteric plexus, resulting in relaxation of smooth muscle involved with peristalsis. This process is blocked by NOS inhibitors, indicating that NO is the nonadrenergic-noncholinergic neurotransmitter of the gut (Bult et al., 1990).

6.7.3 *Vascular Actions of NO*

NO is the chief endogenous vasodilator released from vascular endothelium (Ignarro et al., 1987) and causes vasodilation of the penile deep cavernosal arteries and sinusoids, permitting the increased blood flow necessary for penile erection (Burnett et al., 1992). NO also mediates vasodilation of the cerebral arteries (Faraci, 1992; Toda et al., 1993). The gas NO, together with two neuropeptides (VIP and peptidine histidine isoleucin [PHI] and the classical transmitter ACh, form a controlling group of substances that regulate the flow of blood through the portal vessels between the hypothalamus and pituitary gland, profoundly influencing neuroendocrine systems (Ceccatelli et al., 1992).

6.7.4 *Developmental Effects of NO as Seen in NOS Knockout Mice*

Homologous genetic recombination techniques can disrupt the murine gene encoding neuronal NOS (nNOS) to produce homozygous neuronal "knockout" mice (Huang et al., 1993). Despite the lack of NOS activity and the absence of NOS staining neurons (figure 6.13), there does not appear to be any gross morphological abnormality in the brain or in peripheral tissues. However, the stomach of the nNOS knockout mouse is markedly enlarged and the circular muscle layer of the pyloris is hypertrophied (figure 6.14), supporting the suggestion that lack of NO is involved in the human disorder infantile pyloric stenosis (Vanderwinden et al., 1992). It is also possible to produce mice lacking endothelial NO (eNOS knockouts). From detailed electrophysiological studies of nNOS and eNOS knockout mice, it appears that that it may be the endothelial rather than the neuronal isoform of NOS that is the

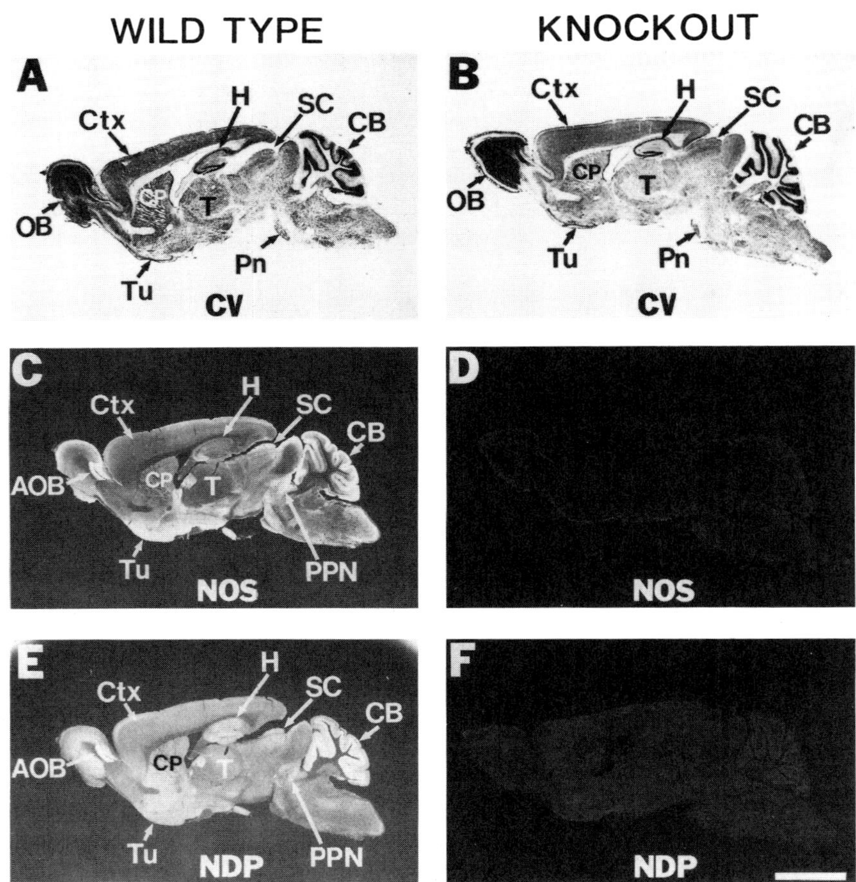

Figure 6.13
Neuronal (n)NOS null mice (KNOCKOUT) are devoid of nNOS immunostaining and do not stain with the special diaphorase stain which marks all NOS neurons. The tissues of these nNOS knockout mice have normal cytoarchitecture. The brains of wild type (normal) mice are depicted in panels (A), (C), and (E), and the brains of the nNOS knockout mice are shown in panels (B), (D), and (F). CV, cresyl violet; NOS, nitric oxide synthase; NDP, NADPH diaphorase staining; AOB, accessory olfactory bulb; CB, cerebellum; CP, caudate putamen; Ctx, cortex; H, hippocampus; OB, olfactory bulb; PPN, pedunculopontine tegmental nucleus; Pn, pontine nuclei; SC, superior colliculus; T, thalamus; Tu, olfactory tubercle. Bar: 2.5 mm. (From Dawson and Dawson, 1994.)

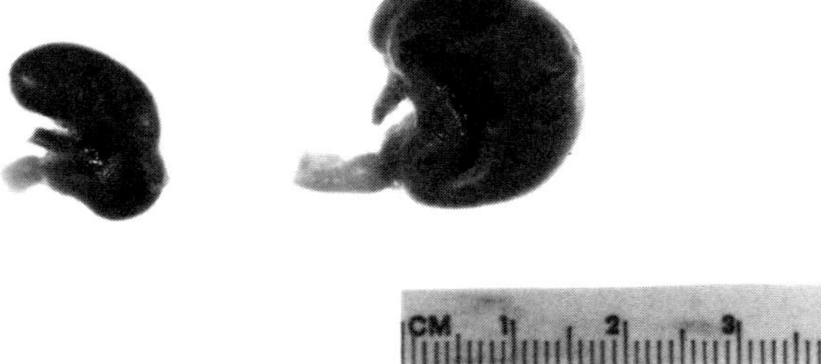

Figure 6.14
Stomach hypertrophy in nNOS knockout mice. A normal stomach is illustrated on the left and the markedly enlarged stomach of a nNOS knockout mouse is shown on the right. (From Dawson and Dawson, 1994.)

major source of NO involved in brain electrophysiological processes, such as long-term potentiation (LTP) in the hippocampus (O'Dell et al., 1994). It is most likely that NO is normally involved in a wide range of processes, including behavioral, since mice lacking the NOS gene become very aggressive and demonstrate immoderate and inappropriate sexual behavior (Nelson et al, 1995).

6.7.5 Neuroprotective and Neurotoxic Actions of NO

Depending on the rate of NO formation, NO may be either neuroprotective or neurotoxic. NOS neurons are resistant to the toxicity of glutamate, acting through NMDA receptors. However, under conditions of focal ischemia, when large amounts of glutamate are released, the resulting excessive release of NO induces neuronal death. NOS neurons are resistant to destruction in Huntington's and Alzheimer's disease and vascular stroke. It has been suggested that NO may possess either neuroprotective or neurodestructive properties depending on its oxidation-reduction status, with NO° being neurodestructive and NO^{+} being neuroprotective (Lipton et al., 1993). The potential involvement of NO in so many serious neurodegenerative diseases opens new possibilities for the development of therapeutic agents, especially of selective neuronal NOS inhibitors (Dawson and Dawson, 1994).

6.8 Significance of Receptor Diversity

There are many possible reasons for the tremendous diversity of neurotransmitter and neuropeptide receptors. Fuxe et al. (1995) suggest that receptor diversity allows the receptors to couple to different types of G proteins, thus permitting the stimulation or inhibition of multiple transduction mechanisms. In different cells a single agonist can stimulate different G proteins to initiate distinct second-messenger responses which, in turn, could result in different gradations of response in different tissues. These dissimilar actions would not be possible through the mediation of a single receptor and single second messenger.

If the receptor subtypes have different affinities for the ligand, it is feasible that the high-affinity receptors permit transmission after low amounts of the ligand. Once the impulse flow has started, it may recruit more distant receptor subtypes with a lower affinity for the ligand, prolonging the effect.

Fuxe et al. also suggest that by recruiting different receptor subtypes, negative or positive cooperativity may develop between the subtypes. *Positive cooperativity* implies that more than one receptor subtype is necessary for the response; *negative cooperativity* suggests that more than one receptor subtype is required to inhibit a response. Further fine-tuning may be through receptor-receptor interactions within the membrane, so that neuropeptide receptors may modulate the desensitization of other receptors by altering their affinities. This could be a mechanism for regulation of the duration of the postsynaptic responses induced by the ligand.

6.9 Regulation of Receptors and Second-Messenger Systems

It has become clear that the intrasignaling network of the cell is extraordinarily complex, with ligands showing extensive redundancy, pleiotropy, and crosstalk between different signaling systems. The specificity of the complex path between stimulus and response is probably dependent on the types, numbers, and affinities of receptors; types of signaling molecules; selectivity of recognition domains; and feedback loops. Ca^{2+} sensitivity or insensitivity of various isoforms of receptors and of second-messenger systems are also important variables. The discovery that these isoforms may be differentially regulated increases logarithmically the possible options for regulation of second-messenger systems.

Another important aspect of receptor regulation is the kinetics of activation of the signaling molecules. The basic concept of the role of kinetics of activation in determining response selectivity is that signaling devices, such as receptors or the downstream signaling molecules, feature not only a switch that turns on the signal after binding with a specific ligand but also a timer that determines how long the switch will stay on. It is the timer, that is, the kinetic aspect of the interaction between receptor and ligand, that will determine how long the switch stays on and thereby may play an important role in choosing between several possible interacting downstream pathways.

A clear example of a timer effect is seen in PC12 cells, a rat pheochromocytoma cell line that possesses receptors for both nerve growth factor (NGF) and epidermal growth factor (EGF). These two neurotrophic factors evoke quite different cellular responses: NGF causes PC12 cells to stop dividing, develop excitable membranes, and differentiate into a sympathetic neuron prototype. EGF, on the other hand, induces cell proliferation. Yet EGF and NGF use the same signaling elements, including tyrosine phosphorylation, 2-deoxyglucose uptake, the Na^+, K^+ pump, and sodium channels. It is the kinetic aspects that determine the final response. NGF induces a sustained activation of MAP (microtubule-associated protein) kinase for at least 90 minutes, whereas EGF stimulates MAP kinase activity to the same level, but only briefly (De Meyts et al., 1995).

6.10 Summary

For neuropeptides to affect their target cells, they must bind to cell surface receptors. They may bind to a variety of receptor types and subtypes, with different degrees of affinity. Receptors are characterized by their affinity for the ligand, reversibility, specificity, number, and saturability. Desensitization of a receptor may occur after continued neuropeptide stimulation: this may be a decrease in receptor number (downregulation) or an increase (upregulation), and may be homologous or more commonly, heterologous, resulting from receptor phosphorylation. Desensitization may also be due to removal of exposed receptors by endocytosis. The many different isoreceptors that form receptor subtypes can be distinguished mainly by specific drug agonists and antagonists. Examples of neuropeptide receptor subtypes are the AVP V1 and V2 receptors, which are differentially distributed in tissues and use different second messengers. Five types of melanocortin receptors have been cloned and the markedly different effects of the melanocortin peptides on the adrenal cortex, melanoma cells, CNS, and peripheral neurons can be explained on the basis of the differential distribution of the receptors in these tissues.

All neuropeptide receptors are proteins, most of which are glycosylated. There are three distinct structural and functional regions of the receptor: the extracellular portion, which contains potential glycosylation sites; the transmembrane region; and the cytoplasmic domain. *G protein–coupled receptors (GPCRs)* are characterized by a core of seven membrane-spanning helices, the length, organization, and amino acid composition of which give each receptor its characteristic specificity. Certain receptors may have several subtypes, resulting in subtle differences in the effects of closely related neuropeptides.

More than 80% of neuropeptide receptors are coupled to G proteins, which are membrane-bound cytoplasmic-facing proteins that bind GTP and act as intermediaries between the receptor and several second-messenger systems. Most GPCRs stimulate adenylate cyclase and cAMP formation, a signaling system in which cAMP is the second messenger. cAMP activates cAMP-dependent kinase, which through its alterations of protein conformation, regulates ion channels, enzyme activity, and structural proteins. Other neuropeptides act through the PI system. Hydrolysis of PIP_2, stimulated by TRH, GnRH, and bombesin, results in the formation of another group of second messengers, diacylglycerol and IP_3. Diacylglycerol activates membrane-bound protein kinase C, a Ca^{2+}-dependent action. IP_3 mobilizes intracellular Ca^{2+}, which stimulates calcium-calmodulin–dependent kinase, resulting in protein phosphorylation. Some GPCRs may activate both second-messenger systems and there may be crosstalk between these different signaling systems.

Another group of neuroptide receptors is coupled to *guanylate cyclase*. Membrane-bound guanylate cyclase forms part of a transmembrane receptor complex for ANH. The ANH receptor has only one membrane-spanning helix and the extracellular binding site for the neuropeptide is directly linked to the catalytic guanylate cyclase domain through this single transmembrane helix.

Tyrosine kinase–coupled receptors do not associate with G proteins and, like the guanylate cyclase receptors, have only a single membrane-spanning helix. The receptors for insulin and several growth factors belong to this class of neuropeptide receptors, most of which are glycosylated. The ligand binds to the extracellular domain of the receptor, initiating a cascade of cytoplasmic phosphorylations that are important during development and growth. The *cytokine receptor family*, which is similar in structure to tyrosine kinase receptors, is represented by the GH and PRL receptors.

Nitric oxide, a free radical gas, acts on a wide variety of physiological processes, including vasodilation, muscle relaxation, and the release of neurotransmitters and neuropeptides. NO activates soluble cGMP and is regulated by nitric oxide synthase (NOS) and inactivated by phosphorylating enzymes. NO may be colocalized with several neurotransmitters and neuropeptides.

The diversity of receptors and their subtypes, with their various affinities for their ligands, permits disparate gradations of responses in different tissues, as well as favoring modulation and interaction of receptors. In this manner, a single message to a receptor may trigger its divergence and the resulting messages may be fine-tuned, enhanced, or eliminated. Receptor regulation depends on a vast number of factors, including types, numbers, and affinities of the receptors, their Ca^{2+} sensitivity, and that of the second messengers. The kinetics of activation can determine which of competing second-messenger systems will be activated by a receptor-ligand complex.

Chapter 7 approaches the problem of whether neuropeptides are neurotransmitters or neuromodulators, and shows that whereas some neuropeptides unequivocally can act as neurotransmitters, they may also act as neuromodulators under different conditions.

Neuropeptides as Neurotransmitters, Neuromodulators, and Neurohormones

7

7.1 Comparison of Neurotransmitters and Neuromodulators

In the preceding chapter, the role of neuropeptides on the transduction machinery of the cell was considered. The end result of the activation of one or several second-messenger systems is a change in the physiological properties of the cell, including membrane permeability, a vital component of the electrical response of the cell. The chemical messages sent by neuropeptides must be decoded by the target cell, often in terms of changes in its electrical properties. In this chapter the effects of neuropeptides on the electrical characteristics of their target cells are considered.

In contrast to the classical transmitters, which produce their membrane effects in milliseconds via changes in membrane conductances, neuropeptides, acting as modulators, may have no membrane effects on their own, or, acting as transmitters, they may produce long-lasting membrane effects: slow excitatory postsynaptic potentials (EPSPs) or inhibitory postsynaptic potentials (IPSPs). *Neuromodulation* may be defined as a change in the electrical properties of a cell, insufficient to evoke a propagated action potential (AP) in the absence of a neurotransmitter but sufficient to alter the response of a cell to the previously or subsequently applied neurotransmitter.

As neuropeptides form an extremely large class of communicating molecules, their effects on the excitability of their target cells is of considerable significance. What will become clear in this rather clouded topic is that the same neuropeptide may act at one site as a neurotransmitter, at another site as a neuromodulator, and at a third site as a neurohormone (figure 7.1). The response of the cell is critically dependent on other factors, such as additional neuronal hormonal inputs, its metabolic state, or the response may be conditional on the presence or absence of a different peptide (Mayer, 1994). Indeed, it is even more complex because the same neuropeptide may

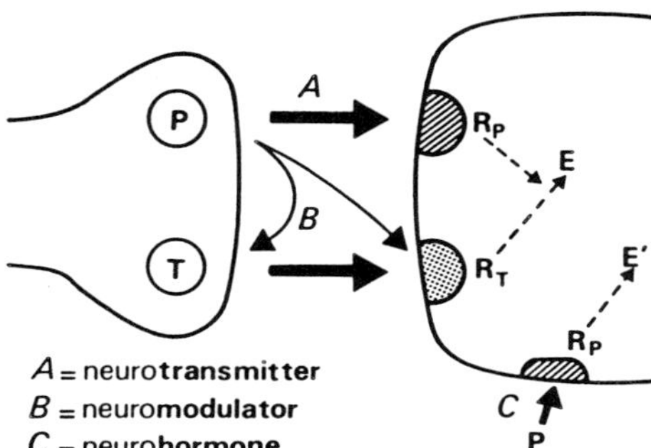

Figure 7.1
Three modes of action of neuropeptides. P, peptide; T, transmitter; R, receptor; E, effect. (From De Graan et al., 1990.)

stimulate one set of cells, inhibit another, and have no effect on a third. As these differences may be due not only to tissue and species-specificity but also to dosage, in vivo vs. in vitro studies, and other experimental variables, it will take time and patience to elucidate the many physiological roles played by the multitudinous neuropeptides.

7.1.1 Classical Neurotransmitters

The classic neurotransmitters include acetylcholine (ACh); the catecholamines epinephrine and norepinephrine (NE); [also known by their European nomenclature as adrenaline (A) and noradrenaline (NA)], and dopamine (DA); the indole amine serotonin or 5-hydroxytryptamine (5-HT), the excitatory amino acids glutamic and aspartic acid; and the inhibitory amino acids γ-aminobutyric acid (GABA) and glycine. Other nonpeptides that are being admitted to this select group as "putative" transmitters include histamine and nitric oxide but they do not fulfill all the properties once deemed necessary to define a neurotransmitter.

7.1.1.1 General Characteristics of Neurotransmitters

Many of these characteristics have been established for neurotransmitters in the peripheral nervous system; it is considerably more difficult to demonstrate them all in the CNS.

1. A neurotransmitter evokes a change in the membrane potential of the postsynaptic membrane of its target cell, either depolarizing (stimulating) or hyperpolarizing (inhibiting) the cell. This is a rapid change when the transmitter uses voltage-gated ion channels, and slower when second-messenger systems are involved.
2. The transmitter is localized mainly in the nerve terminals, preferentially in synaptic vesicles aggregated within the terminals.
3. The transmitter is selectively released by nerve stimulation, with the release being dependent on Ca^{2+} influx.
4. The transmitter reacts specifically with receptors on the postsynaptic or presynaptic membrane, or both. This response is prevented by specific pharmaceutical antagonists, and facilitated by specific agonists which mimic the action of the transmitter.
5. Application of the purified transmitter to the postsynaptic cell evokes the same response as transmitter released by nerve stimulation.
6. An inactivation mechanism (or mechanisms) is present to permit the postsynaptic membrane to return to its resting potential.
7. The structure of the transmitter is constant and consequently its biological activity does not vary with this parameter.

7.1.1.2 Mode of Action of Neurotransmitters

Neurotransmitters are fast-acting agents, opening ionic gates and causing an immediate flow of current through ion channels. The opening of a channel causes a rapid and brief conductance change. These are *ionotropic transmitters* acting through voltage-gated channels. ACh, acting at nicotinic receptors, is such a transmitter. Receptors for ionotropic transmitters may also produce a second messenger, for example, receptors for the excitatory amino acids glutamic or aspartic acid are linked to a Ca^{2+} channel, the NMDA receptor. When this channel opens, intracellular Ca^{2+} is increased and serves as a second-messenger to modulate Ca^{2+}-calmodulin processes.

Other transmitters may cause a slower, longer-lasting change, affecting membrane permeability indirectly through reactions involving second messengers and protein phosphorylation, processes discussed in chapter 6. As these transmitters affect cell metabolism, they are termed *metabotropic transmitters.* NE is an example of a metabotropic transmitter, as is ACh acting on muscarinic receptors.

7.1.1.3 Synthesis, Release, and Inactivation of Neurotransmitters

The classical neurotransmitters are synthesized in the nerve terminals, with the necessary enzymes being transported from the cell body to the terminals. Synthesis is rapid and pools of reserve transmitter may be found in the terminals so that there is little chance of transmitter depletion with prolonged nerve activity. The transmitters are stored in small, clear vesicles, often organized in three dimensions at active sites on the presynaptic membrane. The transmitters may be co-localized with neuropeptides in the same or different vesicles at the nerve terminals (figure 7.2). The release of the transmitter is sparked by Ca^{2+} influx initiated by the AP.

The transmitter binds to specific receptors on the postsynaptic or presynaptic membrane in a spatially focused manner, that is, from nerve terminal to post- or presynaptic membrane. Inactivation is through precise mechanisms which may include extracellular enzymatic inactivation, reuptake into the nerve terminals with subsequent repackaging, intracellular enzymatic inactivation.

7.1.2 Neuromodulators

Contributing to the complexity resulting from the infinite number of structural synaptic combinations, and the great variety of possible chemical transmitters in the CNS, is the delicate fine-tuning of synaptic and nonsynaptic processes by neuromodulators.

7.1.2.1 General Characteristics of Neuromodulators

1. Neuromodulators do not usually evoke an effect on their own but alter the effects of a classical transmitter at the synapse. In such cases they coexist with the classical transmitter in the nerve terminals.
2. They act more slowly and their effects are longer-lasting as they affect G protein–linked receptors and subsequent second messenger systems (see figure 7.2).
3. They are not restricted spatially to the synapse nor are they restricted to the duration of the postsynaptic AP.
4. Their release is dependent on the nerve AP but they may be secreted in a continuous or intermittent process. Neuromodulator release is often dependent on the duration, frequency, and pattern of stimulation.
5. They are effective in very low concentrations (picomolar to nanomolar), that is, they possess high potency.
6. Neuropeptide modulators may contain smaller transmitter substances within their structure such as glutamic acid, GABA, or aspartate. It is not known whether these small molecules are released and function as neurotransmitters.

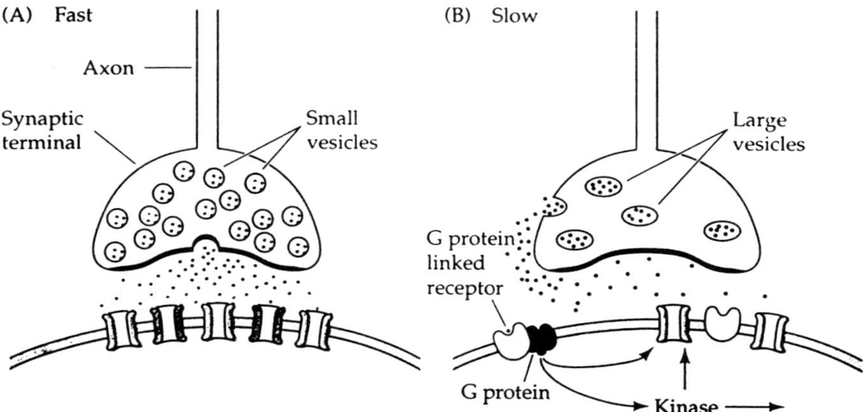

Figure 7.2
Presynaptic and postsynaptic pathways of fast and slow synaptic transmission. (A) Small molecule transmitters are rapidly released from small, clear vesicles at the active zone, act directly on postsynaptic ion channels, and are rapidly removed. (B) Neuropeptides are stored in large, dense-core vesicles, are released from nonspecialized sites, and act on G protein–linked receptors, which influence ion channels and other processes indirectly. At many synapses the two pathways coexist. (From Scheller and Hall, 1992.)

7. No specific inactivating mechanisms have been demonstrated.
8. Neuropeptides may alter their biological activity according to the form of the processed peptide, that is, somatostatin 28, somatostatin 14, and somatostatin 12 may differ considerably in their potencies.

7.1.2.2 Mode of Action of Neuromodulators

The mechanisms of such systems as they affect excitability and firing patterns differ markedly, and in many cases the details are vague or unknown. The possibilities are, however, infinite. Most neuropeptide neuromodulators act through second-messenger systems, utilizing G proteins. Changes in cAMP levels, Ca^{2+}, IP_3 or diacylglycerol will affect membrane permeability to ions and consequently the excitability of the postsynaptic membrane and thus the response of the cell to neurotransmitters. Neuromodulators may affect receptor number, affinity, accessibility, and cross-linking; the receptors may be postsynaptic, presynaptic, or autoreceptors. Neuromodulators may act presynaptically to increase (facilitate) or inhibit the release of another transmitter; or they may may act on presynaptic autoreceptors to facilitate or inhibit their own release.

7.1.2.3 Synthesis, Release, and Inactivation of Neuromodulators

Neuropeptide modulators are synthesized from large precursor molecules on the ribosomes, processed through the ribosomes and post-translationally modified in the Golgi apparatus or in vesicles (see chapter 3). Synthesis is slow and the neuropeptides must then reach the nerve terminals by axonal transport. These are time-consuming processes and neuropeptide stores are likely to be depleted with prolonged stimulation. The time needed for replenishment will be affected by the distance of the terminals from the cell body and the rate of axonal transport. Thus peptidergic neurotransmission may be influenced by events with latencies on the order of hours rather than milliseconds (Lundberg and Hökfelt, 1985).

Neuropeptides are stored in large, dense vesicles and may be colocalized with other neuropeptides or classical transmitters or both (see chapter 4). As with the neurotransmitters, neuropeptide release is Ca^{2+}-dependent, but there does not appear to be any organization of neuropeptide-containing vesicles at the presynaptic membrane prior to release. In fact, neuropeptide vesicles are not always confined to the nerve terminals but may be released at various axonal sites, including axonal varicosities, to diffuse and bind to receptors over a relatively wide region. Inactivating mechanisms include nonspecific proteases and peptidases.

7.2 Evidence for Selected Neuropeptides as Neurotransmitters or Neuromodulators

7.2.1 *Substance P (SP)*

SP was first proposed as an excitatory *neurotransmitter* by Otsuka and Konishi (1976) and this neuropeptide fulfills many of the criteria needed for a neurotransmitter. Referring to the criteria listed above,

1. SP has a marked excitatory effect on spinal motor neurons, and on neurons in sympathetic ganglia, producing slow, noncholinergic EPSPs.
2. SP is present in the terminals of the primary sensory neurons in the dorsal horn of the spinal cord. SP is also present in certain nerve terminals that form axodendritic synapses with spinal neurons in the substantia gelatinosa, and synaptic vesicles contain SP.
3. SP is released from the spinal cord in response to electrical stimulation of sensory nerves, or of preganglionic nerves to sympathetic ganglia, in a Ca^{2+}-dependent manner.
4. SP antagonists prevent the excitatory action of the peptide on spinal motor neurons and on neurons in the sympathetic ganglia. Depletion of SP by capsaicin abolishes the slow, noncholinergic EPSPs.
5. Synthetic SP applied to the isolated spinal cord exerts a powerful excitatory effect on spinal motor neurons, being 1000 to 10,000 times more powerful than the excitatory amino acid glutamate on a molar basis.
6. No specific inactivating mechanism has been demonstrated.

Sensory neurons are also susceptible to excitation by SP as seen by the large, reversible depolarization that brief spurts of SP evoke (figure 7.3). However, in addition to its role as a neurotransmitter, SP can act as a *neuromodulator*. In several sites in the nervous system, SP has no action on its own but modifies the action of ACh on the nicotinic ACh receptor. In sympathetic ganglia SP facilitates both nerve-stimulated EPSPs and the depolarization caused by local application of ACh. It may inhibit or facilitate nicotinic reponses. The neuromodulatory action may be quite specific: electrophoretically administered SP inhibits the ACh-evoked activation of spinal Renshaw cells but has no effect on the excitation of these cells by glutamate (figure 7.4).

7.2.2 *Luteinizing Hormone–Releasing Hormone (LHRH) or Gonadotropin-Releasing Hormone (GnRH)*

The more widely accepted terminology for the hypothalamic hormone that releases LH and FSH from the

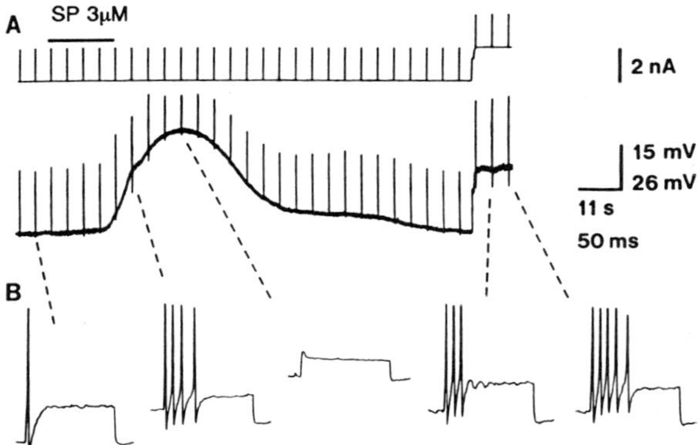

Figure 7.3
Dual effects of substance P (SP) on spike discharge of sensory neurons in the trigeminal root ganglia: excitatory and repetitive. (A) Short (7 seconds) application evoked a large, reversible depolarization. The resting potential was −58 mV in control conditions. Depolarizing steps (100 ms, 3 Hz) were used to elicit a spike before SP application. (B). Selected traces from A (dotted lines) are shown on a larger scale. Note the repetitive discharge during SP-induced depolarization and the absence of spikes during the peak response. Following recovery, repetitive discharge was observed from about the same membrane potential at which repetitive discharge occurred during SP depolarization. (From Spiegelman and Puil, 1991.)

anterior pituitary gland is gonadotropin-releasing hormone, or GnRH. Almost as widely accepted is luteinizing hormone–releasing hormone, or LHRH. However, LHRH does not indicate its role in releasing FSH so this text uses the GnRH nomenclature. There does not seem to be a universal FSH-releasing hormone (FSH-RH). However, as these classical experiments by Jan and Jan (1985) refer to this neuropeptide as LHRH, their terminology has been retained in the following description.

Using frog sympathetic ganglia as their model system, Jan and Jan, in a series of papers commencing in the early 1980s, were the first to demonstrate that an LHRH-like peptide (LHRH-lp) is a *neurotransmitter* at an excitatory synapse in the ganglion, and probably coexists with ACh in the same nerve terminals. They also showed that while both LHRH-lp and ACh are released on nerve stimulation at synapses within the sympathetic ganglia, LHRH-lp diffuses a greater distance than ACh and probably acts on cells distant from the synapse. Their work is clearly summarized in Jan and Jan (1985) and partly illustrated in figure 7.5.

LHRH-lp fulfills most of the criteria for a neurotransmitter. Again, referring to the criteria listed above,

1. LHRH-lp produces a late, slow EPSP, different in its time constants from the nicotinic and muscarinic potentials resulting from ACh release.
2. LHRH-lp is present in the preganglionic nerve terminals of the bullfrog sympathetic ganglia.
3. Stimulation of the preganglionic nerves releases LHRH-lp; section of the nerves depletes the ganglion of LHRH-lp.
4. The late slow EPSP is blocked by LHRH antagonists. These do not block the cholinergic potentials, indicating different receptors for LHRH and ACh.
5. The physiological effects of the late slow EPSP are mimicked by the application of synthetic LHRH in a medium devoid of Ca^{2+}, indicating that LHRH acts directly on sympathetic neurons.
6. Unlike the classical neurotransmitters, there does not seem to be an inactivating mechanism for LHRH-lp, apart from diffusion. Consequently it appears to have a fairly long lifetime (many seconds) after release, which probably accounts for the long duration of the late slow EPSP. In addition, late slow EPSPs can be recorded in cells distant from the LHRH-lp–containing nerve terminals, cells that are

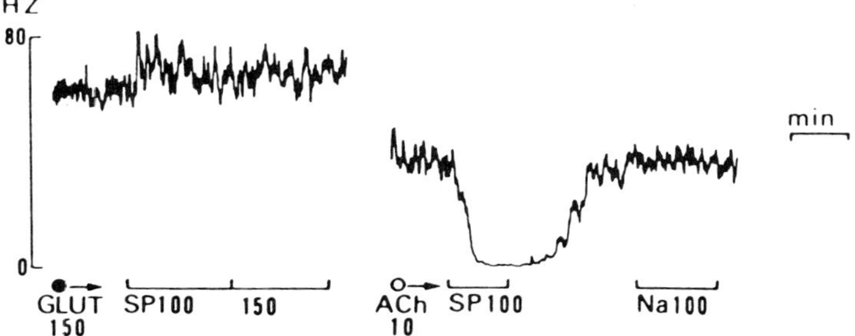

Figure 7.4
Microelectrophoretic administration of substance P (SP) to a Renshaw cell in the ventral horn of the spinal cord. SP had no effect on the excitation maintained by a continuous administration of glutamic acid (GLUT) but abolished the firing evoked by acetylcholine (ACh). A current control ejecting Na^+ had no effect. (From Ryall and Belcher, 1977.)

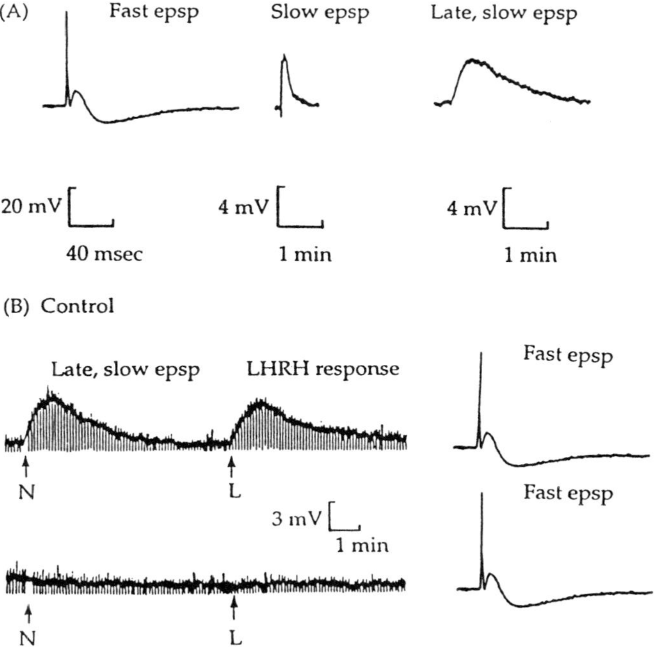

Figure 7.5
(A) In the frog sympathetic ganglia ACh mediates nicotinic fast EPSPs and muscarinic slow EPSPs. Late, slow EPSPs are mediated by a LHRH-like peptide, evoked by nerve stimulation. (B) Bath application of an LHRH antagonist completely blocks the late, slow EPSP (N) and the LHRH (L) response. The antagonist has no effect on the membrane potential, membrane, resistance, or the cholinergic fast EPSPs. (From Jan and Jan, 1982.)

not in synaptic contact with the peptide-containing nerve endings.

7.2.3 Oxytocin (OT) and Vasopressin (VP)

In addition to their endocrine effects, these two neuropeptides are involved in the regulation of several vital CNS functions, such as thermoregulation, cardiovascular regulation, and behaviors such as drinking, learning, maternal, sexual, and social behaviors. Complex neuronal pathways lead from the magnocellular nuclei to widely divergent neuronal networks. Extrahypophyseal pathways with OT or VP, or both, characterized in synaptic vesicles by immunoelectron microscopy, provide morphologic evidence for these hypophyseal neuropeptides as putative *neurotransmitters*. Electrophysiological studies support this concept. Although the electrical responses to OT and VP are somewhat species- and tissue-specific, there are certain dominant patterns that appear, chiefly excitatory, whether the investigations are in vivo or in vitro. Some examples are described below:

OT-containing neurons contact large preganglionic vagal neurons which can be impaled with micropipettes to study the effects of OT on their electrical properties. These brainstem vagal neurons are spontaneously active, firing at a rate of about five spikes per second. OT reversibly depolarizes them, causing a transient increase in their firing frequency, a postsynaptic effect (figure 7.6). This action is through OT receptors rather than V1 or V2 vasopressin receptors (Dreifuss et al., 1992).

Extracellularly, VP generally evokes excitatory responses that are blocked by V1 receptor antagonists. although neurons in some brain regions may be inhibited. The excitatory effect of iontophoretically applied VP in ventral hippocampal neurons is blocked by V1 receptor antagonists. Synaptic transmission is usually facilitated. In the forebrain and brainstem, VP effects are via a postsynaptic receptor; in the spinal cord and peripheral tissue, both presynaptic and postsynaptic receptors appear to be involved. These excitatory actions on CNS neurons are similar for both VP and OT, although the affinity of these peptides for the OT and VP receptors differs markedly (de Kloet et al., 1990).

7.2.4 Somatostatin (SS)

SS, an inhibitory neuropeptide widely distributed thoughout the central and peripheral nervous systems, is best known for its inhibitory action on GH secretion, but SS also inhibits the secretion of insulin, gastrin, glucagon, and TSH. The various somatostatin analogs have differerent potencies on different tissues and in addition, an intriguing example of the role of dosage and duration on neuropeptide effects can be demonstrated. Using small, intermediate, and large doses of SS, applied by pressure ejection to impaled cells, to investigate the responses of neurons in hippocampal slices, Sharfman (1993) showed that the most potent effect appears to be presynaptic. Small dosages of SS decrease the release of the inhibitory transmitter GABA, with which SS is co-localized. Intermediate dosages of SS may induce a combination of depolarization and hyperpolarization of the postsynaptic membrane, depending on the type of cell investigated and the duration of the SS application. Prolonged or repetitive SS exposure may activate second-messenger systems.

Another interesting complication in interpreting the role of SS on central neurons is that different effects are evoked when the neuropeptide is applied to the soma or to the dendritic regions of the cell. This type of painstaking investigation into the electrophysiological responses of single cells to neuro-

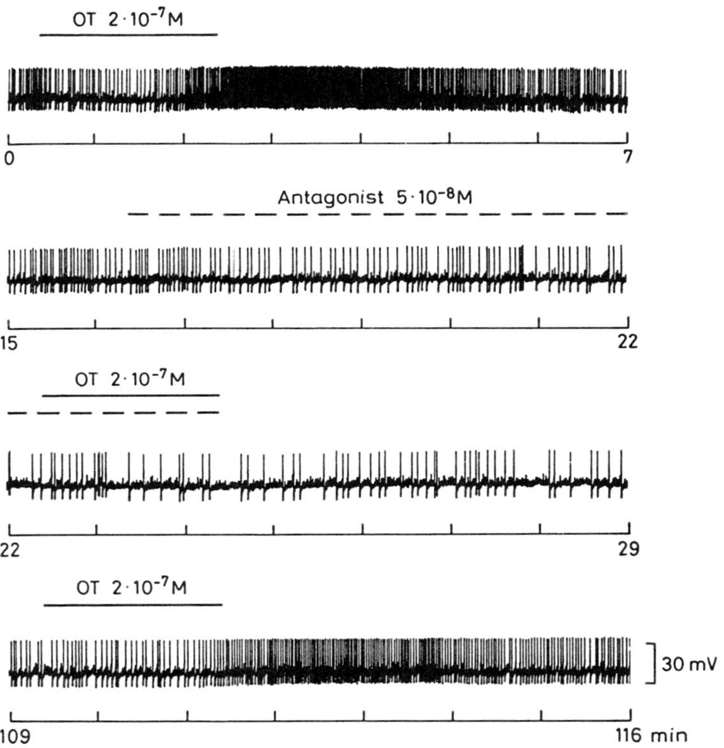

Figure 7.6
Effect of oxytocin on a rat motoneuron and its suppression by a potent antagonist. OT was added to the perfusion solution at 200 nm for the time indicated by the solid bar above each trace. Top trace shows that the OT-induced increase in neuronal excitability is suppressed by the antagonist (third trace); bottom trace shows that following washout of the antagonist, OT partially recovered its excitatory effect. (From Dreifuss et al., 1992.)

peptides is made more accurate by the use of tissue slices or of a monolayer preparation of cells, as illustrated in figure 7.7. In this figure, recording electrode pipettes impale two different neurons, while a third pipette dispenses the drug or neuropeptide under study. When SS is applied in intermediate dosages to the soma of hippocampal pyramidal cells, small depolarizations that could produce AP discharge are briefly evoked by SS 14. When applied to dendritic regions, SS 14 produces depolarizations similar to those seen after somatic applications or hyperpolarizations (figure 7.8). Scharfman and Schwarzkroin, (1988) suggest that the hyperpolarizations are due to excitation of inhibitory neurons that synapse upon the impaled pyramidal cell. Of course, in the intact brain, all these geometric and dosage effects come into play. Most of the electrophysiological evidence indicates that SS acts as a *neurotransmitter* in the CNS.

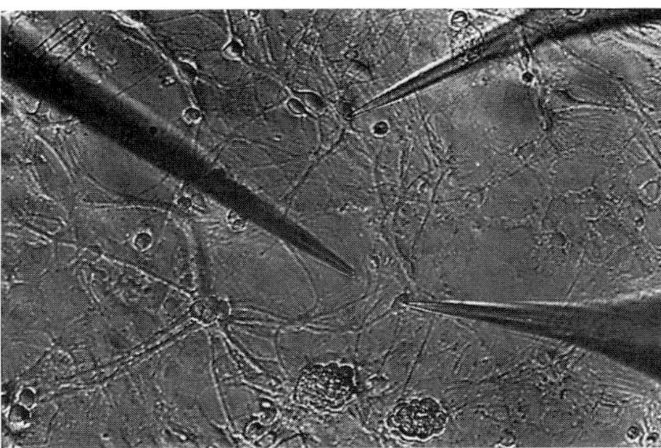

Figure 7.7
Recording from individual neurons is facilitated by monolayer culture. Phase contrast microscopy of cultured rat hippocampal neurons shows two cells under simultaneous recording. The two pipette images at the right are patch pipettes, recording intracellularly from whole cells. The pipette at the left is used to apply specific agents close to the cells under study. (From Barker et al., 1987.)

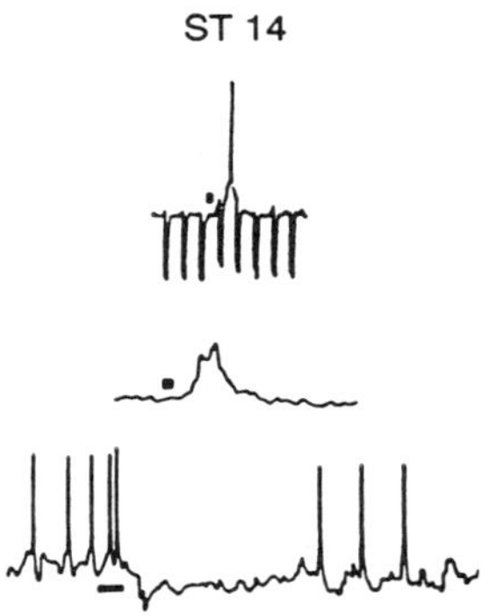

Figure 7.8
Effects of brief pressure applications of somatostatin (ST) on pyramidal neurons in hippocampal slices. (Top) Response of a pyramidal cell as recorded by intracellular electrodes to ejections of ST 14 (1 μM) into the *soma*. Modest depolarizations occur (down deflections) that) sometimes produced an action potential. Middle and lower traces, After ejection of ST 14 on dendrites, pyramidal cells responded with hyperpolarizations or depolarizations. Each trace is from a different neuron. Somatostatin was applied for the duration of the horizontal bar. (From Scharfman, 1993.)

7.2.5 Thyrotropin-Releasing Hormone (TRH)

TRH, in addition to its stimulatory effect on the secretion of TSH and other pituitary hormones, has widespread effects in the CNS. It increases the excitability of motor neurons in the spinal cord. It antagonizes the pharmacological action of barbiturates, including barbiturate depression of respiration. In tissue slice studies, TRH noticeably modulates the discharge pattern of respiratory neurons in the brain stem. Figure 7.9 shows that these neurons fire in an unpatterned way prior to the application of TRH. During exposure to TRH the neurons fire in bursts. Prolonged exposure to TRH evokes a depolarizing afterpotential and bursting firing in the same neuron. These effects indicate both *neurotransmitter* and *neuromodulator* roles for this 3–amino acid peptide.

7.2.6 Vasoactive Intestinal Polypeptide (VIP)

VIP has been shown to excite cells in the CNS and coexists with ACh in both central and peripheral cholinergic synapses. VIP *modulates* cholinergic transmission by a postsynaptic mechanism. Exogenously applied VIP to the intestine converts the subthreshold EPSPs of these cells to propagated APs. In the peripheral nervous system, using the frog neuromuscular junction as a model, Gold (1984) demonstrated that VIP acts as a modulator at this synapse, facilitating neuromuscular transmission while having no direct postsynaptic effect. VIP does not affect miniature endplate potential (MEPP) frequency but increases both the evoked and spontaneous release of ACh.

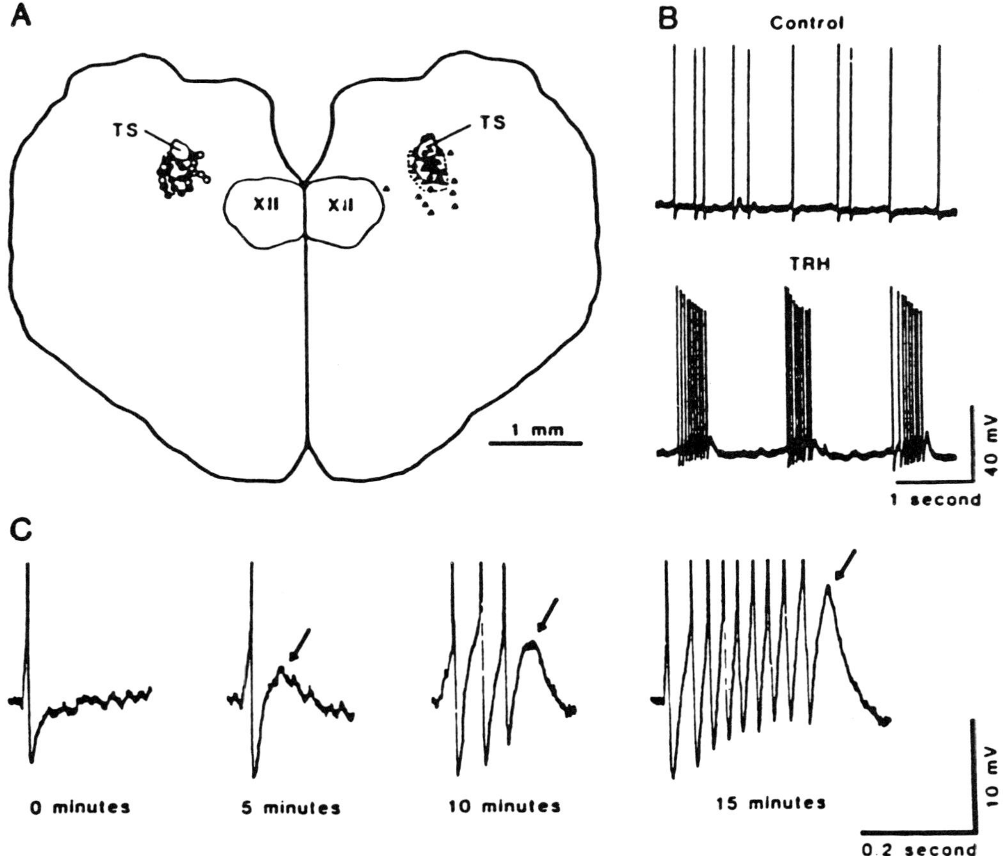

Figure 7.9
Modulation by thyrotropin-releasing hormone (TRH) of discharge pattern of neurons in the nucleus tractus solitarius (TS). (A) diagram of the cross section of the brain stem. The right side depicts a map of the dorsal respiratory group near the TS. Triangles show the distribution of identified respiratory neurons. The left side indicates locations of neurons studied in a slice preparation of the TS; closed circles are cells that responded to TRH; open circles show loci of unresponsive cells. (B) Effect of TRH on neuron firing. Unpatterned activity occurred prior to TRH (control), while phasic bursting was observed during exposure to TRH. (C) A depolarizing afterpotential and bursting in the same neuron was observed during exposure to TRH. (From Dekin et al., 1985.)

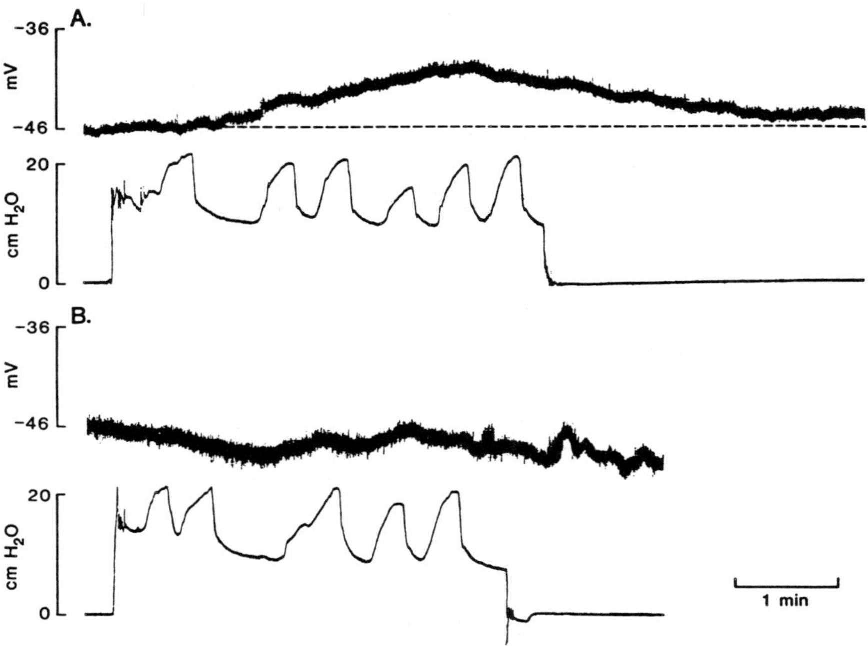

Figure 7.10
(A) Distention of the colon (lower-trace) results in the release of vasoactive intestinal polypeptide (VIP) and the consequent formation of slow, noncholinergic excitatory action potentials, 7 mV in amplitude (upper trace). (B) When VIP antiserum is present, the slow depolarization caused by colonic distention is blocked. Both adrenergic and cholinergic blocking agents were in the bathing solution. Recordings were made from the same neuron. (From Love et al., 1988.)

In the gut VIP acts as a *neurotransmitter*, released from lumbar colonic nerves to evoke slow EPSPs. VIP is the most important neuropeptide with widespread relaxant activity, able to cause relaxation of gastric and intestinal smooth muscle, and of the several sphincters of the gastrointestinal tract (figure 7.10). VIP and its homologs (peptide histidine isoleucine, glucagon and secretin) cause relaxation of these muscle cells via high-affinity VIP receptors and G_s proteins.

Again, in the male and female reproductive systems, VIP may act as a *neurotransmitter*. VIP is present in the male and female genital tracts of all species examined. In both sexes, VIP seems to fulfill some important neurotransmitter criteria (Fahrenkrug et al., 1988): there is dense VIP innervation of the blood vessels and smooth musculature of the vagina and clitoris, the cavernous smooth muscle and blood vessels of the penis, and VIP is stored and released from large spherical dense-core vesicles in the nerve terminals. VIP is released during sexual excitement when the blood flow to these organs is increased due to vasodilation. This relaxation of the vascular smooth muscle is atropine-resistant, that is, noncholinergic.

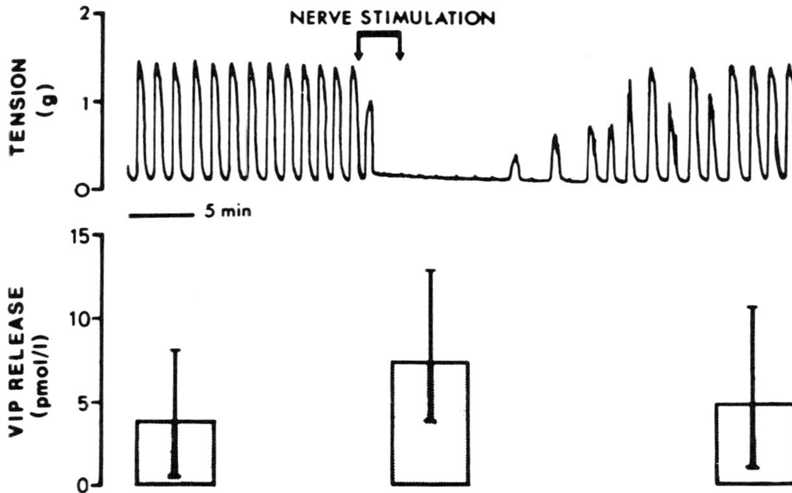

Figure 7.11
Isometric tension recordings from feline myometrial strips in vitro. (Upper trace) The spontaneous contractions of myometrial preparations are abolished by transmural nerve stimulation in the presence of α- and β-adrenoceptor blocking agents, and atropine. (Lower trace) A significant release of vasoactive intestinal polypeptide (VIP) from myometrial nerves accompanied the smooth muscle relaxation. (From Fahrenkrug et al., 1988.)

Similarly, a noncholinergic, nonadrenergic release of VIP is induced by electrical stimulation of the sympathetic nerve to the uterus; VIP released from these nerve terminals causes relaxation of the myometrium (figure 7.11).

7.2.7 *Neuropeptide Y (NPY)*

NPY is widely distributed throughout the peripheral and central nervous systems and modulates neurotransmitter release in a highly selective manner. It is generally co-localized with other transmitters, particularly NE. NPY produces both presynaptic and postsynaptic effects. *Presynaptically*, NPY inhibits the release of classical neurotransmitters such as NE from sympathetic and ACh from parasympathetic neurons through Y_2 receptors. NPY is a powerful inhibitor of SP and ACh release from dorsal root ganglion neurons in culture. The ability of NPY to block neurotransmitter release depends on how strongly the presynaptic neuron is stimulated, and the inhibitory effects of NPY can be overcome by more rapid or longer stimulation (Colmers and Bleakman, 1994). *Postsynaptically*, acting through the Y_1 receptor and in high (micromolar) concentrations, NPY may act directly to evoke a long-lasting constrictor action in vascular beds, but in low nanomolar concentrations it potentiates the action of other vasoconstrictors such as NE or histamine. These effects are illustrated diagramatically in figure 7.12.

7.2.8 *Neurotensin (NT)*

NT was first discovered by Susan Leeman who noticed its ability to cause conspicuous vasodilation. Further studies showed that NT causes contraction of

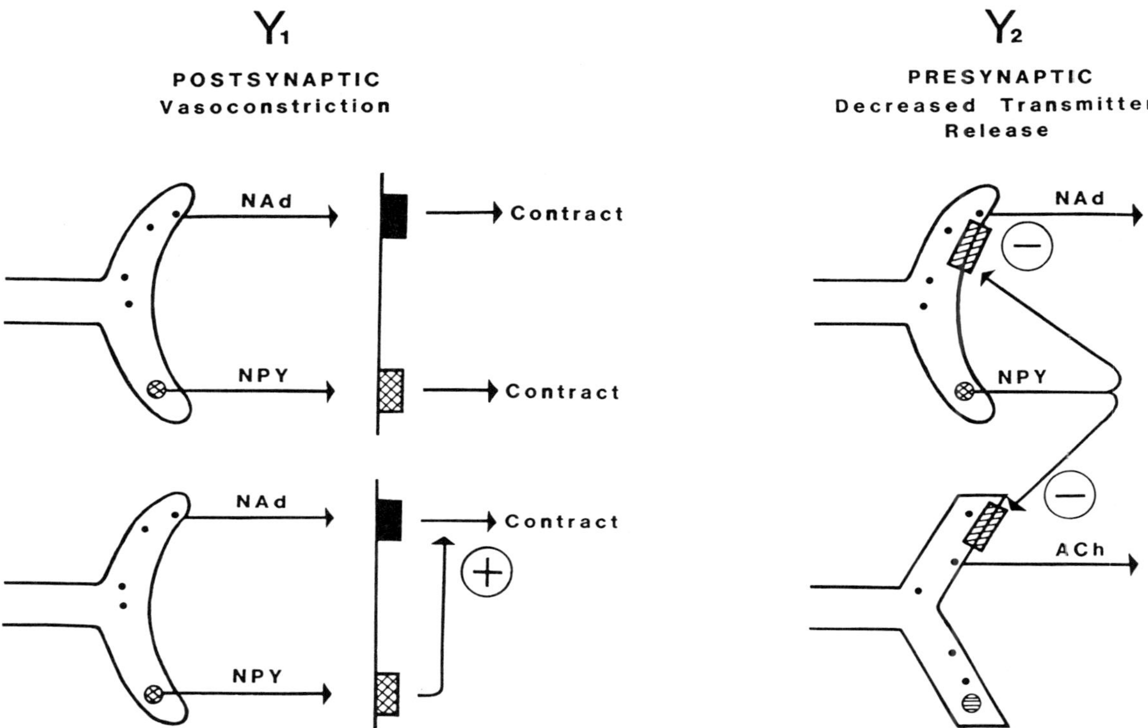

Figure 7.12
Schematic diagram summarizing the actions of neuropeptide Y (NPY) in the autonomic nervous system. (Left top) NPY causes a long-lasting vasoconstriction in some blood vessels mediated by *postsynaptic* Y_1 *receptors*. (Left, bottom) NPY also potentiates the constrictor action of noradrenaline (NAd), also a postsynaptic action. *Presynaptic actions, using* Y_2 *receptors*, are shown at right. In the top trace, NPY inhibits the release of NAd from sympathetic nerves. In the bottom diagram, acetylcholine (ACh) release from parasympathetic nerves is inhibited. Noradrenaline is also norepinephrine. d, direct action. (From Potter and Ulman, 1994.)

intestinal smooth muscle (Carraway and Leeman, 1973) apparently by stimulating the release of ACh from cholinergic nerves and SP from enteric nerves, a *neuromodulatory* effect. Both ACh and SP act as excitatory transmitters in the intestinal tract. However, NT induces a strong relaxation of guinea pig colon, acting directly, that is, as a *neurotransmitter* on high-affinity receptors on smooth muscle cells of the colon. These confusing results appear to be due to a bifunctional effect of NT: it has both a direct relaxant and indirect contractile action (Kitagabi, 1982).

NT also *modulates* the excitation induced by glutamate. In spinal dorsal horn neurons NT decreases glutamate-induced excitation, whereas in the hypothalamus NT potentiates glutamate-induced excitation. In the midbrain NT attenuates DA-induced inhibition, but does not affect glutamate-induced excitation in the same cells. In most other areas studied, NT acts as a *neurotransmitter* causing excitation of the postsynaptic cell (Shi and Bunney, 1992).

7.2.9 *Angiotensin (AT)*

AT II is a powerful vasoconstrictor and cardiac stimulant produced by enzymatic cleavage from a larger precursor AT I, which in turn is the product of the kidney enzyme renin acting on a plasma protein, angiotensinogen (see chapter 18). AT II acts via AT_1 receptors *presynaptically* to *modulate* (increase) NE release from sympathetic nerve terminals and to facilitate *postsynaptic* responses to NE. The several mechanisms by which AT II may increase NE release and effectiveness are illustrated in figure 7.13. AT II also acts directly as a *neurotransmitter* on AT_1 receptors on smooth muscle to cause vasoconstriction (Renaud and Bourque, 1991). It is possible that AT II may also act directly via AT_1 receptors to facilitate the firing of neurons in certain circumventricular organs, with

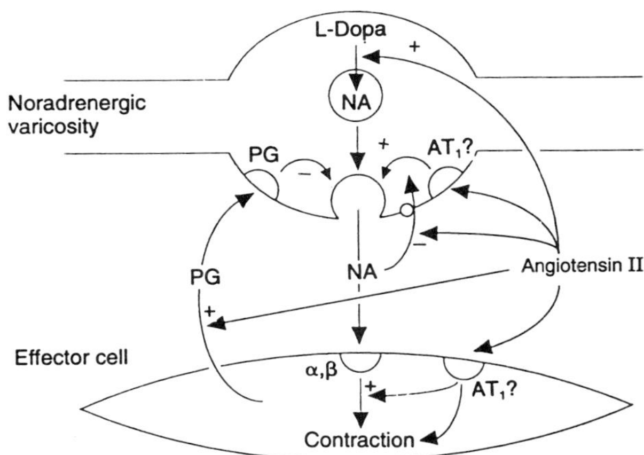

Figure 7.13
The interaction of angiotensin II (AT II) with noradrenergic (NA) neurotransmission. AT II acts directly on smooth muscle to produce contraction, probably through angiotensin I (AT_1) receptors. It also enhances NA transmission by (1) activation of prejunctional receptors on sympathetic nerve terminals to increase NA release; (2) inhibition of NA uptake by nerve terminals; (3) stimulation of NA synthesis from L-dopa; and (4) increasing effector cell responsiveness to NA. Prostaglandins (PG) may act presynaptically to oppose the AT II–mediated NA release. PG release, in turn, is stimulated by AT II. (From Reid et al., 1995.)

consequent changes in drinking behavior, blood pressure, and the release of VP (Renaud and Hu, 1995).

7.2.10 *Melanocortins*

The melanocortins have a *neuromodulating* effect on peripheral and central neurotransmission. In experiments investigating the ameliorative effects of the noncorticotropic fragment ACTH 4–10 on neuromuscular function in hypophysectomized rats, Gonzalez and Strand (1981) showed that this peptide increases MEPP frequency, a presynaptic parameter, while leaving postsynaptic characteristics unchanged.

Similar results were obtained by Johnston et al. (1983) on the frog neuromuscular junction. ACTH 1–39 and several of the smaller melanocortins, including α-MSH, increase endplate amplitude and MEPP frequency, presynaptic events that last several hours. In these experiments, however, ACTH 4–10 was ineffective, a discrepancy that may be attributed to the difference in species.

ACTH, ACTH 4–10, and α- and β-MSH improve neuromuscular efficiency by acting on the presynaptic elements of the neuromuscular junction, presumably by increasing the release of ACh. These potentiating effects are seen only in the developing neuromuscular system of the neonatal animal (figure 7.14), during nerve regeneration, or in the physiologically depressed neuromuscular system of the hypophysectomized rat, emphasizing the concept that neuropeptides may be circumscribed in their action by the physiological or developmental state of the organism (Strand et al., 1993). Similarly, melanocortin peptides modulate cardiac excitability, contractility, and sensitivity to NE, presumably by increasing NE uptake into cardiac sympathetic nerves and increasing Ca^{2+} influx (Zeiler et al., 1982; Strand and Smith, 1986).

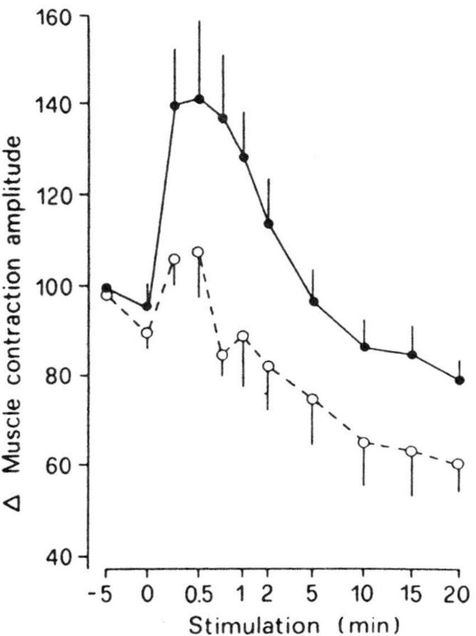

Figure 7.14
Effect of ACTH 4–10 (0.1 μg/kg intraperitoneally) on the contraction amplitude of the extensor digitorum longus muscle of the young rat (9 to 15 days old). Closed circles, peptide-treated animals; open circles, saline-treated controls. (From Smith and Strand, 1981.)

Central effects of the melanocortins indicate that, in general, they act as *neuromodulators*. Krivoy and Zimmermann (1977) showed that β-MSH modulates synaptic transmission in the cat spinal cord, increasing the excitability of neurons in the monosynaptic reflex, without causing spontaneous discharge of α-motor neurons. ACTH and MSH peptides affect several neurotransmitter systems, including cholinergic, dopaminergic, noradrenergic, and serotinergic synthesis and turnover. In the brain, ACTH 1–24 and α-MSH have a modulating effect on dopamine D_2 receptors as shown by their ability to antagonize the stimulus-evoked release of DA and ACh from caudate nucleus slices. These effects are reviewed by De Graan et al. (1990).

Studies of brain wave activity in freely moving, conscious rats administered injections of ACTH or MSH show waves of high-amplitude, slow (4 to 9 Hz) activity (Sandman et al., 1971). In humans, certain aspects of brain wave activity, as measured by computer analysis of the electroencephalogram (EEG) and a more sophisticated technique, the electroretinogram (ERP), which is a temporally structured response of the brain to peripheral sensory stimulation, are affected by ACTH compounds (Beckwith and Sandman, 1982). Although many investigations point to an excitatory effect of melanocortins on EEG parameters, the results vary considerably with the paradigm involved. A detailed description of the complex effects is available in a review by Sandman and Kastin (1987).

7.2.11 Opiates

The three main opiate receptor subtypes, μ, γ, κ, all appear to act as *neuromodulators*, inhibiting the release of many neurotransmitters, including epinephrine, DA, ACh, and SP. The electrophysiological correlates of these presynaptic actions can be investigated by application of the peptide from micropipettes to the target cell while recording from it. The specificity of the response is usually ascertained by administering an opiate antagonist, such as naloxone, which should decrease or eliminate the opiate-induced effect.

In the spinal cord, the effect of enkephalins and morphine is almost always inhibitory, although there are dissimilarities in their effects on different structures. These discrepancies are probably due to different receptor populations. In the upper dorsal horn, enkephalinergic terminals make axodendritic and axosomatic synapses, suggesting that the enkephalins act postsynaptically at these sites (figure 7.15). As the enkephalins are localized in vesicles in nerve terminals and released by depolarization in a Ca^{2+}-dependent manner, enkephalin is probably acting as a *neurotransmitter.* The opiates are discussed in detail in chapter 14.

However, in the retina and olfactory bulb, structures closely associated with sensory processing, enkephalins increase the firing of output neurons. In the hippocampus, enkephalins produce epileptiform elec-

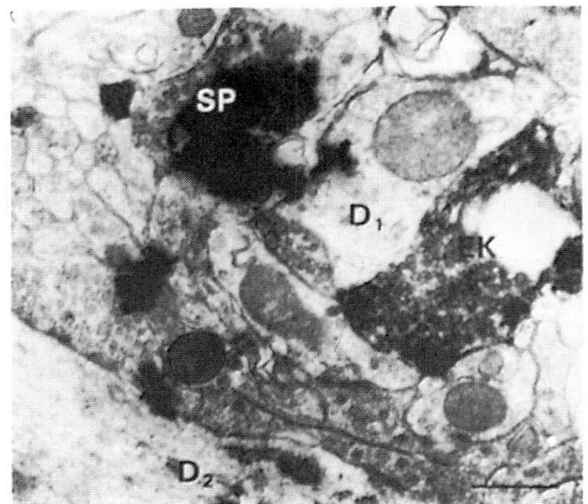

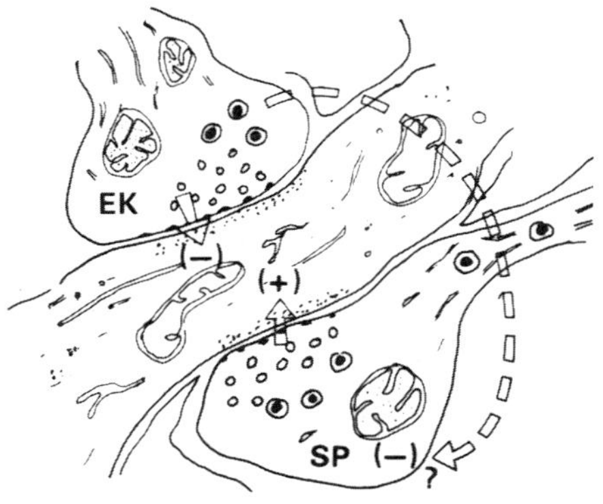

Figure 7.15
Substance P (SP)–containing nerve terminals establish axodendritic synapses in the spinal nucleus of the trigeminal nucleus, demonstrated by radioimmunocytochemistry with internally radiolabeled antibodies. The axons synapse with dendrites (D) of local circuit neurons and of spinothalamic neurons. This is probably an excitatory (+) synapse. Enkephalin-immunoreactive terminals (EK) do not usually synapse with SP fibers but terminate on common dendrites, acting as an inhibitory synapse. Since opiates inhibit release of SP from the trigeminal nucleus and opioid receptors are present in primary sensory fibers, "non-synaptic" interactions (arrows) probably account for the inhibition of SP release by EK. (From Cuello, 1983.)

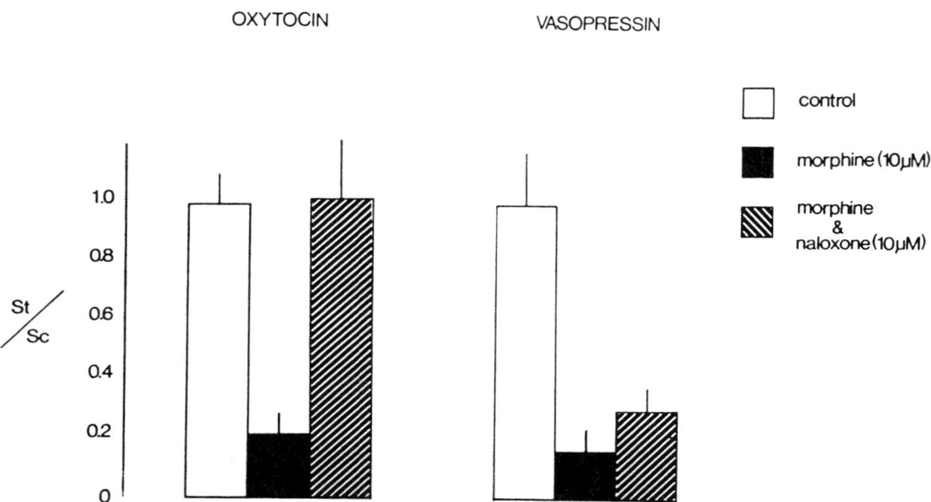

Figure 7.16
Effect of morphine (10 μM) on electrically evoked release of vasopressin (VP) and oxytocin (OT) from the rat intermediate lobe in vitro. Morphine suppresses the release of both VP and OT, but only OT inhibition was reversed by naloxone. (From Clarke and Merrick, 1985.)

trical activity, similar to seizures. This does not appear to be due to the release of an excitatory transmitter but rather to disinhibition, the inhibition of tonically active, adjacent inhibitory interneurons, probably through the suppression of GABA release. The mossy fibers of the hippocampus contain glutamate as well as the opiate peptides enkephalin and dynorphin. These peptides are released only by high-frequency stimulation, consistent with evidence from the peripheral nervous system that high-frequency stimulation is needed for the secretion of peptide cotransmitters (see chapter 4). It is likely that the extended duration of peptide effects contributes to the length of long-term potentiation involved in learning and memory (Morris and Johnston, 1995).

Morphine acts presynaptically on primary afferents, reducing the probability that the terminal will be invaded by an incoming impulse, and thereby induce the release of transmitter. The *neuromodulatory* action of morphine is well illustrated by its ability to inhibit the release of OT and VP from the nerve terminals of the neural lobe of the pituitary gland, a finding that is strongly supported by in vitro experiments (figure 7.16). Naloxone reverses the inhibition of OT release, but inexplicably does not affect the suppression of VP (Clarke and Merrick, 1985). In summary, the action of the opiates on EPSPs or IPSPs in different areas of the brain is primarily inhibitory (Olson et al., 1994, 1995).

7.3 Summary

Neuropeptides may act as neurohormones, neurotransmitters, or neuromodulators. Classical neurotransmitters include ACh, epinephrine, NE, DA,

5-HT, glutamic and aspartic acid, and GABA. Histamine and NO are "putative" transmitters. The characteristics of neurotransmitters include a change in the membrane potential of the postsynaptic cell; release from synaptic vesicles in nerve terminals after nerve stimulation; a Ca^{2+}-dependent response; specific binding to pre- or postsynaptic membrane receptors; the existence of an inactivating mechanism(s). Application of the purified transmitter to the postsynaptic cell evokes the physiological response, which can be blocked by antagonists. Ionotropic neurotransmitters act rapidly, through voltage-gated channels. Metabotropic transmitters act more slowly, through second messengers. Synthesis of transmitters is rapid in the nerve terminals, so depletion of transmitter is unlikely. They are stored in small, clear vesicles in the nerve terminals.

Neuromodulators do not evoke an effect on their own but alter the effects of a classical transmitter at the synapse. Their action is slow and long-lasting as they act through second messengers. They are released in response to an AP but their release requires a longer duration and higher frequency of stimulation. They are effective in very low concentrations but their biological activity may vary according to the length of the processed peptide. There are no specific inactivating mechanisms. Changes in second messengers affect membrane permeability to ions and thus can change the excitability of the postsynaptic membrane to transmitters. Neuromodulators may also affect receptor characteristics, whether the receptors are pre- or postsynaptic, or autoreceptors, and thus can inhibit or facilitate the release of other colocalized transmitters or neuropeptides, or even their own release. Neuropeptides are stored in large, dense vesicles which are not always limited to nerve terminals so that their action may be widespread.

There is convincing evidence for SP and GnRH (LHRH) as neurotransmitters. VP and OT appear to act as excitatory transmitters in the CNS, but also as neuromodulators. Somatostatin may act as either an excitatory or inhibitory transmitter, depending on dosage, type of cell investigated, and the duration of application. TRH has both neurotransmitter and neuromodulator actions. VIP appears to be restricted to neuromodulation at cholinergic synapses, but in the gut and reproductive tract VIP acts as a neurotransmitter. NPY is a neuromodulator, inhibiting the release of NE and ACh and SP in the intestinal tract, except for the colon where it appears to act as a transmitter. In certain areas of the CNS, NT modulates excitation evoked by glutamate and DA-induced inhibition, whereas in other brain regions NT acts as a neurotransmitter. AT II is a neuromodulator at sympathetic nerve endings, presynaptically increasing NE release, but acts directly as a neurotransmitter on AT_1 receptors on smooth muscle to cause vasoconstriction.

The melanocortins are neuromodulators in the central and peripheral nervous systems, generally increasing excitability. They modulate cardiac excitability, contractility, and sensitivity to NE, presumably by increasing NE uptake into cardiac sympathetic nerves and increasing Ca^{2+} influx. Opiates all appear to act as neuromodulators, inhibiting the release of many neurotransmitters, including epinephrine, DA, ACh, and SP. Their effects in the spinal cord are always inhibitory but in many brain regions opiates increase the firing of neurons, probably through disinhibition of tonically active inhibitory interneurons. Enkephalins in the spinal cord probably act as transmitters; again, their action is primarily inhibitory.

Chapter 8, the last chapter in part I, deals with the complex interactions between the neuroendocrine and immune systems, and their involvement in the response of the organism to stress. Just as the nervous and endocrine systems have been shown to be interdependent, the immune system now appears to be part of a triumvirate that regulates physiological responses to internal and external stressors, including bacteria, viruses, tumors, and foreign tissues.

Neuropeptides, Stress, and the Immune System

8

8.1 Integration of the Neuroendocrine and Immune Systems

Several important recent developments have clearly shown that the neuroendocrine and immune systems are closely coordinated and mutually regulated. These developments include techniques that can detect minute amounts of neuropeptides, the discovery that the immune system contains receptors for neuropeptide hormones, and that leukocytes synthesize pituitary and hypothalamic hormones. The immune-derived neuropeptides appear to be biologically active and they, as well as neuropeptides of pituitary and hypothalamic origin, may function as endogenous regulators of the immune system. In addition, activated immune cells produce blood-borne proteins, the cytokines, that bring information concerning foreign bodies, bacteria, viruses, tumors, and toxins to the neuroendocrine system, information that cannot be detected by the nervous system. This information is essential to the coordination of the requisite behavioral, endocrine, and metabolic changes necessary to restore homeostasis following antigen challenge. This information activates the hypothalamic-pituitary-adrenal (HPA) axis, so that exposure to antigens provokes a correlated response of the neuroendocrine system, chiefly through the increased secretion of corticotropin-releasing hormone (CRH), ACTH, and adrenocorticosteroids. These hormones affect metabolism and modulate the immune response. Their interactions are closely involved in adaptive responses to psychobiological states, such as sleep, appetite, libido, and mood (Ader et al., 1991). In turn, abnormalities in the neuroendocrine system are implicated in diseases involving immune system dysfunction, such as the autoimmune diseases. These interactions are considered in this chapter.

The disadvantage of this active new discipline is the assortment of cumbersome names it has attracted, such as neuroimmunoendocrinology, neuroendocrinimmunology, psychoneuroendocrinology, and psychoneuroimmunology.

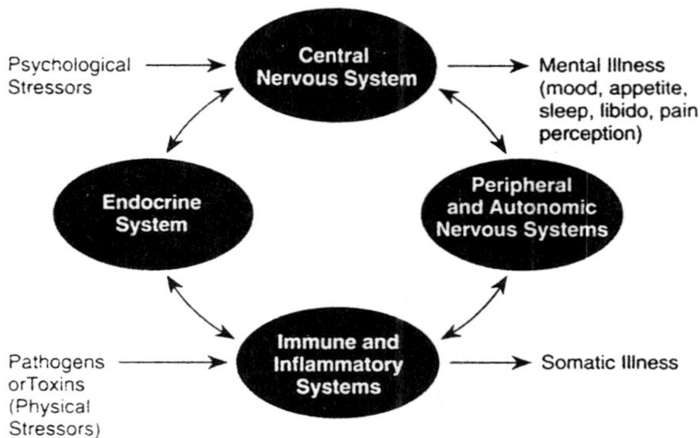

Figure 8.1
Neuroendocrine-immune interactions illustrating the interdependence of the CNS and peripheral and autonomic nervous systems, the endocrine system, and the immune and inflammatory systems. (From Wilder, 1995.)

8.2 Stress and the Hypothalamus

Stress may somewhat ambiguously be defined as a condition in which homeostasis, or the steady state of the internal milieu, is disturbed by a harmful internal or external stimulus. Successful adaptation to stress involves most of the regulatory systems of the organism acting to restore homeostasis to the endangered individual. Thus the response to stress incorporates the cerebral cortex, the autonomic nervous system, the neuroendocrine system, and the immune system (figure 8.1). Hans Selye (1936) realized that a wide variety of noxious stimuli evoked the release of ACTH and corticosteroids in a uniform response he called the *alarm reaction*. This is accompanied by an involution of the thymus and other lymphoid organs and suppression of the immune response; a shift in energy balance from storage in the liver and adipose tissue to readily available energy substrates in the circulation; and the inhibition of costly anabolic processes such as growth and tissue repair, and reproductive functions (Munck et al., 1984). If the stress becomes chronic, however, the depletion of energy stores and the prolonged suppression of reproduction may lead to a wide variety of disruptions of normal physiological processes, including increased anxiety, hypertension, gastrointestinal disorders, muscle weakness, anorexia, impotence, and immunosuppression.

The role of the *cerebral cortex* in emotional stress was first shown by Sherrington (1906) in decorticate animals. Lacking a cerebral cortex, these animals respond to a pleasant stimulus with all the evidence of rage; this is called *sham rage* and only occurs if the hypothalamus has not been destroyed along with the cerebral hemispheres. The normal behavioral response to stress is distinguished by increased arousal and alertness and suppression of sexual and feeding behaviors. The cerebral cortex probably acts as a constant neural inhibitor of the emotional expression of the hypothalamus, acting through the associative cortex. Other brain regions that activate the stress systems include the amygdala, the hippocampus, and the mesocorticolimbic or reward system. In humans, the highly developed cognitive functions of the cerebral cortex result in the increasing importance of psychological stress in the adaptive and nonadaptive defense mechanisms of the integrated stress system.

The hypothalamic area also contains regions that control the sympathetic and parasympathetic nervous systems; stress activates the sympathetic system as seen by increased heart rate and blood pressure, increase in rate and depth of respiration, and dilation of the pupils. Stress activates the neuroendocrine nuclei of the hypothalamus, resulting in the release of CRH and VP, which not only cause the release of ACTH but can also act directly on blood vessels and the kidney to increase blood pressure by vasoconstriction and retention of water. Both the sympathetic and parasympathetic nervous systems, in addition to secreting epinephrine, NE, E and ACh, secrete a variety of neuropeptides, including NPY, somatostatin, enkephalin, neurotensin and galanin (see section 4.2.1 in chapter 4), as well as NO. The neurotransmitter 5-HT, also plays an important role in the function of the stress system. Add to this the action of the cytokines, released from cells of the immune system after exposure to bacteria, viruses, or toxins, and it is apparent that an enormous complex of interactive, mutually regulating loops exists to maintain homeostasis despite insults from the external or internal environment. The HPA axis is the coordinator of stress responses, translating neural, endocrine, and cytokine information into physiological responses. Figures 8.2 and 8.3 depict some of the complex interactions of the central (catecholinergic neurons in the brain stem and CRH neurons in the hypothalamus and brain stem) and peripheral (sympathoneural, sympathoadrenal, and the pituitary-adrenal axis) components of the stress system. Table 8.1 lists the behavioral and physical adaptations that occur in stressed animals (Chrousos and Gold, 1992)

8.2.1 Neuroendocrine Aspects of Stress

The neuroendocrine aspects of stress are coordinated through the sequential stimulation of hypothalamic CRH, which, together with the synergistic action of VP, causes the secretion of pituitary ACTH, MSH, and the endorphins. Responding to ACTH stimulation, the adrenal cortex secretes glucocorticoids which have a major role in suppressing immune functions, including production of cytokines by T cells and antibodies by B cells (see section 8.3). High levels of circulating glucocorticoids exert a negative feedback control on both the hypothalamus and anterior pituitary, terminating the secretion of CRH and ACTH, and consequently the stress response (Munck and Holbrook, 1984; Sapolsky et al., 1984). These feedback mechanisms are discussed in detail in chapter 10. Glucocorticoids do not protect against the source of stress itself but rather against the body's normal reaction to stress. More recently, it has been suggested that glucocorticoids increase resistence to stress through dual reactions involving integrated enhancing or permissive actions, as well as suppressive effects (DeRijk and Berkenbosch, 1994; Munck and Náray-Fejes-Tóth, 1994).

There is also a close connection between stress and *pain suppression*. β-Endorphin is usually released in equimolar quantities with ACTH as a result of their simultaneous processing from POMC. Teleologically, it may be considered that the secretion of the analgesic endorphins during stress permits the stressed animal or human to be oblivious to the pain of trauma

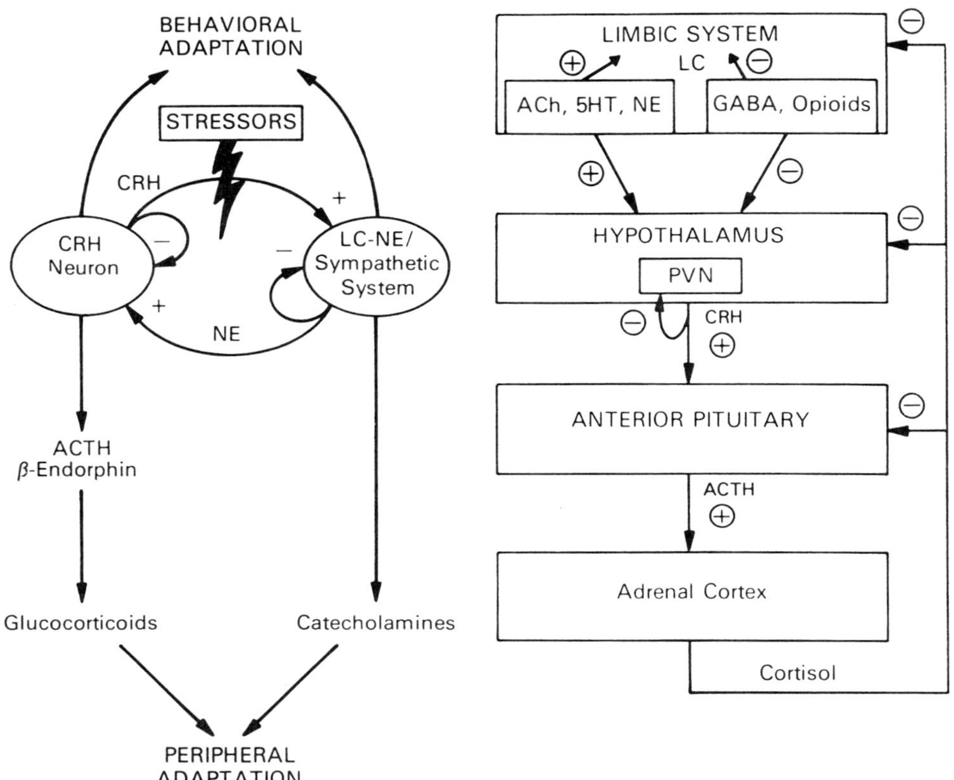

Figure 8.2
The stress system and neurotransmitter as well as neurohormonal control mechanisms modulating corticotropin-releasing hormone (CRH) secretion. (Left) CRH neurons stimulate both pituitary ACTH secretion and the central autonomic arousal system (locus ceruleus-norepinephrine [LC-NE] system), leading, respectively, to glucocorticoid and norepinephrine (NE) secretion. The positiv reverberating loop between the CRH neuron and the autonomic arousal centers is under ultrashort-loop feedback control, respectively, by CRH and NE presynaptic inhibition. Plus signs represent stimulation; minus signs indicate inhibition. (Right) Hypothalamic CRH neurons receive positive NE input from the central limbic system (LC), cholinergic and serotonergic stimulation, and opiate and GABAergic inhibition. Circled plus signs represent stimulatory pathways; circled minus signs, inhibitory pathways. ACh, acetylcholine; 5HT, 5-hydroxytryptamine (serotonin); GABA, γ-aminobutyric acid; PVN, paraventricular nucleus. (From Gold, 1992.)

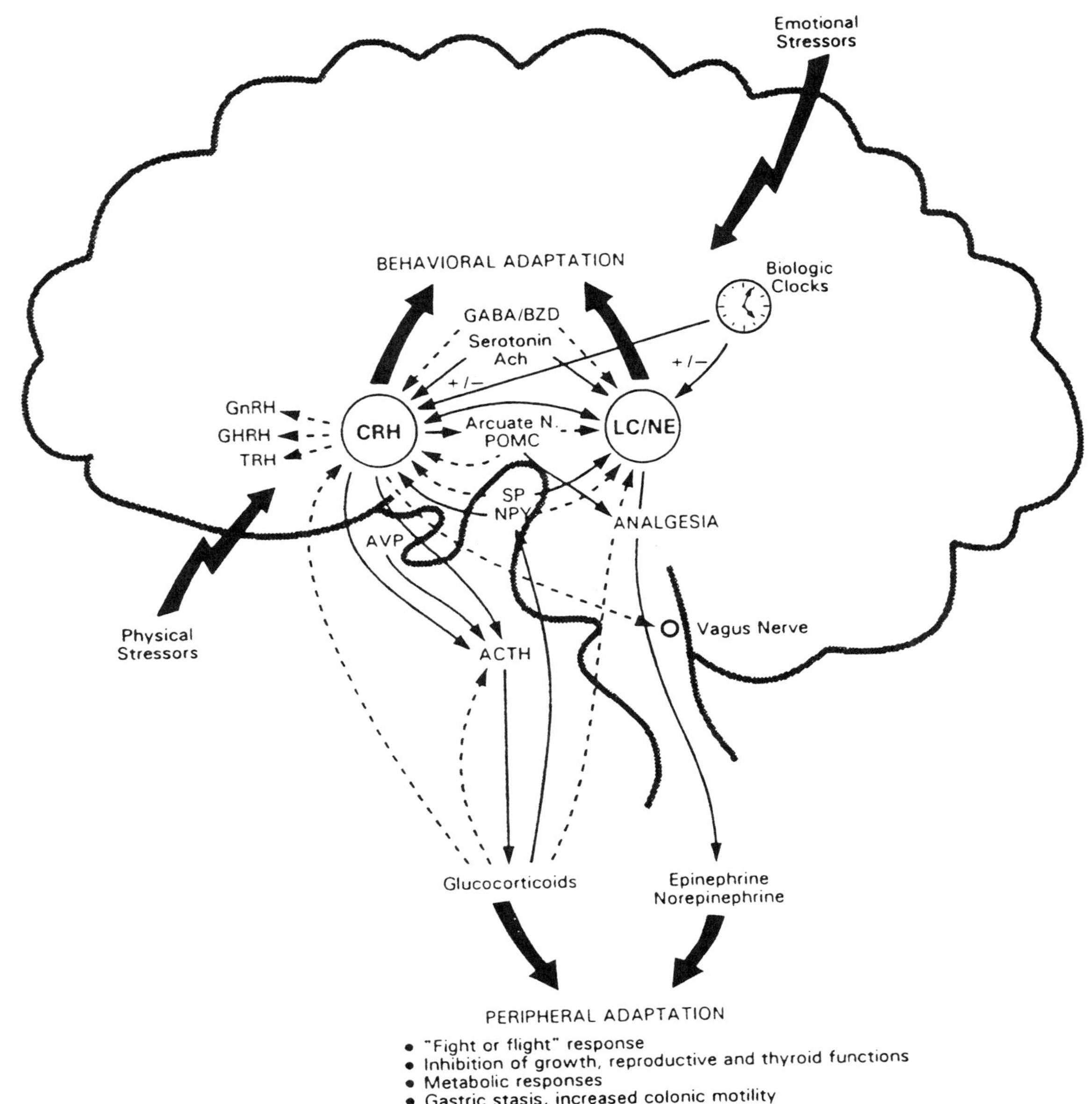

Figure 8.3
A simplified representation of the central and peripheral components of the stress system, their functional interrelations, and their relation to other CNS systems involved in the stress response. Solid lines represent direct or indirect activation and dashed lines represent direct or indirect inhibition. GABA/BZD, γ-aminobutyric acid/benzodiazepine; ACTH, adrenocorticotropic hormone; AVP, arginine vasopressin; CRH, corticotropin-releasing hormone; GnRH, gonadotropin-releasing hormone; GHRH, growth hormone–releasing hormone; TRH, thyrotropin-releasing hormone; LC, locus ceruleus; NE, nor-epinephrine; POMC, pro-opiomelanocortin; SP, substance P; NPY, neuropeptide Y; AVP, vasopressin. (From Stratakis and Chrousos, 1995.)

Table 8.1
Behavioral and physical adaptation during stress

Behavioral Adaptation
Adaptive redirection of behavior
Acute faciliation of adaptive and inhibition of nonadaptive pathways
increased arousal, alertness
increased cognition, vigilance, and focused attention
suppression of feeding behavior
suppression of reproductive behavior
containment of stress response
Physical Adaptation
Adaptive redirection of energy
oxygen and nutrients directed to CNS and stressed body site(s)
altered cardiovascular tone, increased blood pressure and heart rate
increased respiratory rate
increased gluconeogenesis and lipolysis
detoxification from toxic products
inhibition of growth and reproductive systems
containment of stress response
containment of inflammatory/immune response

From Chrousos and Gold (1992).

or the tremendous exertion demanded by "fighting or fleeing," the familiar behavioral and physiological response described by Walter Cannon in the early 1900s. Cannon associated the stress response to the activation of the sympathetic nervous system and the adrenal secretion of catecholamines (Cannon and de la Paz, 1911). Some of the components of this response include cautious avoidance, focused attention, and inhibition of reproductive and feeding behaviors. Similarly, stress-released ACTH and MSH, which increase attention and motivation, also improve neuromuscular performance (see chapter 11), all-important components of the successful response to stress.

8.2.2 The Hypothalamic-Pituitary-Adrenal Axis and the Sympatho-Adrenal-Medullary System

Both the HPA axis and the sympatho-adrenal-medullary (SAM) system are involved in the stress response, a response that is nonspecific despite the multiple stressors that evoke it. The SAM and HPA systems are anatomically and functionally interconnected and during stress they can interact at various levels. The activated HPA axis responds by increased levels of CRH, ACTH, and adrenal corticoids. CRH increases SAM activity as seen by heightened levels of plasma catecholamines. Mobilization of the SAM system activates the HPA axis through NE-increased CRH release (figure 8.4). In addition, the SAM release of catecholamines has a direct inhibitory effect on the immune system, similar to that of the glucocorticoids, inducing leukocytosis, lymphopenia, and inhibition of natural killer cell activity. These responses occur after exposure to infections, accidental or surgical trauma, and stress of various types, such as thermal, exercise-induced, and emotional stress, and increased plasma interleukin levels.

8.2.3 Stress-Related Disorders

There is considerable evidence that stress increases susceptibility to certain diseases, including cancer. Increased levels of glucocorticoids increase the rate of tumor growth. Either over- or understimulation of the HPA axis can have drastic effects. A *hyperresponsive stress system*, with its prolonged exposure to ACTH-evoked glucocorticoids as a result of chronic stress, can cause hypertension and immunosuppression, with consequent vulnerability to inflammatory disease, the accumulation of visceral fat leading to hyperinsulinism and insulin resistance, tachycardia and hypertension, and Cushing's disease. In highly trained athletes of

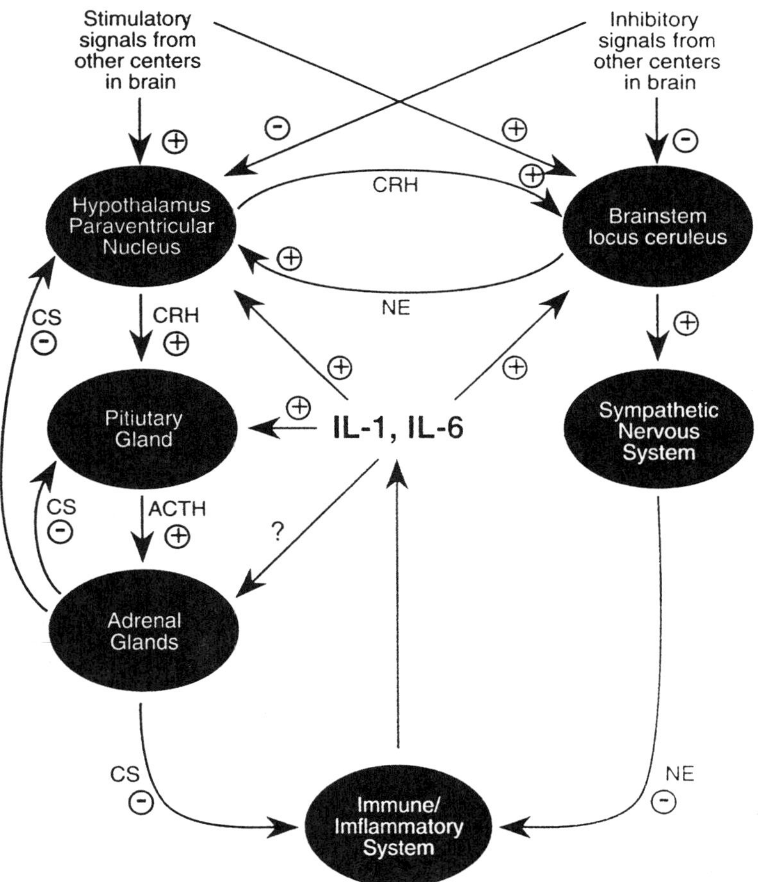

Figure 8.4
Bidirectional feedback regulation of the neuroendocrine-immune network. Starting at the bottom of the figure, the activated immune-inflammatory system (IIS) produces the cytokines, interleukin-1 (IL-1) and interleukin-6 (IL-6), which initiate stimulation of the hypothalamic-pituitary-adrenal axis, which results in corticosteroid (CS) inhibition of the immune-inflammatory system. IL-1 and IL-6 also stimulate the brainstem neurons which, via sympathetic system production of norepinephrine (nNE), inhibit the IIS. CS secretion feeds back to inhibit the pituitary and hypothalamus, and other brain areas may inhibit brainstem neurons. Every positive (+) reaction has a balancing inhibitory (−) reaction. CRH, corticotropin-releasing hormone; ACTH, adrenocorticotropic hormone. (From Wilder, 1995.)

both sexes, chronic HPA activation suppresses the reproductive axis at all levels: GnRH, LH, and FSH and the gonads. Females suffer from amenorrhea, males from low testosterone levels, loss of libido, and impotence. Other disorders arising from a hyperreactive stress system include anorexia nervosa, melancholy, depression, insomnia, chronic active alcoholism, and cognitive dysfunction.

A *hyporesponsive stress system* can be equally devastating, resulting in seasonal depression in the dark months of the year, chronic fatigue, somnolence, and an increased susceptibility to autoimmune and inflammatory diseases such as rheumatoid arthritis (Stratakis and Chrousos, 1995). This long list of diseases or disorders clearly shows the widespread in volvement of the neuroendocrine and immune systems in all physiological functions.

The *hippocampus* is also involved in the control of the HPA axis, exerting a negative influence over pituitary-adrenal function, a control that depends largely on hippocampal glucocorticoid receptors. Prolonged exposure to glucocorticoids reduces the number of hippocampal neurons as does increasing age, with its corresponding increase in glucocorticoid secretion (Sapolsky et al., 1984). Clinically, synthetic glucocorticoids are prescribed in vast quantities for the treatment of arthritis or asthma, the suppression of autoimmunity, or to prevent rejection of tissue transplants. Sapolsky (1994) points out that the numerous deleterious side effects of such therapy may include changes in cognition and emotion and also cause or worsen the degeneration of hippocampal neurons. Such damage impairs the inhibitory role of the hippocampus in turning off glucocorticoid secretion and the prolongation of corticoid secretion creates a vicious circle that further damages hippocampal neurons. In addition, the glucocorticoids reduce cerebral blood flow and brain glucose utilization, with implications for the development of Alzheimer's disease and other neurodegenerative diseases.

8.2.3.1 Individuality of the Stress Response

The response to stress, whether acute or chronic, is also highly individual, which is why the definition of stress in the beginning of this chapter was termed "somewhat ambiguous." What is stressful to a highly stress-sensitive individual is not necessarily stressful to a more stress-resilient person. Genetic factors, gender, and prenatal and early life psychological and physical stress all have profound and long-lasting effects on the basal activity of the stress system.

8.2.3.2 Perinatal Effects of Stress Hormones

Early dysregulation of the stress system may lead to disturbances in growth and development and cause psychiatric, endocrine, or autoimmune diseases during childhood, adolescence, and adulthood (Stratakis et al., 1995). Many endocrine maladaptations may involve the HPA axis: ACTH and α-MSH can exert numerous and long-lasting effects through the action of the adrenal steroids. These include permanent alterations in central neurotransmitter systems, neuroendocrine function, and adult sexual behavior in rats (Segarra et al., 1991; Alves et al., 1993). Some of the changes evoked by the noncorticotropic peptide fragments of ACTH such as ACTH 4–10 and α-MSH are opposite to those induced by glucocorticoids, suggesting that alterations in neural organization during development may be peptidergic rather than solely corticosteroid-induced (Beckwith et al., 1977; Nyakis et al., 1981).

8.3 The Immune System

The immune system may be divided into *primary lymphoid organs* (bone marrow and thymus, and in birds, the bursa of Fabricius), which produce mature lymphocytes, and *secondary lymphoid organs* (spleen, lymph nodes and tonsils, and Peyer's patches in the intestine), which are concerned with immune responses.

8.3.1 The Inflammatory Response

The defense of the mammalian organism against pathogens and transformed host cells depends on the highly specialized immune system, which reacts quickly as soon as injury occurs and initiates a cascade of local events known as the *inflammatory response.* Monocyte phagocytes, including macrophages, monocytes, and neutrophils, are attracted to the site of injury where they phagocytose the bacteria and other invaders.

8.3.2 The Acute Response

In addition to their phagocytic activities, macrophages play a critical role in the recognition of pathogens and the initiation of systemic reactions known as the *acute-phase response.* The acute phase of bacterial infection is initiated by recognition of a component of the bacterial cell wall, a *lipopolysaccharide (LPS).* Injection of LPS into a healthy animal will result in an acute-phase response identical to that produced by the bacteria. The mechanism by which macrophages and monocytes recognize LPS depends upon LPS first binding to a soluble serum protein to form a complex that then binds to a surface receptor on the immune cells (figure 8.5). Once the receptor has bound the LPS complex, the cell produces and releases soluble protein mediators called *cytokines,* which enter the circulation and act on the brain, neuroendocrine system, liver, and other organs to begin the acute phase.

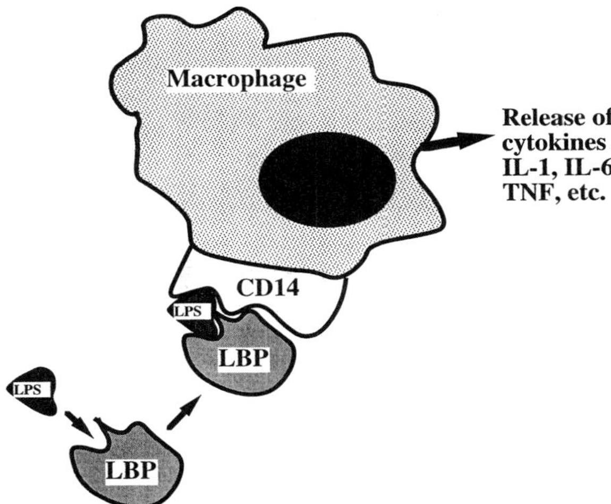

Figure 8.5
Response of macrophages to lipopolysaccharide (LPS). LPS first binds to an LPS-binding protein (LBP). This complex then binds to CD14, a receptor on the surface of macrophages. This stimulates the release of various inflammatory mediators, including interleukin IL-1 and IL-6 and tumor necrosis factor (TNF). These mediators act on target cells throughout the body, including the neuroendocrine system, initiating the acute-phase response. (From Long, 1996).

8.3.3 The Cytokines

8.3.3.1 Immune System–Generated Cytokines

The cytokines form a large group of blood-borne secretory peptides previously classified as lymphokines, monokines, interferons, colony-stimulating factors, or growth factors. A subset of the cytokines are the inflammatory cytokines which include the *interleukins:* interleukin-1 (IL-1), interleukin-2 (IL-2), interleukin-6 (IL-6), and tumor necrosis factor-α (TNF-α). These cytokines, made chiefly by activated macrophages, are pivotal to initiating both local and systemic inflammation in the acute phase. These peripheral reactions evoke central effects, including fever, adrenal activation, decreased plasma iron levels, changes in lipid metabolism, loss of appetitite, and increased sleep. Consequently, messages from the activated immune system must reach and influence the neuroendocrine system, specifically the HPA axis, and it is the cytokines that convey these messages. They represent a diffuse communication network that supplements and interfaces with the nervous system and the endocrine system (Majde, 1994). It has been imaginatively suggested by Blalock (1992) that the cytokines function as a sixth sensory system, transmitting immune signals to the CNS that cannot be detected by the other five sensory organs (figure 8.6).

8.3.3.2 Cytokine Regulation of the Neuroendocrine System

a. Systemic cytokines

If circulating cytokines are to affect behavioral and neuroendocrine actions they should be able to enter the CNS. Banks and Kastin (1994) have successfully shown that IL-1 and TNF-α can penetrate the BBB by selective and saturable transporters, but they probably penetrate in rather low amounts. Cytokines may also reach the CNS through sites with a leaky BBB, such as the circumventricular organs (see chapter 5).

In their systemic role, the cytokines alter neuroendocrine function either through the CNS or through direct action on neuroendocrine cells to stimulate the release of CRH, ACTH, and glucocorticoids. The feedback loop then is completed as the glucocorticoids shut off the immune response that initiated the cycle (see figures 8.4 and 8.7). All four cytokines appear to be able activate the HPA axis at several levels—the hypothalamic, pituitary, and adrenal. However, there are individual differences be-

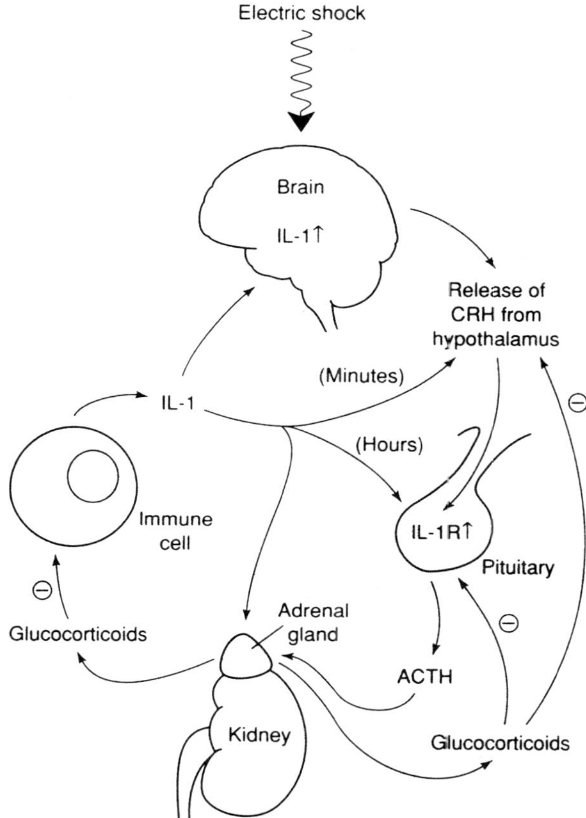

Figure 8.6
Sites of action of interleukin-1 (IL-1) in the hypothalamo-pituitary-adrenal axis. IL-1 or electric shock can act on the brain to elevate endogenous IL-1. IL-1 causes the release of corticotropin-releasing hormone (CRH) from the hypothalamus, which results in the release of ACTH from the anterior pituitary and elevates IL-1 receptor (IL-1R) levels in the pituitary gland. IL-1 then acts directly on the pituitary, prolonging ACTH production. IL-1 also may act directly on the adrenals. The synthesis and release of IL-1 is inhibited by glucocorticoid feedback. Glucocorticoids also inhibit the secretion of hypothalamic CRH and ACTH (not shown). (From Blalock, 1994.)

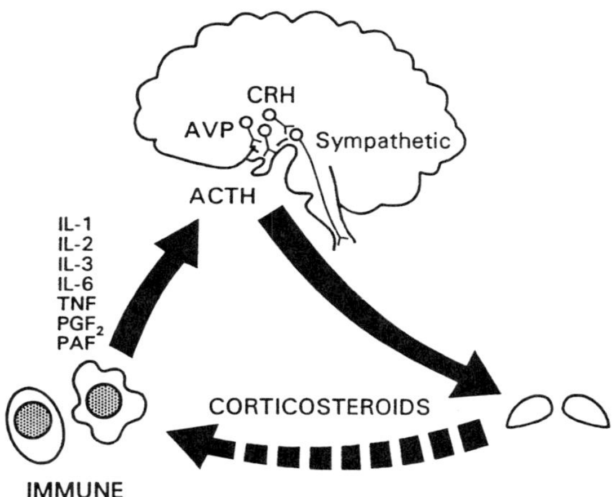

Figure 8.7
The communication pathway between the hypothalamic-pituitary-adrenal axis and the cytokines. Cytokines synthesized by immune cells during inflammation stimulate the hypothalamus to secrete corticotropin-releasing hormone (CRH) and the pituitary to secrete ACTH. The resultant secretion of corticosteroids by the adrenal gland suppresses the immune response that began the cycle. The list IL-1 to PAF on the left are cytokines. IL-1, etc, interleukin-1; TNF, tumor necrosis factor; PGF, prostaglandin F; PAF^2, platelet activating factor; AVP, arginine vasopressin. (From Sternberg and Licinio, 1995.)

tween the various interleukins. IL-1 acts mainly to evoke CRH secretion, and secondarily to sensitize pituitary corticotrophs to CRH action. IL-6 is shown in figure 8.8 to act directly on pituitary secretion of ACTH. Receptors for the cytokines are found on hypothalamic neuroendocrine cells and on pituitary corticotrophs.

However, the actions of the cytokines are probably more complex than this and the immune system may use several pathways and sites of entry to communicate with the brain and to activate the neurons responsible for stimulating the HPA axis. Lee and Rivier (1994) and Rivest (1995) have shown that administration of IL-1 or the endotoxin LPS causes a rapid increase in the expression of the immediate early gene c-*fos* (see chapter 2) in selective regions of the brain (brainstem; medial preoptic area, including the organum vasculosum of the lamina terminalis; the arcuate nucleus and median eminence region; and the PVN). Brainstem activation could involve the noradrenergic and adrenergic pathways to the PVN. In addition, circulating IL-1 may be transduced by sensory components of the vagus nerve to stimulate brainstem nuclei (figure 8.9).

b. Cytokines of central origin

Many of the neural and endocrine cells that have receptors for cytokines, and respond to them, also produce cytokines, which probably act locally by paracrine or autocrine actions, or by a combined action of both. As local neuroendocrine cytokines are present in the hypothalamus and pituitary, they may well have important regulatory effects upon these structures (Spangelo and Gorospe, 1995). Consequently, both systemic and local cytokines coordinate the appropriate neuroendocrine responses to an antigen challenge.

c. Cytokine Production by the sympathetic nervous system

Both the primary and secondary lymphoid organs are densely innervated by sympathetic nerves which reach all peripheral sites of inflammation via postganglionic sympathetic neurons. Activation of the SAM by stress causes systemic secretion of IL-6, which, by triggering the HPA axis, participates in the stress-induced suppression of the immune-inflammatory reactions.

8.3.4 The Thymus

The thymus has been called the master gland of the immune system and, through the action of thymic

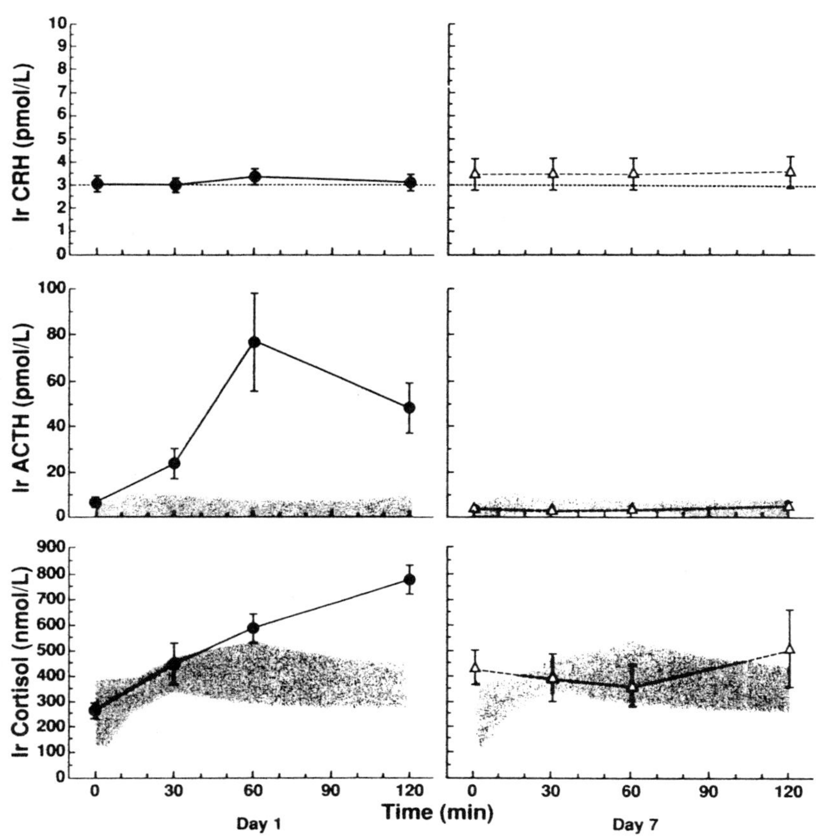

Figure 8.8
Mean ± SE plasma-immunoreactive corticotropin-releasing hormone (IrCRH, top), immunoreactive Ir-ACTH (middle), and cortisol (bottom) responses to a subcutaneous bolus injection of 30 µg/kg interleukin-6 (IL-6) in cancer patients. IL-6 prokes a robust increase in plasma ACTH and cortisol but does not affect CRH. The shaded areas represent the responses of normal, healthy volunteers to a standard dose of 1 µg/kg of ovine CRH and are included for comparison. (From Mastorakos et al., 1993.)

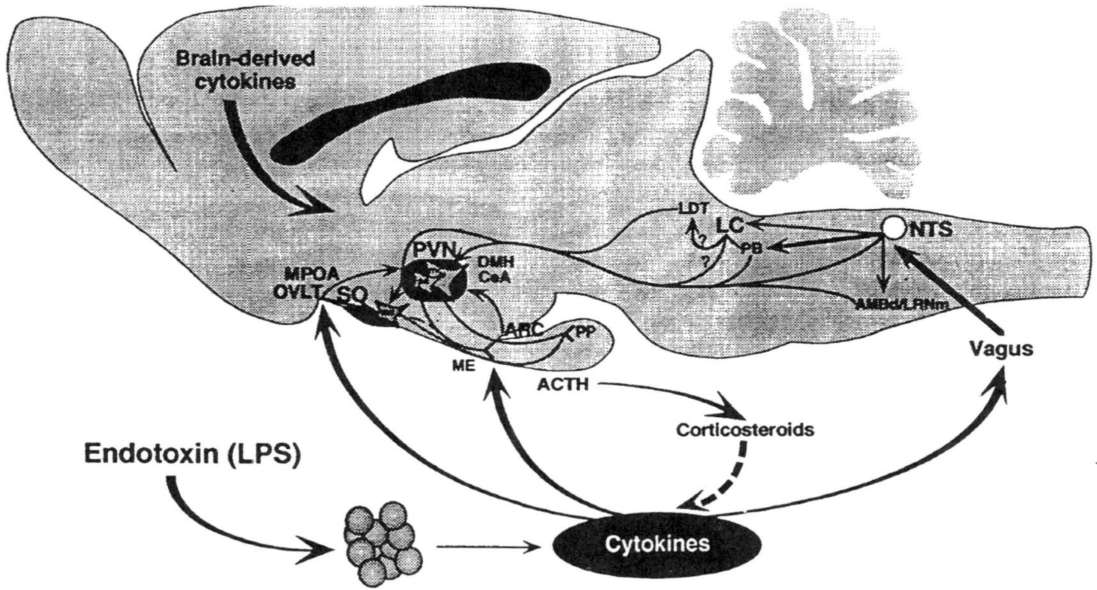

Figure 8.9
Schematic illustration of the possible physiological relevance of the systemic endotoxin-induced immediate early genes expression in selective areas of the rat brain. Cytokines may target the brain at different levels, including the brainstem, medial preoptic area (MPOA), organum vascularis of the lamina terminalis (OVLT), and the arcuate nucleus (ARC) and median eminence (ME) region. AMBd, dorsal division of the nucleus ambiguus; LRNm, lateral reticular medial nucleus; NTS, nucleus of the solitary tract; LDT, lateral dorsal tegmental nucleus; PB, parabrachial nucleus; PP, posterior pituitary; PVN, paraventricular nucleus of the hypothalamus; SO, supraoptic nucleus, DMH, dorsomedial hypothalamus; CoA, anterior commissure. (From Rivest, 1995.)

peptide hormones, is responsible for the differentiation of T lymphocytes and for the stimulation of the immune system. T cells are so named because they mature in the *t*hymus; B cells mature in the *b*one marrow. Both types are derived from stem cells in hemopoietic tissues such as bone marrow. Helper T cells stimulate B cells to proliferate and differentiate into antibody-producing cells. In addition to the thymic hormones and cytokines, the thymus secretes an astonishing variety of important neuropeptides that are immunologically identical to hypothalamic and pituitary neuropeptides. These include the hypothalamic peptides VP, OT, CRH and LHRH, and the pituitary peptides PRL, GH, TSH, ACTH, FSH and LH. Thymic gene expression of substance P (SP), NPY, VIP, β-endorphin, and met-enkephalin has been shown at both the protein and mRNA level (Dardenne and Savino, 1994).

8.3.4.1 Thymic Regulation of Neuroendocrine Function

Not only does the thymus itself produce these neuropeptides but it also regulates the secretion of several

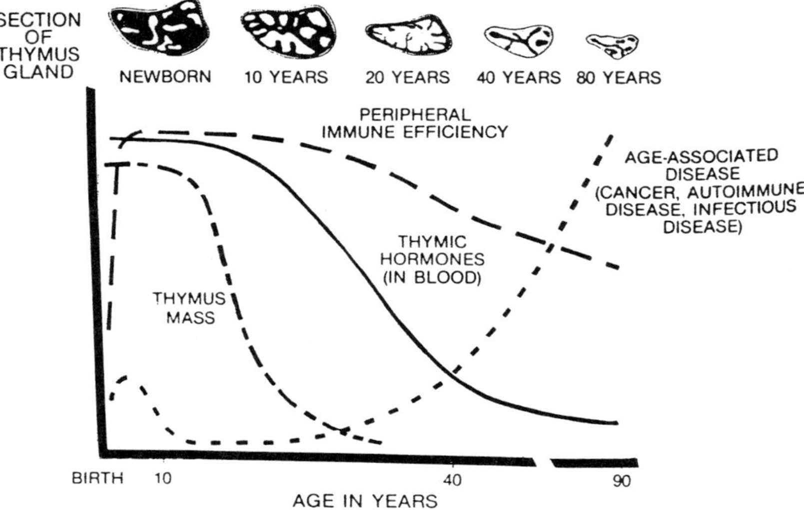

Figure 8.10
Relationship of thymic structure and function to peripheral immune efficiency and age-associated diseases over the life span. (From Fabris et al., 1988.)

pituitary and hypothalamic neuropeptides. One component of the thymic hormone *thymosin*, thymosin β_4, stimulates the release of LH from the pituitary and GnRH from the hypothalamus. Another thymosin component elicits the release of PRL and GH.

8.3.4.2 Neuropeptide Regulation of Thymic Function

The thymus undergoes a progressive deterioration in both structure and function with age (figure 8.10). It reaches its maximum size at puberty, after which it begins to involute and to be replaced by fat. This structural deterioration is accompanied by a decline in its production of thymic hormones, which are required for proliferation and differentiation of T cells and thus of T cell–dependent functions. *Glucocorticoids* are the major cause of thymic involution through the activation of the genetically programmed suicide pathway (apoptosis). In addition to glucocorticoids, the thymus is under complex neuroendocrine control (figure 8.11; see also section 8.4), with hypothalamic and pituitary neuropeptides using the classic endocrine route, whereas locally produced neuropeptides use paracrine and autocrine pathways. Functional receptors for many of the pituitary and hypothalamic hormones are present on thymic cells.

8.4 Regulation of the Immune System

The type of stimulus appears to determine the particular hormone that immune cells will synthesize. The B cell mitogen LPS stimulates leukocytes to produce ACTH 1–39 and β-endorphin, whereas a T cell mitogen stimulates lymphocytes to produce TRH but not ACTH. LPS induces the production of ACTH 1–25 and γ-endorphin. Important to note is that the ACTH secreted by activated lymphocytes is bioactive and able to stimulate corticosterone secretion by adrenal cells (Clarke and Bost, 1989). Almost all the known neuropeptides are produced by the cells of the immune system but the stimuli that evoke their expression vary.

8.4.1 Self-Regulation by the Immune System

The immune system may regulate itself in a manner similar to that of hypothalamic regulation of pituitary hormones. Lymphocyte-derived CRH or VP can induce ACTH secretion by lymphocytes or by the pituitary gland. Similarly, immune-derived GHRH can elevate lymphocyte GH. However, the production of ACTH by lymphocytes takes a different route from the neuroendocrine pathway of hypothalamic stimulation of pituitary POMC and ACTH. In the immune system, CRH (whether of hypothalamic or immune system derivation) causes IL-1 production by macrophages, and IL-1 elicits POMC production by B cells (Blalock, 1992). Another difference lies in the way glucocorticoids block POMC synthesis. In the neuroendocrine system, these steroids block the HPA axis via negative feedback on CRH and ACTH secretion. In the immune system, glucocorticoids block macrophage production of Il-1, thus indirectly blocking B cell synthesis of POMC (figure 8.12). Blalock (1994) cites several other important differences between pituitary hormone production and that of the immune system. There is no storage of these hormones in the immune system, so that there is a delay before the hormones become available (see figure 8.6); synthesis of immune-derived neuropeptides requires induction; lymphocytes produce much less neuropeptide than neuroendocrine cells but they are far more numerous and also more mobile, so that the hormone can be delivered locally, using paracrine or autocrine approaches, or both. Table 8.2 lists the neuropeptides presently identified in immune cells.

8.4.2 Immune System Homeostasis: Immunosuppressive Neuropeptides

Neuropeptides regulate several important immune functions. These include antibody formation, lymphocyte cyotoxicity, lymphokine production, hypersensitivity, and macrophage and neutrophil activation and chemotaxis. The hypothalamic-pituitary axis plays a key role in immunoregulation. A proper balance must be maintained between the immunosuppressive (adrenocortical hormones) and the immunostimulatory (PRL and GH). Other hormones play a modulatory role (table 8.3). It is likely that the immunosuppressive role of ACTH may be through cleavage of MSH from ACTH, with the consequent antipyretic and immunosuppressive actions due to MSH (Smith et al., 1992).

8.4.2.1 Corticotropin-Releasing Hormone

CRH is the principal regulator of the stress response, stimulating the release of ACTH from the pituitary and consequently the secretion of glucocorticoids from the adrenal gland, with subsequent suppression of the immune reponse. CRH inhibits the pituitary-gonadal and pituitary-thyroid axes and suppresses pituitary secretion of GH and PRL. In addition to this neuroendocrine role, CRH modulates stress-related immunosuppression independent of corticosteroids, as shown by the retention of the immunosuppressive actions of CRH in adrenalectomized animals (Jain et al., 1991). All this is strong evidence for an major role for CRH in the integration of the activities of the nervous, endocrine, immune, and inflammatory systems.

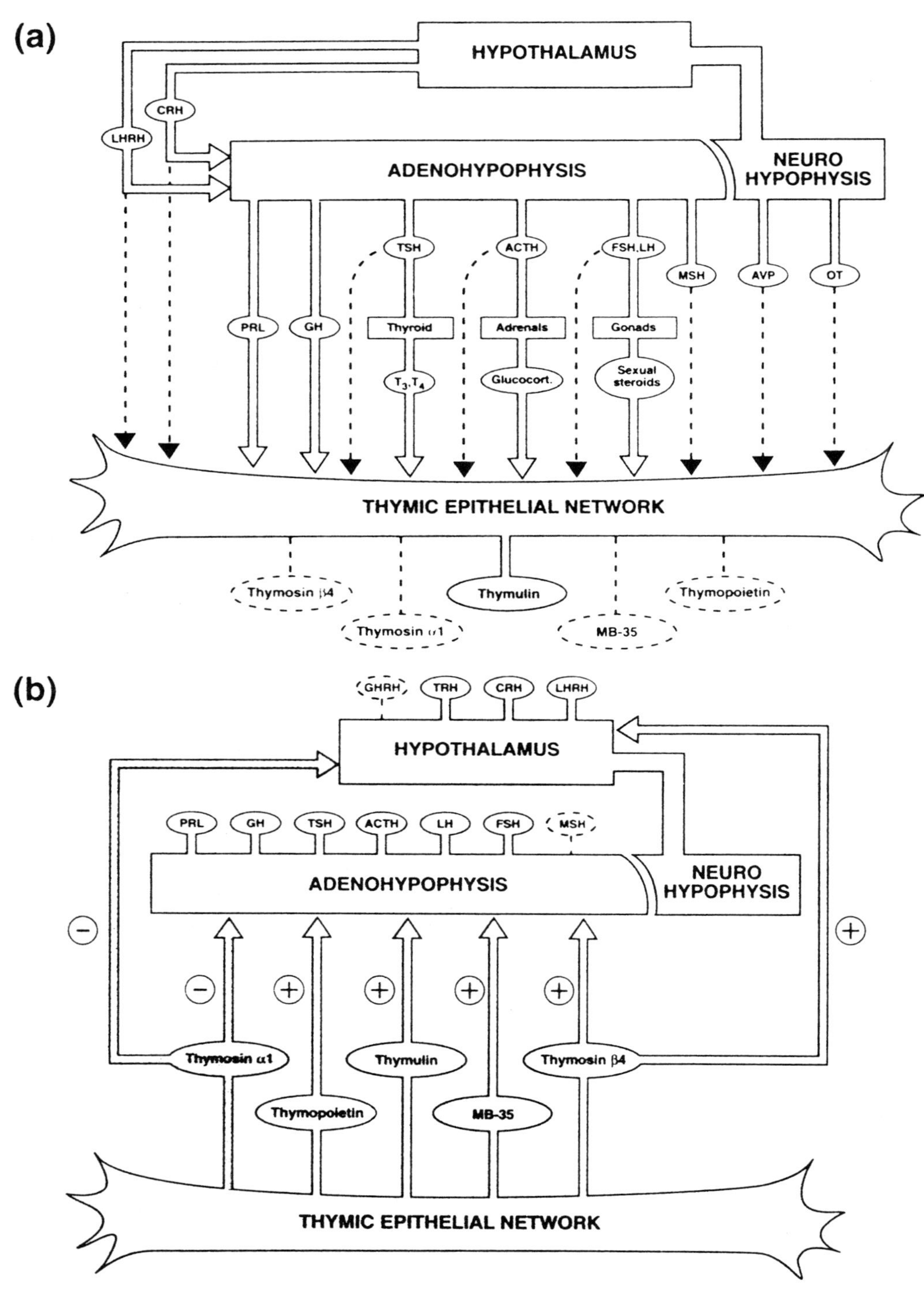

(a)
HYPOTHALAMUS
CRH
LHRH
ADENOHYPOPHYSIS
NEURO HYPOPHYSIS
TSH
ACTH
FSH,LH
MSH
AVP
OT
PRL
GH
Thyroid
Adrenals
Gonads
T3,T4
Glucocort.
Sexual steroids
THYMIC EPITHELIAL NETWORK
Thymosin β4
Thymulin
Thymopoietin
Thymosin α1
MB-35
(b)
GHRH
TRH
CRH
LHRH
HYPOTHALAMUS
PRL
GH
TSH
ACTH
LH
FSH
MSH
ADENOHYPOPHYSIS
NEURO HYPOPHYSIS
Thymosin α1
Thymulin
Thymosin β4
Thymopoietin
MB-35
THYMIC EPITHELIAL NETWORK

Strangely, CRH may have a proinflammatory action. Peripherally secreted CRH, indistinguishable from hypothalamic CRH, is found in acute and chronic inflammatory sites, including synovial fluids and tissues from patients with rheumatoid arthritis. In these sites it appears to act as an autocrine or paracrine proinflammatory mediator, in contrast to the glucocorticoid-mediatiated anti-inflammatory effects that result from activation of the HPA axis.

A line of transgenic mice has been developed that have abnormalities of the HPA axis with chronic overproduction of CRH. These mice express a chimeric CRH transgene containing the mMT-1 promoter upstream of the rat CRH genomic gene (see chapter 2) These mice also have elevated ACTH and glucocorticoid levels and constitute an excellent model for the study of chronic stress (Stenzel-Poore et al., 1996). In these animals, the proportion of B cells is markedly reduced, both in the bone marrow where B cells begin their development, and in the spleen where further maturation occurs. B cell function is

Figure 8.11
Bidirectional hormonal interactions involving the thymic epithelium and the hypothalamic-pituitary-adrenal (HPA) axis. (a) *The influence of HPA-derived neuropeptides on thymic endocrine activity* as fully demonstrated (solid arrows) or partially demonstrated (dotted arrows). These interactions may occur directly on thymic epithelial cells (TECs) or via target glands that release their hormones to act on TECs. Other thymic hormones (in dashed ellipses) may also be under endocrine control. (b) *The influence of thymic hormones on the HPA.* Thymic peptides can exert direct effects on both hypothalamic and pituitary cells, either positive (+) or negative (−), depending on the thymic peptide. Effects on melanocyte-stimulating hormone (MSH) or growth hormone–releasing hormone (GHRH) (shown in dashed ellipses) are putative. T_3, triiodothryonine; T_4, thyroxine; MB 35, peptide component of thymosin; other abbreviations as in appendix A. (From Dardenne and Savino, 1994.)

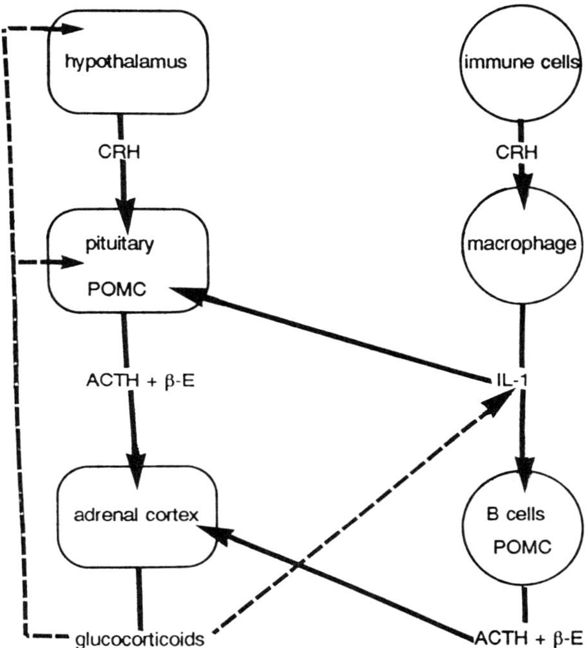

Figure 8.12
Similarities and differences between regulation of the hypothalamic-pituitary-adrenal axis and the immune systems. On the left of the diagram, the hypothalamus produces corticotropin-releasing hormone (CRH) which stimulates anterior pituitary corticotrophs to synthesize and process pro-opiomelanocortin (POMC) to ACTH and β-endorphin (β-E). ACTH stimulates the adrenal cortex to secrete glucocorticoids. On the right of the diagram, immune system cells produce CRH which stimulates macrophages to produce the cytokine interleukin-1 (IL-1), which then activates B cells to synthesize and process POMC to ACTH and β-E. B cell–derived ACTH is capable of stimulating adrenal secretion of glucocorticoids. Glucocorticoids, however, inhibit IL-1 production by macrophages, and consequently *indirectly* inhibit B cell production of ACTH and β-E. In addition, glucocorticoids *directly* inhibit the hypothalamic CRH, thus effectively suppressing the immune response in two ways.

Table 8.2
Cellular sources of neuropeptides in the immune system

Source	Peptides or Proteins
T lymphocytes	ACTH, endorphins, TSH, HCG
	PRL, met-enkephalin, PTH-rP, IGF-1
B lymphocytes	ACTH, endorphins, GH, IGF-I
Macrophages	ACTH, endorphins, GH, SP, IGF-I, ANH
Splenocytes	LH, FSH, CRH
Thymocytes	CRH, GnRH, VP, OT, PRL, GH, TSH, ACTH, LH
Mast cells and PMN cells	VIP, somatostatin
Megakaryocytes	NPY

Adapted from Blalock (1994).
Abbreviations not previously defined: ANP, atrial natriuretic hormone; PMN, polymorphonuclear; PTH-rP, parathyroid hormone–related protein.

Table 8.3
Hormonal suppression, stimulation, and modulation of immune system homeostasis

Immuno-suppressive	Immuno-stimulatory	Immuno-modulatory
CRH	GHRH	GnRH, sex steroids
ACTH,	GH	TSH, thyroxine
α-MSH	PRL	Endorphins
glucocorticoids		VP, OT
somatostatin		SP
		VIP

CRH, corticotropin-releasing hormone; GHRH, growth hormone–releasing hormone; GnRH, gonadotropin-releasing hormone; ACTH, adrenocorticotropic hormone; GH, growth hormone; TSH, thyroid-stimulating hormone; MSH, melanocyte-stimulating hormone; PRL, prolactin; VP, vasopressin; OT; oxytocin; SP, substance P; VIP, vosoactive intestinal polypeptide.

Table 8.4
Endocrine and physical changes shared by humans with Cushing's disease and corticotropin-releasing hormone (CRH) transgenic mice

Cushing's Disease	CRH Transgenic Mice
cortisol ↑[a]	corticosterone ↑[a]
ACTH ↑	ACTH ↑
muscle wasting	muscle wasting
obesity	obesity
thin skin	thin skin
amenorrhea	fertility ↓

From Stenzel-Poore et al. (1996).
↑, increased; ↓, decreased.
[a] Cortisol and corticosterone are the human and rodent glucocorticoids, respectively.

also diminished, with a marked decrease in the response to immune challenge, both in the primary (8 days) and memory (about 1 year) response. This defective memory response may indicate the seriousness of chronic CRH overproduction and chronic HPA activation on immune function. In table 8.4 the endocrine features and physical characteristics of CRH transgenic mice are compared to those in humans with Cushing's disease in which pituitary hypersecretion of ACTH is usually the cause: only rarely is there overproduction of CRH.

8.4.2.2 Adrenocorticotropic Hormone and α-Melanocyte–Stimulating Hormone

Apart from its role as a stimulus to the secretion of glucocorticoids, the effects of which are discussed below, ACTH has direct effects on lymphoid cell proliferation and ACTH suppresses the antibody response. Investigations on spleen cells in vitro show that these are direct effects of ACTH 1–39 cells that cannot be duplicated by ACTH peptide fragments such as ACTH 1–24; α-MSH (ACTH 1–13, acetylated or nonacetylated); or CLIP (ACTH 18–39). Similarly, only ACTH 1–39 can suppress the production of the immunoregulatory lymphokine interferon-γ (INF-γ). This suggests that there is a remarkable dissociation of the immunoregulatory and steroidogenic effects of ACTH 1–39 (Johnson et al., 1992).

The amino acid and nucleotide sequences of spleen and pituitary ACTH are identical. Full-length POMC transcripts and β-endorphin immunoreactivity are detectable by in situ hybridization and immunonohistochemistry in some lymphoid cells. Specific, high-affinity ACTH receptors are found on both B and T cells. The mechanism for ACTH stimulation of lymphocyte receptors is similar to ACTH stimulation of steroidogenesis in adrenal cells, that is, cAMP and mobilization of Ca^{2+} are involved.

While α-MSH is ineffective on spleen cells, it has certain immunosuppressive actions such as antagonizing several effects of IL-1, including pyrogenicity, thymocyte proliferation, the induction of acute-phase proteins, and of prostaglanin E in fibroblasts. These effects are not mediated by classical α-MSH receptors (Cannon et al., 1986).

8.4.2.3 Glucocorticoids

The adrenal glucocorticoids represent the end product of HPA activation. They are major regulators of carbohydrate and lipid metabolism, and through their catabolic effects on lymphoid tissue and suppression of antibody formation, they are potent anti-inflammatory and antiallergic agents. All the lymphoid organs and leukocytes have glucocorticoid receptors, the number of which is markedly increased in stimulated lymphocytes. Corticosteroids inhibit almost every component of the immune and inflammatory response, including thymic growth and differentiation, and also inhibit practically all the functions of the monocyte macrophage cell. This means that cell metabolism, chemotaxis, phagocytosis, and cytotoxic reactions, the capacity to present antigen, secrete cytokines, and produce enzymes, are all inhibited by glucocorticoids. In this manner, glucocorticoids return immune system perturbations to normal, preventing an excessive response to the stress that could produce selfinjury, that is, autoimmune disease.

8.4.2.4 Opiate Neuropeptides

Lymphoid cells and monocyte macrophages have receptors for opiate peptides, some of which are inhibited by the opiate antagonist naloxone. Lymphocyte opiate receptors can be defined by the same four classes as in neuronal tissue and their receptors appear to share many of the unique characteristics of neuronal opiate receptors, including molecular size, immunogenicity, and signaling pathways (Carr, 1991). Opiates influence immune function by affecting antibody production; IL-1, IL-2, and prostaglandin synthesis; as well as acting indirectly through the brain (Plotnikoff et al., 1986). α-Endorphin (amino acids 61–76 of β-lipotropin) is a potent inhibitor of antibody production by mouse spleen cells and binds to receptors on the spleen cells that are similar to those of brain opiate receptors. The specificity of the opiate effects is shown by the very slight effect of the related β- and γ-endorphins, with leu- and met-enkephalin being intermediate to the two endorphins in their antibody suppressive effects. These endorphins are discussed as immune system modulators in section 8.4.4.4.

8.4.2.5 Somatostatin

Somatostatin is a hypothalamic neuropeptide that is also found in the central and peripheral nervous systems. Its actions are extensive in that it inhibits the secretion of GH, VIP, TSH, glucagon, insulin, secretin, gastrin, and CCK. Somatostatin secretion is evoked by CRH, and like CRH, it has potent inhibitory effects on the immune system, such as T cell proliferation and other immune responses. Immune cells have receptors for somatostatin.

8.4.3 Immune System Homeostasis: The Immunostimulatory Hormones

8.4.3.1 Growth Hormone and Prolactin

Cell proliferation in both the primary and secondary lymphoid tissues is dependent on pituitary GH and PRL which control the expression of growth-regulatory genes (proto-oncogenes). Essential growth factors, such as the thymic hormones and insulin-like growth factor (IGF), are also dependent on PRL and GH. This growth-promoting action is opposed by the ACTH-adrenocorticoid axis. Defects in this regulatory circuit may lead to serious consequences to either the immune system or the neuroendocrine system (Berczi, 1994).

GH and PRL receptors are present on monocytes and lymphocytes and both these neuropeptides have a direct mitogenic effect on lymphoid cells. They increase IL-1 and IL-2 production and potentiate the induction of TNF-α. GH stimulates DNA and RNA synthesis in the spleen and thymus and affects hematopoeisis by stimulating neutrophil differentiation. Overall, injections of GH increase thymic size, stimulate thymocyte production, augment antibody synthesis and skin graft rejection, and reverse the leukopenia caused by stress. Mice injected with antibody to GH develop thymic atrophy. As very low levels of GH are produced by lymphocytes, lymphocyte-derived GH probably acts in a paracrine or autocrine manner.

Dwarf mice lack both PRL and GH and are immunodeficient: treatment with GH or PRL restores immune function to normal (Berczi, 1994). The significance of GH in immune function was at one time seriously compromised by the fact that human pituitary dwarfs do not show major symptoms of immunodeficiency, until it was found that human dwarfs have adequate levels of PRL, which permits normal immune function. It seems that normal immune function can be attained through the actions of either PRL or GH, a not surprising observation considering the close homology of these two ancient neuropeptides (Weigent and Blalock, 1995).

The hypothalamic-pituitary, PRL, and GH systems are also profoundly affected by stress. Although acute stress may increase production of GH, chronic stress is associated with inhibition of GH, secondary to CRH-stimulated somatostatin secretion. This syndrome is seen in children who fail to grow when exposed to chronic stress, a syndrome dramatically described in the novel by Günther Grass *The Tin Drum*.

8.4.3.2 Growth Hormone–Releasing Hormone

GHRH is a hypothalamic neuropeptide that stimulates the release of GH and consequently has an indirect stimulatory action on the immune system. GHRH is also produced by lymphocytes, and lymphocyte GHRH-related RNA is similar in size and properties to hypothalamic GHRH.

8.4.4 Neuroendocrine Modulators of the Immune System

8.4.4.1 Gonadotropin-Releasing Hormone

GnRH is synthesized in the hypothalamus, gonads, mammary glands, placenta, spleen, and thymus.

GnRH plays a key role not only in regulating reproductive function through its activation of pituitary secretion of FSH and LH and the resulting secretion of sex steroids but also in immune function. Experiments on castrated, autoimmune disease–prone mice demonstrate that GnRH has a direct effect on autoimmune disease, independent of gonadal secretion. (Jacobson et al., 1994). T cells in the thymus synthesize GnRH and T cells have GnRH receptors. The complementary DNA (cDNA) sequences of hypothalamic and lymphocyte GnRH are identical (Weigent and Blalock, 1995). Biologically active LH and FSH are also found in lymphocytes in response to GnRH stimulation.

8.4.4.2 Interaction Between the Hypothalamic-Pituitary-Adrenal and Hypothalamic-Pituitary-Gonadal Axes

Activation of the stress response inhibits the hypothalamo-pituitary-gonadal (HPG) axis at multiple levels. CRH suppresses secretion of GnRH in the hypothalamic arcuate nucleus either directly or indirectly via stimulation of β-endorphin or corticosteroids. Corticosteroids also directly inhibit the pituitary release of LH and the gonadal production of sex steroids, estrogen, progesterone, and testosterone. The linkage of the HPG and HPA axes, and the sex-related functional differences in the responsiveness of these systems, have important implications for understanding the development of autoimmunity. Females have a more active HPA axis than males, that is, stress induces higher glucocorticoid levels. The ontogeny of the immune system appears to be linked to the ontogeny of the reproductive system, and autoimmune diseases flare up or subside during periods in which the reproductive system is undergoing pronounced changes, such as puberty, in the postpartum period, or in menopause. In general, estrogen and progesterone are immunostimulatory rather than immunosuppressive and autoimmune diseases are much more common in females than in males. The female-to-male ratio of autoimmune thyroiditis is 19:1; of rheumatoid arthritis, 3:1 to 4:1. Moreover, autoimmune diseases tend to increase with age and to parallel the age-related changes in the endocrine system: the activity of both the HPA and HPG axes dwindles as people age, whereas autoantibody formation increases markedly with increasing age (Marchetti et al., 1991).

8.4.4.3 Hypothalamic-Pituitary-Thyroid Axis

The HPT axis is modulated by thyroid hormones, which probably increase its activity. TRH stimulates the production of antibodies, increasing lymphocyte TSH and TSH mRNA. Some lymphoid cells express TSH receptors, the synthesis of which is increased by exposure to bacterial endotoxins.

The *HPT axis* has been shown recently to exert both positive and negative immunoregulatory effects on intestinal lymphocytes. The intestinal mucosa separates the external environment formed by the gut from the internal milieu; the extremely large surface area provided by the intestinal microvilli, while a superb arrangement for absorption, is not the most efficient barrier against toxins and infectious agents. The intraepithelial lymphocytes of the intestinal mucosa act as a primary lymphoid organ, representing a pool of cells as great as that of the peripheral lymphocytes in the spleen. Almost all these intestinal intraepithelial cells are T cells. Administration of either TRH, or TSH itself, promotes the development of the intraepithelial lymphocytes, whereas thyroxine has an immunosuppressive effect. What is surprising is that thyroxine has little or no effect on other lymphocytes outside the intestine so that it appears that the regulatory effects of TRH or TSH are independent of thyroxine. The concept is that TRH acts on specific TRH receptors on intestinal cells to cause the release of TSH, which then activates TSH receptors on the intraepithelial cells to stimulate the release of cytokines. This would represent a paracrine network of hormonal regulation of the intraepithelial cells (Wang et al., 1997).

8.4.4.4 Endorphins

The endogenous opiates, the β-, γ-, and α-endorphins, modulate the activity of cells in the immune system. These peptides are amply produced in response to stress as cleavage products from POMC. β-Endorphin may enhance or suppress T cell proliferation and IL-2 production. These endorphins increase the natural cytotoxicity of lymphocytes and macrophages toward tumor cells and inhibit major histocompatibility class II antigen expression.

8.4.4.5 Vasopressin and Oxytocin

VP is a hypothalamic octapeptide that is transported to the posterior pituitary for release into the circulation. As the main stimuli for VP release are changes in plasma osmolality, blood pressure, and blood volume, stressors such as hemorrhage, plasma hypertonicity, or water loss increase VP levels. In addition, surgical stress, nausea, and insulin-induced hypoglycemia also increase plasma VP levels. However, VP release is not affected by many stressors that activate the HPA and SAM axes, such as immobilization, cold, ether, and footshock.

VP modulates the stress response both directly, by stimulating ACTH release, and indirectly, through augmenting CRH release. The VP receptor on lymphocytes does not appear to be of the V1 or V2 type: they are V1-like but novel. VP provides a positive signal for induction of IFN-γ, as compared to the negative signal of ACTH.

OT, like VP, travels from the hypothalamus to the posterior pituitary and its main role is in labor and lactation. Both hypothalamic neuropeptides may reach the anterior pituitary via the capillary plexus shared with the posterior pituitary gland, and influence ACTH release. However, many of the stressors that do not affect VP release result in increased OT secretion. These include immobilization, stress, ether, and hypoglycemia. OT may modulate lymphocyte function.

8.4.4.6 Substance P

SP is a member of the tachykinins, sensory neuropeptides which cause tachycardia by lowering peripheral blood pressure. SP is widely distributed in the CNS and in peripheral tissues where it plays an important role in pain. SP modulates the activity of cells involved in inflammation. It is a chemoattractant for immune cells, influences their metabolism, and stimulates chemotaxis and lysosomal enzyme secretion by neutrophils (Johnson et al., 1992). SP also stimulates T cell proliferation and immunoglobulin production by B cells. About 10% of T cells express specific SP receptors. Through its ability to increase microvascular permeability SP probably facilitates cell traffic to local sites of inflammation.

8.4.4.7 Vasoactive Intestinal Polypeptide

VIP has partial sequence homology to GHRH but has an inhibitory action on a number of immune responses. It inhibits mitogen-stimulated proliferation of T lymphocytes without affecting B lymphocytes. VIP modulates cytokine production by inhibiting the generation of IL-1 from lymphocytes, and may modulate lymphocyte traffic by inhibiting egress from lymph nodes. Receptors for VIP are present on a number of immune cells.

8.5 Summary

The information required to maintain physiological homeostasis in response to many stressors is sent to the CNS through the nervous and neuroendocrine systems. However, information concerning foreign bodies, bacteria, viruses, tumors, and toxins can only be sent via blood-borne proteins, the cytokines, that are produced by activated immune cells. Cytokines stimulate the HPA axis which, through the secretion of CRH, ACTH, and glucocorticoids, modulates or suppresses the immune reaction. The hypothalamus is the chief integrating organ of the HPA axis, receiving input from the cerebral cortex and the limbic system, and activating not only the neuroendocrine response but also the sympathetic nervous system, which releases catecholamines and also several other neuropeptides. The catecholamines, in turn, stimulate the release of CRH, which further increases catecholamine secretion. This coordinated response is the alarm reaction. When the stressor mobilizes the immune system, then the cytokines are additional catalysts for HPA activation. As endorphins as well as ACTH are released during processing of POMC, pain suppression may accompany the acute phase of stress.

Whereas the alarm reaction is a protective mechanism, a hyper- or hyporesponsive stress system increases susceptibility to many diseases. Overstimulation of the HPA axis due to chronic stress can lead to hypertension, immunosuppression, anorexia nervosa, and several other disorders. A hyporesponsive HPA axis can result in increased susceptibility to autoimmune and inflammatory diseases, chronic fatigue, and somnolence. The hippocampus normally exerts an inhibitory influence on CRH secretion, but prolonged exposure to glucococorticoids, due to stress or age, decreases the number of hippocampal neurons and correspondingly prolongs glucocorticoid secretion. The response to stress is highly individual and may be influenced by perinatal exposure to stress or stress hormones.

The immune system reacts to pathogens and foreign bodies by a local inflammatory response and a systemic acute-phase response, which results in the production of cytokines by immune cells. The inflammatory cytokines include the interleukins IL-1, IL-2, and IL-3 and TNF-α which reach the CNS through the BBB and the circumventricular organs. They activate the HPA axis at all levels and probably influence many other brain regions, although there are individual differences in cytokine efficacy. Cytokines are also produced by central neural and endocrine cells, and by lymphoid organs innervated by sympathetic nerves, so that both local and systemic cytokines coordinate the appropriate neuroendocrine response to an antigen challenge.

The thymus produces thymic hormones which are essential for the differentiation of T lymphocytes and for immune cell stimulation. In addition, the thymus secretes cytokines and a vast number of neuropeptides, immunologically identical to the neuroendocrine peptides. Components of a thymic hormone regulate hypothalamic and pituitary secretion of some neuropeptides. The thymus is under complex neuroendocrine control, both from HPA axis hormones, especially glucocorticoids, and from its own, locally produced neuropeptides. Both glucocorticoids and age cause thymic involution.

The immune system is regulated by the neuropeptides it produces as well as by neuropeptides from the hypothalamus and pituitary. However, the production of ACTH by lymphocytes differs from that of the neuroendocrine system in that CRH causes IL-1 production by macrophages, which then elicits POMC production by B cells. There are several other differences between pituitary hormone production and neuropeptide production by the immune system. Neuropeptides, in turn, regulate the immune system and a balance must be maintained between the immunosuppressive hormones (CRH, ACTH, glucocortiocids, and somatostatin) and the immunostimulatory hormones (PRL, GH, and GHRH). Other neuropeptides have a modulatory action on the immune system. The HPG axis is generally immunostimulatory and is suppressed in stress by CRH and corticosteroids. There are sex-related differences in immune system responsiveness, and changes during the reproductive life of females are correlated with the occurrence of autoimmune diseases. Both the HPA and HPG axes decline with age and autoantibody formation increases correspondingly. Other neuropeptides that modulate the immune system are TSH, endorphins, VP and OT, and SP and VIP.

In part II of this text, families of neuropeptides are discussed and the processes by which they regulate and integrate physiological systems examined.

Neuropeptide Families: The Regulatory Role of Neuropeptides

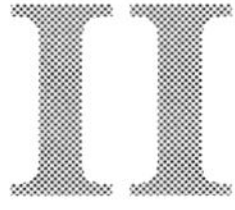

Characteristics of Hypothalamic Regulatory Neuropeptides

9

9.1 Concept of Hypothalamic Regulation of Pituitary Tropic Hormones

9.1.1 Classical Hypothalamic Regulatory Neuropeptides

Our understanding of the relationship between the hypothalamus and the anterior pituitary gland developed chronologically in the reverse order of that of the actual control mechanisms. In the early 1900s the concept developed that the anterior pituitary gland was the "master gland" controlling the endocrine system. This derived from clinical studies which related acromegaly (continued growth of the extremities after maturity due to hypersecretion of growth hormone, or GH) to adenomas of the anterior pituitary gland, and from animal experiments which demonstrated that the stunting of growth after hypophysectomy could be reversed by extracts of the pituitary gland. The pituitary hormones were identified (GH, ACTH, TSH, FSH, LH and PRL), and as they stimulated target tissues elsewhere in the body, they were named *tropic hormones*.

Evidence that the pituitary was not the independent, autonomous ruler of the endocrines, but that the hypothalamus potently influenced pituitary secretion, began to accumulate in the 1940s with Harris's experiments, discussed in chapter 5, which demonstrated that electrical stimulation of the hypothalamus induced ovulation in rabbits, and that the route for such influence was through the portal vessels linking the hypothalamus with the anterior pituitary. The pioneering studies of McCann and Brobeck, (1954), Guillemin and Rosenberg (1955), and Saffran and Schally (1955) provided direct evidence for the first hypothalamic-releasing factor, corticotropin-releasing factor (CRF), which regulated the production of ACTH. Since the structure of this molecule has been determined (Vale et al., 1981), it is more appropriate to name it corticotropin-releasing hormone (CRH).

Following this fundamental discovery, the other hypothalamic regulatory hormones were identified in rapid succession and named the *hypophysiotropic hormones*. Enormous numbers of sheep hypothalami were processed to identify these hypothalamic neuropeptides; the extremely small amounts of active substances derived from tissue is strong evidence of the potency of these neuropeptides, which do not have to be diluted in the systemic circulation but have ready access to the pituitary through the portal vessels via the median eminence (ME) (see chapter 5). The ME provides a link between the brain and the pituitary and as there is no BBB in this structure the hypothalamic peptides can easily cross, in both directions, the basement membrane of the fenestrated capillaries.

More than 40 neuropeptides and other chemical messengers have been localized in the ME but to qualify as a classical hypothalamic regulatory hormone, the following criteria should be met (Merchenthaler, 1991):

1. The messenger should be present in the nerve terminals of the external zone of the ME, the region that consists of the special vasculature and the nerve endings of the hypothalamic neurons.
2. The messenger should be present in higher concentrations in the portal blood than in peripheral plasma.
3. Specific receptors for the messenger should be present on anterior pituitary cells.
4. Anterior pituitary secretion should be affected by the messenger at concentrations found in portal blood.

Only the classical hypothalamic neuropeptides fulfill all these criteria. These are the *release-stimulating hormones* (*-RH*) and the *release-inhibiting hormones* or *factors* (*-IF*). The release-stimulating hormones include CRH, GnRH (first believed to be two hormones LHRH and FSH-RH), thyrotropin–releasing hormone (TRH) and growth hormone–releasing hormone (GHRH). It is uncertain whether there is a MSH releasing hormone separate from CRH. There is also some evidence for several PRL-releasing factors, including oxytocin (OT) and several other neuropeptides. For some time VP was believed to be the corticotropin-releasing factor, but its effects are secondary, or complementary, to those of CRH.

Somatostatin—also called somatotropin release-inhibiting factor (SRIF)—was the first release-inhibiting hormone to be purified, isolated, its structure determined (Brazeau et al., 1973), and its inhibitory action on the production of pituitary growth hormone (somatotropin) demonstrated. There is also evidence for a peptidergic prolactin-inhibiting factor (PIF). The neurotransmitter DA, included in the list of classical hypothalamic messengers, is a potent prolactin inhibitor and is probably the major hypothalamic inhibitor of MSH secretion, although a peptide MSH-inhibiting factor (MIF) has been postulated.

9.1.2 Nonclassical Hypothalamic Regulatory Neuropeptides

In addition to the classical hypothalamic regulatory messengers, there are several putative ones that fulfill some, but not all of the criteria listed above. These include galanin, NPY, β-endorphin, and VIP. These and many other neuropeptides found in the ME may be added to the list of classical regulatory hormones as new techniques for analysis and identification are developed.

In addition, most hypothalamic hormones affect more than one pituitary hormone: TRH stimulates

PRL as well as TSH secretion; somatostatin inhibits not only GH secretion but that of most other pituitary hormones if the dosage is high enough. Several non-hypophyseal neuropeptides may affect pituitary hormone secretion. For example, angiotensin II increases plasma levels of ACTH, PRL, GH, and TSH, but not LH or FSH.

9.1.3 Extrapituitary Functions of Regulatory Neuropeptides

All the neuropeptides that regulate the release of the anterior pituitary hormones have functions apart from their regulatory activities. They may act as neurotransmitters or neuromodulators influencing many physiological functions, as will become clear in the discussions of the individual regulatory neuropeptides later in this chapter.

9.1.4 Localization of Regulatory Neuropeptides

The classical regulatory neuropeptides are found in well-defined areas of the brain: CRH in the PVN; GHRH in the arcuate nucleus; somatostatin in the anterior periventricular area; TRH in the PVN. The catecholamine DA is found in the A12 region of the hypothalamus and the A2 and A4 regions of the brainstem. Almost 70% of the LHRH-immunoreactive neurons are in the septum, preoptic, and suprachiasmatic areas (Merchenthaler, 1991).

Most of the hypothalamic regulatory neuropeptides are colocalized with other neuropeptides and classical neurotransmitters but as far as the present evidence shows, there is no coexpression of more than one classical hormone in one neuron.

9.2 Feedback Controls

9.2.1 Long, Short, and Ultrashort Feedback Loops

9.2.1.1 Long Feedback Loop

Sayers and Sayers (1947) were the first to show that the corticosteroids could exert a negative feedback action on the anterior pituitary and this important concept was extended by Moore and Price (Price, 1975) who demonstrated that the gonadal steroids could suppress the release of hypophyseal FSH and LH. Subsequently, it was shown that the adrenal glucocorticoids suppressed ACTH secretion by inhibiting the release of CRH by the hypothalamus, as well as by depressing ACTH secretion by corticotrophs of the anterior pituitary. This inhibition of pituitary and hypothalamic hormones by the hormones of the target organ is known as the *long-loop negative feedback* and has been well documented for glucocorticoids, ACTH, and CRH, and for thyroxine, TSH, and TRH.

The picture is less clear for the gonadal steroids. The long-standing belief that estrogen, progesterone, and androgen exert inhibitory feedback effects on LH secretion by suppressing the release of hypothalamic GnRH has not been experimentally confirmed despite much effort expended on this problem over the last two decades. These steroids appear to act by diminishing the ability of GnRH to evoke LH secretion from the pituitary gonadotrophs. There is even considerable evidence that the gonadal steroids facilitate the release and synthesis of GnRH, depending upon the stage of the estrous cycle. It is clear that estradiol exerts a profound positive feedback effect on the sensitivity of pituitary LH to GnRH to effect the crucial LH surge prior to ovulation (Kalra and Kalra, 1994).

9.2.1.2 Short Feedback Loop

In addition, many of the pituitary hormones suppress their own release without circulating through the systemic circulation. These hormones reach the hypothalamus to inhibit the relevant releasing hormones either through retrograde transport in the portal system or via the CSF. This is the *short-loop negative feedback* (Motta et al., 1965). The short loop is used by LH, FSH, ACTH, PRL, and GH, and probably also by TSH.

9.2.1.3 Ultrashort Feedback Loop

The *ultrashort negative feedback loop* refers to the hypothalamic or pituitary neuropeptide directly inhibiting its own release, occurring at the site of its production. This may happen as a direct recurrent inhibition or through an interneuron that affects the rate of discharge of the hypothalamic neuron. The ultrashort-loop negative feedback has been shown for the hypothalamic hormones somatostatin, GHRH, and GnRH (McCann and Krulich, 1989), and for the pituitary hormones ACTH and GH. These three forms of negative feedback are illustrated in figure 9.1

9.2.2 Involvement of Additional Neuronal Circuits, Neuropeptides, and Neurotransmitters

The description of the classical feedback loops simplifies an exceedingly complex situation. The neuronal circuitry within the hypothalamus involved in the regulation of GnRH and LH incorporates other neuropeptides and amino acids as well as NO (figure 9.2). This holds true for the regulation of CRH, which is modified by the combined activities of many neuronal pathways that project to the PVN and the ME. Neural input from the limbic system is stimulatory, whereas input from the hippocampus is inhibitory. These neuronal messages work in concert with circulating factors, such as the glucocorticoids and the cytokines.

9.2.3 Dependence on Neuronal Sensitivity

The sensitivity, and consequently the responsivity, of the hypothalamic neurosecretory neurons is profoundly affected by corticosteroids, especially under stressful conditions. Figure 9.3 exemplifies the many elements that impinge on the PVN to regulate its secretion of CRH.

9.3 Regulation of Synthesis of Hypothalamic Regulatory Neuropeptides

Some hormones act directly on the firing of hypothalamic neurons, some on electrical activity and G protein–coupled mechamisms. Hormones can activate or inhibit specific genes. The rate of transcription may be increased, the half-life may be increased or decreased, as evidenced by changes in mRNA accumulation. For example, the ventromedial nucleus (VMN) of the hypothalamus, the primary site of control for female reproductive behavior, responds to estradiol with induction of ribosomal RNA formation, induction of receptors for progesterone and oxytocin, as well as by increased synaptogenesis (McEwen, 1991). To complicate matters, the responsiveness of the brain to the same hormone differs in males and females. Estradiol induces more progesterone receptors in the female hypothalamus than in the male, and induces a dramatic increase in synapse formation in the female VMN but fails to induce synaptogenesis in the male VMN despite the presence of estrogen receptors in this structure (Corini and McEwen, 1990),

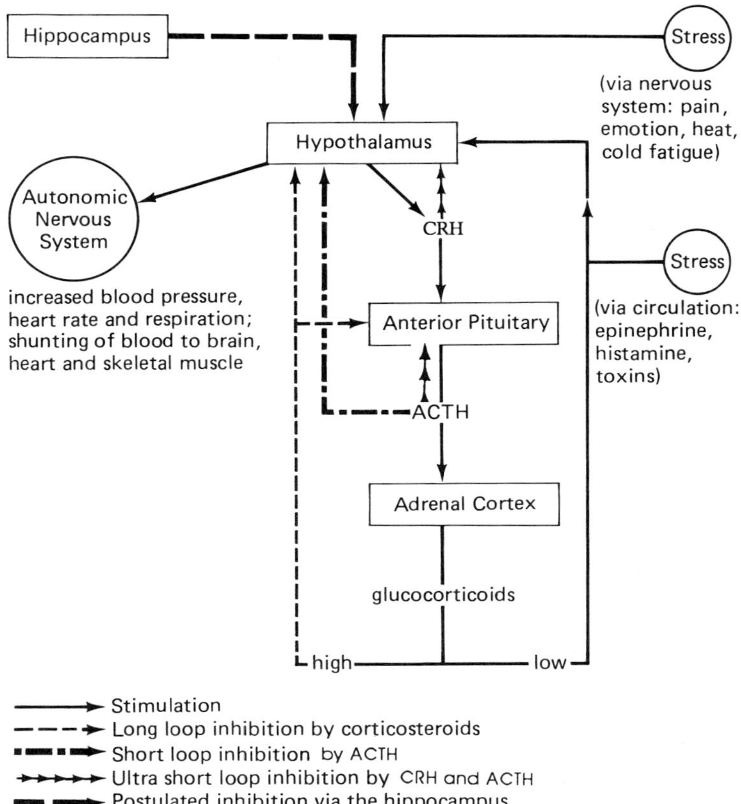

Figure 9.1
Stress causes the secretion of releasing hormones by the hypothalamus. Secretion may be inhibited by various negative feedback mechanisms: a long loop, a short loop, and an ultrashort loop. The ultrashort loop shown is the inhibition of corticotropin-releasing hormone (CRH) on its own secretion by the hypothalamus; the inhibition by ACTH on pituitary corticotroph secretion of ACTH is not shown. Only the release of CRH is depicted but other hypothalamic hormones (thyrotropin-releasing hormone, melanocyte-stimulating hormone, vasopressin, oxytocin, and β-endorphin) may be secreted depending upon the specific type of stress.

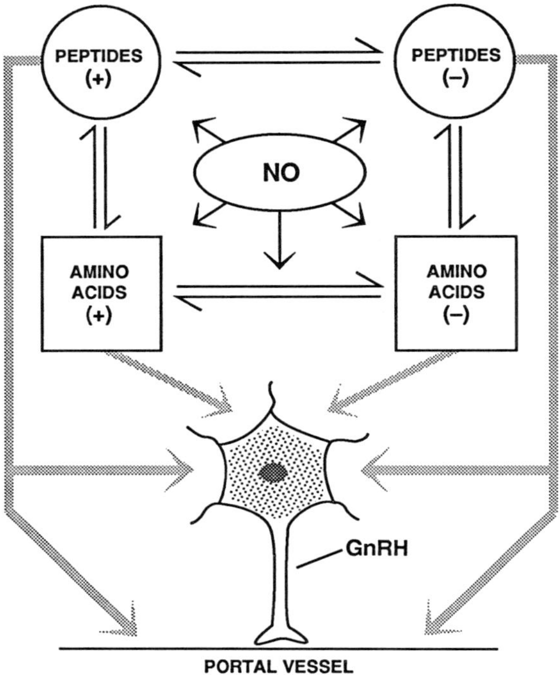

Figure 9.2
Diagrammatic representation of gonadotropin releasing hormone (GnRH) pulse-generator circuitry in the hypothalamus. The core network in this circuitry is composed of neurons that produce peptides and amino acids which exert either excitatory (+) or inhibitory (−) influences on luteinizing hormone (LH) secretion. Nitric oxide (NO) modulates GnRH release either directly or indirectly or via the inhibitory or excitatory messengers. Components of this circuitry appear to communicate with each other, which is crucial in sustaining the episodic basal and cyclic GnRH discharge. These signals are also released in the hypothalamus and into the hypophyseal portal system. There are therefore two sites of action, one in the hypothalamus to modulate GnRH secretion into the portal system and another at the level of the pituitary gonadatrophs to modify GnRH-induced LH release. Interactions between these messengers, at the level of both the hypothalamus and the pituitary gonadotrophs, are regulated by gonadal steroids (not shown). (From Kalra and Kalra, 1994.)

Second-messenger systems and their ligands are coupled to activation of the genes involved in the synthesis of the releasing hormones and the release-inhibiting hormones. The hypothalamic neurons must have multiple receptors for a wide variety of ligands since so many hormones and transmitters affect their secretion. For example, the CRH gene may be activated by a series of different ligands, including catecholamines, 5-HT, ACh, IL-1, and IL-6, and the expression of the CRH gene is inhibited by glucocorticoids, GABA, SP, ANH, opiate peptides, and precursors of NO. These ligands usually act through protein kinase A, protein kinase C, or the glucocorti-

Figure 9.3
Schematic representation of the integrated neuroendocrine control of ACTH secretion. Corticotropin-releasing hormone (CRF) cells in the paraventricular nucleus (PVN) receive afferents from other hypothalamic (hpt) neurons, limbic structures, the subfornical organ, brainstem, and the PVN itself. Excitatory amino acids of unknown origin and humoral factors such as glucocorticoids, interleukins, growth factors, and so forth, directly influence the activity of CRF neurons. Some of these act through specific receptors on the perikarya or nerve terminals. CRF neurons co-express a variety of chemical messengers, including arginine vasopressin (AVP), enkephalins (ENK), angiotensin II (ANG), neurotensin (NT), cholecystokinin (CCK), peptide histidine isoleucine (PHI), vasoactive intestinal polypeptide (VIP), and γ-aminobutyric acid (GABA). CRF and the coexpressed substances are transported from the perikarya by axoplasmic transport to nerve terminals in the median eminence, where they are released into capillaries of the portal system, from whence they reach the sinusoids of the anterior pituitary. CRF stimulates the secretion of ACTH into the systemic circulation. In the adrenal cortex, ACTH stimulates the secretion of glucocorticoids, which, in turn, inhibit CRF production by the PVN and ACTH secretion by the pituitary. POMC, pro-opiomelanocortin; NPY, neuropeptide Y, NE, norepinephrine; GAL, galinin; E, epinephrine; 5HT (serotonin). (From Petrusz and Merchenthaler, 1992.)

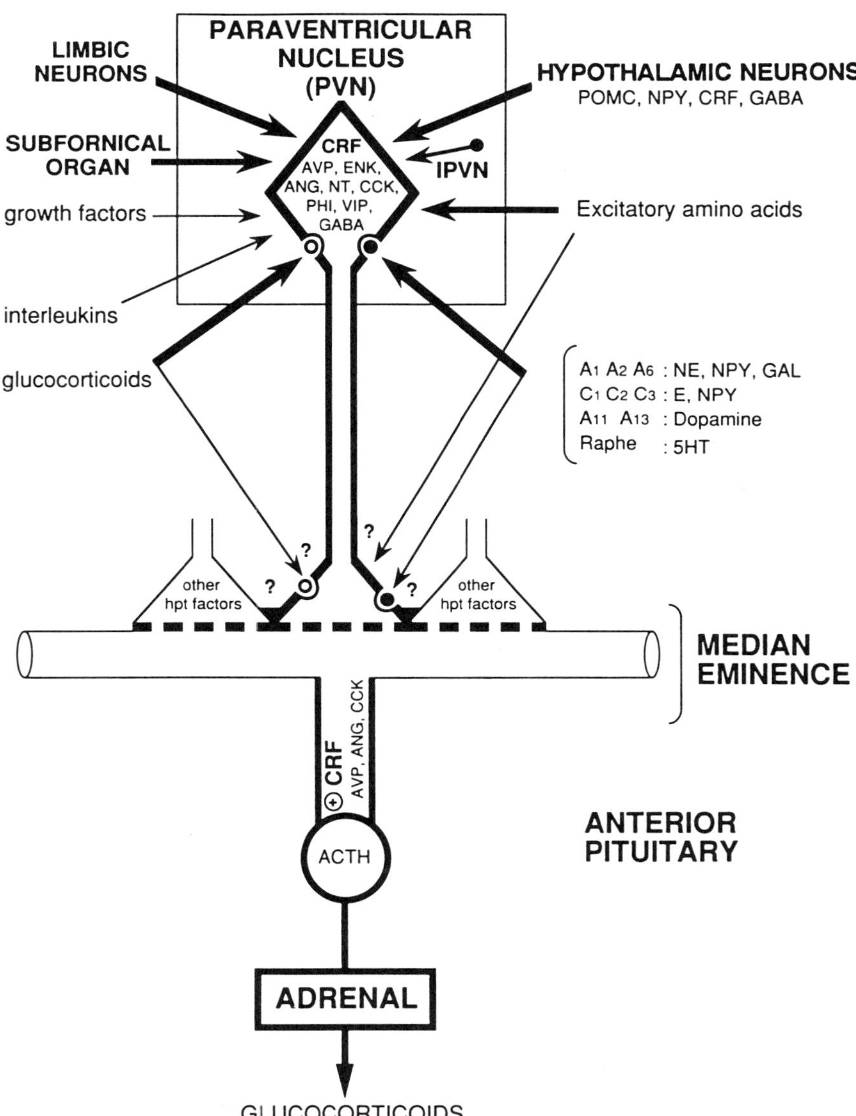
PARAVENTRICULAR NUCLEUS (PVN)
LIMBIC NEURONS
HYPOTHALAMIC NEURONS
POMC, NPY, CRF, GABA
SUBFORNICAL ORGAN
CRF
AVP, ENK, ANG, NT, CCK, PHI, VIP, GABA
IPVN
growth factors
Excitatory amino acids
interleukins
glucocorticoids
A1 A2 A6 : NE, NPY, GAL
C1 C2 C3 : E, NPY
A11 A13 : Dopamine
Raphe : 5HT
?
other hpt factors
MEDIAN EMINENCE
CRF
AVP, ANG, CCK
ANTERIOR PITUITARY
ACTH
ADRENAL
GLUCOCORTICOIDS

coid second-messenger systems (Majzoub et al., 1993). It should be realized that hormones rarely act alone and gene induction is often the cumulation of many interacting factors.

9.4 Mechanism of Action of Hypothalamic Regulatory Neuropeptides

Neuropeptides act by combining with highly specific receptors on their target cells and activating second-messenger pathways (see chapter 6). The second-messenger system used by the pituitary cells in response to hypothalamic stimulation or inhibition varies with the pituitary cell type. CRH stimulation of ACTH release appears to be mediated by cAMP in the corticotrophs; GHRH stimulates the somatotrophs to activate the cAMP pathway for LH release, but cAMP is of considerably less importance for gonadotroph production of FSH. Prostaglandins can activate the production of cAMP and seem to be involved in the release of GH and ACTH. Some pituitary cell types may utilize the phosphoinositol system. Calcium is essential to the releasing process, both extracellular Ca^{2+} and Ca^{2+} mobilized from intracellular stores. The hypothalamic inhibiting hormones, somatostatin and PIF, probably act by inhibiting adenylate cyclase and also by decreasing the availability of Ca^{2+} to the cell (McCann, 1991).

The regulatory hypothalamic neuropeptides act very rapidly on the pituitary cells to promote or inhibit pituitary hormone release and it appears that the release itself acts a stimulus to synthesis of the specific pituitary hormone involved. Increased synthesis is correlated with an increase in mRNA, which may be secondary to the release process.

9.5 Modification of the Adult Hypothalamus by Perinatal Influences

Exposure of the fetus or neonate to stressors or changes in sex steroids can permanently affect the HPA or HPG axes.

9.5.1 *Effects of Perinatal Exposure to Sex Steroids*

9.5.1.1 Normal Development of the Sexual Hypothalamus

Perinatal exposure of the CNS to gonadal steroid hormones results in both biochemical and morphological changes, termed *sexual dimorphisms*, among CNS neurons. Sexual dimorphisms have been demonstrated in many brain regions involved with reproductive function, including the VMN, suprachiasmatic nucleus, preoptic area (POA), arcuate nucleus, and amygdala. These changes result in sexually differentiated behaviors in adult life (Goy and McEwen, 1980; Arnold and Gorski, 1984; Toran-Allerand, 1984). This organizational effect of the sex steroids sets the stage for the development of either an "acyclic" hypothalamus in the male or a "cyclic" hypothalamus in the female (McEwen et al., 1977; McEwen, 1978, 1983). The basic or "default' neuronal pattern in the developing brain is believed to be "female-like." It is the presence of a fetal or early postnatal testosterone surge during this *critical period of* ontogeny that ultimately leads to the formation of the acyclic hypothalamus in which GnRH, LH, and FSH and the testicular androgens are secreted in a tonic manner. This hormonal sequence is essential to normal adult male sexual behaviors (interest in a receptive female, mounting, and intromission), behaviors that are referred to as the *activational effects* of the sex steroids.

Similarly, the estrous or menstrual cycle of the normal adult female depends on the cyclic production of GnRH, FSH, estradiol, LH, and progesterone. The proper sequence of these activational hormones is essential to ovulation, preparation of the uterus for implantation, and, at least in rodents, to almost all aspects of female sexual and maternal behavior. The primary hormonal control site in the female is the VMN of the hypothalamus; for the male it is the POA of the hypothalamus.

9.5.1.2 Sex Hormone Modification of the Developing Hypothalamus

Genetic males castrated in the first few days after birth (the critical period) are permanently feminized and demasculinized in adulthood (Grady et al., 1965). Absence of testosterone at the stage of hypothalamic differentiation leaves both males and females sensitive to female hormones, so both display female behavior (Levine, 1966). A single injection of testosterone to a female rat during the first few days of life irreversibly masculinizes her: her hypothalamus becomes acyclic, and if primed with sex steroids in adulthood, she is unable to ovulate or express normal female behavior, such as receptivity (lordosis) to a sexually active male.

9.5.2 Effects of Perinatal Exposure to Stress or Stress Hormones

In rats, male offspring of stressed mothers are particularly susceptible to prenatal stress and display poor male sexual behavior as adults (Ward, 1972). This is due to the increased levels of maternal ACTH, which curtail fetal androgen levels necessary during this critical period for the development of an acyclic hypothalamus. Male rats exposed during the critical perinatal period to stress hormones, such as ACTH or corticosterone, or to nicotine, which evokes endogenous ACTH secretion, undergo a similar disruption in the masculinization of the hypothalamus, manifested by a dramatic decrease in male sexual behavior (Rhees and Fleming, 1981; Segarra and Strand, 1989; Segarra et al., 1991. Studies by Alves et al. (1993) indicated that whereas female rats are less susceptible to perinatal stress, there is a decreased lordotic response and delayed vaginal opening (a sign of delayed reproductive maturation). Coupled with these changes is an increase in the maturation of the monoamine systems that innervate the hypothalamus (figure 9.4). Both 5-HT and DA are believed to be involved in the control of reproductive processes in the female rat.

The type of stress to which neonates are exposed influences their subsequent sensitivity to stress. Neonatal rats exposed to brief handling, to maternal separation for 3 hours, or left totally undisturbed, were compared as adults in terms of their pituitary-adrenal reponsiveness to restraint stress. As illustrated in figure 9.5, the maternally separated group reacted with a high level of ACTH and corticosterone, whereas the briefly separated animals responded with a 40% reduction in corticosteroid secretion as compared to the nonhandled rats. These differences among the groups were correlated with differences in ME content of CRH and VP, and with differences in hypothalamic CRF mRNA, which was lowest in the handled rats and highest in the maternally separated animals (Plotsky et al., 1993).

Sexual orientation, that is, heterosexuality or homosexuality, has been related to sex differences in the hypothalamus. Many factors may determine sexual orientation, such as genetic factors, sex hormones, and maternal stress, the latter being thought to increase human homosexuality both in males and females. The stages in dvelopment at which sex steroids determine sexual differentiation of the human brain are in the first half of gestation when the genitalia are being

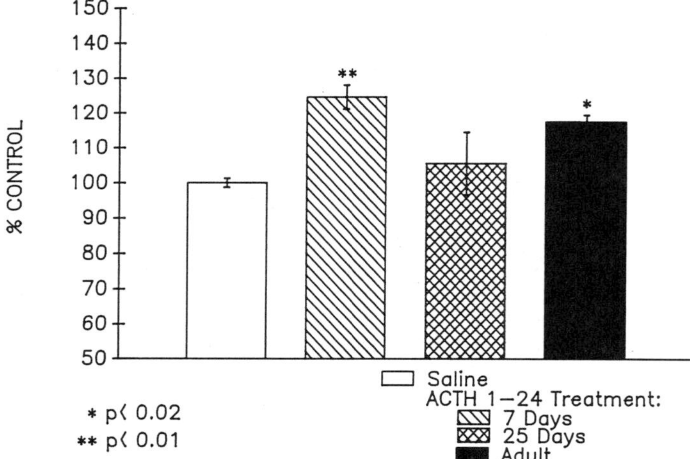

Figure 9.4
Changes in high-affinity specific serotonin (5-HT) uptake (percent of control) in the hypothalamus of 7-day, 25-day, and adult (80- to 90-day) rats following daily ACTH 1–24 injections (0.5 mg/kg subcutaneously) during the first week of postnatal life. Values for saline-treated animals (control) at each age were normalized to 100% and are represented by one bar (error bar is the mean of the errors over the three time points). There is a significant increase in 5-HT uptake at 7 days, which, although not evident at 25 days, reappears in adulthood. (From Alves et al., 1993.)

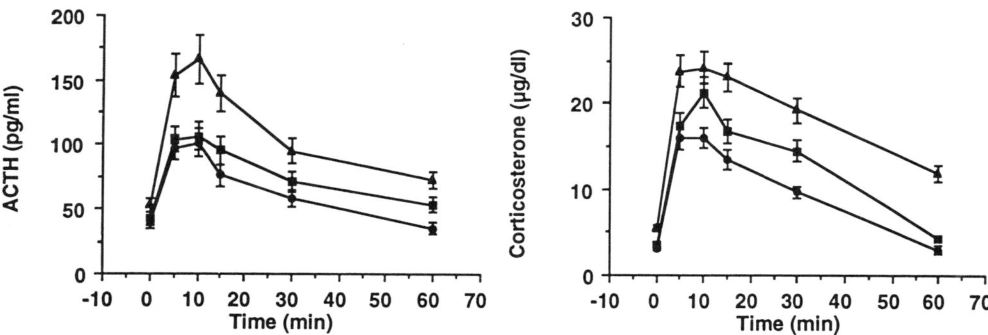

Figure 9.5
Effect of neonatal environmental experience on adult ACTH and corticosterone secretory responses to restraint. As neonates the rats were subjected to one of three treatments. (1) nonhandled (NH) rats (squares) were left undisturbed; (2) briefly handled (H) rats (circles) were separated from the dam for 15 minutes daily; (3) maternal separation (MS) rats (triangles) were separated from the dam for 3 hours daily. All groups showed significant stressor-induced pituitary-adrenal secretory responses as adults. Furthermore, the ACTH responses of the NH and MS groups were significantly different from one another ($P < .05$). Error bars represent SEM. (From Plotsky et al., 1993.)

formed, during the perinatal period, and during puberty. This controversial topic is very well reviewed by Swaab and Hofman (1995).

9.5.3 Perinatal Influences in Primates, Including Humans

The long-term effects of neonatal stress on the regulation of the HPA axis is not confined to rodents. The offspring of rhesus monkeys stressed during pregnancy show enhanced HPA axis reponsivity to stressors later in life and the most profound effects were from stress early in gestation (Clarke et al., 1994). The appalling consequences of maternal deprivation in rhesus monkeys separated from their mothers at birth have been dramatically described in the work of the late psychologist Harry F. Harlow (1986). These young monkeys become withdrawn, fearsome, and aggressive.

There may be considerable relevance of these animal studies to humans. Exposure of the human fetus to nicotine as a result of maternal smoking can influence both the HPG and the HPA, with unknown consequences to subsequent sexual behavior and susceptibility to stress. The animal experiments with nicotine were equivalent to the amount of nicotine absorbed by a woman smoking one cigarette a day. Maternal stress during pregnancy has been shown to affect human infants.

In humans, infant and childhood separation stress is identified with a permanent increase in β-endorphin and cortisol, and a marked increase in adult psychopathology (Breier, 1989). Maternal psychosocial stress during the third trimester is associated with increased maternal plasma levels of ACTH and cortisol, amplified by placental release of CRH. Precocious elevation of CRH levels increases the risk of premature delivery and decreased birth weight. These observations show the close linkage between the HPA axis and birth outcome (Sandman et al., 1997). Childhood trauma has been linked to many cases of child aggression, and of the many forms of abuse and neglect, maternal deprivation is perhaps the most damaging to a child (Ferris, 1996).

9.6 Summary

Hypothalamic regulatory neuropeptides stimulate or inhibit the secretion and release of the anterior pituitary tropic hormones, so named because they stimulate peripheral target organs. The regulatory hormones reach the anterior pituitary gland through the portal vessels in the ME. The criteria required for classical hypothalamic neuropeptides include the presence of the neuropeptide in the nerve terminals in the ME; a higher concentration of the neuropeptide in portal blood than in plasma; specific receptors for the neuropeptide on anterior pituitary cells; and the ability to affect anterior pituitary cells at physiological concentrations. In addition to their effects on the pituitary, the hypothalamic regulatory peptides affect many other physiological functions.

Hypothalamic release–stimulating neuropeptides are CRH, GnRH, TRH, and GHRH, which cause the release of ACTH and MSH, LH and FSH, and TSH and GH respectively. The only uncontested hypothalamic release–inhibiting hormone is somatostatin although there is a putative peptidergic PRL–inhibiting factor (PIF) and a putative MSH–inhibiting factor (MIF). The neurotransmitter DA probably is the physiological hypothalamic inhibitor of both PRL and MSH. Many other neuropeptides affect anterior pituitary secretion but do not fulfill all the criteria listed above for the classical hypophyseal regulatory neuropeptides.

There are several negative feedback controls that mediate the release of the hypothalamic and anterior pituitary neuropeptides. Hormonal secretions by the target organ, for example, adrenal glucocorticoids, inhibit the release of both the hypothalamic (CRH) and pituitary (ACTH) neuropeptides by a long feedback loop. Direct local suppression of pituitary secretion by its own hormones is the short feedback loop, and the direct local suppression of hypothalamic neuropeptides on their own release forms the ultrashort negative feedback loop. In addition, complex neuronal circuits, hormones, and neurotransmitters are involved in modifying hypothalamic neurosecretion. This may be through electrophysiological changes, activation or inhibition of specific genes, alterations in neuronal sensitivity, and differential sexual responses. The second-messenger system activated by the pituitary cells in response to hypothalamic stimulation varies with the cell type.

Exposure of the fetus or neonate to stressors or changes in sex steroids at critical periods in development permanently affects the adult hypothalamus. The organizational effect of the sex steroids determines the development of the "acyclic" male hypothalamus or the "cyclic" female hypothalamus. This is fundamental for the development of female estrous or menstrual cycles and the later appropriate female or male sexual behaviors when activated at puberty by the sex steroids. Similarly, exposure to maternal stress, smoking, or ACTH during the perinatal period negatively affects subsequent sexual behavior, especially in males. The harmful effects of stress, especially the stress of maternal deprivation, can be seen in rhesus monkeys and in human infants.

Chapter 10 discusses the individual hypothalamic hormones that regulate the secretion of pituitary hormones. Other non-hypothalamic neuropeptides that may act on pituitary secretion are considered briefly.

Hypophysiotropic Neuropeptides: TRH, CRH, GnRH, GHRH, SS, PACAP, DSIP

10

10.1 Hypothalamic Releasing Hormones

10.1.1 Thyrotropin-Releasing Hormone (TRH)

10.1.1.1 Historical Significance

It has been suggested that the discovery of TRH was the single most important event in the development of the discipline of neuroendocrinology, for it succeeded in legitimizing the field in the face of a host of skeptics who believed the hypothalamic releasing factors were figments of the imagination. It makes a fascinating story and the intense scientific rivalry between Roger Guillemin and Andrew Schally, who shared the Nobel prize for medicine or physiology in 1977 (with Rosalyn Yalow) for the elucidation of the chemical structure of this tripeptide, is dramatically described by Reichlin (1989). Their success encouraged other neuroendocrinologists to continue their efforts to isolate the other, far more complex regulating hormones.

Guillemin finally obtained 1 mg of material from 300,000 sheep hypothalami and showed TRH to be composed of only three amino acids, glutamine, histidine, and proline, with a molecular weight of 362. Six isomeric tripeptides of these three amino acids were synthesized and tested for biological activity after treatment with acetic anhydride to reproduce the blocked N-terminus of the natural TRH. None of the untreated tripeptides had any biological activity and only one of the treated tripeptides, H-Glu-His-Pro-OH, showed some TRH activity. Full potency for this tripeptide required amidation of the C-terminus (Burgus et al., 1970). The structure of the active TRH may be represented as pyro-Glu-His-Pro-$CONH_2$.

10.1.1.2 Phylogenetic Distribution

Although TRH is found in large quantities in the hypothalamus and brain of submammalian vertebrates, including amphibians and fish, it does not stimulate pituitary-thyroid function in species lower than Aves. TRH appears to have its first action on the pituitary in amphibians, in which it stimulates PRL secretion. The tripeptide is not species-specific: Schally showed that porcine TRH has the same structure as ovine TRH (Nair et al., 1970). The role of TRH in the regulation of pituitary-thyroid function appears late in evolution, representing an example of an old hormone acquiring a new function, in addition to its several other roles as a neural peptide.

10.1.1.3 Anatomical Distribution

TRH is present in large amounts in axons originating from neurons in the medial parvocellular portion of the PVN, and terminating in the ME in close apposition to the portal capillary system, to form the *PVN-tuberoinfundibular system* regulating TSH release. Some axons terminate in the posterior pituitary, which may provide an alternative route by which TRH can regulate anterior pituitary secretion through the blood vessels that connect the two structures. TRH-containing neurons are found in many other regions of the hypothalamus, such as the arcuate and tuberomammillary nuclei, but as they do not project to the ME they probably are not involved in the hypothalamus-pituitary-thyroid (HPT) axis (Lechan and Toni, 1992).

Almost 70% of the total TRH is found outside the hypothalamus, although concentrations in these areas are not as high as in the hypothalamus, except for the spinal cord, in which levels are comparable to that of the hypothalamus. TRH-secreting neurons are distributed to structures related to the limbic system (amygdala, nucleus accumbens, olfactory lobe), to the septum, to the spinal cord and medulla oblongata, including the dorsal motor nuclei of the vagus, and in the spinal vestibular nucleus. TRH-containing neurons in the PVN are unique in that they are rarely associated with another neuropeptide (Ceccatelli et al., 1989), but most TRH-containing fibers of the spinal cord and medulla oblongata and neurons in the motor nuclei contain both TRH and SP. There seems to be a functional interaction between TRH and 5-HT since most 5-HT terminals contain TRH (Arvidsson et al., 1992). TRH is also present in the anterior lobe of the pituitary, with a subpopulation of somatotrophs (which secrete GH) possessing pro-TRH mRNA and TRH, as well as GH (Bruhn et al., 1994).

TRH is present throughout the gastrointestinal tract, especially in the cecum and in the islets of Langerhans of the pancreas. Lesser amounts are found in almost all peripheral tissues, including the placenta. The widespread distribution of TRH to so many neuronal and non-neuronal structures provides an anatomical basis for its many physiological functions, apart from its actions as a hypothalamic regulatory neuropeptide.

10.1.1.4 Synthesis and Inactivation of TRH

TRH is *synthesized* according to the classical peptide biosynthetic pathway from a larger preprohormone molecule that is post-translationally cleaved, processed, and packaged into secretory granules. Prepro-TRH of the rat is a 255–amino acid protein with a molecular size of 26 kD. It contains five copies of the sequence Gln-His-Pro-Gly, with at least two flanking-region peptides (Lechan et al., 1986), whereas the human TRH genome contains a sixth copy of the TRH coding sequence at its C-terminal end. Human prepro-TRH has about 60% amino acid homology with that of the rat. The rat TRH transcriptional unit extends 2.6 kb and has three exons interrupted by two introns (figure 10.1). The 5′-untranslated region of the mRNA is encoded by exon 1; the signal sequence and most of the N-terminus is encoded by exon 2. The remainder of the translated sequence of proTRH is encoded by exon 3.

Pro-TRH undergoes differential proteolytic processing in various tissues to generate not only the genuine TRH and the connecting peptides but also several other novel peptides. TRH is cleaved first as a tetrapeptide before it enters axonal processes and then is cyclized at the glutamine residue to form pyroglutamic acid. Finally, there is an exchange of glycine for NH_2 (Sevarino et al., 1989). Connecting peptides are colocalized with TRH in nerve endings in the ME and coreleased through a mechanism involving voltage-operated Ca^{2+} channels. The connecting peptide Ps4 potentiates the action of TRH on TSH release in the pituitary, demonstrating that these two peptides, which originate from a single multifunctional precursor, may function synergistically to promote hormonal secretion (Ladram et al., 1994). There is a daily rhythm in TRH and TRH mRNA in the hypothalamus, with basal TRH release peaking at 7 A.M.

TRH is inactivated by the TRH-degrading ectoenzyme, a peptidase with a very high degree of substrate specificity, and which is regulated at the pituitary level by both estradiol and thyroid hormones. Substrate specificity is unusual for neuropeptide inactivation, since they are generally inactivated by nonspecific proteolytic enzymes. TRH is unique in that it has a cyclized

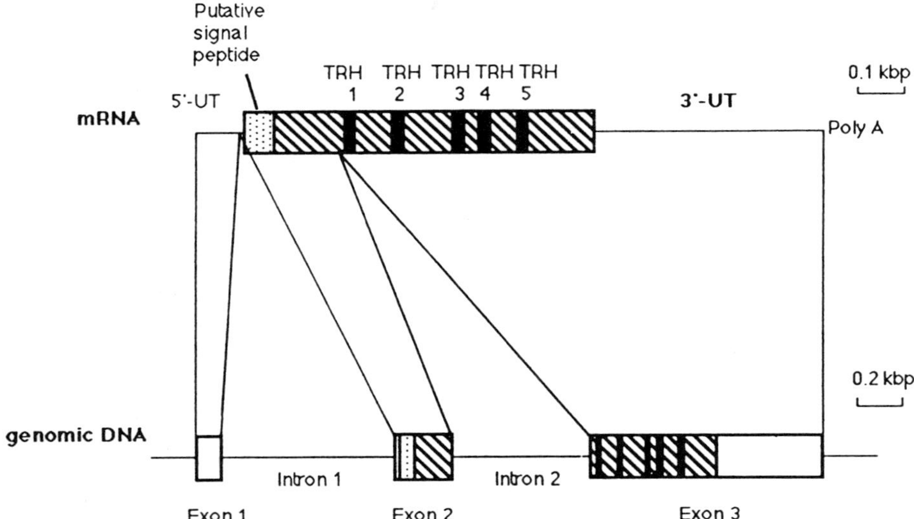

Figure 10.1
Structure of the rat preprothyrotropin-releasing hormone (TRH) gene: schematic diagram of the messenger RNA (mRNA) (top line) and genomic DNA (bottom line). The 5′-untranslated region (5′UT) and 3′-untranslated region (3′-UT) are shown by the solid line (top) and open boxes (bottom). The signal peptide is indicated by a stippled box. The striped boxes indicate connecting and terminal peptides. The solid boxes indicate the TRH-coding regions. (From Lee et al., 1989.)

N-terminus, an amidated C-terminus, and an internal proline residue: consequently it is not degraded by aminopeptidase, carboxypeptidase, or by nonspecific peptidases such as pepsin. Only the TRH-degrading ectopeptidase can hydrolyze TRH by cleaving the pyroGlu-His bond (Bauer, 1995).

10.1.1.5 Regulation of TRH Synthesis and Actions

a. Long-loop negative feedback on the hypothalamus by thyroid hormone

The synthesis of TRH in PVN neurons is regulated by circulating thyroid hormone. TRH neurons in the medial and periventricular subdivisions of the PVN contain functional thyroid hormone receptors which respond to thyroid hormone through a decrease in TRH gene expression and a fall in TRH synthesis. Thyroidectomy or the oral administration of thioamines results in hypothyroidism and a consequent increase in pro-TRH mRNA in the PVN. The administration of high doses of thyroid hormone prevents the hypothyroid-induced rise in TRH (Segerson et al., 1987). This feedback regulation of TRH by thyroid hormone is a direct effect, apparently mediated by the active form of the hormone, triiodothyronine (T_3). T_3 also decreases TRH secretion into the hypophyseal portal blood (Wang et al., 1994). TRH secretion by other PVN neurons and by other brain TRH neurons is not regulated in this manner.

b. Long-loop negative feedback of thyroid hormones on the anterior pituitary

Both thyroid hormones, T_3 and thyroxine (T_4), exert a negative feedback effect on the thyrotrophs of the anterior pituitary. TRH also has a negative effect on the anterior pituitary cells as TRH receptors on pituitary cell membranes are downregulated by increasing TRH concentrations, decreasing the number of receptors but not their affinity.

c. Ultrashort loop negative feedback of TRH

There is probably an ultrashort feedback regulation of TRH by its own secretion. Many TRH-containing neurons from other brain areas impinge on the TRH neurons of the HPT axis.

d. Regulation by humoral and external factors

TRH neurons in the PVN are crowded together with other neuropeptide-containing neurons such as neuropeptide Y (NPY) and somatostatin, which have an inhibitory effect on TRH secretion. TRH neurons receive a dense input from neurons originating in other brain areas, which release *catecholamines* at their synaptic contacts with the cell bodies and dendrites of TRH-containing neurons. Epinephrine and NE stimulate TRH secretion, whereas DA is probably inhibitory. The actions of 5-HT are not clear. The catecholamines primarily affect the secretion of TRH into the portal vessels rather than acting on TRH gene expression.

Many factors in addition to thyroid hormones affect the sensitivity of anterior pituitary cells to TRH. *Growth hormone* influences the TSH response to TRH: humans administered GH have a diminished TSH response to TRH and may develop hypothyroidism as a result of the GH therapy (Root et al., 1970). Reports on the effects of glucocorticoids are conflicting, depending on whether the experiments are done in situ

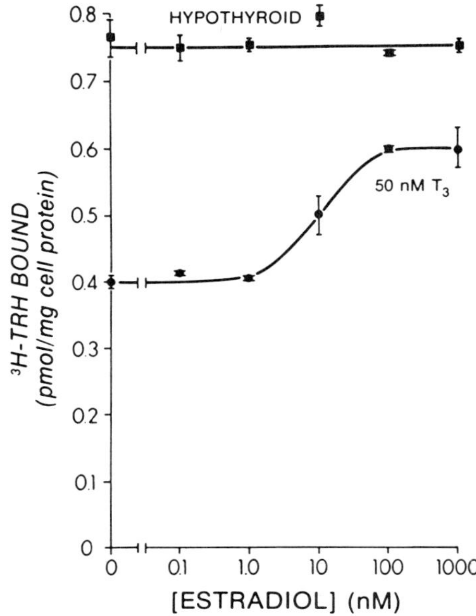

Figure 10.2
The effect of estradiol on binding of [^{3}H]–thyrotropin-releasing hormone (TRH) to TRH receptors on growth hormone cells in the presence and absence of triiodothyronine (T_3). (From Perrone et al., 1980.)

or on cultured cells. Glucocorticoids inhibit the HPT axis in both rat and humans, most probably by an indirect effect on the TRH neuron since glucocorticoids have the opposite effect on cultured hypothalamic cells, stimulating the expression of TRH peptide and TRH mRNA (Luo et al., 1995). T_3 increases pro-TRH gene expression in cultured anterior pituitary cells and glucococorticoids potentiate this effect. Estrogens also increase TRH receptor number in cultured cells, but this effect is dependent upon the presence of T_3 in the growth medium (figure 10.2). Acute cold stimulus causes a rapid increase in plasma TSH after 15 minutes exposure to 4°C and an increase in hypothalamic TRH mRNA.

10.1.1.6 TRH Receptors and Second Messengers

The TRH receptor is restricted to a small fraction of the anterior pituitary cells, that is, the thyrotrophs and mammotrophs (PRL-secreting cells), and to a much lesser extent, to some somatotrophs (GH-secreting cells). These cells contain high-affinity binding sites for TRH and have a high degree of specificity. The TRH receptor exhibits strict structural specificity in all three amino acid positions. Substitution of the N-terminal pGlu with a noncyclic Gln decreases binding affinity 200-fold, for example (Hinkle, 1989). A potent TRH analog, *N*-methyl-TRH, has a greater affinity for TRH receptors that TRH itself and is more potent in stimulating TSH and PRL secretion. Several TRH receptor isoforms have been identified: TR $\alpha 1$, TR $\beta 1$, and TR $\beta 2$; the first two receptor types are most prevalent on TRH cells in the PVN (Lechan et al., 1994).

TRH effects on pituitary cells are mediated by an increase in intracellular Ca^{2+} concentration or through a Ca^{2+}-independent protein kinase activation: these events then involve the phosphatidylinositol second-messenger system (Gershengorn and Thaw, 1985) and result in increased TSH secretion and exocytosis. Interestingly, G proteins mediate the response of hypoglossal motor neurons to TRH: these excitatory responses are apparently independent of activation of protein kinase C or adenylate cyclase and do not involve increases in intracellular inositol triphosphate and Ca^{2+} concentrations (Bayliss et al., 1994). It is probable that the second-messenger pathways used by TRH on neurosecretory cells differ considerably from those used by excitatory neurons.

10.1.1.7 Functions of TRH

The most important physiological role of TRH is the *stimulation of TSH secretion*. The response of the pituitary thyrotrophs is rapid: in humans an i.v. dose of 75 ng/minute brings peak TSH secretion in 20 to 30 minutes; in rats an i.v. bolus of 50 ng brings plasma TSH to a peak in 5 minutes. In addition to its well-defined role as a thyroid-stimulating hormone, *TRH promotes PRL secretion* but does not appear to play a dominant role in the physiological control of PRL release.

TRH acts as *neurotransmitter* and *neuromodulator* (see chapter 7). In the hypothalamus or in spinal cord slices, TRH can act as a neurotransmitter, evoking an early, brief neuronal excitation or a late, longer-lasting modulation of neuronal responses to transmitters or both (figure 10.3). The excitatory and the modulatory actions of TRH are independent of each other and may be mediated by different subcellular mechanisms (Kow and Pfaff, 1996).

TRH has marked *behavioral* and *vegetative effects*. TRH antagonizes some of the effects of opiates, and is involved in thermoregulation, increasing body temperature when injected into the preoptic region and attenuating the hypothermic effects of pentobarbital, ethanol, and several other peptides. TRH has potent neurotrophic activity. Some of these actions of TRH are summarized in table 10.1. Many of these effects have been studied using TRH analogs that have a potency similar to, or greater than, that of natural TRH but which have been modified to prolong the plasma half-life of the peptide.

10.1.1.8 Clinical Implications of TRH

Patients with hypothyroidism due to hypothalamo-pituitary disorders may secrete TSH with a reduced biological activity, failing to bind to thyroid receptors. As oral administration of TRH restores TSH activity to normal, it is inferred that there is a defect in endogenous TRH production (Beck-Peccoz et al., 1985). Unsatisfactory results have been obtained using

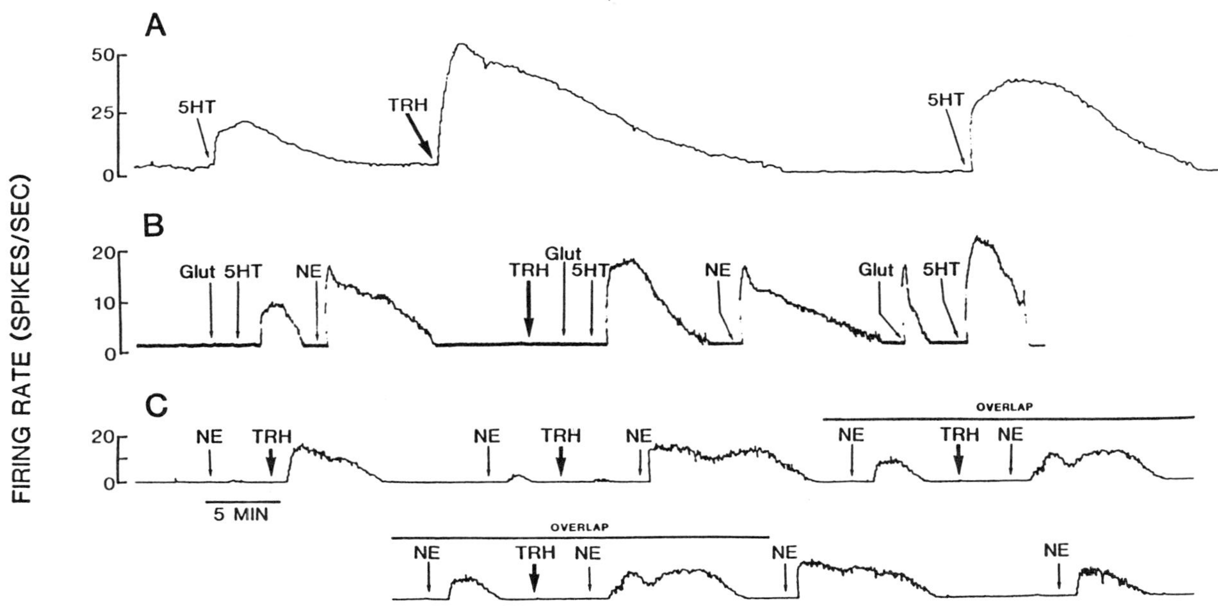

Figure 10.3
Excitatory and modulatory effects of thyrotropin-releasing hormone (TRH): neuronal responses to repeated applications of neurotransmitters and neuropeptides. Each trace is the firing rate histogram obtained from a single spinal neuron. The arrows represent the time points at which the agent was applied. (A) TRH causes both excitation and potentiation. The excitation occurred with short latency, but lasted for an atypically long time. Note the serotonin (5HT) response was potentiated for a long time (>40 minutes) after TRH application. (B) TRH did not excite neuronal activity but potentiated neuronal responses. Note, glutamate (Glut) remained ineffective right after TRH application but became excitatory in the next application, and the potentiation of the 5-HT response grew from the first to the second post-TRH application. This unit was lost halfway through recovery from the last 5-HT response. (C) A long recording split into two traces to show the effect of repeated applications of TRH. As the excitatory response to TRH desensitized, the potentiation of the norepinephrine (NE) response became stronger. At the end of this recording, the NE response appeared to be recovering from the potentiation. (From Kow and Pfaff, 1996.)

TRH therapy in patients with psychiatric disorders. TRH does appear to ameliorate some motor neuron disorders, with intrathecal infusion of TRH or its analog RX 77368 slowing the rate of deterioration in patients with amyotrophic lateral sclerosis (ALS) (Guiloff and Eckland, 1987; Munsat et al., 1989). TRH has also been tried, with varied success, on patients with spinal muscular atrophy, brain and spinal injuries, epilepsy, and shock.

10.1.2 Corticotropin-Releasing Hormone (CRH)

10.1.2.1 Structure and Phylogenetic Distribution

As described in chapter 9, the first concrete evidence for the existence of a hypothalamic releasing factor came from the independent discovery by Guillemin and Schally in 1955 that stress-induced corticosteroid secretion was dependent upon a hypothalamic factor.

Table 10.1
Extrapituitary actions of thyrotropin-releasing hormone (TRH)

Arousal effects of centrally administered TRH
Antagonizes the sedative effects of barbiturates, chloral hydrate, chlorpromazine, and alcohol
Antagonizes the effects of opiates (not analgesia)
Antagonizes the hypotensive effects of neurotensin
Antagonizes natural states of CNS depression
Arouses hibernating ground squirrels
Increases locomotor activity
Produces “wet dog shakes” similar to those observed after morphine withdrawal
Autonomic effects of centrally administered TRH
Increases mean arterial pressure and respiratory rate
Increases blood flow in thyroid, adrenal cortex, and gastrointestinal tract
Increases gastrointestinal motor activity
Stimulates gastric volume and acid secretion
Increases pancreatic secretion of amylase
Blocks glucagon-induced hyperglycemia
Neuromodulatory effects
Increases muscle action potential number and muscle tonus
Weakly excites spinal alpha motor neurons
Facilitates dorsal horn excitability
Increases turnover of dopamine, norepinephrine, and acetylcholinc
Potentiates serotonin effects
Effects on hypothalamic functions
Produces hyperthermia in rabbits and mice, but hypothermia in cats
Suppresses drinking and feeding
Neurotrophic effects (in vitro)
Stimulates axonal growth of motor neurons
Stimulates myelination
Increases choline acetyltransferase activity
Neurotrophic effects following trauma
Increases survival after anaphylactic or hemorrhagic shock
Improves recovery from spinal cord injury
May ameliorate certain degenerative neurological disorders

It was not until 1981 that Vale and his co-workers isolated, sequenced, synthesized, and identified the biological activity of a 41–amino acid ovine hypothalamic CRH. The structure of CRH is species-specific but the biological activity is not, that is, CRH from one species will induce ACTH secretion in other species. CRH has been immunocytochemically identified in annelids, insects, fish, amphibians, reptiles, and birds, as well as mammals. Human, rat, canine, and equine CRH are identical, but human CRH differs from that of the sheep by 7 amino acids in positions 2, 22, 23, 25, 38, 39, and 41. The amino acid sequence of CRH is remarkably similar to that of amphibian sauvagine, fish urotensin, and a newly identified mammalian peptide, urocortin (Vaughan et al., 1995). All these neuropeptides evoke ACTH secretion. In the CRH sequence below, residues identical to those of sauvagine are shown in italics.

H-Ser-Gln-Glu-*Pro-Pro-Ile-Ser*-Leu-*Asp-Leu*-Thr-Phe-His-*Leu-Leu-Arg*^{16}-Glu-Val-Leu-*Glu*-Met-Thyr-*Lys*-Ala- Asp-Gln-Leu-Ala-*Gln-Gln-Ala*^{31}-His-Ser-*Asn-Arg*-Lys-*Leu-Leu-Asp*-Ile-Ala-$NH_2{}^{41}$

Ovine CRH has a molecular weight of 4670 and the full C-terminal region is required for biological activity. Deamination of the C-terminus reduces biological activity to 0.1%. Deletion of the N-terminal part produces peptides that act as competitive inhibitors of CRH activity in vitro, whereas substitutions of amino acids affecting the α-helical structure of the CRH molecule double the potency of the parent peptide (Rivier et al., 1984).

10.1.2.2 Anatomical Distribution of CRH Neurons

Immunocytochemical studies show CRH to be widely distributed within the CNS as well as in other tissues. Most CRH is found in neurons in the hypothalamic nuclei involved in the control of ACTH release from the anterior pituitary, that is, the parvicellular neurons of the PVN, the axons of which terminate in the external zone of the ME for CRH release into the portal capillaries. These form the *CRH-tuberoinfundibular system* regulating ACTH release. While it is well known that the magnocellular neurons of the PVN synthesize VP, it is only recently that is was realized that approximately half of the parvicellular CRH neurons of the PVN also contain VP, which can interact with CRH to stimulate ACTH secretion.

Many CRH-containing neurons of the PVN also express additional neuropeptides, mainly ATII, CCK, and enkephalin, and to a lesser extent neurotensin and VIP. Other CRH neurons in the PVN are colocalized with OT and project to the posterior pituitary. CRH-containing neurons from the SON also contain OT and project to the ME, where CRH is released into the portal system, whereas other SON axons that contain both OT and CRH terminate in the posterior pituitary gland.

Extrahypothalamic sites of CRH within the CNS include the limbic system, especially the amygdala, areas in the brainstem, and the spinal cord. Many of the CRH-containing neurons of Barrington's nucleus, a pontine nucleus implicated in micturition, project to the periaqueductal gray and dorsal motor nucleus of the vagus, where they may be involved in behavioral or autonomic aspects of stress reactions. Their projections to the spinal parasympathetic nucleus that innervates the bladder may account for the proposed role of CRH in micturition (Valentino et al., 1995).

Peripheral tissues that show CRH-like immunoreactivity include the placenta, where the very high levels of CRH may be involved in the cascade of events involving ACTH, prostaglandins, and glucocorticoids that culminates in parturition. CRH is also found in the lung; the gastrointestinal tract; the pancreas; testis; ovary; immune system; adrenals; and heart.

10.1.2.3 Neural and Humoral Input to the PVN

CRH is an important coordinator of the endocrine, neuroendocrine, autonomic, and behavioral responses to stress (see figure 9.3), and the innervation of the PVN reflects the extensive afferent input necessary for such integrated action. Through neural input from visceral, somatic, and special sensory systems, the CRH neuron in the PVN becomes the center of an information highway bringing data about a variety of stresses. Information from blood-borne molecules also is received by these cells. The sources of this information have been grouped into four major classes (Sawchenko et al., 1993):

1. *Visceral information* is gated through the nucleus of the solitary tract by catacholinergic pathways.
2. Information about the *osmotic composition of blood* is carried by AT II and plasma ions, through cells of the lamina terminalis, the rostral margin of the third ventricle, which lie outside the BBB.
3. *Central integration of the HPA axis* with other neuroendocrine, autonomic, and behavioral regulatory mechanisms is provided by neurons in the hypothalamus and preoptic area that send projections into the PVN.
4. *Inhibitory influences* are routed from cells in the limbic region of the telencephalon, including the hippocampus, amygdala, and septum, that send projections to the PVN both directly and indirectly through the stria terminalis.

10.1.2.4 Synthesis, Inactivation, and regulation of CRH

The *CRH gene* has been highly conserved through evolution, with gene sequences encoding human and rat CRH showing 94% homology. The human CRH gene is on chromosome 8. A detailed description of the structure and cloning of the rat CRH gene is given by Thompson et al. (1987). The precursor molecule, *prepro-CRH,* for human CRH contains 196 amino acids, ovine pro-CRH contains 190 amino acids, and the signal peptide regions for these two prohormones are highly homologous (about 92%). The C-terminus of the precursor has the CRH peptide sequence preceded by a pair of basic amino acids, and followed by a Gly-Lys (figure 10.4). The 41–amino acid neuropeptide CRH is cleaved at a pair of dibasic amino acids from its larger precursor molecule, *pro-CRH,* by the action of endopeptidases. There are additional pairs of basic amino acids within the prohormone and they indicate potential sites of proteolytic cleavage which may produce novel peptides. There is some evidence that pro-CRH may be biologically active, that is, capable of stimulating ACTH release from cultured anterior pituitary cells (Morrison et al., 1995). No specialized inactivating mechanism for CRH has been found.

a. *Regulation of CRH synthesis and actions*

The PVN is the principal source of CRH in hypophyseal portal plasma and CRH mRNA and CRH content in PVN neurons is regulated negatively by glucocorticoids and positively by a wide variety of physical and emotional stresors. The HPA response to different types of stressors varies with the type of stressor, its duration and pattern of stimulation, the age and sex of the individual, its perinatal experience, and its dominance position within a social group.

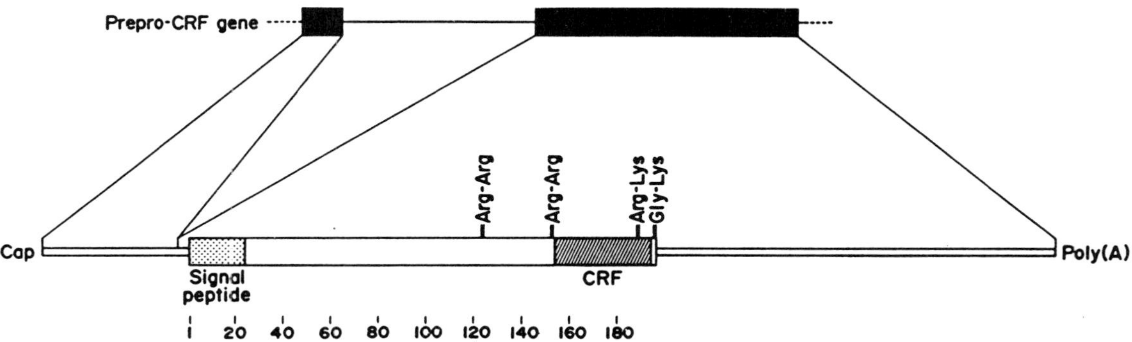

Figure 10.4
Schematic representation of the structures of preprocorticotropin-releasing factor (CRF) and its gene. The schemes are based on data taken from Shibahara et al. (1983). The gene is shown above: the exons are indicated by black boxes, the intron by a solid line, and the flanking regions by dashed lines. The topology of the mRNA is shown in the lower portion; the thick portion represents the protein-coding region; the capping site has been tentatively assigned. The locations of CRF and the signal peptide, as well as characteristic amino acid residues, are indicated. Amino acid numbers beginning with the initiative methionine are given. (From Numa, 1985.)

b. *Long-loop negative feedback*

Traditionally, inhibition by glucocorticoids on the CRH neurons of the PVN is considered to be the predominant regulator of CRH release by PVN neurons (figure 10.5). Iontophoretic application of glucocorticoids inhibits the *activity* (Saphier and Feldman, 1988) and decreases CRH mRNA levels of CRH neurons in the PVN in a dose-dependent manner, and in vitro experiments indicate that glucocorticoids inhibit the release of secretogogues (both CRH and VP) from neurosecretory axons in the ME. Adrenalectomy, which removes glucocorticoid inhibition, results in a considerable increase in ACTH secretion, an increase that can be blocked by replacement glucocococorticoids (figure 10.6). Both physical and psychological stressors produce a marked increase in CRH mRNA.

A long-loop negative feedback loop at the level of the corticotrophs of the anterior pituitary is supported by evidence that prior glucocorticoid treatment diminishes the pituitary secretion of ACTH in response to stressors. Glucocorticoids downregulate pituitary CRH receptors, decrease CRH receptor binding, and cause a rapid decrease in POMC gene transcription. This representation may be an oversimplification since glucocorticoid negative feedback can act in a stimulus-specific manner: physical stressors such as hemorrhage are relatively resistant to glucocorticoid feedback actions in contrast to the susceptibility to such negative feedback following emotional stress (Plotsky et al., 1989).

c. *Short and ultrashort feedback loops*

These two regulatory loops, involving ACTH inhibition of hypothalamic CRH, and CRH augmentation of its own secretion by an intrahypothalamic ultrashort-loop positive mechanism, play a role in controlling CRH release (Ono et al., 1985). ACTH

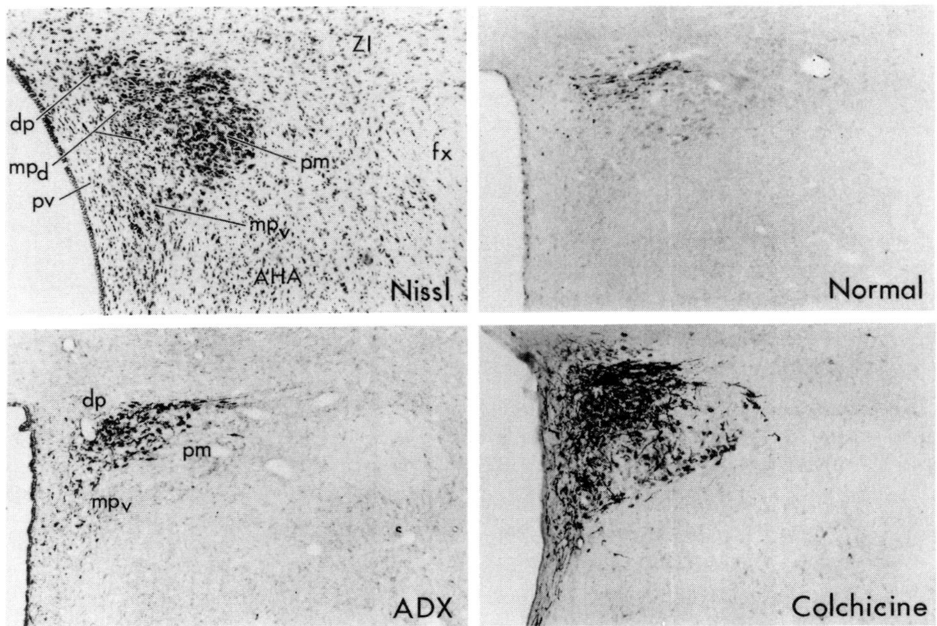

Figure 10.5
Corticotropin-releasing factor (CRF) immunostaining in the paraventricular nucleus showing CRF-immunoreactive neurons in untreated (Normal), adrenalectomized (ADX), and colchicine-pretreated rats. A Nissl-stained section is shown for reference. In normal animals, the relatively few CRF-immunoreactive cells are detected principally in the dorsal aspect of the medial parvocellular subdivision of the nucleus (mp$_d$). In response to removal of steroid feedback (ADX), the number and staining intensity of immunoreactive neurons increases in this division. Nonspecific enhancement of perikaryal staining by colchicine reveals a more expansive distribution of CRF cells, including the magnocellular division (pm) and autonomic-related projection neurons (dp, mp$_v$). AHA, anterior hypothalamic area; dp, dorsal parvocellular part; fx, fornix; mp$_d$ dorsal medial parvocellular part; mp$_v$, ventral medial parvocellular part; pm, posterior magnocellular part; pv, periventricular part; ZI, zona incerta. (From Sawchenko et al., 1993.)

and ACTH-related peptides, such as α-MSH, ACTH 1–13, inhibit release of CRH from hypothalamic explants and, in humans, ACTH suppresses plasma CRH. ACTH acts on the ACTH receptor on CRH neurons to block the release of CRH, decreasing ACTH levels in the ME (Lyson and McCann, 1994.) This appears to be a short negative feedback on CRH release which is independent of glucocorticoids.

d. Role of the limbic system in CRH inhibition

In addition to the direct action of glucocorticoids on CRH neurons in the PVN, a considerable portion of this inhibition is indirect, mediated by activation of the *limbic system*, especially the hippocampus and amygdala, an important site for the control of emotional and autonomic responses to stress (Endröczi et al., 1959; Sapolsky et al., 1991). Lesions of the limbic

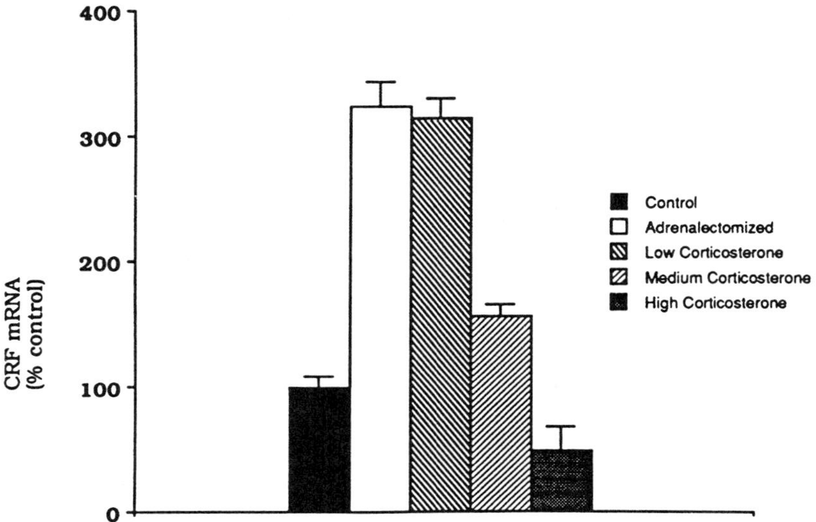

Figure 10.6
Levels of mRNA, measured by quantitative in situ hybridization, for corticotropin-releasing factor (CRF) in the parvocellular division of the paraventricular nucleus in sham-adrenalectomized (control) rats, adrenalectomized rats given 0.9% saline, and adrenalectomized rats given corticosterone in 0.9% saline for 1 week after surgery. Low dose, 2.5 mg/L; medium dose, 25 mg/L; high dose, 125 mg/mL. Error bars represent SEM. (From Lightman and Harbuz, 1993.)

system nuclei or of the pathways from the limbic system to the hypothalamus prevent glucocorticoid feedback onto the HPA axis. The amygdala contains high levels of CRH, and glucocorticoids can augment their inhibitory action by increasing CRH mRNA expression in the amygdala, while reducing CRH mRNA in the PVN (Makimo et al., 1994).

The amygdala is a prime candidate as a pathway for communication between the neuroendocrine and immune systems as it responds to cytokines released from immune cells (see chapter 8). IL-2 induces CRH release from both the hypothalamus and amygdala (Raber et al., 1995). NPY is also involved in the regulation of responsiveness to stress, possibly through an interaction of the CRH and NPY systems in the amygdala.

e. ***Basal vs. stress regulation: involvement of VP***
Stress results in a rapid response of immediate early genes in the PVN, followed by activation of CRH, VP, enkephalin, and other mRNA transcripts. CRH is the predominant transcript to be activated in acute stress, but the pattern of mRNA activation varies according to the stimulus. Under basal conditions, some CRH neurons co-express VP, but the number of neurons coexpressing both neuropeptides increases after stress, indicating that the role of VP appears to be limited to corticotropin response to stress, a fine example of functional plasticity in the neuroendocrine system (Paulmyerlacroix et al., 1995). VP mRNA is preferentially activated in response to chronic immunological stresses (Lightman, 1994). Osmotic stress

increases VP secretion by the magnocellular neurons, which causes an inhibition of parvicellular CRH.

As might be expected from the rich innervation of CRH neurons in the PVN, CRH release from the hypothalamus is also influenced by several neurotransmitters, including ACh, 5-HT, NE, and GABA. The catecholamines have little or no effect on basal CRH gene expression but are important in the rapid induction of transcription in response to stressful stimuli (Lightman and Harbuz, 1993).

f. Circadian rhythm of CRH secretion

CRH, and consequently ACTH and corticosteroids, is secreted on a circadian basis, with levels in the human generally rising on arousal and peaking in the early morning, with a decline over the remainder of the 24-hour period. For nocturnal animals, such as rodents, the HPA hormones peak in the early evening. Careful investigators always take measurements of these hormones at the same time, to eliminate variations due to the marked periodicity of their secretion. The suprachiasmatic nucleus (SCN) is believed to be the source of this biological clock. It is possible that CRH may play a pivotal role in brain activation and the regulation of sleep-wake cycles.

10.1.2.5 CRH Receptors and Second Messengers

The CRH receptor is a member of the class of seven transmembrane helix G protein–coupled receptors. It mediates ligand-dependent stimulation of intracellular cAMP in response to physiological concentrations of CRH and to the related frog skin peptide, sauvergine. The molecular mass of the CRH receptor varies according to the tissue and species from which it is derived, from about 58 to 75 kD. The receptors are glycosylated and the heterogeneity between brain and pituitary CRH receptors results from different post-translational glycosylation of the native protein; the functional significance, if any, of this difference is not known. CRH receptors in the brain, pituitary, and spleen are high-affinity membrane receptors with similar kinetic and pharmacological properties.

a. CRH receptor distribution

Identification of the cDNAs encoding the human and rat CRH receptor has permitted the mapping of the distribution of cells expressing CRH receptor mRNA in brain and pituitary by in situ hybridization. CRH receptors are widely distributed in the CNS, being most highly concentrated in the anterior and intermediate lobes of the pituitary, olfactory bulb, cerebral cortex, amygdala, and cerebellum. CRH receptor expression is generally low in the hypothalamic region. In the brainstem, high expression of CRH receptors is found in nuclei associated with somatic, visceral, auditory, and vestibular systems.

b. Receptor subtypes

The recent cloning of the CRH_1, CRH_{2a}, and CRH_{2b} receptor subtypes facilitates the separation of the many physiological effects of this neuropeptide. The anatomical distribution of these receptor types is quite different. CRH_1 receptor mRNA is most abundant in neocortical, cerebellar, and sensory structures. On the other hand, CRH_2 receptors are found mainly in subcortical structures, particularly in the lateral septal nuclei, the ventromedial hypothalamic nuclei, and the PVN. It has been suggested that the anxiogenic and anorectic actions of CRH in these nuclei are CRH_2-mediated (Grigoriadis et al., 1996). In addition, CRH_1 and CRH_2 receptors differ markedly in their structures, pharmacological profiles, and their regulation in response to a variety of stressors.

The spleen, an important source of immune cells, is also well supplied with CRH receptors, which are restricted to the macrophage-rich regions, further reinforcing the importance of CRH in the integration of the responses of the CNS, endocrine, and immune systems to stress (Grigoriadis et al., 1993).

c. Regulation of CRH receptors

CRH receptors in the pituitary, but not in the brain, are affected by changes in the HPA axis. This differential regulation of brain and pituitary CRH receptors is mystifying. Following adrenalectomy and chronic stress, conditions in which endogenous ACTH levels are high, there is a loss of pituitary CRH receptors due to the coordinated actions of CRH and VP. Glucocorticoid administration causes a downregulation of CRH receptors concomitant with the inhibition of ACTH secretion. None of these manipulations appear to affect brain CRH receptors.

d. Second messengers

CRH activates the adenylate cyclase complex, stimulating adenylate cyclase activity and activating cAMP-dependent protein kinase at concentrations in the range of its ACTH-stimulating activity. The binding of CRH to pituitary membranes is inhibited by guanyl nucleotides, a charcteristic of receptors that are coupled to adenylate cyclase by a guanyl nucleotide regulatory protein. Other second-messenger systems are probably also involved, including calcium and arachidonic acid and its metabolites. The interaction of CRH with VP is important, for the VP second-messenger pathway involves calcium and phospholipid-dependent mechanisms, with stimulation of protein kinase C. CRH is the most potent secretogogue for ACTH release, whereas VP is only a weak agonist but can be shown to facilitate CRH activity, especially in chronic stress.

10.1.2.6 CRH-Binding Protein

It has been suggested that a 38-kD peptide-binding glycoprotein inactivates CRH and prevents pituitary-adrenal stimulation when CRH levels are substantially elevated (Suda et al., 1989). The CRH-binding protein inhibits the ACTH-releasing characteristics of CRH in an in vitro pituitary bioassay, and has been identified and cloned from sheep brain. Maternal plasma concentrations of CRH in the later phases of pregnancy are extremely high, matching the levels found in hypothalamic portal blood, yet there is only a moderate increase in maternal ACTH. If, as has been suggested, elevated levels of "free" CRH are reponsible for parturition, and that CRH-binding protein levels are low in women suffering from pre-eclampsia and preterm labor, the binding protein may be acting as a placental clock, controlling the length of human pregnancy (Behan et al., 1996).

10.1.2.7 Functions of CRH

The most important function of CRH is its role in initiating stress-induced ACTH secretion, which results in the adrenal release of glucocorticoids. An additional neuroendocrine function is its modulating effect on other hypothalamic neuropeptides. CRH stimulates the secretion of somatostatin and β-endorphin, and inhibits the release of GnRH, GH, OT, and VP.

a. CRH acts as a major inhibitor of reproductive function

Through its central inhibitory effects on GnRH and LH, CRH suppresses reproductive functions, including sexual behavior, but it also acts as a direct inhibitor of testicular function. CRF is secreted by the Leydig cells of the testis and acts as a potent inhibitor of LH action. CRH also stimulates Leydig cells to secrete β-endorphin, which then inhibits FSH action on the Sertoli cells of the tubules (Dufau et al., 1959).

b. CRH acts as a neurotransmitter and neuromodulator

In addition to its endocrine functions, CRH may act as a neurotransmitter or neuromodulator in extrahypothalamic circuits to integrate the multisystem responses to stress. The wide spectrum of autonomic, electrophysiologic, and behavioral effects of this neuropeptide are consistent with this concept. Central administration of CRH produces behavioral activation, increased wakefulness as seen in lightening of EEG-monitored sleep, and at high doses, evokes kindling, a model of partial complex seizures. CRH has a mainly excitatory effect on the electrical activity of neurons in the limbic system, hippocampus, cortex, some regions of the hypothalamus, and the locus ceruleus, a possible integrating center in the pons which provides noradrenergic input to many CNS structures. Ultrastructural studies show that axon terminals containing immunoreactive CRH (CRH-ir) directly contact catecholamine-containing dendrites in the locus ceruleus and may presynaptically modulate other afferents (Vanbockstaele et al., 1996). In a few regions, such as the PVN and lateral septum, CRH has an inhibitory effect.

c. Behavioral, autonomic, and immune effects

CRH neurons in the PVN have distinct activating effects on behavior, reinforcing behavioral responses to stressors. CRH injected into the brain increases arousal as measured by locomotor activation and increased responsiveness to stressful stimuli. This arousal can be shown to be independent of the pituitary-adrenal axis and is reversed by specific and selective CRH antagonists (Koob, 1992). In a transgenic mouse model of CRH overproduction, endocrine abnormalities develop involving the HPA axis, such as elevated levels of ACTH and glucocorticoids. These animals develop an anxiogenic behavioral state, as

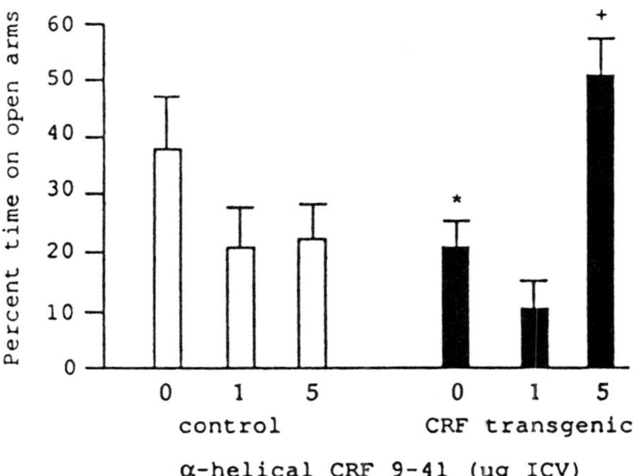

Figure 10.7
Mean (±SEM) percent time spent on the open arms during a 5-minute test on the elevated plus-maze. Corticotropin-releasing hormone (CRH) antagonist (α-helical CRH 9–41) was infused into the lateral cerebral ventricles. Mice were placed in the maze 5 minutes after infusion and monitored through the use of computer-interfaced, infrared photobeams that measure the time spent in each enclosed compartment. $^{*}P < .05$ vs. vehicle-treated control group. $^{+}P < .05$ vs. vehicle-treated transgenic group. (From Stenzel-Poore et al., 1994.)

seen by the decreased time spent on the exposed arms of an elevated plus-maze, a reaction that is reversed by the administration of a CRH antagonist (figure 10.7). Other indications of anxiety in rodent animal models include decreased sleeping, enhanced fear responses, decreased food intake, increased head shakes and grooming, and suppressed sexual behavior. Similar responses are evoked by the icv administration of CRH, which mobilizes autonomic and behavioral responses to stress, activating locomotor reactions, lowering body temperature, and regulating food intake. The reduction in food intake has been specifically localized to the PVN as it is evoked by microinjection of CRH into the PVN, but not into other brain regions. CRH also plays a major role in the immune response to stress, a topic that was discussed in detail in chapter 8. A dissociation of the behavioral, endocrine, and autonomic activity of CRH and CRH-derived peptides is correlated with the structure of these molecules (Diamant and De Wied, 1993).

Human sleep is characterized by the cyclic occurrence of rapid eye movement (REM) and non-REM periods and by distinct patterns of hormonal secretion. Neuropeptides play a key role in sleep regulation. CRH inhibits slow wave sleep and GH release, whereas GHRH has the opposite effect. An inbalance of these neuropeptides in favor of CRH may contribute to the disturbed sleep that occurs during normal aging and depression (Steiger, 1995).

CRH is involved in the physiological regulation of the autonomic nervous system, modifying the sympathetic and parasympathetic efferent systems, including adrenomedullary activity (Brown and Fisher, 1990). These sympathetic effects are mediated by CRH-evoked epinephrine and NE secretion. CRH (given icv) acts on the parasympathetic nervous system by inhibiting the vagus nerve. In the cardiovascular system this results in an elevation of arterial pressure due mainly to an increase in cardiac output resulting from increased venous return and an elevated heart rate. High levels of the circulating catecholamines probably contribute to this effect. In the gastrointestinal tract, CRH inhibition of the vagus diminishes gastric secretion. In addition, CRH induces hyperglycemia characterized by an increase in plasma glucagon and a suppression of insulin secretion.

This extensive range of CRH effects permits this neuropeptide to dominate a generalized adaptive response to various types of stress and the PVN is anatomically and physiologically placed as a central integrating unit to unify these adaptive reactions.

10.1.2.8 Clinical Implications of CRH

Clinically, the most common test used for determining abnormal HPA function is an alteration in the negative feedback control of the HPA axis, using the dexamethasone suppression test. Dexamethasone, a synthetic glucocorticoid, suppresses cortisol secretion in normal persons. Patients with Cushing's disease, characterized by excessive cortisol secretion due to ACTH-secreting pituitary tumors, show a much reduced suppression, or no suppression. These patients do not show a diurnal variation in their ACTH or cortisol levels, leading to the suspicion that the primary source of the disease in some patients may be a CNS disturbance involving CRH.

In line with animal models involving over- or underproduction of CRH in maladaptation to stress, dysfunction of the HPA axis in humans possibly may underlie many other pathological disorders (see also chapter 8). Overproduction of CRH has been implicated in affective disorders such as depression, anxiety, and anorexia nervosa. CRH overproduction at peripheral inflammatory sites, such as synovial joints, may contribute to autoimmune diseases such as rheumatoid arthritis. A decrease in CRH, accompanied by an increase in CRH receptor number in affected brain regions in Alzheimer's patients, is highly correlated with the extent of the decrease in choline acetyltransferase activity, suggesting that the CRH and ACh systems may interact (De Souza, 1995). Abnormal changes in CRH have also been associated with other neurodegenerative diseases, such as Parkinson's disease and progressive supranuclear palsy. The potential of CRH to evoke spontaneous seizure activity in rats may indicate some involvement with epileptic seizures. CRH, the preeminent mediator of the mammalian stress response, is under intensive investigation in the search for pharmacological tools that may help

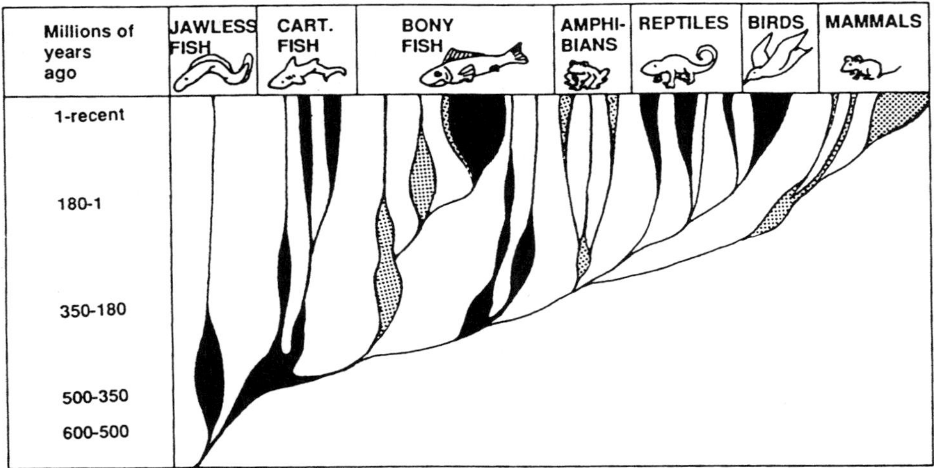

Figure 10.8
Scheme for the evolution of the human form of gonadotropin-releasing hormone (GnRH). Vertebrate classes with animals containing the human form of GnRH (mammalian GnRH) are shown by dotted areas. (From Sherwood et al., 1993.)

relieve the causes and symptoms of these debilitating diseases.

10.1.3 Gonadotropin-Releasing Hormone

10.1.3.1 Structure and Phylogenetic Distribution

McCann et al. (1960) provided the first evidence for LH releasing activity in hypothalamic extracts. Subsequently, GnRH, a hypothalamic neuropeptide, was isolated and characterized by Schally et al. (1971) and Guilleman (see Amos et al., 1971). GnRH is a decapeptide, pGlu-His-Trp-Ser-Tyr-Gly-Leu-Arg-Pro-Gly-NH_2, which releases both LH and FSH from the anterior pituitary gland in a pulsatile fashion. For some time it was believed that two different GnRHs, LHRH and FSH-RH, were required for hypothalamic stimulation of the pituitary gonadotropins. Currently, the consensus is that only the LHRH factor is required so most investigators prefer the more encompassing term *GnRH.*

Only one form of GnRH is found in placental mammals, but nine different forms of GnRH have been found in nonmammalian vertebrate brains, in the lamprey, cartilaginous fish, bony fish (salmon), amphibians, reptiles, and birds (chick). Some of these lower vertebrates produce two types of functionally equivalent GnRH, encoded by different genes, indicating that gene duplication has occurred at least twice during evolution and has existed for at least 500 million years (Miyamoto et al., 1984). Figure 10.8 shows a scheme for the evolution of the human GnRH. All of the vertebrate GnRHs stimulate gonadotropin secretion but there are differences in receptor specificity. In mammals, only mammalian GnRH exhibits full activity, whereas, with the exception of the lamprey, the lower vertebrates respond to all forms of GnRH.

10.1.3.2 Anatomical Distribution and Morphology of GnRH Neurons

Using immunocytochemical methods, the GnRH neuronal system has been mapped out in detail. GnRH neurons are arranged in loose networks rather than in discrete nuclei, with marked differences in their distribution in mammalian species. In primates the GnRH neurons are found in the medial basal hypothalamus (MBH) and the arcuate nucleus of the hypothalamus. In the rodent, the GnRH neurons form a loose network stretching through the septo-preoptico-infundibular pathway, a telencephalic-diencephalic continuum (Silverman, 1988).

Most of the GnRH neurons project to the ME, the final common path to the anterior pituitary, but some GnRH fibers continue down the infundibular stalk to enter the posterior pituitary. Cells of the septal-preoptic area also innervate the organum vasculosum of the lamina terminalis, one of the circumventricular organs. There are several other extrahypothalamic GnRH terminals: some innervate the epithalamus and perhaps the pineal; others enter the stria terminalis and project into the amygdala, the mammillary complex, and the ventral tegmental area of the midbrain. Figure 10.9 illustrates the widespread distribution of GnRH fibers in the brain.

Olfactory stimuli play an important role in reproductive physiology and behavior and GnRH cell bodies are found in many olfactory structures, including the main and accessory olfactory bulbs, the anterior olfactory nucleus, and olfactory portions of the limbic system. During early development, cords of GnRH cells migrate from the olfactory pit and nasal septum to the POA. GnRH is also produced in peripheral organs, including the ovary, testis, placenta, and lactating mammary gland.

The *morphology* of most GnRH neurons is simple, being oval or fusiform with a diameter of 10 to 20 μm, and with simple unbranched dendrites and an axon. The population of GnRH cell bodies and terminals forms a dynamic system, varying with the hormonal state. Most GnRH neurons are smooth early in life but develop spines at the time of puberty. Other GnRH cells are more complex, and they receive axosomatic or axodendritic synapses from other GnRH cells, as shown in figure 10.10, providing an anatomical basis for the pulsatility of GnRH upon which the pulsatile release of the gonadotropins is dependent (Silverman, 1988). GnRH neurons or their dendrites are closely apposed to the basement membrane of brain capillaries, which may expedite the passage of the gonadal steroids which regulate GnRH secretion.

Afferent input to GnRH neurons is sparse but physiological and microscopic studies indicate that many neurotransmitters, including catecholamines, 5-HT, GABA, and aspartate regulate GnRH neurons. In addition, many neurons containing neuropeptides such as CRH and neurotensin (NT), NPY, SP, and ACTH or β-endorphin make synaptic contact with GnRH neurons and presumably are capable of influencing GnRH synthesis and release. *Colocalization* of GnRH with ACTH 17–39 and β-endorphin in both the arcuate nucleus and preoptic area may correlate with the importance of opiates in the regulation of gonadotropin secretion.

10.1.3.3 The GnRH Gene and Processing of GnRH

The GnRH gene in neural tissue has four exons, the first of which contains the 5′-untranslated region. Exon 2 codes for the signal peptide, the GnRH decapeptide, the enzymatic amidation site, and the precursor processing site. Exon 2 also codes for the N-terminal 11 amino acids of a second, 56–amino acid GnRH-associated peptide (GAP), which is contained

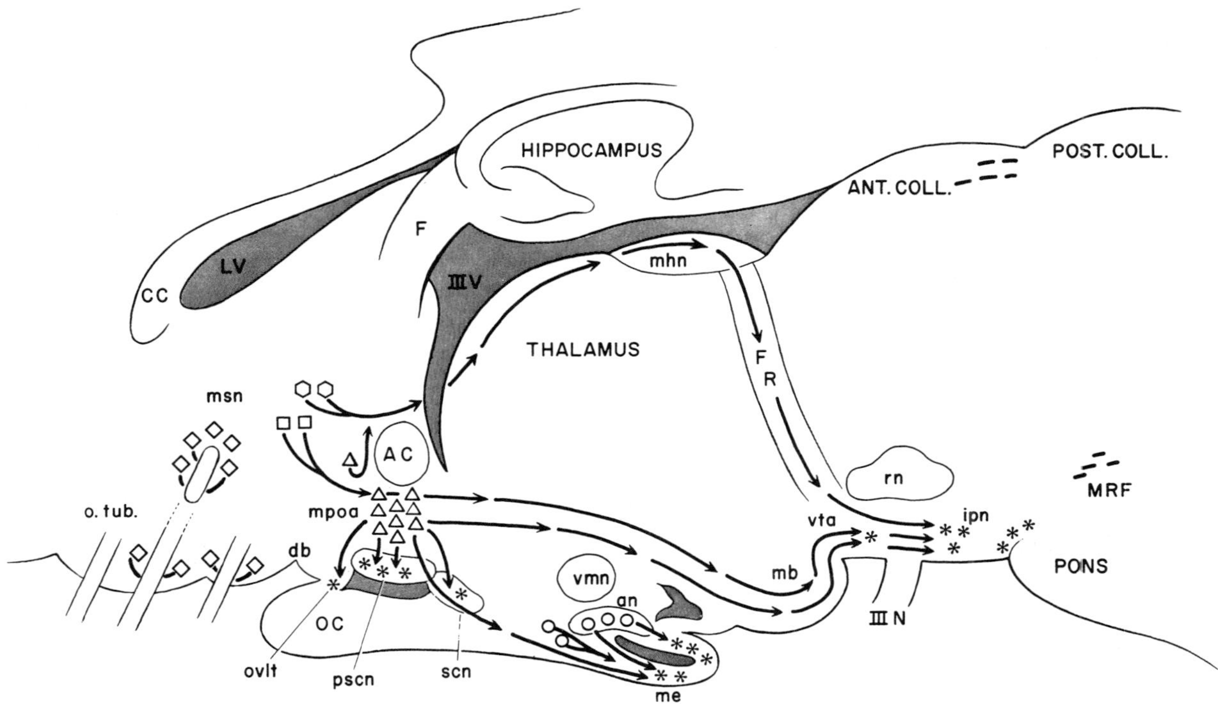

Figure 10.9
Midsagittal plane of the guinea pig brain from the level of the septum rostrally to the pons posteriorly. Different groups of gonadotropin-releasing hormone (GnRH) cells are indicated by the geometric symbols, fiber pathways are indicated by arrows, and terminal fields are indicated by asterisks. The subchiasmatic pathway is not indicated. It is not known whether any GnRH cells have more than one projection. AC, anterior commissure; an, arcuate nucleus; ANT. COLL., anterior colliculus; CC, corpus callosum; db, diagonal band of Broca; F, fornix; FR, fasciculus retroflexus; ipn, interpeduncular nucleus; LV, lateral mb, mammillary body, medial division; me, median eminence; mhn, medial habenula; mpoa, medial preoptic area; MRF, medial reticular formation; msn, medial septum; OC, optic chiasm; o.tub., olfactory tubercle; ovlt, organum vasculosum of the lamina terminalis; POST. COLL., posterior colliculus; pscn, preoptic suprachiasmatic nucleus; rn, red nucleus; vmn, ventromedial nucleus; vta, ventral tegmental area; IIIV, third ventricle; III N, oculomotor nerve. (From Silverman, 1988.)

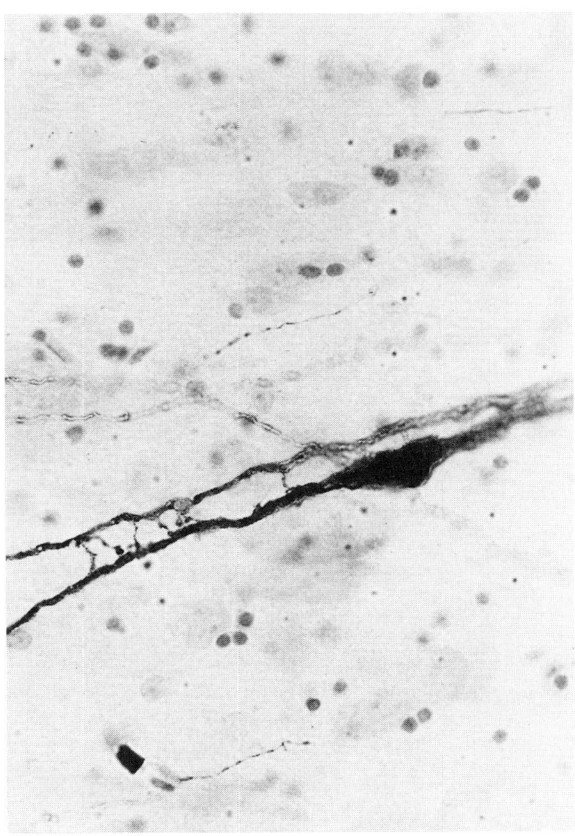

Figure 10.10
Two neighboring gonadotropin-releasing hormone (GnRH) neurons in the monkey hypothalamus appear to share numerous bridges. (From Hoffman et al., 1992.)

within the prepro-GnRH (figure 10.11). Exon 3 codes for the next 32 GAP residues. Exon 4 codes for the last 13 amino acids of GAP, the termination codon, and the 3′-untranslated region of the mRNA (Adelman et al., 1986). Figure 10.12 compares the GnRH genes of the human, rat, and salmon.

The importance of the GnRH gene and its products is exemplified in the dependence of mammalian reproductive functions on the integrity of the gene. The *hypogonadal (hpg) mutant mouse* has a defect in the gene that results in a deletion in the mRNA of two exons. As a result the hpg mouse completely lacks GnRH neurons and the consequent absence of GnRH prevents the maturation of the infantile reproductive tract. Implantation of normal fetal or neonatal septal-preoptic tissue into the third ventricle of the hpg mouse can partially restore reproductive function to both males and females. However, introduction of the wild-type mouse GnRH gene into the mutant mouse germ line completely restores reproductive capacity (Mason et al., 1986).

GnRH is synthesized in humans and rats as part of a large precursor protein pro-GnRA, of 92 amino acids (90 in mice), which yields a 69–amino acid prohormone after removal of the signal peptide. Cleavage of the signal peptide occurs at an unusual cleavage site—Ser-Gln. The sequences upstream of this cleavage site are highly conserved. The processing events within the GnRH neuron occur mainly in the soma and the cleavage products are then transported to the nerve terminals.

Cleavage of the prohormone yields the mature GnRH decapeptide, with blocked termini after C-terminal amidation, and GAP. GAP was initially thought to inhibit the secretion of PRL (Nikolics et al., 1985) but this is debatable and the biological function of GAP is not clear (Thomas et al., 1988). It

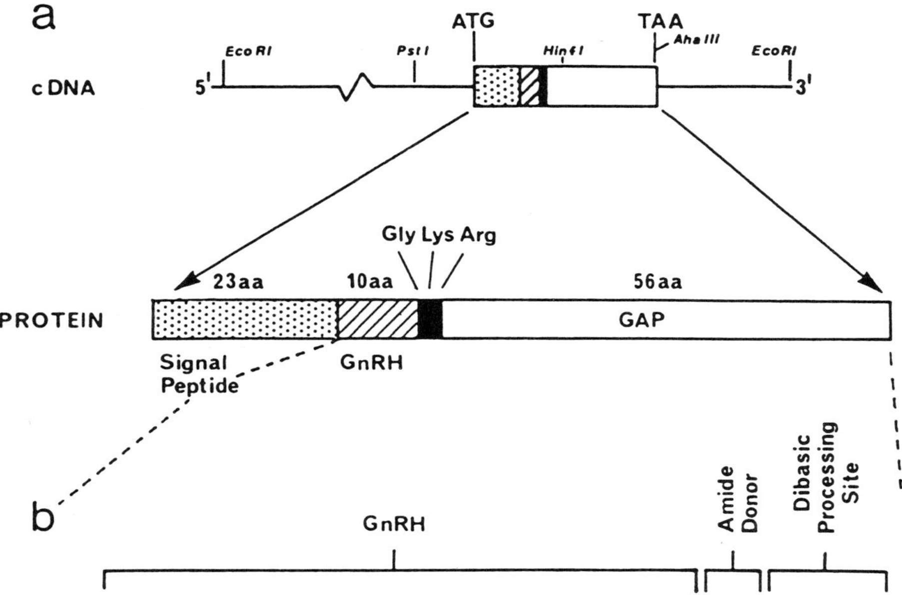

Figure 10.11
Complementary DNA (cDNA) and precursor protein for human gonadotropin-releasing hormone (GnRH). The coding region is located between the initiation codon for protein synthesis ATG and the termination codon TAA. Schematic representation of the encoded protein identifies the three domains, namely signal peptide, GnRH, and GnRH-associated peptide (GAP) with the respective sizes in amino acid (aa) residues. (From Nikolics et al., 1985.)

may be that GAP is involved in the correct processing and packaging of the active hormone.

The small size of the GnRH molecule has made it possible to synthesize many analogs, which have been used to demonstrate many of the structural and functional properties of the molecule. Substitution of D-Lys^6 for Gly^6 increases its biological potency, apparently by stabilizing a β-turn needed to maintain the active conformation of the peptide. Studies of various GnRH analogs show that Arg^6, or at least a basic amino acid, is essential to GnRH activity in mammals but not in birds, reptiles, amphibians, or fish (Millar and King, 1988).

10.1.3.4 GnRH Receptors and Second Messengers

The presence of at least two molecular forms of hypothalamic GnRH in most vertebrates suggests the existence of different GnRH receptor subtypes. The N- and C-terminal sequences are important for receptor binding and the N-terminal sequence contains information involved in receptor activation. The pituitary GnRH receptor has a molecular weight of 60 K, when determined on denatured samples prepared for sodium dodecyl sulfate–polyacrylamide gel electrophoresis (SDS-PAGE). When the molecular weight is determined for the receptor within the gonadotroph plasma membrane, the estimate is 136 K,

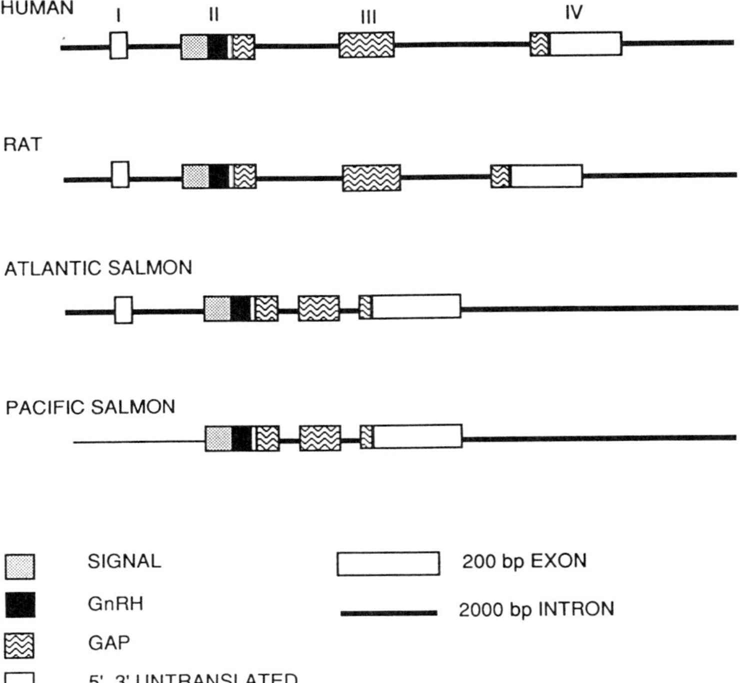

Figure 10.12
Comparison of the gonadotropin-releasing (GnRH) genes of human, rat, Atlantic salmon, and Pacific salmon. Exons I, II, III, and IV are labeled. Untranslated regions and the processing site following GnRH are shown as open boxes. The 5′-portion containing exon I has not been reported for Pacific salmon. GAP, GnRH-associated peptide. (From Sherwood et al., 1993.)

suggesting that the receptor may exist in the membrane as a multisubunit complex (Conn and Venter, 1985).

During the estrous cycle, pituitary GnRH receptor concentrations and GnRH mRNA levels rise on the morning of proestrus and fall rapidly on the afternoon of proestrus, coincident with the preovulatory surge of gonadotropins. These changes can be mimicked by estradiol administration indicating that estrogen regulation of GnRH receptors is through changing levels of GnRH receptor mRNA (Jinnah and Conn, 1988; Quinonesjenab et al., 1996). Male concentrations of GnRH receptors approximate those of females in metestrus.

GnRH regulates its own receptors, which are initially downregulated by continuous administration of GnRH, followed by a recovery and upregulation. The dependence of this autoregulation on Ca^{2+} was shown in figure 6.3. GnRH receptors are also found in the gonads, as is GnRH. The presence of GnRH receptors on gonadal cells permits the direct inhibitory action GnRH exerts on ovarian and testicular function, bypassing the stimulatory actions of FSH and LH on these organs.

The *second messenger* for GnRH is the phosphatidylinositol system. Binding of GnRH to its receptor initiates Ca^{2+} influx and coupling with the second messenger, resulting in the further release of Ca^{2+} from the endoplasmic reticulum.

10.1.3.5 Pulsatile Secretion of GnRH

Secretion of GnRH is pulsatile and the pattern of the pulses is dictated by a pulse generator which has its origin in the vicinity of the mediobasal hypothalamus and arcuate nucleus (Knobil, 1989). The electrophysiological correlates of the GnRH pulse generator are steep rhythmic multiunit volleys, which are rapidly followed by pulses of LH release (figure 10.13). The release of LH and FSH is almost completely dependent upon the pulsatile release of GnRH; continuous infusion of GnRH suppresses LH and FSH secretion (figure 10.14). The pulse generator can function autonomously but it is normally modulated by ovarian steroids, neuropeptides, and neurotransmitters (discussed below). In addition, GnRH may influence its own release via either a short C- or ultrashort-loop feedback mechanism.

10.1.3.6 Regulation of GnRH Secretion by Gonadal Steroids

In both sexes the neural signal from the pulse generator to the GnRH neurons occurs daily, but is modified by the ovarian steroids, the endogenous opiates, and several other factors in the female during reproductive cycles. Basal GnRH release in both males and females is kept relatively low owing to the long-loop *negative feedback* of the gonadal steroids. The inhibition is most probably directly on the anterior pituitary, and indirectly on the hypothalamus, since the GnRH neurons lack receptors for the gonadal steroids (Shivers et al., 1984). Removal of the negative feedback (in castrated male and female rodents and primates, postmenopausal women, and hypogonadal men) evokes chronic hypersecretion of both LH and FSH, and a resulting hypothalamic pulse generator operating at about 1 cycle/hour (Plant et al., 1989). Currently, it is believed that regulation of GnRH secretion is through an intricate communication system between the hypothalamus and the anterior pituitary, and involves other neuropeptides, amino acids, steroids, and neurotransmitters.

10.1.3.7 The LH Surge

a. Positive feedback of gonadal steroids on GnRH in late proestrus

Ovulation in most mammals occurs spontaneously and is induced by a *positive feedback cascade* that involves the ovary; the CNS, especially the hypothalamus; and the anterior pituitary gland. In the female, there is an abrupt and steep rise in GnRH secretion just prior to ovulation, followed by a rapid fall to baseline levels. The abrupt escalation of GnRH secretion is initiated by the rise in estradiol levels toward the end of proestrus (figure 10.15). The massive release of GnRH is followed by a dramatic rise in LH levels, the *LH surge*, which peaks to 100 times basal levels, and is essential to ovulation. At the same time the pituitary gonadotrophs become more sensitive to GnRH, probably owing to progesterone secreted during the luteal phase and to the priming effect of GnRH on GnRH neurons by which a pulse of GnRH increases pituitary responsiveness to a second pulse.

b. Switch to negative feedback on GnRH in the luteal phase

The preovulatory surge in LH is a singular endocrine event that involves a switch from the negative feedback effect of estrogen to a positive feedback effect,

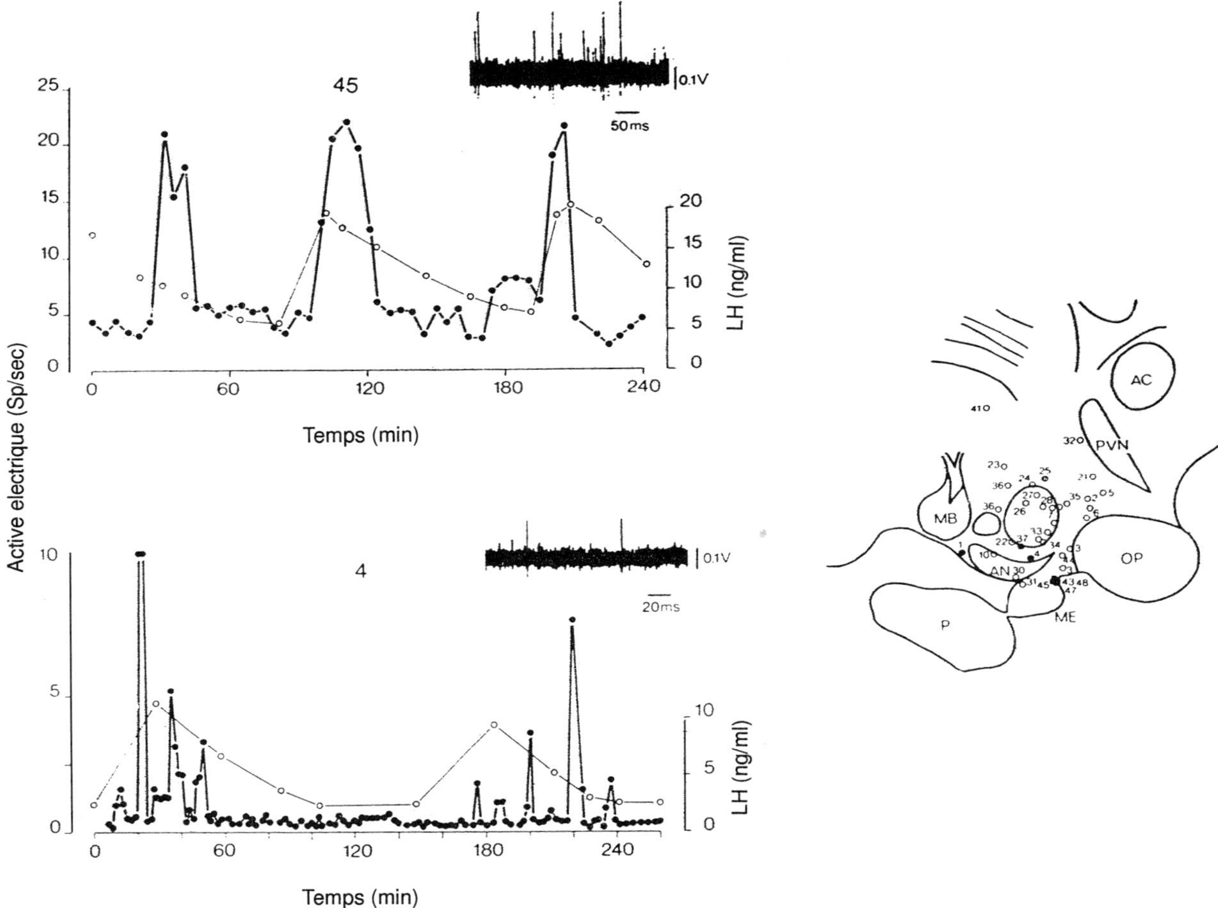

Figure 10.13
Electrical activity (spikes/second) recorded in various hypothalamic sites and plasma levels. (Top panel) Example (one of four) of multiunit activity recorded in the median eminence (ME). The recording site (45) is represented on the schematic diagram on the right. (Bottom panel) Example (one of three) of the unit activity of a neuron, the approximate location of which (4) is represented on the schematic diagram. Dark symbols represent recordings which showed a correlation with plasma luteinizing hormone (LH) levels. Dark squares, multiunit activity; dark circles, single unit. AC, anterior commissure; AN, arcuate nucleus; PVN, paraventricular nucleus; MB, mammillary body; ME, median eminence; OP, optic chiasma; P, pituitary. (From Dufy et al., 1979.)

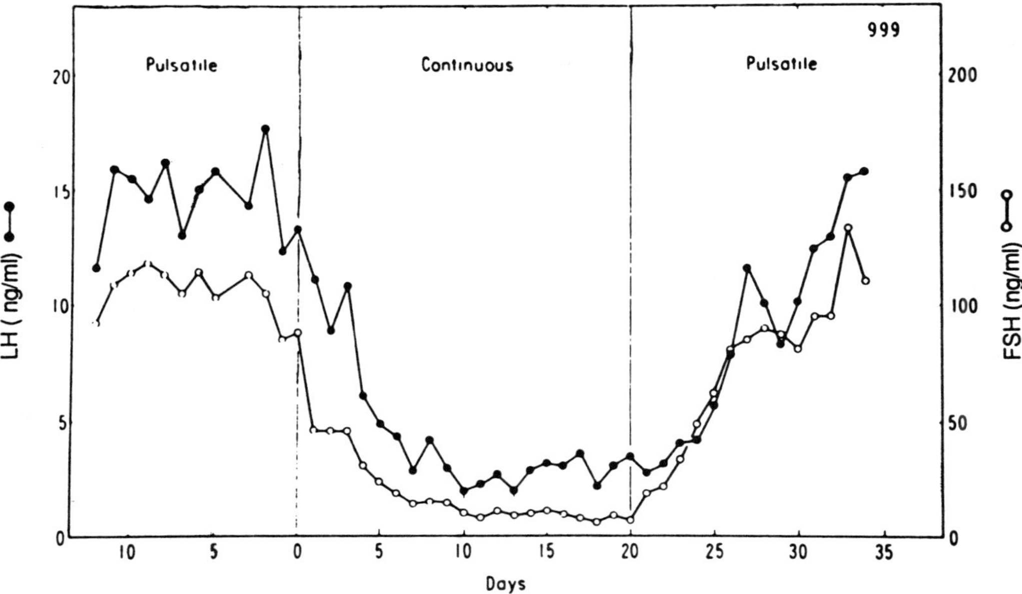

Figure 10.14
Comparison of plasma luteinizing hormone (LH) and follicle-stimulating hormone (FSH) after pulsatile vs. continuous administration of gonadotropin-releasing hormone. Gonadotropin secretion is markedly inhibited by continuous infusion, but is reestablished when pulsatile infusion resumes. (From Belchetz et al., 1978.)

changes that involve both the hypothalamus and the pituitary gland. This involves disinhibition of negative inputs to the GnRH neurons as well as activation of positive inputs. The positive feedback of estradiol in proestrus, and the negative feedback of the synergistic action of estradiol, progesterone, and the opiate system in the luteal phase, are integrated and synchronized with the neural input into an intricate positive and negative feedback cascade that regulates GnRH secretion. These hormonal changes have been extensively studied in the estrous cycle of the rat, which has hormonal profiles similar to those of the menstrual cycle in women (figure 10.16).

The male does not have an LH surge because the amounts of estrogen produced by the male are too low to stimulate the hypothalamus, and in addition, the male has been exposed to androgens during the critical developmental period (see chapter 9, section 9.5.1). Consequently the male acyclic hypothalamus lacks an estrogen-sensitive central GnRH pulse generator. In primates, however, including humans, an LH surge can be induced by estrogen.

c. *Role of neuropeptide Y and galanin*

The innate pulsatile secretory pattern of the GnRH pulse generator network in the hypothalamus is strongly modified by two hypothalamic neuropeptides, NPY and galanin, which are secreted concomitantly with LHRH and amplify the preovulatory LH surge. Secretion of these neuropeptides is in-

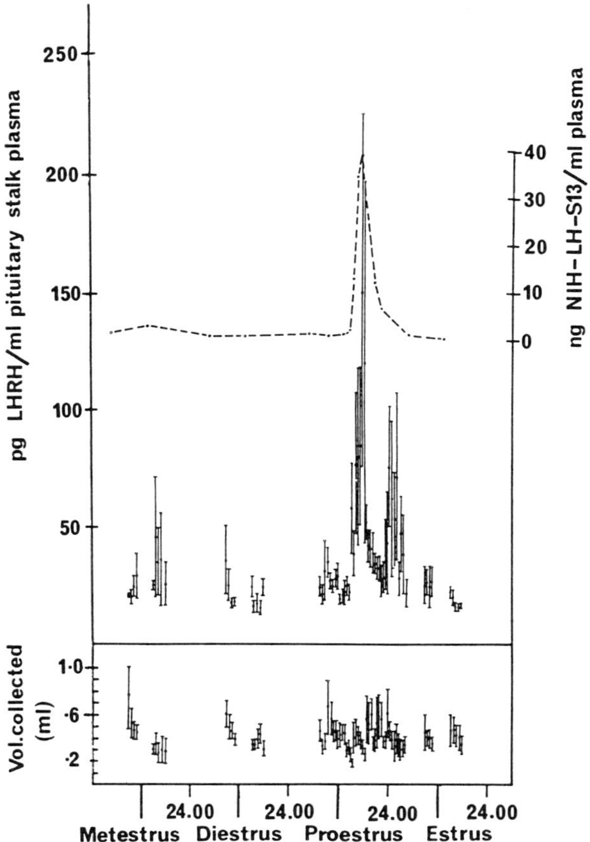

Figure 10.15
Mean (±SEM) concentrations of luteinizing hormone–releasing hormone (LHRH) (top panel) and volumes (bottom panel) of 30-minute collections of pituitary stalk blood during the estrous cycle. Most means are based on 5 to 15 samples; a few are based on 3 to 4 samples. Broken line represents mean concentrations of plasma LH. MH-LH (Abbott Laboratories, Chicago). (From Sarkar et al., 1976.)

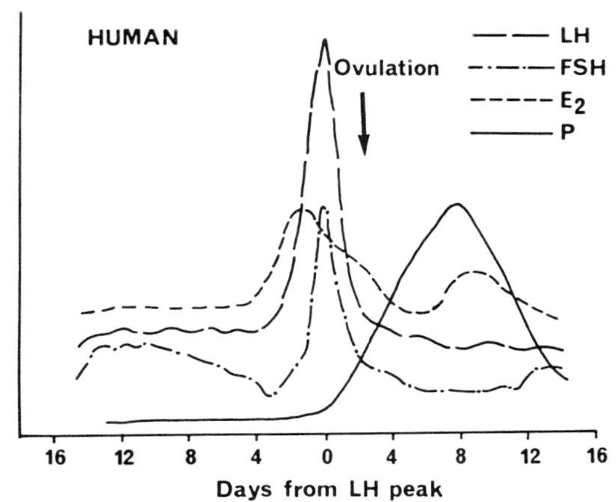

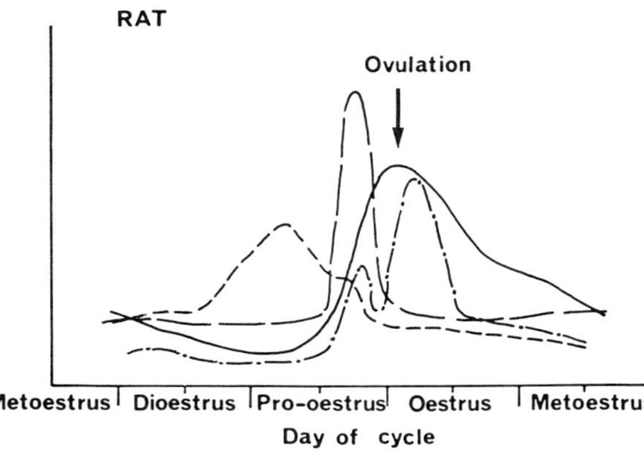

Figure 10.16
Schematic diagram of the key hormonal changes during the human menstrual cycle and the rat estrous cycle. Ovulation is preceded by a surge of luteinizing hormone (LH), which is triggered by a surge of estradiol-17β (E_2) and accompanied and followed by a surge of progesterone (P). In the human, the timing and magnitude of the follicle-stimulating hormone (FSH) surge are less consistent than that of the LH surge. (From Fink, 1988.)

creased by estradiol and progesterone, which appear not be able to affect GnRH neurons directly. This view relegates the ovarian steroids to providing an optimal environment for the prolonged GnRH, NPY, and galanin hypersecretion, rather than direct steroidal augmentation of either the synthesis or release of GnRH. This optimal environment includes not only the activation of excitatory, synergistic signals (NPY, galanin, NO etc.) but also the "disinhibition" of inhibitory signals (opiates and GABA), permitting a functional link with a timing device to accelerate GnRH and LH in the afternoon of proestrus (Kalra and Kalra, 1994).

GnRH may modulate its own release through an ultrashort-loop feedback mechanism (autoregulation). Synaptic contacts between fibers from neurons in the SCN, the biological clock, and GnRH cells in the POA may provide an anatomical basis for integration of circadian signals and GnRH release. Also to be considered in this system is the substantial influence of external factors (e.g., light) and internal factors (e.g., emotions, stress) on GnRH release.

d. Opiate inhibition of GnRH release

This is an important factor in GnRH regulation. β-Endorphin is found in portal blood and its concentration is inversely correlated with preovulatory LH release (Hulse et al., 1984). β-Endorphin suppresses GnRH release into portal blood from GnRH nerve terminals and thereby inhibits both the pulsatile release and preovulatory release of the gonadotropins. As GnRH neurons in culture possess opiate receptors, opiates may act directly on GnRH neurons to suppress release of the decapeptide (Maggi et al., 1995). Opiate inhibition may be activated by aspartate, which has an inhibitory effect on GnRH release (Giri et al., 1996).

e. Neural structures

Neural structures crucial for the GnRH surge include the medial preoptic area and SCN, hypothalamic areas which contain the cell bodies of many GnRH neurons crucial to the GnRH surge. Surgical separation of these regions from the rest of the brain still permits the anterior hypothalamus to generate LH surges, but the estrous cycles are irregular and their frequency varies from that of normal animals. It is highly probable that the normal activity of the GnRH surge generator is dependent on inputs to the hypothalamus from the limbic system, which plays an important part in emotions and conveys the olfactory signals that influence reproductive behavior.

10.1.3.8 Regulation of FSH Secretion

FSH secretion is regulated differently from LH and involves the peptide hormone inhibin. As this FSH-inhibin feedback mechanism probably is directly on the anterior pituitary and does not involve the hypothalamus, it is discussed in chapter 13, section 13.2. There are marked differences in the pulsatile release of FSH and LH. The FSH surge in women usually accompanies the LH surge, but its magnitude and precision are far less than that of the LH surge. In the rat the peak of the FSH surge occurs about 11 hours after the LH surge, indicating a dissociation betwen LH and FSH secretion. If, as is supported by most experimental evidence, there is only one GnRH, this dissociation may be due to differential pituitary FSH responsiveness to FSH and LH, or to other factors, such as inhibin, which may cause a separation in the timing of release of these two gonadotropins.

10.1.3.9 Reflex-Induced GnRH Secretion

This is a mechanism used by reflex ovulators, as in the rabbit, which ovulates after coitus, assuring a very high fertility rate. The reflex consists of vaginal stimulation which activates the GnRH cells in the brain resulting in a GnRH surge, followed by an LH surge. Suckling initiates GnRH release independent of the ovarian steroids and directly suppresses the GnRH pulse generator neurons in the MBH (Maeda et al., 1995).

10.1.3.10 Regulation by Neurotransmitters, Neuropeptides, and Melatonin

NE is also a potent simulator of GnRH pulses and the pulsatile release of NPY and NE coincides or precedes GnRH pulses. NE and glutamate stimulate GnRH release via NO release from NOergic neurons in the arcuate nucleus. NO also amplifies the magnitude and duration of the LH surge induced by estrogen acting via NPY (Bonavera et al., 1996). Inhibitory and excitatory amino acid neurotransmitters participate in the feedback actions of estradiol on LH secretion, acting on GnRH cell bodies and dendrites in the POA, but not on their nerve terminals (Jarry et al., 1995). DA has a stimulatory effect, although this has been debated.

Melatonin, produced by the pineal gland at night, inhibits GnRH-induced release of LH (Vanecek and Klein, 1995), accounting for the depressive effect of melatonin on reproduction in circadian and photoperiodic rhythms. Melatonin may be involved in long-term reproductive rhythms such as seasonal reproductive activities, which are highly sensitive to the the light-dark cycle, and the onset of puberty.

10.1.3.11 GnRH in Puberty and Menopause

a. Puberty

Pulsatile GnRH-gonadotropin secretion is high in the first year of life and then declines gradually in the human to hypogonadal levels. Pituitary responsiveness to exogeneous GnRH is also low at this time. As there is little or no ovarian function until puberty, inhibition of GnRH secretion must be central. As puberty approaches, GnRH neurons undergo morphological changes and the number of GnRH receptors in the pituitary increases. At the onset of puberty the GnRH pulse generator becomes activated resulting in a diurnal pattern of pulsatile GnRH and LH release. This pubertal increase in LHRH release appears to be due to the removal of tonic inhibition from GABA neurons and a subsequent increase in the stimulatory inputs of NPY and NE neurons to GnRH neurons (Terasawa, 1995).

In the female the ovary becomes mature enough to secrete adequate amounts of estradiol to initiate the first preovulatory LH surge and the ovary becomes more sensitive to the action of LH and FSH. Similar central and gonadal changes occur in males, with the testis probably increasing its sensitivity to hypothalamic-pituitary stimulation. Several suggestions as to the activator of the GnRH pulse generator have been proposed, such as the catecholamines, the excitatory neurotransmitter aspartate, and the endogenous opiates (Plant et al., 1989), but despite decades of investigations the specific initiator(s) of the onset of puberty is still unknown.

b. Menopause

A gradual decline in ovarian function occurs before the onset of menopause. Since the endocrine changes in menopause are equivalent to castration, eliminating the negative feedback influence from gonadal steroids, it is not surprising that GnRH, LH, and FSH levels increase. FSH increases more than LH because of the decrease in the specific FSH inhibitor, inhibin. The disappearance of opiate influence on GnRH secretion adds further to the increased activity of the GnRH-gonadotropin axis. It is remarkable that the hypothalamic nuclei do not degenerate with age, with the exception of the SCN the sexually dimorphic nucleus, which is twice as large in adult men as in women (Swaab, 1995).

Men usually do not have these abrupt neuroendocrine changes, during midlife or later, but testosterone levels, spermatogenesis, and fertility decline. It is unclear whether this is an age-related change in the brain-pituitary axis or a change in gonadal function.

10.1.3.12 GnRH as a Neurotransmitter and Neuromodulator

The presence of GnRH in neurons not directly involved in the hypothalamic-hypophysial system indicates a possible neurotransmitter or neuromodulatory role. GnRH is found in neurons near the olfactory bulb and may transduce olfactory stimuli to reproductive behavior. GnRH nerve terminals in the retina may modulate visual responsiveness from olfactory stimuli. In the sympathetic nervous system GnRH produces late, slow EPSPs, as was convincingly demonstrated by Jan and Jan (1982; see chapter 7) in postganglionic neurons of bullfrog lumbar sympathetic ganglia. GnRH may regulate the activity of dopaminergic, opiate-, NPY-, or galanin-containing neurons, all of which participate in the control of GnRH release from the ME in an intracerebral feedback loop system in which GnRH neurons project to the arcuate nucleus (Jennes and Woolums, 1994).

10.1.3.13 Functions of GnRH

Pituitary-gonadal effects involve the essential regulation by GnRH of LH and FSH secretion during reproductive life. GnRH plays a central role in the ontogeny and regulation of pituitary-gonadal function during fetal life since the synthesis and secretion of gonadotropins in the fetus is critically dependent upon GnRH production by the fetal hypothalamus. GnRH is the pulse generator involved in puberty, in the endocrine changes during the estrous and menstrual cycles.

Extrapituitary effects include a direct inhibitory action by circulating systemic GnRH on the gonads, acting on specific GnRH receptors. In addition, GnRH or a GnRH-like peptide is present in the ovary and testis, and in the testis inhibits LH-stimulated testosterone production, acting as a paracrine messenger between the Sertoli and Leydig cells.

GnRH is also implicated as a paracrine regulator of thymic cell function, involving a putative reproductive-immune interconnective pathway which may involve GnRH as a major factor in reproductive senescence (Marchetti et al., 1991).

Behavioral effects of GnRH are clearly shown by its induction of mating behavior in many species, including primates. This is a direct effect since the gonadotropins alone have no effect on mating behavior, and GnRH can induce this behavior even in hypophysectomized animals (Millar and King, 1988). GnRH is very likely involved in coordinating other behavioral patterns involved in reproduction in both females and males through its widespead neural connections in the CNS, especially the olfactory system. An especially interesting observation is that a fragment of GnRH (AC-GnRH-(5–10) is behaviorally active but does not affect LH release (Dudley and Moss, 1988).

10.1.3.14 Clinical Implications of GnRH

Owing to the large number of GnRH analogs available, GnRH agonists and antagonists can be used in a wide variety of clinical conditions involving reproduction. These include activation of the pituitary-gonadal axis in cases of hypogonadism or delayed puberty, and in the treatment of endometriosis, benign uterine tumors, and, together with an androgen blocker, prostatic cancer.

GnRH can be used to increase fertility, but it must be administered in a pulsatile manner, once every 60 to 90 minutes. Hourly injections over the course of several weeks are impractical, but long-lasting depot compounds, nasal sprays, and programmable minipumps are feasible alternatives (Jacobs et al., 1984). Various treatment combinations using GnRH analogs and ovarian steroids are used to retrieve a preovulatory oocyte for in vitro fertilization (Diedrich and Schmutzler, 1991).

In patients with Kallmann's syndrome, there is an absence of GnRH and a resulting hypogonadism and accompanying anosmia, believed to be due to a failure of GnRH neurons to migrate from the olfactory tract to the hypothalamus. Deletion of a gene, the KAL gene, in the X chromosome, near the tip of the short arm, is responsible for the syndrome. The infertility can be successfully reversed by treatment with a pulsatile GnRH pump.

GnRH as a contraceptive device is not satisfactory in males or females since it requires continuous administration in high dosages to induce receptor downregulation and inhibit the release of FSH and LH. This method, while preventing ovulation and spermatogenesis, eliminates sex steroid production and must be combined with sex steroid replacement therapy.

10.1.4 Growth Hormone–Releasing Hormone

GHRH regulates the secretion of GH by anterior pituitary somatotrophs, through complex interactions with somatostatin, also called somatotropin-release inhibiting hormone, or SRIH (see section 10.2.1), and the mediation of many neurotransmitters and neuropeptides acting at the hypothalamic level. In the absence of hypothalamic GHRH, the synthesis and secretion of GH is suppressed and growth is severely retarded. Lesions in the arcuate nucleus of the hypothalamus, or administration of a GHRH antibody, abolish or depress GH secretory pulses, a deflation that is reversed by GHRH administration (Tannenbaum and Ling, 1984). GHRH-producing tumors cause acromegaly in human patients.

10.1.4.1 Structure and Anatomical Distribution

GHRH was first isolated from human pancreatic tumors by Guillemin et al. (1982) and by Rivier et al. (1982) in two forms, as GHRH (1–40)-OH and GHRH (1–44)-NH_2 amino acid polypeptides. Both variants are generated from the same precursor (prepro-GHRH), with the full biological activity residing in the first 29 amino acids. Hypothalamic and pancreatic GHRH appear to be identical. GHRH belongs to the secretin-glucagon family, which also includes VIP. GHRH shares nine residues with VIP, with the greatest similarities occurring in the N-terminal regions of the peptide. The structure of human pancreatic GHRH is

Tyr-Ala-Asp-Ala-Ile-Phe-Tyr-Asn-Ser-Tyr^{10}Arg-
Lys-Val-Leu-Gly-Gln-Leu-Ser-Ala-Arg^{20}-Lys-Leu-
Leu-Gln-Asp-Ile-Met-Ser-Arg-Gln^{30}-Gln-Gly-Glu-
Ser-Asn-Gln-Glu-Arg-Gly-Ala^{40}Arg-Ala-Arg-
Leu^{44}-NH_2

Most GHRH neurons are found in the arcuate nucleus of the hypothalamus and the pituitary stalk, but the periventricular area and the SON and PVN also contain significant amounts of GHRH. The perikarya are mostly fusiform and bipolar and release GHRH into the pituitary portal system from nerve terminals in the ME.

There is close apposition of somatostatin fibers and varicosities with GHRH neurons in the arcuate and ventromedial nuclei, and also dense and overlapping innervation of somatostatin and GHRH projections into the ME (Leshin et al., 1994). Other nerve terminals impinging on GHRH perikarya contain the neuropeptides SP and met-enkephalin. In addition, GHRH is *colocalized* with one or more other neuropeptides, including NT, α-MSH, somatostatin, SP, NPY, TRH, galanin, and enkephalin. Colocalization with the neurotransmitters DA, ACh, or GABA can also be shown. This rich distribution of neuropeptides and neurotransmitters permits the complex regulatory control evident for GHRH.

Extrahypothalamic fibers containing GHRH extend through the limbic area, the cerebral cortex, and the hindbrain region. GHRH is also present in the peripheral nervous system and in most other tissues, including the gastrointestinal tract, the pituitary, gonads, adrenal, thyroid, lung, and kidney. It is found in tumors, which may cause excessive GH secretion with resulting acromegaly.

10.1.4.2 The GHRH Gene; GHRH Processing, Secretion, and Inactivation

The GHRH gene is located on chromosome 20. The gene spans over 9 kb and contains five exons and four introns. The GHRH sequence is followed by a single Arg residue which serves as a signal for proteolytic processing. Rat GHRH has a free C-terminus but all other GHRHs are C-terminally amidated. Another peptide of 29 or 30 amino acids follows the Arg residue.

Prepro-GHRH, a 107– or 108–amino acid precursor, is processed in the same way as other polypeptide precursors, by cleavage and amidation. The processing of GHRH precursor is variable and tissue-specific. Both forms of the precursor are present in the hypothalamus in equal amounts, with comparable potency for the physiological regulation of GH secretion. In addition to the 1–40 (rat) and 1–44 (human) forms of GHRH, a 29– or 30–amino acid peptide is cleaved from the precursor and co-released into the portal vessels. The function of this peptide is not known.

GHRH is inactivated by peptidases which remove the N-termimal peptide (Tyr-Ala) and cleave GHRH at positions 2 and 3 to produce a biologically inactive peptide GHRH(3–44)-NH_2 (Frohman et al., 1989).

10.1.4.3 GHRH Receptors and Second Messengers

High-affinity, low-capacity binding sites for GHRH are present on hypothalamic and anterior pituitary cells, but not on on other brain neurons tested. It is interesting that only partial occupation is needed for optimal GH release. The number of GHRH receptors is reduced with aging, and also in the obese Zucker rat, in which GH secretion is diminished. Glucocorticoids and estrogen are physiological regulators of GHRN receptor gene expression: administration of estradiol or glucocorticoids decrease GHRH receptor mRNA and oophoerectomy or adrenalectomy increases it (Lam et al., 1996).

GHRH receptors are coupled via G proteins to several intracellular signal transduction systems: the adenylate cyclase system, the phosphatidylinositol system, the Ca^{2+}-calmodulin system, and the arachidonic acid–eicosanoid system. These complex interacting messenger systems are reviewed by Harvey (1995).

Continuous instead of pulsatile administration of GHRH attenuates the pituitary response to the polypeptide and may be explained by the uncoupling of the adenylate cyclase system from GHRH receptors, as well as by the downregulation of the receptors. This desensitization of GHRH receptors is prevented by somatostatin even though somatostatin inhibits GHRH.

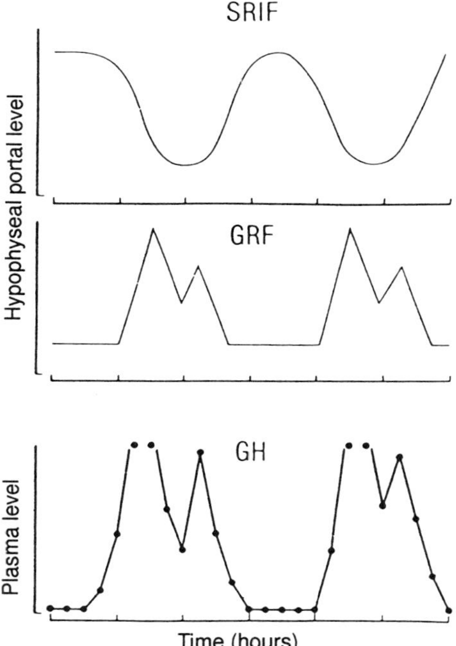

Figure 10.17
Schematic representation of the postulated rhythmic secretion of somatostatin (SRIF) and growth hormone–releasing hormone (GRF) into hypophyseal portal blood with the resulting alterations in growth hormone (GH) secretion as observed in plasma. (From Tannenbaum and Ling, 1984.)

10.1.4.4 Pulsatile Secretion of GHRH

The pulsatile secretion of GHRH develops slowly in the postnatal period in parallel with the dual network of GHRH and somatostatin hypothalamic neurons and is reflected in the pulsatile response of pituitary somatotrophs and the consequent release of GH. This is accompanied by a reduction in hypothalamic secretion of somatostatin, as depicted in figure 10.17. In growing children, GH is secreted approximately every 3 hours. There is a sexually dimorphic pattern of pulsatile GHRH release which is the result of sex differences and age-dependent changes in the expression of the GHRH and somatostatin genes (Argente et al., 1991).

10.1.4.5 Regulation of GHRH

The mechanisms regulating central GHRH secretion are not clearly understood. GHRH is inhibited by a short-loop feedback action of GH on hypothalamic GHRH neurons. This involves the induction of *c-fos* mRNA, primarily in neurons in the arcuate nucleus that are neither GHRH nor somatostatin neurons. Lam et al. (1996) suggest that these unidentified neurons are directly involved in transducing the effects of GH in the brain. GHRH mRNA in the MBH is markedly increased after hypophysectomy, a rise that can be reversed by treatment with GH, indicating a negative feedback mechanism between GH and GHRH synthesis (Muller et al., 1988), a concept supported by the observed increase in the expression of the GHRH gene in GH-deficient mice. A direct suppression of the GHRH gene by GH is indicated by studies on transgenic mice expressing a tyrosine hydroxylase–human GH fusion gene in the hypothalamus. The resulting GH deficiency and dwarfism is a consequence of impaired GHRH production due to the locally produced human GH in the hypothalamus (Szabo et al., 1995).

The neuronal network for GHRH regulation involves somatostatin, the noradrenergic and cholinergic systems, and neuropeptides. The adrenergic systems appear to have dual effects on GHRH secretion, with α-adrenergic neurons inhibiting GHRH release and the β-adrenergic system exerting an inhibitory influence. DA inhibits GHRH release, presumably through dopaminergic stimulation of somatostatin (Kitajima et al., 1989). Opiates and serotonin may act to stimulate GHRH release, whereas GABA probably inhibits it.

Many hormones affect GHRH stimulation of pituitary GH. Testosterone increases GHRH-induced GH secretion, as do the thyroid hormones. Glucocorticoids enhance GH gene transcription and increase GHRH receptor synthesis, However, excess glucocorticoids inhibit normal growth in all species studied through a mechanism that increases hypothalamic somatostatin and enhances β-adrenergic reponsiveness of the neurons (Devesa et al., 1995). Glucocorticoids change the responsiveness of the producing neurons from α_2-adrenoreceptors to that of β-adrenoreceptors. There may be a negative feedback loop between insulin-like growth factor and GHRH.

10.1.4.6 Development, Maturation, and Aging

Fetal and neonatal GHRH appear to be necessary for GH production during development. The synthesis, content, and release of GNRH increase postnatally and at puberty, at which time GHRH neuronal function becomes markedly sexually dimorphic (Argente et al., 1991). Hypothalamic GHRH levels are higher in the adult male than in the adult female, a testosterone-dependent discrepancy.

Neonatal and juvenile animals are more responsive to GHRH than are adult or aging animals and humans. GHRH concentrations in the plasma decline with aging, apparently due to a degeneration of GHRH neurons. Similarly, the normal feedback regulation of GH on GHRH and somatostatin neurons in the hypothalamus disappears with age.

10.1.4.7 Growth Hormone–Releasing Peptide (GHRP-6)

GHRP-6 (His-D-Trp-Ala-Trp-D-Phe-Lys-NH_2) is a synthetic hexapeptide that causes the release of GH in a specific and dose-related manner. GHRP-6 is more potent than GHRH and acts synergistically with GHRH to provoke a strong GH response. Although GHRP-6 acts on the pituitary, its main action is at the hypothalamic level. The receptor for this synthetic GH secretogogue has been cloned and it is distinct from the GHRH receptor, indicating that there is a second route for GH regulation, apart from GHRH and somatostatin. (Conn and Bowers, 1996). GHRP-6 also stimulates the release of ACTH and cortisol in normal men (Frieboes et al., 1995).

10.1.4.8 Functions of GHRH

Pituitary actions of GHRH include not only the *stimulation* of GH synthesis and release but also the *proliferation* and *differentiation* of the pituitary somatotrophs during ontogeny and puberty.

Sleep is regulated by GHRH and GHRP-6, affecting the sleep EEG and nocturnal hormonal secretion. GHRH causes an increase in slow wave sleep and in GH secretion, while blunting ACTH and cortisol release. The sleep-onset GH pulse decreases with age and may be correlated with the shortened sleep periods of senescence. Both in rats and in humans, the time of day at which GHRH is administered is an important variable. Both GHRH and GHRP-6 promote sleep, but GHRH increases slow wave sleep, whereas GHRP enhances stage 2 sleep and does not affect slow wave sleep. These different actions indicate that the two peptides act on different receptors (Frieboes et al., 1995). The balance between GHRH and CRH in sleep regulation is discussed in section 10.1.2.

Food intake is stimulated by GHRH in a circadian phase–dependent manner that involves the SCN (Vaccarino et al., 1995).

Behavior is modified by GHRH which modulates long-term memory as well as the extinction reponse, but the effect varies with the age of the animal.

10.1.4.9 Clinical Implications of GHRH

Retarded growth due to lack of GH is usually caused by a hypothalamic deficiency of GHRH, and as the pituitary somatotroph is capable of responding to exogenous GHRH, a logical therapy for GH-deficient children would be administration of GHRH. Clinical studies indicate an acceleration of growth in children when GHRH is given in a pulsatile manner, but growth slows considerably after a year of therapy (Vance and Thorner, 1988).

If an oral version of the synthetic GHRP were to be successfully developed, it would provide a valuable clinical alternative to the expensive and difficult (by injections three times a week) administration of GH in GH-deficient children and in the elderly (Conn and Bowers, 1996). See also section 13.5.5.

Although acromegaly may be caused by excess secretion of GHRH, clinical treatment usually involves reducing GH secretion by increasing somatostatin levels, through the administration of a long-acting SS analog such as octreotide or DA agonists such as bromocriptine.

10.2 Hypothalamic Release Inhibiting Hormones

10.2.1 Somatostatin

The presence of a GH release–inhibiting substance in hypothalamic extracts was first reported by Kruhlich et al. (1968) and subsequently isolated, characterized, and named somatotropin-release inhibiting factor (SRIF), then renamed somatostatin by Guillemin's group (Brazeau et al., 1973). Somatostatin not only inhibits the release of GHRH but is a multifunctional hormone, inhibiting the release of many other pituitary, pancreatic, and gut hormones, as well as the exocrine secretions of the gastrointestinal tract. Somatostatin also has an effect on the development of the brain and a maintenance role in the adult and aging brain. Consequently, yet another name may be found for it because somatostatin is too restrictive a term.

10.2.1.1 Structure and Anatomical Distribution

The structure of the tetradecapeptide somatostatin is

H-Ala-Gly-Cys-Lys-Asn-Phe-Phe-Trp-Lys-Thr-
Phe-Thr-Ser-Cys-OH.

This cyclic peptide has a disulfide bond between residues 3 and 14 giving it the ring structure essential to biological activity. Multiple N-terminally extended forms exist, such as mammalian somatostatin-28, fish somatostatin-22, -25, and -28, and lamprey somatostatin-34 and -37. These somatostatins have been isolated from hypothalamic, pancreatic, and gastrointestinal tissues and are found in a wide variety of other tissues.

In the mammalian CNS, somatostatin neurons are concentrated mainly in the periventricular preoptic area and the anterior hypothalamus, with fewer cells in the arcuate and ventromedial nuclei. The SS neurons have relatively long projections to the ME and to limbic structures and the brainstem. There is considerable overlap with GHRH neurons and projections in the hypothalamus and ME (see 10.1.4.1). Somatostatin is present in some cerebral cortical and autonomic nervous system neurons (Elde and Hökfelt, 1979) supporting its importance in central autonomic regulations. Other somatostatin neurons are interneurons involved in local regulatory circuits. Many somatostatin interneurons co-express NPY, as well as GABA, indicating a functional role for somatostatin in GABA inhibitory circuits. The somatostatin

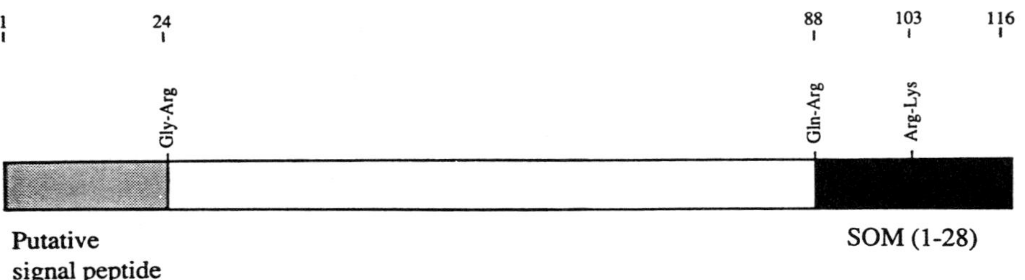

Figure 10.18
Structure of the human and rat preprosomatostatin-116 molecule. The putative signal peptide extends from amino acids 1–24 and is indicated by the gray area. Somatostatin (SOM)-28 extends from amino acid 88 and SOM-14 extends from amino acid 103. Amino acid sequences where cleavage takes place are indicated. There is a high degree of homology between human and rat preprosomatostatin, with only 4 amino acid substitutions. (From Meister and Hökfelt, 1992.)

system of neurons and fibers is among the earliest of the transmitter systems to be established in the visual cortex and suggests a role for the peptide in cortical organization as well as visual processing (Feldman et al., 1990).

Extraneuronal somatostatin is extensive throughout the gastrointestinal tract in mucosal D cells and in myenteric neurons, and in the D cells of the pancreas where it affects the secretion of insulin and glucagon. In some pancreatic islet cells, somatostatin is colocalized with NO. Somatostatin is also found in the thyroid and heart, and in the salivary glands of some species.

10.2.1.2 The Somatostatin Gene; Somatostatin Processing, Release, and Inactivation

Somatostatin is an ancient peptide, being found in single-cell protozoa. It may be considered to be a member of a *multigene family* of peptides, with two important biologically active products, somatostatin-14 and -28. In rats and humans, somatostatin molecules are derived from a single gene, but in several teleost species there are two distinct and active genes. Gene I codes for somatostatin-14, which is constant for all vertebrates except the lamprey. Gene II codes for the various extended forms. Both the human and the rat genes consist of two exons and one intron. In exon 1, in addition to an untranslated region, the final portion corresponds to 46 amino acids of preprosomatostatin. Exon 2 starts with the rest of the prosequence, followed by the coding sequence for somatostatin-28, which is itself terminated by the 14 amino acids of somatostatin-14.

In general, somatostatin-28 is the more potent variant for inhibiting GHRH, GH, PRL, TSH, and insulin secretion, whereas somatostatin-14 is selective in its inhibitory actions on glucagon secretion, gastric exocrine secretion, splanchnic blood flow, and intestinal motility.

Processing of somatostatin may occur in a tissue-specific manner. Preprosomatostatin, a 116–amino acid peptide, contains both the somatostatin-14 and somatostatin-28 forms (figure 10.18). It is synthesized in the endoplasmic reticulum, the signal peptide removed and prosomatostatin translocated to the Golgi system. Prosomatostatin can be cleaved post-translationally in secretory granules to generate the two mature forms, somatostatin-14 and somatostatin-

28, and the latter can also be subsequently processed to somatostatin-14 (Patel, 1987). In fish, however, there are two separate and independent products, one from prosomatastatin I (somatostatin-14) the other from prosomatostatin II (somatostatin-28).

The *release of somatostatin-14 and -28* into the ME occurs in amounts proportional to their intracellular content, a ratio of somatostatin-14 to somatostatin-28 of approximately 3:1. Although the amount of somatostatin-28 released is less that that of somatostatin-14, it is three to eight times more potent in evoking GH release and it also binds better to somatostatin receptors. Consequently, somatostatin-14 and -28 may have equally important roles in the inhibition of GH.

Inactivation of somatostatin occurs very rapidly, the plasma half-life being less than 3 minutes. The synthesis of long-acting somatostatin analogs such as octreotide (SMS 201-995), an octapeptide, extends the half-life of this potent inhibitory hormone and makes feasible the therapeutic use of somatostatin.

Independence of the brain and gut somatostatin systems is shown by the lack of effect of hypothalamic lesions on pancreatic somatostatin.

10.2.1.3 Somatostatin Receptors and Second Messengers

Somatostatin-14 receptors are generously distributed in all major brain regions, with the highest concentration in the cerebral cortex, intermediate concentrations in the hypothalamus, thalamus, amygdala, and hippocampus, and the lowest concentrations in the mid- and hindbrain. Somatostatin-14 receptor concentrations in the anterior pituitary, the zona glomerulosa of the adrenal cortex, and the exocrine pancreas are almost as high as in the cerebral cortex (Patel, 1987). Somatostatin receptors are present on the delta cells (somatostatin-producing), beta cells (insulin-producing), and alpha cells (glucagon-producing) of the pancreatic islets, with the receptors on the alpha cells present in the greatest concentration.

Somatostatin receptors are heterogeneous: at this time, five different types have been determined (1–5) (Epelbaum et al., 1994). Genes for all five high-affinity receptors have recently been cloned. The different subtypes vary in size but almost all have the same intronless organization. All receptors identified so far bind somatostatin-14 and somatostatin-28 with high affinity and are coupled to G proteins and inhibit adenylate cyclase and Ca^{2+} fluxes. In the *pituitary*, the somatotrophs, thyrotrophs, and lactotrophs have a single class of binding sites with a nanomolar affinity, whereas the *brain* has multiple subtypes. Receptor subtypes 1 and 2 are involved in the neuroendocrine regulation of GH secretion in both sexes (Beaudet et al., 1995). Subtype 3 is found in the motor neurons of the spinal cord and motor nuclei of the brainstem, as well as in the sensory neurons of the spinal ganglia, implying a possible role for these receptors in motor and sensory functions (Senaris et al., 1995). Subtype 5 receptors are involved in insulin secretion, and subtypes 2 and 5 are probably the receptor subtypes in somatostatin-susceptible cancers.

10.2.1.4 Pulsatile Secretion of Somatostatin

Pulsatile secretion of somatostatin occurs in coordination with GHRH and GH secretion, as shown in figure 10.17. GHRH stimulates the peaks of GH secretion at times when somatostatin concentration is low, and when levels rise, peripheral GH levels drop. The inhibition of GH secretion by somatostatin is accompanied by a positive role as somatostatin prepares the somatotroph to respond optimally to the new pulse of hypothalamic GHRH (Turner and Tannebaum, 1995). Elimination of endogenous somatostatin by long-term immunoneutralization markedly reduces GHRH responsiveness, an indication that somatostatin antagonizes GHRH centrally, as well as acting on the pituitary gland. Obviously, a precise balance between GHRH, GH, and somatostatin is required for their proper pulsatile release.

10.2.1.5 Regulation of Somatostatin

The *ultrashort-loop negative feedback*, as propounded by McCann and his colleagues (Samson et al., 1988), involves an autoregulation of somatostatin through the local release of somatostatin onto somatostatin-producing neurons in the hypothalamus, inhibiting further somatostatin release. A *positive ultrashort loop* may also be used for the stimulation of somatostatin release by GHRH. Anatomical support for this concept comes from the presence of axon collaterals from peptide-containing cells that terminate in the tuberoinfundibular region. A *short-loop positive feedback* system may also exist, by which somatostatin release is stimulated by GH from the pituitary.

Several neuropeptides that affect GH release may do so through an action on hypothalamic somatostatin neurons, whereas glucocorticoids increase the hypothalamic content of somatostatin. POMC- and galanin-containing interneurons also participate in the regulation of somatostatin and GHRH neuronal activity, and to add further complexity to this system, sex steroids affect the expression of somatostatin directly in PVN neurons (Bertherat et al., 1995).

Neurotransmitters play an important role in the control of GH release and the site of action appears to be mainly at the hypothalamic level. 5-HT decreases somatostatin release, and both DA and adrenergic stimulation increase somatostatin release. However, the adrenergic transmitters have complex effects, with stimulatory and inhibitory actions mediated by different receptors. Stimulation of the α_1- and β-adrenoreceptors probably increases somatostatin release. Cholinergic systems are important regulators of GH release, probably through the inhibition of somatostatin release rather than stimulation of GHRH release (Richardson et al., 1980). However, stimulation of somatostatin release by ACh has been reported by Peterfreund and Vale (1983).

10.2.1.6 Somatostatin as a Neurotransmitter and Neuromodulator

Somatostatin hyperpolarizes cell membranes by opening various K^+ channels, a common method for inhibition by neurotransmitters. Somatostatin also selectively inhibits high voltage–activated Ca^{2+} channels in hippocampal pyramidal neurons (Ishibashi and Akaike, 1995). Owing to the widespread distribution of somatostatin, its inhibitory effects are extensive. Some examples include the inhibition of spontaneous firing of locus ceruleus neurons by the direct activation of somatostatin receptors, inhibition of medial amygdala neuron firing, and the hyperpolarization of pyramidal neurons in the ventral subiculum. In addition to its inhibitory effects on pituitary cells and hypothalamic GHRH, somatostatin modulates the release of 5-HT in the hypothalamus and facilitates DA release in the nucleus accumbens and striatum. Its action on DA neurons may account for the hyperlocomotor activity in the rat after central applications of an analog.

Peripheral neurotransmitter and neuromodulatory actions of somatostatin include a potent negative inotropic effect on the atria, and inhibition of neurogenically induced contractions in the guinea pig ileum, actions resulting from somatostatin-induced hyperpolarizations.

10.2.1.7 Functions of Somatostatin

The main function somatostatin is *inhibitory*. It suppresses the secretion of GH, TSH, and PRL by the anterior pituitary. In addition it suppresses the secretion of insulin and glucagon by the endocrine pancreas, as part of an intrinsic paracrine control system. Somatostatin inhibits gastric acid and secretin secretion, indirectly though its inhibitory action on gastrin, and is probably an intrinsic paracrine regulator of all internal and external secretions of the gastrointestinal tract (see chapter 17, section 17.6).

Somatostatin has *neurotrophic effects*, probably starting in ontogeny as a regulator of neuroblast proliferation during brain maturation, initiating neurite outgrowth. Somatostatin then contributes to the maintenance of neuronal health in the adult and aging brain. This inference is based on the selective and specific decrease in somatostatin concentrations and high-affinity somatostatin type 1 receptor binding sites in the neocortex, hippocampus, and CSF of patients with Alzheimer's disease (Epelbaum, 1986). In addition, decreased levels of somatostatin correlate with the distribution of senile plaques and neurofibrillary tangles.

Somatostatin has numerous effects on the release and metabolism of other neuropeptides and neurotransmitters (see review by Epelbaum, 1986). Consequently, there are diverse *autonomic* and *behavioral* effects ascribed to somatostatin, including control of body temperature, blood pressure, hunger and satiety, nociception, the acoustic startle response, and learning and memory. The *analgesic* effect of somatostatin, intrathecally or epidurally administered, may be due to an interaction with opiate receptors.

Somatostatin has potent *oncological effects*, suppressing the growth of certain tumors. Neuroblastomas, menangiomas, and low-grade gliomas have somatostatin receptors and some somatostatin analogs can inhibit their proliferation.

Sleep is affected by somatostatin, which increases REM sleep without affecting other phases. *Cortistatin*, a peptide with strong structural similarities to somatostatin, a product of a different gene, depresses neuronal electrical activity, but unlike somatostatin, induces low-frequency waves in the cerebral cortex (Delecea et al., 1996).

10.2.1.8 Clinical Implications of Somatostatin

As somatostatin inhibits GH secretion, somatostatin analogs have been used for the control of acromegaly. Octreotide, the long-acting somatostatin analog, has been succesfully used to decrease GH-secreting pituitary tumors as well as pituitary tumors that secrete TSH. However, the analog has no effect on PRL- and ACTH-secreting pituitary tumors. Somatostatin analogs may also be useful in the treatment of diseases of the gastrointestinal tract and pancreas, and of hormone-sensitive tumors, such as breast and prostatic cancer.

The correlation of somatostatin changes with pathological alterations in the brain, suggests that somatostatin analogs may be useful in treating Alzheimer's disease, epilepsy, Huntington's disease, and similar neurodegenerative diseases.

10.2.2 Hypothalamic Inhibition of Prolactin Release

PRL is an ancient hormone that has developed many functions over the course of evolution. These include reproduction and the nurturing of the young, osmoregulation, growth, support of metabolism, metamorphosis, and in mammals, milk production. PRL is produced by the lactotrophs of the anterior pituitary, which are under constant inhibition, which keeps their secretory activity low. As there is no endocrine target organ to exert a negative feedback control over the lactotrophs, the tonic inhibition is provided by the hypothalamus. There is no evidence for the postulated peptidergic PRL-inhibiting factor (PIF). Instead, there is much support for hypothalamic DA as the physiological PIF.

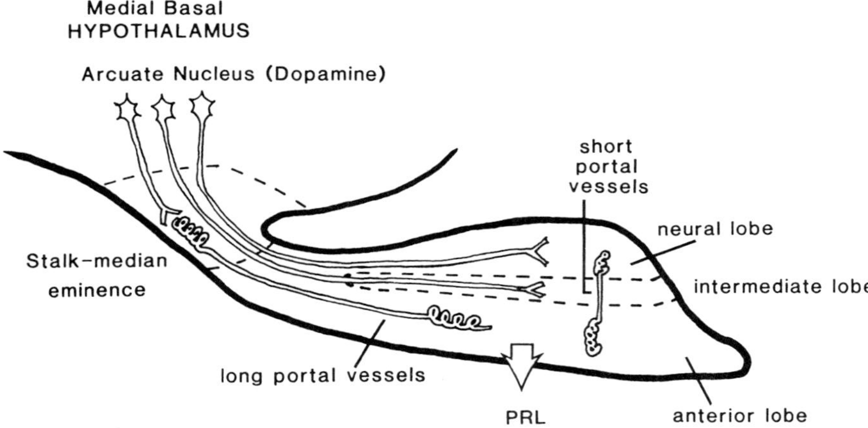

Figure 10.19
Schematic representation of the hypothalamic-pituitary complex. The long portal vessels connect the hypothalamus and the anterior lobe and the short portal vessels connect the posterior and anterior lobes. The dopamine neurons have perikarya in the arcuate nucleus and terminals in the median eminence (tuberoinfundibular dopaminergic neurons) and neural and intermediate lobes (tuberohypophyseal dopaminergic neurons). PRL, prolactin. (From Ben-Jonathan, 1990.)

10.2.2.1 Tonic Inhibition of Prolactin by Dopamine

There are two dopaminergic systems emanating from the hypothalamus that maintain *tonic inhibition* over PRL secretion. The tuberoinfundibular system, located entirely within the MBH, provides the major DA input to the anterior pituitary via the long portal vessels. The other DA system is the tubero hypophyseal system with terminals in the posterior and intermediate lobes of the pituitary. From this system DA reaches the anterior lobe via the short portal vessels that connect the neural, intermediate, and anterior lobes of the pituitary (figure 10.19).

10.2.2.2 Factors That Suppress Dopamine Inhibition

A small peptide, *PRL-releasing factor (PRF)*, was first identified by Ben-Jonathan in 1982, as described in the review (Ben-Jonathan, 1990). PRF is present almost exclusively in the neurointermediate lobe, localized within non-neural cells. The synthesis and release of PRF are subjected to a short-loop negative feedback by PRL, and tonic inhibition by DA (Ben-Jonathan et al., 1991). When this hypothalamic inhibition is overcome, by suckling, estrogen, or other agents, PRF is released and transported via the short portal vessels to the anterior pituitary lactotrophs to stimulate PRL secretion and release.

a. *Suckling-induced PRF release*

Suckling is the most potent physiological stimulus to PRF release. The long-held view is that via a neural route from the nipples to the hypothalamic-hypophyseal complex via the spinal cord and midbrain, suckling suppresses DA release and releases one or more putative PRL-releasing factors such as TRH or VIP. These neuropeptides, acting through the long portal vessels to the anterior pituitary, stimulate the lactotrophs to increase PRL secretion. There is a long list of other endogenous compounds believed to release PRL by a direct action on the anterior pituitary. These include estrogen, the opiate peptides, GnRH, and 5-HT.

This dominant view of anterior pituitary control is too simple since removal of the neurointermediate lobe completely abolishes the suckling-induced rise in PRL. Nor is the fall in DA and the rise in TRH or VIP great enough to account for the striking increase in lactotroph responsiveness and resulting massive PRL discharge. Thus much of the dramatic change in responsiveness and rise in PRL induced by suckling must be attributed to PRF release and delivery to the anterior pituitary through the short portal vessels. The neural lobe is further implicated in PRL release as suckling induces the release of OT which further augments PRF release. Some of the neural and humoral connections regulating PRL are schematically outlined in figure 10.20.

b. Is α-MSH the common pathway?

Another possibility is that the agent that increases responsiveness is α-MSH, a neuropeptide produced in large amounts in the intermediate lobe. The secretion of α-MSH is tonically inhibited by DA derived from the tuberoinfundibular system. Some of the arguments in favor of this theory are that neurointermediate lobe stores of α-MSH are rapidly depleted within minutes of suckling and antibodies to α-MSH severely diminish the PRL response to suckling. It is possible that both PRF and α-MSH are involved in the amplified response to suckling (Frawley, 1994).

c. Estradiol

Estradiol is a natural stimulus to PRL secretion and probably acts at variable levels: hypothalamic DA and anterior pituitary lactotrophs, as well as PRF. Rising blood levels of estradiol just prior to proestrus and the LH surge trigger a surge of PRL and an increase in circulating α-MSH, which in turn induces the recruitment of additional PRL cells into the secretory pool. Thus α-MSH could be the active principle responsible for both the increased responsiveness and increased recruitment of PRL cells resulting from suckling and from estrogen treatment (figure 10.21).

10.2.2.3 Clinical Implications of Dopamine Inhibition of Prolactin

Hyperprolactinemia resulting from pituitary tumors is considerably reduced by the administration of bromocriptine, a DA agonist. The agonist mimics the action of the endogenous DA, shrinking the tumor.

10.3 Pituitary Adenylate Cyclase–Activating Polypeptide (PACAP)

The regulation of the activities of the anterior pituitary gland is not completely accounted for by the classical group of hypothalamic releasing and release-inhibiting neuropeptides. A PRL-releasing hormone is still missing and many other aspects of anterior pituitary control, growth, and differentiation are unexplained. In view of this, Arimura and his collegues set out to find other hypothalamic releasing hormones that might affect the anterior pituitary. This work is described by Arimura and Shioda (1995). They discovered two substances with adenylate cyclase–stimulating activity in rat pituitary cell cultures: these substances were isolated in a pure form from ovine hypothalamus and identified as a 38-residue peptide (PACAP 38) and a 27-residue peptide (PACAP 27).

10.3.1 Structure and Distribution of PACAP

PACAP is a widely distributed, biologically active peptide of either 27 or 38 amino acids, similar in

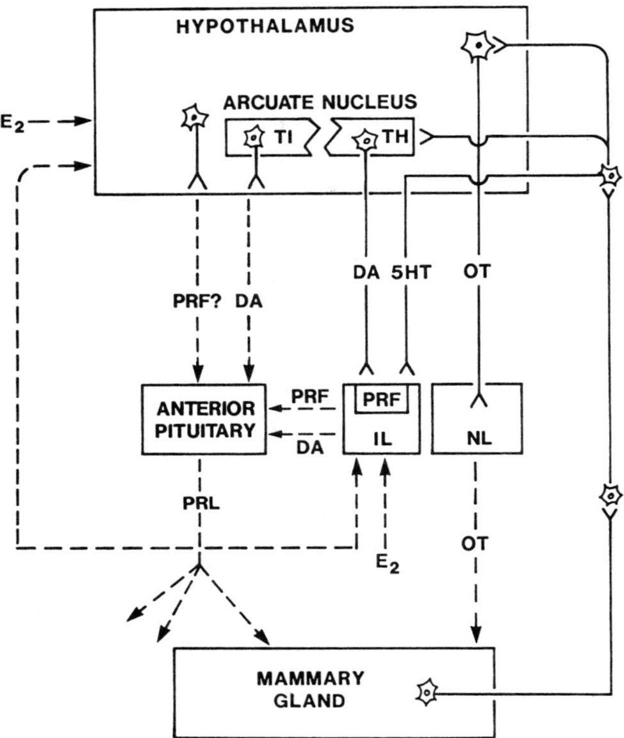

Figure 10.20
A model depicting the neuroendocrine regulation of prolactin secretion. See text for explanation. TH, tuberohypophyseal; TI, tuberoinfundibular; OT, oxytocin; E_2, estradiol; 5HT, serotonin; DA, dopamine; PRF, prolactin-releasing factor; IL, intermediate lobe; NL, neural lobe; PRL, prolactin. Connecting and interrupted lines are neural and humoral communications, respectively. (From Ben-Jonathan et al., 1991.)

structure to the members of the secretin-glucagon-VIP family, but with the greatest similarity in structure and actions to VIP.

The structure of *PACAP 38* is

His-Ser-Asp-Gly-Ile-*Phe-Thr-Asp*-Ser-*Tyr*-Ser-*Arg*-Tyr-*Arg-Lys-Gln-Met-Ala-Val-Lys-Lys-Tyr-Leu*-Ala-Ala-Val-*Leu*^{27}**-Gly-Lys-Arg-Tyr-Lys-Gln-Arg-Val-Lys-Asn-Lys**^{38}-NH_2

PACAP 27 lacks the last amino acids shown in **bold** above. The amino acid residues shown in *italics* are common to PACAP 38, PACAP 27, and VIP (Arimura and Shioda, 1995).

Like VIP, PACAP affects many tissues, stimulating adenylate cyclase not only in anterior pituitary cells but also in many other endocrine cells, especially the adrenal medulla and endocrine pancreas, the nervous system, and several peripheral organs. PACAP is

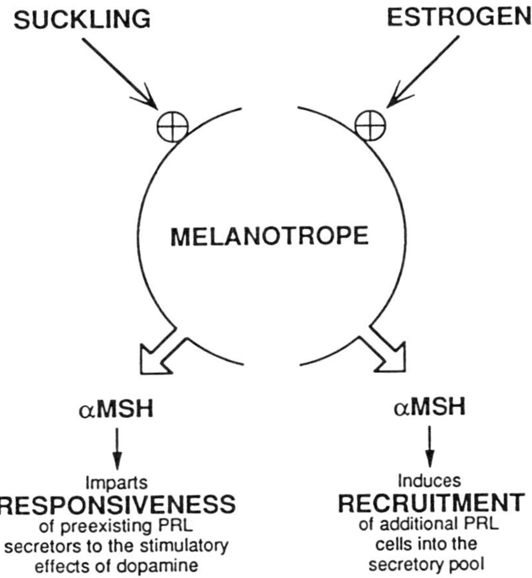

Figure 10.21
Dual roles of α-melanocyte–stimulating hormone (αMSH) in the dynamic release of prolactin (PRL). (From Frawley, 1994.)

found in the highest concentration in the hypothalamus, especially in the ME and posterior pituitary, but also in many other tissues, especially the testes, which contain more PACAP in total than the whole of the brain (Arimura et al., 1991).

10.3.2 The PACAP Receptor

PACAP receptors are 437– to 495–amino acid proteins, with the seven transmembrane domains characteristic of G protein–coupled receptors. These receptors are capable of differential coupling to intracellular signaling cascades and their extensive distribution in a variety of tissues accounts for the many actions of PACAP and VIP. PACAP receptors are expressed in the brain during early embryonic development and increase in number up to the early postnatal period.

There are three types of PACAP receptors, types 1, 2, and 3. *PACAP receptor type 1* is the predominant form in the pituitary, brain, adrenal, and testis, and there are four or five isoforms of the PACAP type 1 receptor produced by alternative splicing of the precursor RNA. Type 1 receptor is PACAP-specific. PACAP 1 receptors are selectively expressed in B and T lymphocytes from the spleen and other lymphoid organs and are likely to mediate many of the purported effects of PACAP and VIP on the immune system (Washek et al., 1995).

PACAP receptor type 2 has a similar distribution to that of the VIP receptor (see chapter 16) and has a binding site that PACAP shares with VIP.

PACAP receptor type 3 has recently been isolated from insulin-secreting cells of the pancreas (beta cells). This receptor has binding properties similar to those of the type 2 receptor, binding PACAP and VIP equally well (Inagaki et al., 1996). PACAP receptor type 3 is a protein of 437 amino acids that has a 50% identity with the other two PACAP receptors and is coupled to adenylate cyclase and calcium mobilization from intracellular Ca^{2+} stores. The high expression of PACAP 3 receptor in pancreatic islets and in insulin-secreting cell lines suggests that PACAP and VIP may play a physiological role in insulin secretion.

10.3.3 Actions of PACAP

10.3.3.1 The Pituitary Gland

In the *anterior pituitary*, PACAP stimulates PRL gene expression and POMC gene transcription via cAMP-dependent protein kinase activation. LH secretion is also stimulated by PACAP, acting directly on the gonadotrophs (Leonhardt et al., 1995). PACAP not only stimulates gonadotropin release from pituitary cells but sustained exposure to PACAP for several hours modulates GnRH-stimulated LH release, increasing the amplitude of LH responses to pulsatile GnRH (Culler and Paschall, 1992). However, a recent report by Anderson et al. (1996) suggests that PACAP acts in the arcuate nucleus region of the MBH to inhibit PRL and LH secretion.

In the *intermediate lobe* melanotrophs express PACAP receptor type 1 isoforms that transduce through the cAMP and inositol phosphate pathways. Both forms of PACAP stimulate α-MSH excytosis and POMC gene transcription in melanotrophs, via receptors coupled to the adenylate cyclase pathway, whereas PACAP 38 may act additionally through the inositol phosphate pathway (René et al., 1996).

10.3.3.2 The Gonads

PACAP stimulates cAMP accumulation and secretory function in Sertoli cells of the testis and in ovarian granulosa cells. This is a specific action of PACAP on PACAP 38 receptors and not via VIP receptors (Heindel et al., 1996). PACAP is synthesized within the seminiferous tubules and probably acts as an autocrine or paracrine regulator of the developing germ cells, or as both.

10.3.3.3 PACAP as a Growth Factor

PACAP acts as a neurotrophic factor, preventing natural neuronal cell death in the dorsal root ganglia in the chick embryo and increasing spinal motor neuron survival (Arimura et al., 1994) and is suspected of being active in some forms of tumor growth. PACAP and VIP are important developmental regulators, and are present in the nervous system, including the sympathetic nervous system, at critical periods of cell proliferation and differentiation. This topic is discussed in more detail in chapter 16 where the actions of VIP are considered.

10.3.3.4 The Gastrointestinal Tract

PACAP causes a neurogenic contraction of the guinea pig ileum that is more potent than that evoked by VIP, but both neuropeptides act by releasing ACh and SP from postganglionic cholinergic and peptidergic nerves. In all other gastrointestinal preparations, and in all other species, PACAP and VIP cause relaxation (Katsoulis and Schmidt, 1996).

10.4 Other Neuropeptides Regulating Anterior Pituitary Hormones

In addition to the hypothalamic regulatory neuropeptides, there are many CNS neuropeptides, some originally identified in the gut or the peripheral nervous system, that have consequential effects on pituitary hormones. As a warning it must be mentioned that many of these effects depend on the dosage and experimental circumstances, and are by no means as clear as the actions of the hypothalamic regulatory neuropeptides. Müller and Nisticò (1989) discuss these variables in detail. A brief list of these neuropeptides indicates the scope of their influence.

10.4.1 Delta Sleep–Inducing Peptide (DSIP)

DSIP is a nonapeptide found in many areas of the brain, including the hypothalamus and pituitary; in peripheral tissues, especially the adrenal medulla; and in plasma, milk, and urine. DSIP induces sleep in many species of mammals, and has been reported to be associated with suppression of slow wave and REM sleep. However, Friedman et al. (1994) found that whereas in humans the diurnal rhythm of DSIP may be directly coupled to body temperature, there was no correlation between DSIP, REM, and slow wave sleep. The effects on sleep as reported by many investigators are variable and not particularly convincing; DSIP probably acts as a modulator of many other sleep-inducing factors (Graf and Kastin, 1986). It has been suggested that DSIP has been misnamed, as have so many other neuropeptides, leading to a false concept of its action (Kastin et al., 1984).

DSIP has extrasleep activities that imply that DSIP may influence the activity of the HPA axis (Kastin et al., 1980). DSIP is colocalized with TSH in the pituitary and GnRH in the hypothalamus. DSIP is colocalized with NE in the adrenal medulla and adrenalectomy increases levels of DSIP in the pituitary and plasma after adrenalectomy (Bjartell et al., 1991). DSIP stimulates the release of ACTH and GH, reduces CRH-induced corticosterone release, and increases SP levels in the hypothalamus. It may have completely different functions in lower vertebrates as DSIP is present in a cartilaginous fish and in the frog (Vallarino et al., 1992).

10.4.2 A Melange of Neuropeptides

SP affects the release of GnRH, PRL, and GH with the effects being stimulatory or inhibitory depending on the dosage. *VIP* increases the release of both PRL and LH, and, under certain circumstances, of GH. *AT II* causes the release of ACTH and β-endorphin, probably through AT II–evoked release of VP from the ME. AT II also is a potent releaser of PRL in cells in culture but not in vivo. In vivo, AT II depresses PRL and GH, while increasing LH. *NPY* inhibits the release of LH and GH, probably through its effects on GnRH and GHRH neurons. Bombesin stimulates PRL and GH release. β-Endorphin stimulates PRL, GH, and ACTH secretion, but inhibits TSH secretion and release. Studies of the individual effects of these extrahypothalamic neuropeptides cannot provide a comprehensive evaluation of the complex situation in the intact organism.

10.5 Summary

Thyrotropin-releasing hormone is composed of only three amino acids—glutamine, histidine, and proline—and amidation of the C-terminus is required for full potency. Isolation and characterization of the tripeptide TRH as a hypophysiotropic neuropeptide was convincing proof of the existence of hypothalamic releasing factors. TRH and all the other hypothalamic neuropeptides are synthesized according to the classical peptide biosynthetic pathway from a large preprohormone that is post-translationally cleaved, processed, and packaged into secretory granules. Also common to all the neuropeptides are receptors that have seven transmembrane domains and are coupled to G proteins (see chapter 6).

In mammals, TRH is present in highest amounts in axons from neurons in the parvocellular PVN which terminate in the ME to form part of the HPT axis. TRH-secreting neurons are in structures related to the limbic system and neurons associated with motor pathways, in the gastrointestinal tract, and in many peripheral tissues, including the placenta. Synthesis of TRH is regulated by circulating thyroid hormone via a long-loop negative feedback on hypothalamic neurons and on the thyrotrophs of the anterior pituitary. Additional regulation of TRH is exerted by many other hormones such as NPY, somatostatin, glucocorticoids, and estrogens, and by catecholamines. Acute cold is a specific stimulus to an increase in hypothalamic TRH mRNA. The TRH receptor is found mainly on thyrotrophs and mammatrophs and uses as second messengers intracellular Ca^{2+}, or a

Ca^{2+}-independent protein kinase activation. Unlike other neuropeptides, TRH is degraded only by a specific TRH-degrading ectopeptidase.

The most important function of TRH is stimulation of TSH, but it also stimulates PRL secretion, and acts as a neuromodulator and neurotransmitter in the CNS, with potent neurotrophic activity. TRH antagonizes some opiate effects and is involved in thermoregulation.

Corticotropin-releasing hormone was first identified through its ability to cause stress-induced corticosteroid secretion. CRH is a 41–amino acid peptide, identified throughout the animal kingdom, with little alteration in amino acid residues. The full C-terminus is essential to biological activity and deamination of this terminus almost completely destroys its activity. CRH is most concentrated in the parvocellular neurons of the PVN, the axons of which terminate in the ME to form part of the HPA axis. Almost half of these neurons also contain VP, which can interact with CRH to stimulate pituitary corticotrophs to secrete ACTH. There are many other CNS sites for CRH, and many peripheral tissues, especially the placenta, contain CRH. Extensive afferent input to the PVN supplies the CRH neuron with information needed for the HPA axis to coordinate endocrine, neuroendocrine, autonomic, and behavioral responses to stress.

CRH is regulated negatively at both the hypothalamic and pituitary level by glucocorticoids (long-loop), by short-loop inhibition by ACTH on CRH, and regulated positively by CRH stimulation of its own secretion (ultrashort loop). The limbic system exerts a inhibitory influence on CRH neurons in the PVN. Stress activates not only mRNA for CRH but also the mRNA for several other neuropeptides, mainly VP. CRH, ACTH, and the corticosteroids are secreted on a circadian basis, peaking in humans in the early morning, and in rodents in the early evening.

CRH receptors are widely distributed in the CNS, mainly in the anterior and intermediate lobes of the pituitary for the release of ACTH and MSH. There are three CRH subtypes which vary in their structure, distribution, and regulation in response to a variety of stressors. The main second-messenger system is the cAMP pathway, but calcium and arachidonic acid and its metabolites are probably also involved. A CRH-binding protein may inactivate CRH when CRH levels are too high.

The most important function of CRH is the initiation of stress-induced ACTH secretion and the consequent release of glucocorticoids. Additionally, CRH increases the secretion of somatostatin and β-endorphin, but inhibits the release of GnRH, GH, OT, and VP. CRH inhibits reproductive functions, acts as a neurotransmitter and neuromodulator in the CNS, modifies the actions of the autonomic nervous system, and activates behavioral responses to stress.

Gonadotropin-releasing hormone is encoded by a gene that has probably duplicated at least twice during evolution. GnRH, a decapeptide, is present in all verte brate brains in different forms, but there is only one GnRH in placental mammals. GnRH stimulates the secretion of both LH and FSH from pituitary gonadotrophs. In primates GnRH neurons are in the MBH and the arcuate nucleus, most of which project to the ME, but there are several other extrahypothalamic projections to different brain areas. GnRH cell bodies are in olfactory structures, reflecting the importance of olfactory stimuli in reproductive physiology. Deletion of two exons from the GnRH gene results in mutants that lack GnRH neurons and fail to develop a mature reproductive tract. Many analogs of the GnRH molecule have been synthesized, with substitution of D-Lys^6 for Gly^6 increasing biological potency.

GnRH receptors are found not only on pituitary gonadotrophs but also on gonadal cells, permitting a direct inhibitory action of GnRH on ovarian and testicular function, bypassing the stimulatory actions of LH and FSH. GnRH regulates its own receptors, which use the phosphatidylinositol system of second messengers. Secretion of GnRH is pulsatile, regulated by a pulse generator in the MBH and arcuate nucleus, which in turn is modulated by gonadal steroids, neuropeptides, and neurotransmitters. The LH surge is initiated by rising estradiol levels at the end of proestrus (positive feedback), followed by negative feedback due to the synergistic action of estrogen, progesterone, and the opiate system in the luteal phase. NPY and galanin are additional important regulators of the GnRH pulse generator, as is input to the hypothalamus from the limbic system.

The GnRH pulse generator is inactive after the first year of life in humans, then is activated at puberty, possibly due to removal of tonic inhibition by GABA neurons and an increase in stimulatory input from NPY and NE neurons. In menopause, GnRH levels increase due to the decline in ovarian steroids and the consequent removal of negative feedback on GnRH neurons. The most important function of GnRH is the regulation of pituitary gonadal function during reproductive life, and in the ontogeny and regulation of pituitary-gonadal function during fetal life. GnRH acts as a neurotransmitter and neuromodulator in the CNS and has a direct inductive effect on mating behavior.

Growth hormone-releasing hormone regulates the secretion of GH through complex interactions with somatostatin. GHRH is present in two forms, GHRH 1–40-OH (rat) and GHRH 1–44-NH_2 (human), both derived from the same precursor, with full biological activity in the first 29 amino acids. GHRH belongs structurally to the VIP-secretin-glucagon family. Most GHRH is in the arcuate nucleus and pituitary stalk, with lesser amounts in the SON and PVN, and GHRH is released into the ME to reach pituitary somatotrophs to stimulate GH release. GHRH is colocalized with many other neuropeptides and neurotransmitters which mediate the complex regulatory control over GHRH. GHRH is inactivated by peptidases to GHRH (3–44-NH_2).

GHRH receptors are regulated by glucocorticoids and estradiol, and are decreased in number in senescence and in mutants in which GH secretion is diminished. The GHRH receptors are coupled to several signal transduction systems, including cAMP, phosphatidylinositol, Ca^{2+}-calmodulin, and arachidonic acid–eicosanoid systems. GHRH is secreted in a pulsatile manner essential to full pituitary response, which is a result of the stimulatory effect of GHRH and the inhibitory action of somatostatin. GHRH is important during fetal development and is increased postnatally and at puberty, at which time it becomes markedly sexually dimorphic, being higher in the male than in the female. GHRH secretion decreases with age.

GHRH secretion is inhibited by a short-loop feedback action of GH on GHRH neurons mediated by unidentified neurons in the arcuate nucleus. Transgenic mice with impaired GHRH production fail to grow. Regulation of GHRH secretion is through poorly understood interactions with somatostatin, adrenergic and cholinergic systems, DA, and 5-HT, as well as through other neuropeptides.

The chief function of GHRH is the regulation of GH secretion and release, but it also stimulates the proliferation and differentiation of pituitary somatotrophs. GHRH regulates slow wave sleep, stimulates food intake in a circadian phase–dependent manner, and modulates long-term memory.

Somatostatin is a multifunctional inhibitor, not only of GH but of many other pituitary, pancreatic, and gut hormones, as well as exocrine secretions. Somatostatin also has an effect on the development of the brain and a maintenance role in the adult and aging brain, indicating that its name is too restrictive. In mammals the most common forms are somatostatin-14 and somatostatin-28, but multiple N-terminally extended forms of somatostatin-14 exist. Somatostatin has a disulfide bond between residues 3 and 14 which provides the ring structure essential to biological activity. Most central somatostatin neurons are in the periventricular preoptic area and the anterior hypothalamus, with long projections to the ME. Some somatostatin is in the cerebral visual cortex and autonomic neurons, and in interneurons. Somatostatin is present extensively in the gastrointestinal tract and pancreas.

Somatostatin is found in single-cell protozoa and throughout the animal phyla. In mammals, including humans, somatostatin-24 and somatostatin-28 are derived from a single gene and a processed from a single preprohormone but from two separate prohormones. Generally somatostatin-28 is the more potent neuropeptide for the inhibition of pituitary hormones, whereas somatostatin-14 has selective inhibitory actions on gut and pancreatic secretions, splanchnic blood flow, and intestinal motility.

Somatostatin-14 receptors are heterogeneous, with five different subtypes, differentially distributed and consequently with different functions. Subtypes 1 and 2 are distributed throughout most brain regions and are involved with the regulation of GH secretion. Subtype 3 is present in motor neurons of the brainstem and spinal cord, and subtype 5 is involved in insulin secretion and somatostatin-susceptible cancers. All the receptors bind to G proteins and inhibit adenylate cyclase and Ca^{2+} fluxes.

Somatostatin release is pulsatile and is coordinated in precise balance with GHRH for appropriate pulsatile secretion of GH. Release is regulated by a negative ultrashort loop of locally secreted somatostatin inhibiting hypothalamic somatostatin neurons. GHRH may provide a positive ultrashort loop by stimulating somatostatin release and GH may stimulate release by a positive short-loop feedback. Adrenergic stimulation and DA increase release; 5-HT and glucocorticoids inhibit release and the effects of ACh are controversial. Somatostatin is a hyperpolarizing neurotransmitter with extensive inhibitory effects on the neuroendocrine system and gastrointestinal tract secretions. Its effects on the autonomic nervous system are many, including control of body temperature, blood pressure, appetite, learning, and memory. Somatostatin has neurotrophic effects during development, has inhibitory effects on certain tumors, and increases REM sleep.

Hypothalamic inhibition of prolactin release. There is little evidence for a peptidergic PRL-inhibiting factor (PIF) but there is much support for hypothalamic DA as the physiological inhibitor of tonic secretion of PRL from the pituitary. DA reaches the anterior pituitary through the tuberoinfundibular system and the portal vessels, and the intermediate and posterior lobes of the pituitary through the tuberohypophyseal system. DA inhibition is overcome by suckling or estrogen, which permit the release of PRF, a small peptide in the intermediate lobe. PRF reaches the pituitary lactotrophs to stimulate PRL secretion and release. Suckling also causes the release of OT, which further augments PRF secretion. α-MSH has been implicated in the release of PRF.

Pituitary adenylate cyclase-activating polypeptide was first identified in the hypothalamus as a compound able to stimulate adenylate cyclase in anterior pituitary cells. PACAP is a widely distributed neuropeptide of either 27 or 38 amino acids, similar in structure to the VIP-secretin-glucagon family, but with the greatest similarity to VIP. PACAP is present in highest concentrations in the hypothalamus, the ME, and the posterior pituitary, and is also found in many peripheral tissues, especially the testis. There are three types of PACAP receptors: Type 1 receptor is PACAP-specific, is found in lymphoid organs, and probably mediates PACAP effects on the immune system. Type 1 receptors are also present in the gonads. Type 2 receptors share a binding site and distribution pattern with VIP. Type 3 receptors bind PACAP and VIP equally well and are found in insulin-secreting cells of the pancreas.

PACAP stimulates adenylate cyclase in anterior pituitary cells and in many other endocrine organs. In the pituitary, PACAP stimulates PRL gene expression and POMC gene transcription, α-MSH exocytosis, and FSH and LH release. PACAP synthesized in the gonads acts as an autocrine or paracrine regulator of the germ cells. In the spinal cord PACAP is a neurotrophic factor during periods of cell differentiation and proliferation. In the gastrointestinal tract, PACAP releases ACh and SP causing relaxation of the ileum.

Delta sleep-inducing peptide, a nonapeptide found in the brain, adrenal medulla, milk, and plasma, induces sleep in many species of mammals. DSIP has been reported to be associated with suppression of slow wave and REM sleep, although this correlation is controversial. However, the diurnal rhythm of DSIP in humans may be directly coupled to body temperature. DSIP probably acts in a modulatory manner, rather than directly, to induce sleep. DSIP is colocalized with TSH in the pituitary, with GnRH in the hypothalamus, and with NE in the adrenal medulla, suggesting that this peptide may have effects on the activity of the HPA axis.

A melange of neuropeptides affects the release of the anterior pituitary neuropeptides, both positively and negatively. These neuropeptides include SP, VIP, AT II, NPY, bombesin, and β-endorphin, some of which may exert their regulatory effects indirectly rather than directly. Studies of the individual effects of these extrahypothalamic neuropeptides cannot provide a comprehensive evaluation of the complex situation in the intact organism.

Chapter 11 is the first of three chapters on the pituitary hormones. Chapter 11 discusses the neuropeptides of the posterior pituitary lobe, oxytocin and vasopressin. Chapter 12 considers the neuropeptides derived from POMC, and chapter 13 discusses the anterior pituitary peptides belonging to the glycoprotein and growth families, and a novel neuropeptide, secretoneurin.

Hypothalamic-Neurohypophyseal Hormones: VP and OT

11

11.1 The Hypothalamic-Neurohypophyseal System

11.1.1 History

Research on the hypothalamic-neurohypophyseal system (HNS) is more than a century old. In 1895 Oliver and Schaefer described the vasopressor effects of posterior pituitary extracts, and named the potent extract *vasopressin* (VP). This was followed in the next few years by descriptions of the activities of the posterior pituitary extracts, *antidiuretic hormone* (*ADH*) and *oxytocin* (*OT*). Clinical studies on patients with diabetes insipidus ascertained that the diuresis was alleviated by neurohypophyseal extracts and in 1947 Verney published a historic paper reporting that injections of hypertonic saline into the internal carotid artery in conscious dogs with water diuresis reduced urine flow. This did not occur if the neurohypophysis were ablated and the antidiuretic effect only developed if the hypertonic saline reached the anterior hypothalamus. With remarkable insight, Verney suggested that the hypothalamus contained "osmoreceptors" which acted as sensors of blood tonicity. Specific evidence that the target of ADH was the distal convoluted tubule of the kidney was provided by Homer Smith (1952) whose experiments clearly demonstrated increased water reabsorption following ADH administration.

OT was the first peptide hormone to have its structure completely elucidated, and the first to be chemically synthesized (du Vigneaud et al., 1953), achievements for which Vincent du Vigneaud was awarded the Nobel prize in chemistry in 1955. At that time OT functions were believed to be restricted to reproductive processes in the female, such as the induction of parturition and milk ejection during lactation. It is now known that OT is involved in female maternal, sexual, and social behavior, has a limited role in male sexual behavior, and has an integrative function in cardiovascular, renal, and immune functions.

As the posterior pituitary gland does not have secretory cells but consists of neural elements, it took the demonstration by Bargmann and Scharrer (1951) to convince the numerous doubting endocrinologists that indeed the posterior pituitary contained hormones but that the site of origin was the hypothalamus. This gave credence to the rapidly growing field of neuroendocrinology. The determination of the molecular structure and the synthesis of both OT and VP followed in the same decade. Since then, investigation into the basic neurobiology of OT and VP has accelerated enormously, elucidating the many endocrine, peripheral, and behavioral functions of these nonapeptides.

11.1.2 Evolution and Structure of Oxytocin and Vasopressin

OT and VP are are members of a family of highly related peptides found throughout the animal kingdom, both vertebrate and invertebrate. In chapter 1 the evolution of neuropeptide hormones was discussed and the hypothalamic-neurohypophyseal hormones OT and VP presented as an excellent example of gene duplication. The gene duplication that led to the formation of the VP-OT two-gene family occurred early during vertebrate evolution and most vertebrate species possess both peptides. They are nonapeptides built on the same basic plan: a ring structure formed by a sulfur bridge connecting two conserved cysteine residues and a C-terminal tripeptide (Hruby and Chow, 1990). The substitution of amino acids in the 3rd and 8th positions is responsible for both quantitative and qualitative differences between these hypothalamic neuropeptides. Figure 11.1 shows the structure of three nonapeptides. *Arginine VP (AVP)* has phenylalanine in position 3, arginine in position 8. *Oxytocin* differs in having isoleucine in position 3, leucine in position 8. A few mammals, for example, the pig and hippopotamus, have *lysine VP (LVP)*, with lysine in position 8. (In this text *VP* refers to *arginine vasopressin*). It is evident that isoleucine in position 3 is

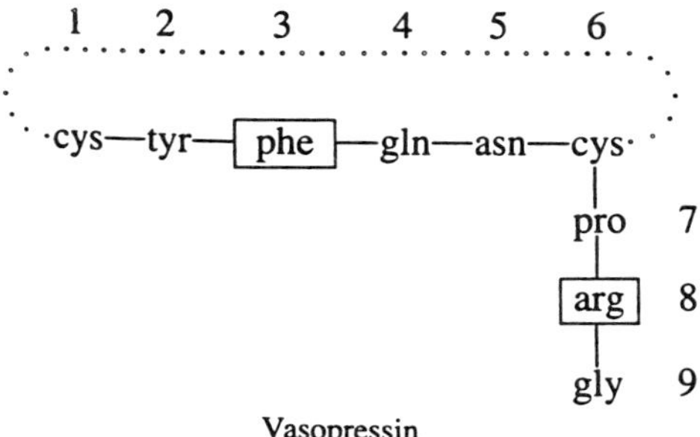

Vasopressin

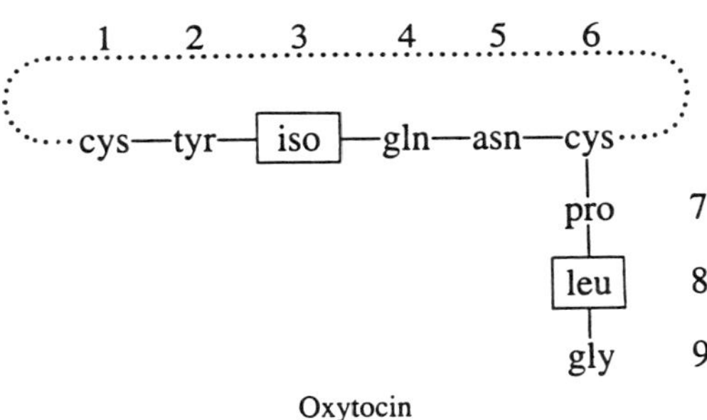

Oxytocin

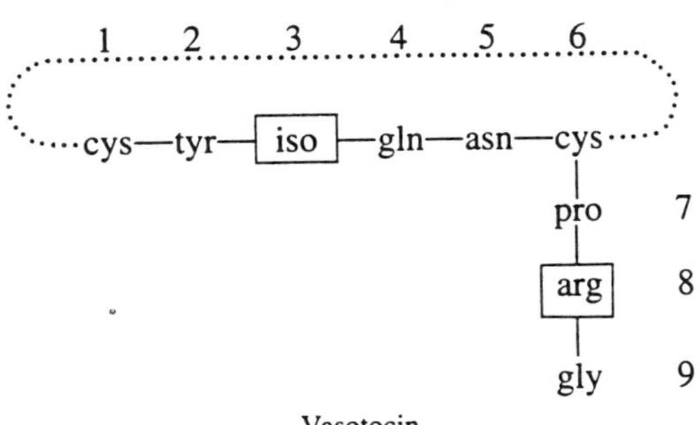

Vasotocin

Figure 11.1
Structure of related hypothalamic neurohypophyseal hormones.

essential to stimulation of OT receptors, and arginine or lysine in position 8 is required for action on VP receptors. *Vasotocin*, a nonapeptide found in lower vertebrates from the primitive *cyclostomes* (lamprey) to the frog, has isoleucine in position 3, arginine in position 8, and as a result has properties in between those of OT and VP. Vasotocin probably was the precursor of the two hormones of higher vertebrates.

Because only a single peptide, either vasotocin [Ile^3]-VP, or [Arg^8]-OT, has been found in the most primitive *cyclostomes*, it is assumed that a primordial gene duplication with subsequent mutations gave rise to the two lineages about 700 million years ago (Acher at al., 1995). The remarkable evolutionary stability of these nonapeptides suggests a strict co-evolution of messenger-receptors, including precursors and processing enzymes. A few groups, such as cartilaginous fishes and marsupials, have two or more peptides of the same type, cartilaginous fishes having six to eight oxytocin-like peptides (Chauvet et al., 1994). Invertebrates contain only a single member of this family, a VP-related peptide *conopressin*, which has the behavioral characteristics of OT, indicating that, in this early evolutionary nonapeptide, the nature of the amino acid at residue at position 8 does not influence its function (Vankesteren et al., 1995). Differences in the structures of these hypothalamic-neurohypophysial hormones throughout phylogeny are shown in figure 1.3. The biological activities of some of the vertebrate neurohypophyseal hormones are listed in table 11.1.

11.1.3 *The Neurophysins*

Neurophysins are small, acidic proteins 93 to 95 residues long, about 10 times the length of OT or VP, and they exist in 1:1 molar noncovalent complexes with the hormones, or as part of the precursor as

Table 11.1
Biological activities of some vertebrate neurohypophyseal hormones

	Activities (IU/μmol)			
	Rat			Rabbit
	Uterine contraction	Increase blood pressure	Anti-diuresis	Milk ejection
Oxytocin[a]	450	5.0	5.0	450
Mesotocin[b]	291	6.0	1.0	330
Isotocin[c]	145	0.06	0.18	290
Vasotocin[d]	120	225.0	260.0	220
Vasopressin[e]	17	412.0	465.0	69
Lysipressin[f]	5	285.0	260.0	63

Adapted from Acher et al. (1995).
Note the oxytocic properties of oxytocin, mesotocin, and isotocin, the vasopressor and antidiuretic activities of vasopressin and lysipressin (Lys-vasopressin), and the dual activities of vasotocin.
Position of residues:
[a] 3 Ile, 8 Leu; placentals, some marsupials.
[b] 3 Ile, 8 Ile; nonmammalian tetrapods, marsupials, lungfishes.
[c] 3 Ile, 8 Ile; bony fishes.
[d] 3 Ile, 8 Arg; nonmammalian vertebrates.
[e] 3 Phe, 8 Arg; mammals.
[f] 3 Phe, 8 Lys; pig, hippopotamus.
All residues in position 4 are Gln, except for isotocin, in which it is Ser.

dimers or even higher oligomers. They were isolated from the neurohypophysis, hence their name. In tetrapods, the neurohypophyseal-neurophysin precursors are encoded by three-exon genes, one coding for the hormone, the signal peptide and the first nine residues of neurophysin, the second exon coding for the central residues (10–76) and the third exon for the C-terminal part (residues 77–105 or 77–145) (Acher and Chauvet, 1995). Figure 11.2 shows the dissociation of the precursor "mother molecule" by countercurrent distribution, into VP, OT, and neurophysins (which can be separated into two highly homologous components, I and II). The neurophysin associated with OT is neurophysin I, whereas neurophysin II is associated with VP. Provasopressin has a third domain, a 39-residue C-terminal glycopeptide *copeptin*, which is cut off from neurophysin II and is found separately in the secretory granules. Consequently, neurophysins are excised by a two-step procedure for provasopressin and by a single-step process for pro-oxytocin.

The function of the OT- and VP-associated neurophysins is still debatable, and the only established role is that of hormone storage within neurosecretory granules. This limits the biological role of neurophysins to that of inactive carriers for OT and VP. However, mammalian neurophysins contain several disulfide bonds and any disruption of the structure or conformation of the neurophysin may disrupt the binding and activity of the endopeptidase responsible for cleaving off the active molecule. The neurophysins probably ensure the correct conformation to permit access to sites by specific processing enzymes. They may also protect the active hormone from enzymatic destruction (Legros and Geenen, 1996). In mutations resulting in hereditary diabetes insipidus, a defect in the neurophysin-encoding sequence completely interferes with normal processing (see section 11.3.3).

11.1.4 The Oxytocin and Vasopressin Genes

The common evolutionary origin of vertebrate VP and OT precursors is supported by the similar structural organization of their genes (figure 11.3). In all mammals, both peptide hormone genes are close together on the same chromosome (in the human on chromosome 20) and are oriented in opposite

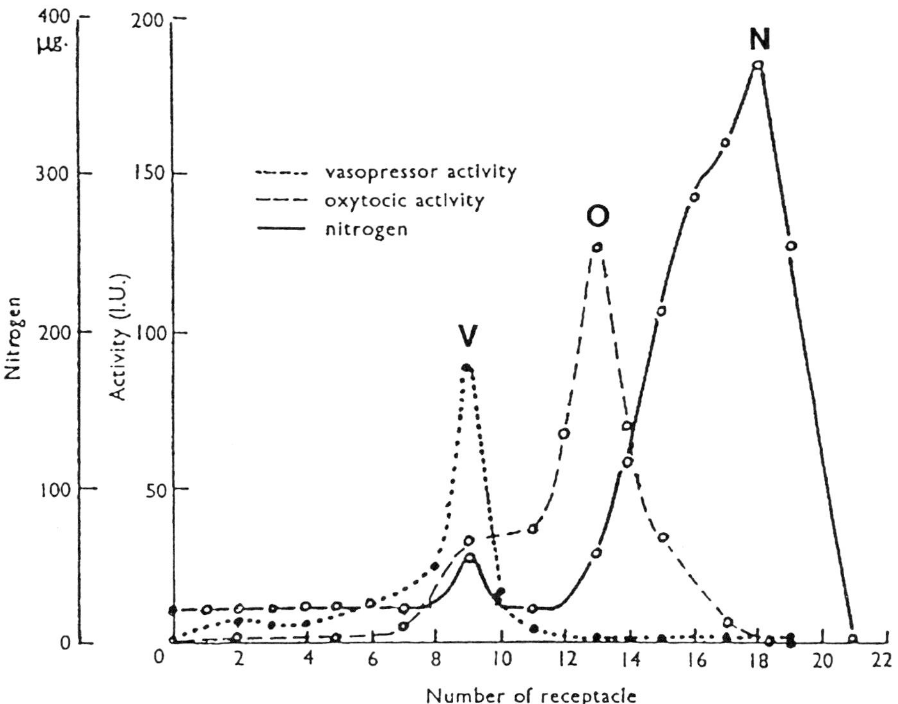

Figure 11.2
Dissociation of the "mother molecule" into vasopressin (V), oxytocin (O), and neurophysins (N). (From Acher and Fromageot, 1957.)

transcriptional directions (Hara et al., 1990). The presursors are encoded by three exons with two intervening sequences interrupting the coding regions at homologous positions, but with different lengths of intergenic sequences ranging from 3.5 kb in the mouse to 11 kb in the rat (figure 11.4).

Expression of the OT gene is confined to anatomically defined groups of magnocellular neurons in the SON and PVN. VP is also expressed in magnocellular neurons of the PVN and SON, but VP and OT are rarely expressed in the same cell. The OT gene is also expressed in a number of peripheral tissues, but there is a marked species difference in peripheral gene expression patterns.

Transgenic mice have been used to target cell-specific expression of the OT gene. The constructs shown in figure 11.5 contain both the entire OT and VP exon and intron structures, and about four times as much 5′ upstream flanking region for the VP gene vs. the OT gene. However, only the OT gene is expressed in the hypothalamic-neurohypophyseal system. Figure 11.5 also shows the minimal construct after removal of bases from the 5′ end of the VP gene that still permits cell-specific expression selectively to

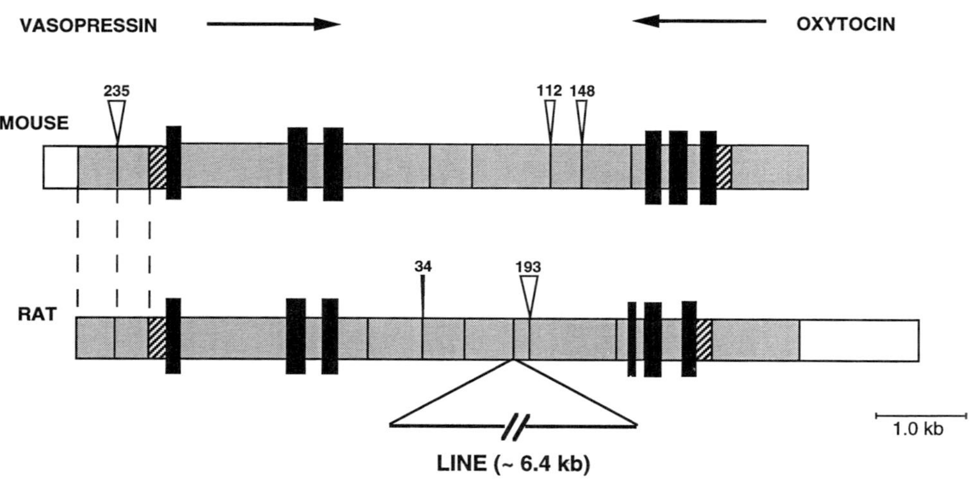

Figure 11.3
Oxytocin and vasopressin gene structures in the mouse and rat. As in all species these genes are on the same chromosomal locus but are in opposite transcriptional orientations (arrows) with each gene containing three exons (black rectangles). The regions separating the genes (intergenic region, IGR) in the mouse is about 3.5 kb vs. about 11 kb in the rat. The rat IGR contains a long interspersed repeated DNA element (LINE) about 6.4 kb long, which is not present in the mouse IGR. Although most of the IGR shows high homology between the rat and mouse genes (shaded regions), there appears to be several unique inserts in both genes (illustrated by triangles with the number of bases shown above). (From Gainer et al., 1995.)

OT neurons (Gainer et al., 1995). Close linkage of the two genes is functionally important for cell-specific expression of OT. As the OT and VP genes are not coexpressed in the same cell, it is possible that one gene in this linked structure is coupled to repression of the other, preventing coexpression (Gainer and Wray, 1992).

11.1.5 Anatomy of the Neurohypophysis (Posterior Lobe)

The neurohypophysis consists of three parts: the median eminence of the hypothalamic tuber cinereum; the infundibular stem (pituitary stalk), which is surrounded by the pars tuberalis of the anterior pituitary; and the pars nervosa (posterior lobe) (figure 11.6). The posterior lobe of the pituitary is derived from the diencephalic neural ectoderm of the floor of the forebrain. A pouchlike recess, Rathke's pouch, forms in the ectodermal roof of the stomodeum and contacts the diencephalon. The pouch is pinched off by surrounding mesoderm and the diencephalic neural outgrowth forms the infundibulum.

11.1.5.1 Hypothalamic Connections

The main neural connection from the hypothalamus to the neurohypophysis is via the supraoptico-hypophyseal tract, which arises in the SON, and the paraventriculo-hypophyseal tract, which arises from the PVN. The SON and PVN are clearly defined hy-

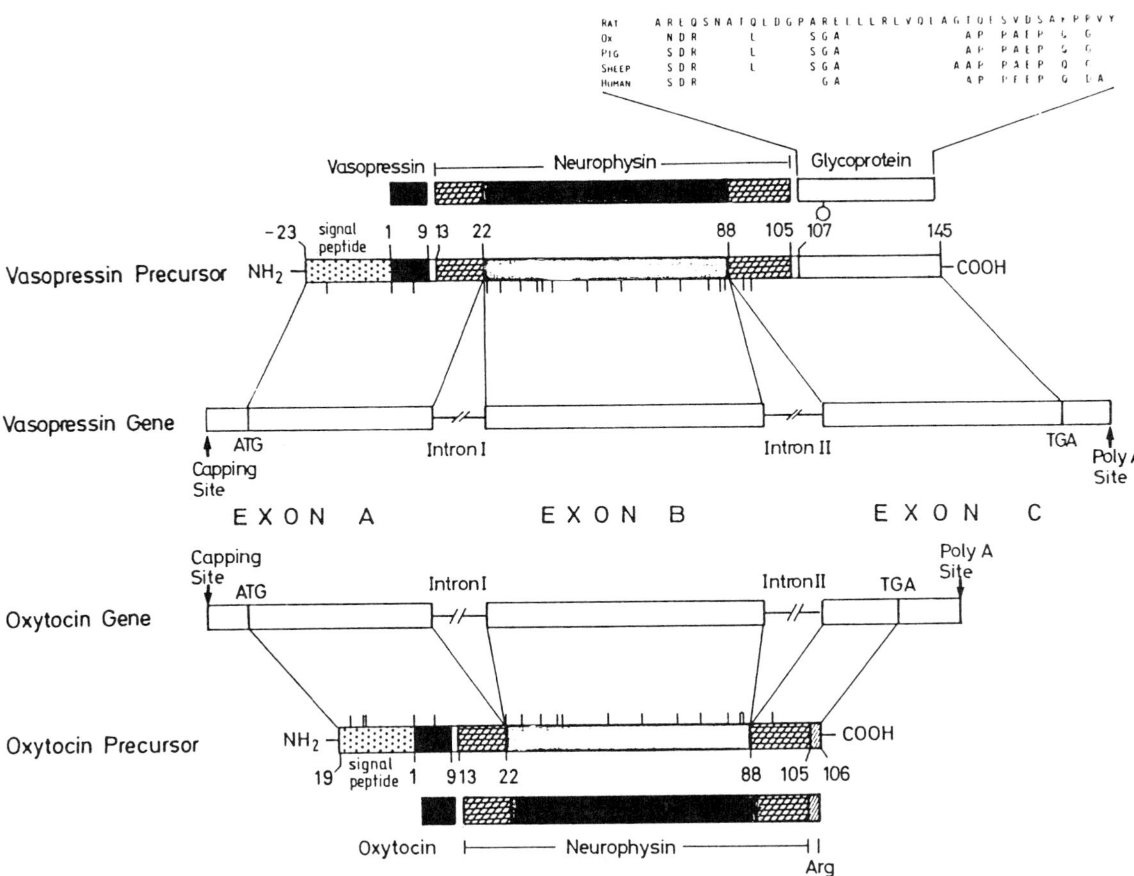

Figure 11.4
Comparison of the structural organization of the oxytocin and vasopressin genes and the deduced protein precursors from the rat. Cysteine residues are marked by vertical lines under the protein precursor. The sites of capping, translational initiation, termination, and the poly (A) site are indicated. (From Richter, 1985.)

A. OT-SPECIFIC RAT GENE CONSTRUCT

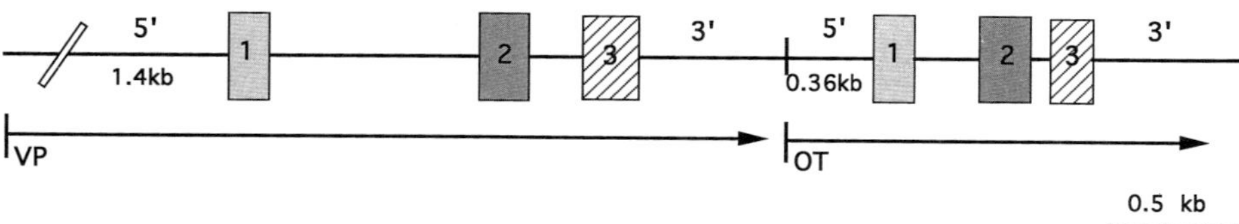

B. "MINIMAL" OT- SPECIFIC RAT GENE CONSTRUCT

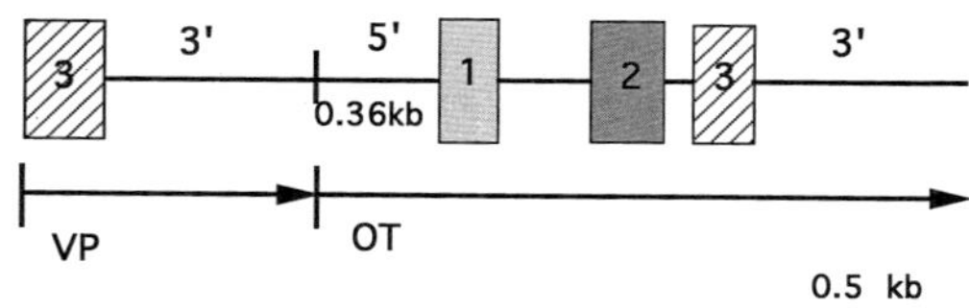

C. "MINIMAL" VP-SPECIFIC RAT GENE CONSTRUCT

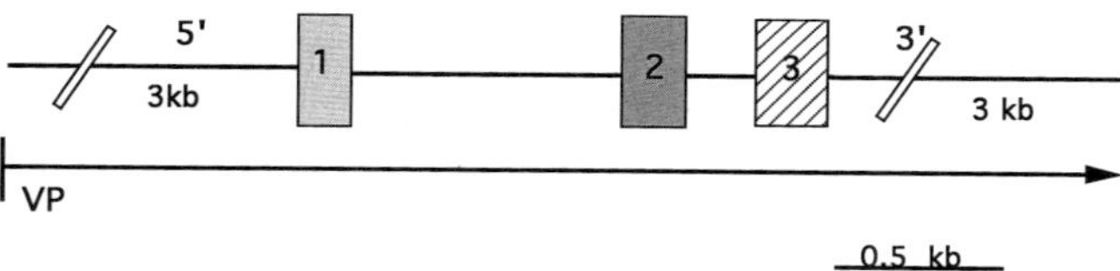

Figure 11.5
Gene constructs showing cell-specific gene expression in the hypothalamic-neurohypophyseal system (HNS) in transgenic mice. A, This construct, which showed cell-specific expression in oxytocin (OT) cells contained the intact vasopressin (VP) and OT genes fused in tandem in the same transcriptional orientation with 1.4 kb and 0.36 kb of the 5′-upstream flanking region of the rat VP and OT genes respectively. B, Systematic removal of bases from the 5′-end of the VP gene in the construct A showed that this truncated ("minimal") construct still produced cell-specific expression selectively to OT neurons in the HNS. C, Cell-specific gene expression of the rat VP gene can be obtained in transgenic rodents with about 3 kb of 5′-upstream flanking region and 3 kb of 3′-downstream untranslated region. (From Gainer et al., 1995.)

pothalamic nuclei and contain 30,000 to 50,000 large, magnocellular neurons as well as many smaller, parvocellular neurons. OT and VP are synthesized in the magnocellular neurons of both the SON and PVN, but not in the same neurons. Within the PVN there is a differential distribution of the two nonapeptides, with the larger VP-containing cells located more medially in the mid and caudal regions of the PVN than the OT-containing neurons (Ginsberg et al., 1994). The axons of these neurons terminate in the perivascular spaces of the neural lobe near blood capillaries, which have a fenestrated endothelium to facilitate diffusion and are surrounded by the supporting cells, the *pituicytes*. Thus the hypothalamic-neurohypophyseal peptides do not use a vascular route to reach the posterior pituitary, but are transported directly, via axons from the magnocellular nuclei, to be released as hormones into the extracellu-

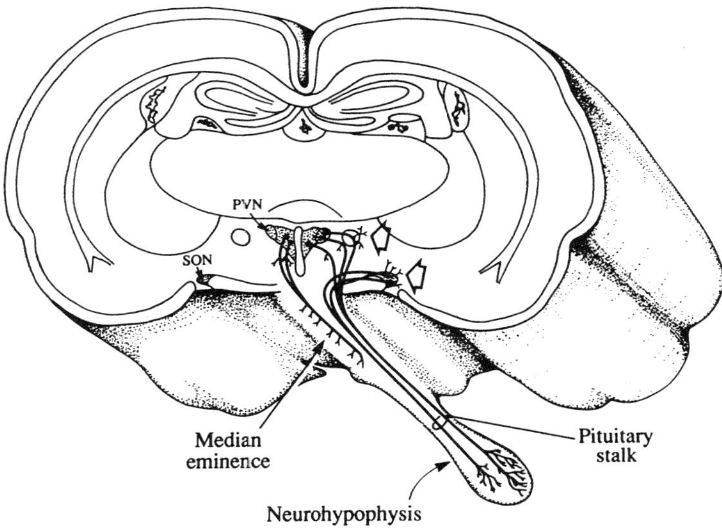

Figure 11.6
Diagram of a rat brain cut away at the level of the supraoptic (SON) and paraventricular (PVN) nuclei showing the main projections of the magnocellular neurons to the neurohypophysis. Also shown are the projections to the median eminence and the axon collateral inputs to the lateral hypothalamus (open arrows). (From Hatton et al., 1992.)

lar or perivascular space. The neuropeptide hormones then cross the perivascular basement membrane and enter the systemic circulation through the fenestrated capillary endothelium.

Collateral axons of the magnocellular neurons are also widely spread throughout the CNS, including the spinal cord, permitting the important interaction of OT and VP with other neural systems, such as the autonomic cardiovascular responses to stressful and osmotic stimuli. These axons deliver the nonapeptides to various brain regions, where they act as *neurotransmitters* or *neuromodulators*. A third role for these peptides is a *paracrine or autocrine* one: OT and VP are also released from the dendrites and cell bodies of the SON and PVN and presumably act on neighboring neurons or on the magnocellular neurons themselves.

In addition to OT and VP, the magnocellular nuclei secrete several other neuropeptides but in much smaller amounts than OT and VP. These peptides include dynorphin, enkephalins, galanin, CCK, TRH, CRH, NPY, VIP and SP.

VP and OT are also produced peripherally. OT mRNA is present in uterine epithelium and in the ovary, and VP is expressed in many of its target peripheral organs.

11.1.5.2 Input from Olfactory Systems

Both the main and accessory olfactory systems provide important routes for stimulation of the SON. Anatomical studies show a direct synaptic input from the olfactory bulbs to the SON (Hatton et al., 1992), thus providing an anatomical basis for the important role of olfactory stimuli in OT- and VP-influenced rodent behaviors.

11.2 Oxytocin

11.2.1 Oxytocinergic Pathways

In addition to the main pathways to the neurohypophysis from the axons of magnocellular neurons in the SON and PVN, OT fibers also innervate β-endorphin neurons in the arcuate nucleus of the hypothalamus, permitting interaction of OT with the endogenous opioid systems of the brain (Csiffary et al., 1992). Oxytocinergic neurons are present in the medial preoptic area (MPOA), a region which concentrates estrogens, and which is an important site for the coordination of reproductive behaviors and ovulation. The MPOA is a likely site for estrogen activation and coordination of OT systems (Caldwell, 1992).

11.2.2 Regulation of the Oxytocin Gene

Several regions regulate the expression of the OT gene. In the proximal 5′ flanking region of both the OT and VP genes are distinct DNA sequences that have been conserved among species. These regulatory elements are targets for transcription factors of the nuclear hormone receptor family. Through these elements the OT gene of rat and humans is responsive to estrogen, thyroid hormones, and retinoids. Using 5′-deletion mutants of the rat OT gene, an estrogen-response region that confers estrogen responsiveness to the OT promoter has been located between the nucleotides 171 to 148 from the transcription initiation site, and contains nucleotides 168 to 156 (Burbach et al., 1992, 1995). The same sequence has been defined in the human OT gene. Other regions of the OT gene provide structural information for hormonal activity and for the correct sorting out of gene products into the regulatory secretory pathway. The overall regulation of the OT gene is a composite of multiple interacting enhancers and repressors.

Physiological conditions dramatically control OT gene expression. These conditions include development, puberty, the various reproductive states of the female, the response to thyroid hormones, and variations in plasma osmolarity. These changes are described in detail by Burbach et al., (1992) and briefly outlined below:

11.2.2.1 Development and Puberty

The OT gene is strongly activated around birth as indicated by levels of OT mRNA in the hypothalamus, and is influenced by sex steroids. During normal postnatal development of female and male rats, OT mRNA content per neuron rises considerably until puberty. This increase is eliminated by gonadectomy and restored by subsequent treatment with estrogen or testosterone.

11.2.2.2 Female Reproductive State

In the adult female rat, OT mRNA levels are highest at estrus and lowest at metestrus. In the pregnant rat, OT mRNA levels rise strikingly in both the magnocellular and parvocellular neurons of the PVN and SON toward the end of gestation, to peak just before parturition, and again during lactation. This hypothalamic augmentation of OT is accompanied by a parallel rise in neurohypophysial OT levels and an increase in OT receptors in the myometrium and mammary gland. Estrogens act as a strong inducer of uterine OT gene expression, an effect potentiated by concomitant progesterone administration. However, estrogen regulation of the OT gene requires priming first by estrogen and progesterone, followed by the subsequent withdrawal of progesterone. Rising levels of estradiol are generally considered to be implicated in the enhanced OT gene expression, but this may not be a direct effect on OT neurons, which lack estrogen receptors and do not concentrate estradiol-17β. Burbach et al. (1992) suggest that paracrine influences from neighboring estrogen-sensitive neurons may mediate actions of estrogen on OT neurons.

OT mRNA levels in the rat uterine epithelium increase more than 150-fold during pregnancy and at term exceed hypothalamic mRNA by a factor of 70 (Zingg et al., 1995). Accordingly, there is close synchrony between the hypothalamic hormones and preparation of the uterus for delivery and of the mammary glands for lactation. During lactation, the OT mRNA levels in the hypothalamic nuclei are dramatically increased, a change reflected in the increase in OT synthesis. At this time the pituitary release of OT increases, and OT plasma levels are elevated.

11.2.2.3 Thyroid Hormone

Thyroid hormone receptors are present on OT neurons and thyroid hormones may be involved in the increase in OT gene expression during development, when thyroid hormones are of particular significance.

11.2.2.4 Plasma Osmolality

Hypothalamic OT neurons are highly responsive to osmotic changes. Hyperosmolality induced by drinking 2% saline or by dehydration induces a two- to fourfold increase in OT mRNA content of SON and PVN neurons. Conversely, hyponatremia is accompanied by a decrease in OT mRNA. It is uncertain whether these changes in OT gene expression are evoked by direct sensoring of osmolality by OT neurons or indirectly via neural pathways, perhaps from osmoreceptors in the carotid arteries and sinus, or from the subfornical organ which can sense changes in blood volume and osmolality and is sensitive to AT II.

11.2.2.5 Circadian Rhythms

OT secretion in the rat, a nocturnal animal, increases during the day, to fall at night, in both females and males. There is some evidence that humans secrete OT with a diurnal rhythm.

11.2.3 Synthesis, Storage, Release, and Inactivation

Pro-oxytocin, the precursor molecule, contains both the biologically active OT nonapeptide and the protein neurophysin I that associates with OT (figure 11.7). OT is produced, packaged in neurosecretory granules, and released by the classic regulated secretory pathway.

11.2.3.1 Changes During Reproductive Events

The OT and VP mRNAs in the rat are subjected to unusual *post-transcriptional modification* during preg-

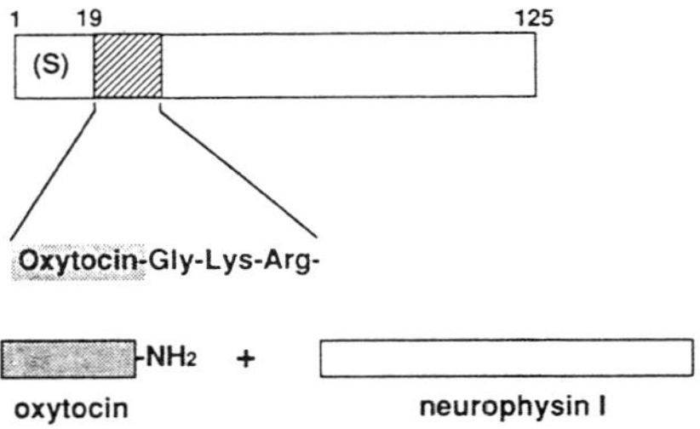

Figure 11.7
The oxytocin precursor prepro-oxytocin is processed to yield the neuropeptide oxytocin and its binding protein neurophysin I by cleavage at the Lys-Arg site. S, signal sequence. (From Mizuno and Matsuo, 1994.)

nancy, lactation, and dehydration. Following these stimuli, there is an increase in OT mRNA size, probably due to the larger poly-A tail of new transcripts (Carter and Murphy, 1991). As might be expected from the physiological conditions that regulate OT mnRNA levels, the synthesis and release of OT in general parallels these controls. OT is released peripherally during reproductively important events such as coitus, parturition, and nursing. OT is also released centrally during social and sexual interactions.

a. Coitus

Vaginocervical stimulation occurs during mating or during the birth of pups, and potently evokes OT release by a reflex pathway which is dependent on prior priming with estrogen and progesterone (figure 11.8). Other neuropeptides released as a result of such stimulation are PRL and LH.

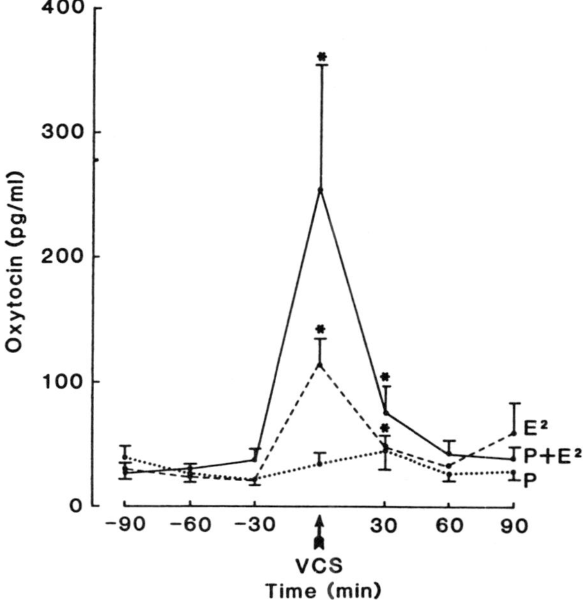

Figure 11.8
Measurement of oxytocin release in the ventromedial nucleus of eight sheep using microdialysis sampling. Vaginocervical stimulation (VCS) fails to increase release when the animals are primed with progesterone (P) alone but provokes significant release following treatment with estradiol alone (E) and this is potentiated by priming with P ($P + E^2$). (From Kendrick and Keverne, 1992.)

b. Pregnancy and parturition

Estrogen stimulates OT synthesis and secretion, whereas progesterone inhibits both these functions. Consequently, as the levels of both these hormones increase during pregnancy, OT levels remain relatively constant until just prior to parturition when progesterone levels fall, permitting a dramatic rise in OT (figure 11.9). By the end of pregnancy, pituitary stores of OT are about 30% higher than in the non-pregnant female, but this store rapidly disappears by the end of parturition as the neurohypophysis releases OT into the blood.

The uterus is protected from high OT levels until parturition by other mechanisms which prevent premature delivery. OT secretion during late pregnancy is limited by *endogenous opioid imhibition.* The opiates are probably coproduced by the OT neurons themselves and act on OT terminals in the posterior lobe. *Uterine sensitivity to OT* does not increase until just before delivery as it is only at this time that the uterine OT receptor number increases.

During parturition, uterine contractions and cervical dilation reflexly increase OT release through the activation of catecholaminergic neurons in the nucleus of the tractus solitarius and in the ventrolateral medulla that may form an afferent pathway to the preoptic area and hypothalamus (Luckman, 1995). This release is triggered during delivery by an increase in the synchronous bursting electrical activity of the magnocellular OT neurons.

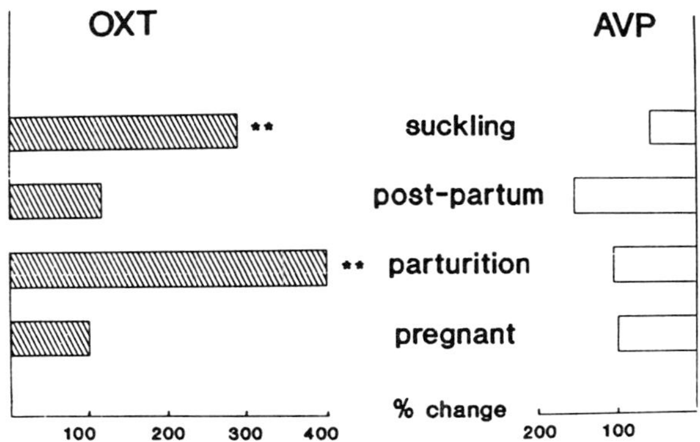

Figure 11.9
Release of both oxytocin (OXT) (n = 6) and vasopressin (AVP) within the supraoptic nucleus of pregnant (=100%) parturient, postparturient, and suckled rats. Measurements were made on microdialysis perfusates. $^{**}P < .01$ vs. pregnant. (From Landgraf et al., 1992.)

c. *Lactation*

Lactation demands a chronic release of OT and pituitary stores are depleted as a result. The release of OT in response to suckling is coupled to electrical activation rather than to sex hormone levels. Stimulation of nerve endings in the nipples results in a reorganization of the pattern of electrical activity of hypothalamic neurons into a brief, high-frequency discharge followed by a relatively extended quiet period, a pulsatile response that results in the release of OT by neurohypophyseal nerve endings (Bourque and Renaud, 1990). This electrical activity is accompanied by a marked increase in immunostaining in the SON of lactating female rats, clearly correlating function with anatomy (figure 11.10). The circulating OT causes contraction of the myoepithelial cells of the mammary gland and consequent milk ejection. During lactation, PRL can increase OT mRNA content in the hypothalamus by a direct action on the hypothalamic-neurohypophyseal system (Ghosh and Sladek, 1995).

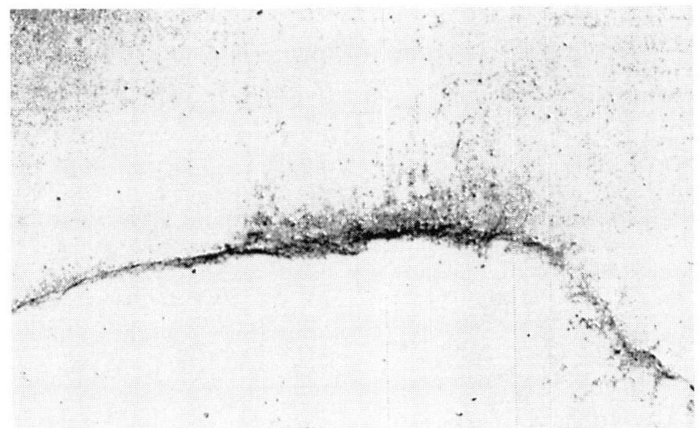

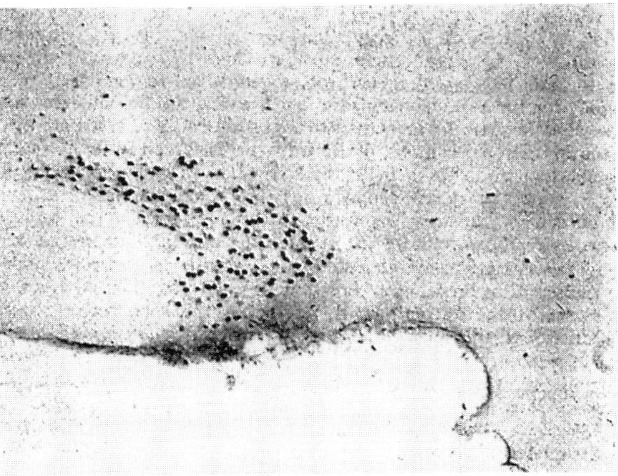

Figure 11.10
Fos-immunostaining in the supraoptic nucleus of lactating female rats under sodium pentobarbital anesthesia. (Top) Lactating rat in which a stimulating electrode was placed on the pituitary stalk and left in position for 90 minutes. No electrical stimulation was given. (Bottom) Lactating rat given 60-minute stimulation of the pituitary stalk (1 mA biphasic pulses at 10 Hz, 10 seconds on, 10 seconds off) in order to activate magnocellular neurons antidromically. The increase in *fos* immunostaining is clear. (From Leng et al., 1993.)

Maternal behavior provides a positive feedback on central OT release. Pup-sniffing and pup retrieval are strong stimuli to the main olfactory bulb. Anogenital licking of the young stimulates the accessory olfactory bulb and this input can be relayed directly from these olfactory systems to the SON to increase OT release.

11.2.3.2 Positive Feedback of Oxytocin on Its Synthesis

During parturition and suckling, OT is released within the SON to act as a positive feedback signal, amplifying its own local or neurohypohyseal release. This local infusion of OT within the SON is important for further OT secretion and milk ejection during suckling. Several factors contribute to this positive feedback mechanism:

a. *Plasticity of the SON neurons*

The stimulus of parturition and then of suckling releases OT both from the dendrites of SON cells and from the neural lobe. Dendritic OT causes plastic changes in the morphology of the magnocellular neurons, remodeling synapses to bring the oxytocinergic neurons closer to each other, which increases the sensitivity of the system to OT. This rearrangement occurs very rapidly during parturition and suckling. Positive feedback is dependent on suckling. When suckling ceases, local release of OT diminishes and the system returns to the basic state. This feedback loop requires the hormonal background of late pregnancy (figure 11.11).

b. *Autoreceptors for OT*

Autoreceptors for OT are present on the axons and dendrites of the PVN and SON in lactating rats, but are not found on the axonal terminals in the posterior lobe. These autoreceptors probably mediate the facilitatory effect of OT on its own release from the dendrites of the magnocellular neurons during the milk ejection reflex (Freund-Mercier and Stoekel, 1995).

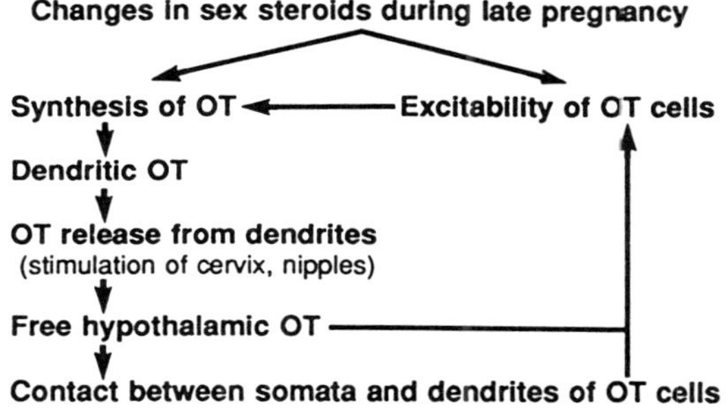

Figure 11.11
Proposed scheme for interactive effects of sex steroids and the dendritic release of oxytocin (OT) in a positive feedback loop which causes and maintains the increased contact between OT cells that occurs during parturition and lactation. Note that the positive feedback loop is broken when suckling ceases. (From Morris and Pow, 1993.)

c. *Sex steroid involvement*

Sex steroids are essential to this local release of OT. Morris and Pow (1993) suggest that during the latter part of pregnancy, rising levels of sex steroids increase OT synthesis and the sensitivity of OT-synthesizing cells, further increasing OT synthesis.

11.2.3.3 Release of Oxytocin by Osmotic Stimuli

Osmotic stress causes the release of OT as well as of VP. Using the immediate early genes as markers of neuronal activity, mRNA and its protein product accumulate specifically in the magnocellular nuclei (Sharp et al., 1991). Excitatory amino acids, such as glutamate, released by glutaminergic interneurons, may be the intermediary system by which hypertonic saline activates magnocellular neurons. As might be expected, GABA inhibits both the electrical and secretory activity of OT and VP neurons following osmotic stimulation.

11.2.3.4 Inactivation of Oxytocin

The kidney, liver, and small intestine are the major sites of whole-body clearance of OT. OT is also degraded in the brain but this plays a lesser role. In the kidney, the chemical degradation of OT probably occurs in the lumen of the proximal convoluted tubule after filtration. During pregnancy, OT is destroyed by a circulating vasopressinase-oxytocinase originating from the placenta. Four major sites of OT cleavage have been identified. The tail portion is cleaved between positions 7 and 8 by a serine protease, and between positions 8 and 9 by a carboxypeptidase. The disulfide bond in the ring portion is cleaved by a thiol:protein disulfide oxidoreductase and an aminopeptidase cleaves between positions 1 and 2 in the ring (Claybaugh and Uyehara, 1993). Several biological functions for the various metabolites resulting from these cleavages have been suggested, but none of these are firmly established.

11.2.4 Oxytocin Receptors and Second Messengers

There appears to be only one type of OT receptor, in contrast to the two main VP receptor subtypes (see table 6.1). However, for all three receptor subtypes, the interaction between position 8 of the ligand and a residue in the first extracellular loop of the receptor is crucial to receptor specificity (Chini et al., 1995).

11.2.4.1 Distribution of Oxytocin Receptors

An unusual aspect of the distribution of OT receptors is their species diversity: OT receptor distribution varies from species to species. The distribution described here is for the rat. Specific high-affinity binding sites for OT are present in several different functional subsystems of the CNS. These include the olfactory system, basal ganglia, limbic system, thalamus, hypothalamus, some cortical regions, the brainstem, and spinal cord. There is a high density of OT receptors in the ventromedial hypothalamus, a target of estrogen action. Whereas OT receptors are recognized with high affinity by VP as well as OT, OT binding sites differ markedly from those for VP and those that are present in the same brain area are found in different parts of the structure (Tribollet et al., 1992).

Receptors for OT are also present in a large number of peripheral tissues, including some endocrine glands (ovary, testis, and adrenal), as well as the uterus, mammary gland, liver, and fat cells. The affinity and ligand specificity of OT-binding sites in these tissues are the same as for OT receptors in the brain. Many receptors for OT recognize VP.

11.2.4.2 Second Messengers

OT receptors belong to the family of *G protein–associated receptors*. Peripheral OT receptors are coupled to *inositol phosphates*: the second-messenger system for brain OT receptors is not known.

11.2.4.3 Regulation of Oxytocin Receptors

OT receptors are differentially regulated in different areas of the brain, and during different physiological conditions. Some receptors appear only transiently during early postnatal life when many systems are maturing, and neonatal OT may be associated with infant behavior such as suckling or with brain differentiation. Some OT receptors are under the control of gonadal steroid hormones and vary with reproductive cycles and behavior. In a few brain areas, OT receptors remain constant. Mating increases both OT receptor affinity and density in estrogen and progesterone-treated animals. Pregnancy is associated with a marked increase in OT receptor number and affinity. In males, OT binding in the ventromedial hypothalamus is regulated not only by estrogen but also by testosterone and its metabolites, through an apparent synergistic mechanism.

11.2.5 Oxytocin as a Neurotransmitter and Neuromodulator

Both morphological and electrophysiological data establish the existence of OT-containing synapses. Electrophysiological studies of large preganglionic vagal motor neurons, which are innervated by OT-containing axons from PVN neurons, show that OT increases the firing frequency of impaled vagal motor neurons. The excitation is due to the generation of a persistent, voltage-gated current which is sodium-dependent, insensitive to tetrodotoxin, and is modulated by divalent cations (Dreifuss et al., 1992). This excitatory action of OT is due to interaction with OT receptors, as it is suppressed by a selective OT antagonist (figure 11.12). Iontophoretic application of OT to cells in the amygdala activates spontaneous firing and potentiates glutamate-induced activation, implying that OT acts as a neuromodulator and neurotransmitter to regulate autonomic functions (Condés Lara et al., 1994). OT also modulates the release of ACh and NE in certain brain regions.

11.2.6 Physiological Functions of Oxytocin

11.2.6.1 Parturition

Parturition occurs as a result of phasic regular uterine contractions, which are dependent on an increase in intracellular Ca^{2+} to activate the actomyosin system. OT stimulates phospholipase C to produce inositol 1,4,5-triphosphate (IP_3), which releases Ca^{2+} from intracellular stores and thereby enhances uterine con-

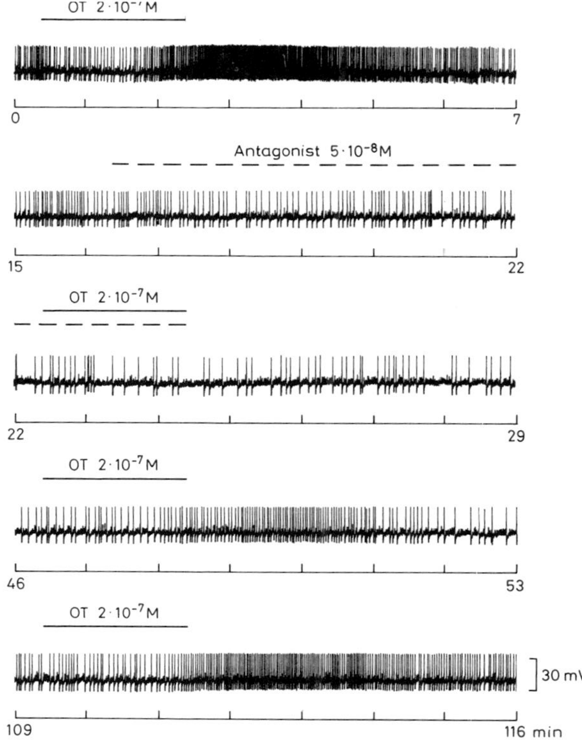

Figure 11.12
Effect of oxytocin (OT) on a rat vagal motorneuron and its suppression by a potent, selective OT antagonist. The traces show the membrane potential; the amplitude of the action potentials was reduced by the low-frequency response of the pen recorder. OT was added to the perfusion solution at 200 nM for the time indicated by the solid line above each trace. The broken line indicates the time during which the antagonist, at 50 nM, was present in the perfusion solution. Note that the OT-induced increase in neuronal excitability (top trace) was suppressed by the antagonist (third trace); following washout, OT partially recovered its excitator effect (bottom trace). (From Dreifuss et al., 1992.)

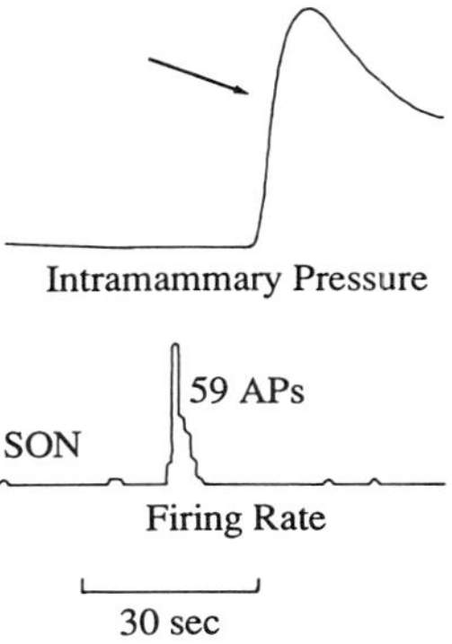

Figure 11.13
Relationship between electrical activity of one supraoptic (SON) cell (lower trace) and intramammary pressure (upper trace) in a suckling mother rat. Note sharp rise in intramammary pressure (arrow) at about 15 seconds after the onset of the burst of action potentials (APs). (From Hatton et al. 1992.)

tractility. OT probably increases uterine prostaglandin synthesis, which would further increase contractility. The sensitivity of the uterus to OT is associated with the level of spontaneous contraction.

11.2.6.2 Milk Ejection Reflex

The lactating mother receives almost constant stimulation from the suckling young. After several minutes of this stimulation, there is a sudden rise in intramammary pressure caused by contraction of the mammary myoepithelial cells (figure 11.13). This is due to a secretion of 1 to 2 ng of OT into the posterior pituitary circulation, calculated as the output of 4500 or more oxytocinergic neurons. The reflex is initiated by stimulation of nerve endings in the nipples, through ascending somatosensory pathways in the spinal cord and brainstem and via indirect multisynaptic pathways to the hypopthalamus. This reflex may be triggered by conditioned stimuli, such as the sight of the offspring, activities associated with nursing or suckling in animals and humans. The reflex is easily inhibited by emotional stress.

11.2.6.3 Modulation of Anterior Pituitary Hormones

OT is not only released into nerve terminals in the posterior lobe but also into the portal vessels that connect the hypothalamus to the anterior lobe, which also has OT receptors. The source of OT terminals in the ME is the PVN, but it is not clear from which group of PVN cells they derive. There is some evidence that OT acts as a modulator of neuroendocrine regulation of PRL, ACTH, and LH.

11.2.6.4 Salt and Water Homeostasis

OT produces natriuresis in mammals, a relic, perhaps, of its derivation from more ancient molecules in nonmammalian species, where OT-related peptides are important regulators of salt and water homeostasis (Zingg et al., 1995).

11.2.6.5 Facilitation of Nociceptive Spinal Reflexes

OT administered intrathecally facilitates the spinal nociceptive flexor reflex, possibly through activation of spinal OT receptors which excite the spinal cord. (Wiesenfeld-Hallin, 1995; Xu and Wiesenfeld-Hallin, 1994).

11.2.6.6 Integration with Other Systems

Local secretion of OT may influence parvocellular neurons of the PVN which project to cortical, brainstem, and spinal neurons, and thus play a role in the integration of cardiovascular and endocrine responses to both stressful and osmotic stimuli. As mentioned in section 11.2.2, OT nerve fibers project to the β-endorphin cells in the arcuate nucleus and influence opiate systems. OT produces an increase in pain threshold (hot plate test) through the action of specific receptors and an involvement with endogenous opiate systems. Opiates, in turn, limit OT secretion during pregnancy by presynaptic inhibition of input to OT neurons. This inhibition is abruptly removed just prior to parturition, permitting OT levels to rise and stimulate myometrial contractions. Progesterone appears to be involved in this elaborate mechanism: high progesterone levels induce β-endorphin secretion, which inhibits OT release. When progesterone levels drop in late gestation, opiate secretion falls and the inhibitory effect on OT secretion is removed (Douglas et al., 1995).

11.2.6.7 Neurotrophic Actions

The transient expression of OT receptors during development is regulated at the transcriptional level in many brain regions, implying that it may be involved in brain maturation.

11.2.6.8 Testicular Function

OT is present in the testis and OT modulates testosterone production and assists sperm transport.

11.2.7 Behavioral Effects of Oxytocin

A potent role for OT has been established for a variety of sexual and social behaviors, not only in mammals but also in avian and reptilian species, in which vasotocin, the evolutionary precursor to OT and VP, is the active nonapeptide. Consequently, OT, VP, and other neuropeptides coordinate physiological, behavioral, and psychological responses to conditions essential to individual and species survival.

11.2.7.1 Reproductive Behaviors

OT facilitates all aspects of reproductive behavior in mammals, including female receptive behavior, maternal behavior, and male mounting behavior. OT effects have been localized to neurons within CNS areas known to control reproductive behaviors (the VMN in the female and the PVN in the male): many of these areas have OT receptors and receive OT projections. The olfactory bulb is also an important site of OT induction of maternal behavior. Social behaviors, which are intimately involved in reproductive behavior, are also regulated by OT. It must be emphasized that all OT-influenced behaviors are dependent upon priming by gonadal steroids and, in turn, OT plays a major role in mediating gonadal steroid influences on such behaviors (Pedersen, 1992).

a. Female sexual and maternal behavior

Both sexual and maternal responses in female rodents are absolutely dependent upon estrogen but are facilitated by OT. *Female sexual receptivity* (lordosis) in rodents is enhanced by OT, which is released during mating, and inhibited by an OT antagonist or by the infusion of antisense oligonucleotides to the 5′ region of the human OT receptor mRNA into the VMN of estrogen-primed rats (McCarthy et al., 1994). Threshold levels of gonadal steroids are essential to this response and the mechanism for estrogen facilitation of sexual response appears to be the induction of OT receptors in the VMN. Mating also induces the immediate early gene product in oxytocinergic neurons, especially in the PVN and near the VMN.

Maternal behavior, which includes anogenital licking of the pups, retrieval of pups into the nest, response to pup ultrasound vocalizations, and crouching in a suckling position, is designed to keep the infants warm, safe, and fed. These responses require a prior exposure to estrogen and can be facilitated by exogenous OT. That endogenous OT plays a physiological role is demonstrated by the blockage of maternal behavior by icv administration of an OT antagonist or antiserum to OT into the ventral tegmental area or the MPOA (Pedersen at al., 1985). There is also an endocrine feedback derived from the behavior of the mother toward her pups: such maternal behavior results in morphological changes in OT neurons in the SON important for lactation.

b. Separation distress and maternal behavior

Central OT may arouse positive feelings of social strength and comfort when evoked by peripheral stimuli, such as nursing. Similarly, centrally administered OT alleviates separation distress, which is measured by the frequency with which isolation calls are emitted by young animals forcefully separated from their mothers. OT levels are high in the first hour after giving birth (also in human), and this coincides with the "sensitive period" during which bonding between mother and infant supposedly occurs.

c. Oxytocin as the "satisfaction" hormone

This rather vague nomenclature is based on several observations that may involve OT. These include the experience of satisfaction from a physiological event such as the obvious satisfaction of a satiated infant after nursing; the ability of OT to substitute for morphine in ameliorating morphine withdrawal; and the evidence that infusion of OT into the brain produces feelings of satiety (Caldwell, 1992).

Other hormones are also involved in female sexual and maternal behavior: lordosis is activated by LHRH, and estrogen-induced maternal behavior requires PRL and the decline of progesterone.

d. Male sexual behavior

Penile erection is induced by i.c.v. administration of nitric oxide donors, such as sodium nitroprusside, which activate central OT transmission in the PVN by a cGMP-independent method. OT itself, administered i.c.v., is one of the most potent methods to induce penile erection in the rat and some other species. OT activation of NO synthase in the PVN is the mechanism involved. This response is completely blocked by morphine.

In copulation, OT shortens ejaculation latency and postejaculation interval, indicating sexual stimulation. OT is released during mating in males as well as in females, and increases the peristaltic contractions of the seminiferous tubules, semen output, and sperm concentration. The mechanism involves the activation of specific OT receptors in the brain, as selective OT antagonists, delivered i.c.v., completely block this facilitation. As in all behaviors, the effectiveness of the hormone depends on the age, previous experience, and hormonal background of the animal.

11.2.7.2 Social Behaviors

a. Male-female pair bonding

Whereas rats fail to establish selective social bonds, the monogamous prairie vole (*Microtus ochrogaster*) has been intensively studied to determine the genetic or hormonal basis for this behavior. Monogamy is rare in mammals and is defined by the presence of long-term male and female associations, nest sharing, male parental care, incest avoidance, and sexual exclusivity. The montane voles, in contrast, are polygymous.

Adult prairie voles form pair bonds after mating and OT is released during mating. OT is necessary and sufficient for partner preference formation, which begins the process of pair bonding. What is surprising is that there is a gender-specific mechanism for pair bonding—in males it is VP and in females it is OT that is necessary for pair bonding (Insel et al., 1995).

In female prairie voles, OT infusions can hasten the formation of partner preference and increase parental behavior (Carter et al., 1992). Recently, an important genetic component of parenting has been discovered in mutant knockout mice that lack an immediate early gene *fos*B. These mutants are completely deficient in maternal behavior—they do not gather the newborns to keep them warm, nor do they suckle or protect them (figure 11.14). Consequently, all the neonates die. If these litters are removed from the mutant mothers immediately after birth and placed with a normal lactating mouse, they thrive. The neuroendocrine route is perceived as being initiated by the smell of the newborns activating an olfactory pathway to the early gene *fos*B in the hypothalamus, which may turn on additional genes that increase brain sensitivity to other hormones such as OT that enhance nurturing behavior. Other hypothalamic-controlled processes, such as adaptation to cold, locomotor activity, eating, and sexual behavior, appear to be quite normal in these early gene *fos*B mutants, suggesting that the defect in nurturing behavior is quite specific (Brown et al., 1996).

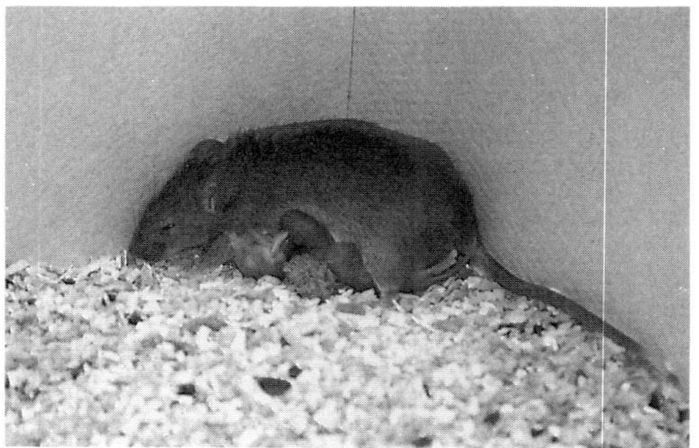

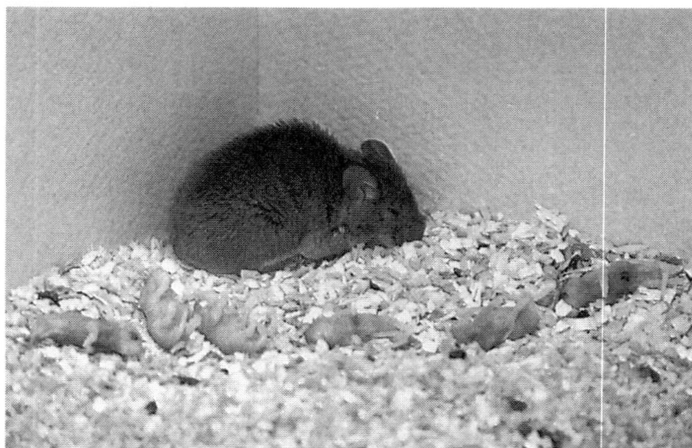

Figure 11.14
A defect in nurturing mice lacking the immediate early gene *fos*B. The upper holograph shows normal maternal behavior—gathering the pups into the nest and suckling them. The lower picture shows the result of the missing gene: the mother ignores the pups, which are left widely scattered in the cage. (From Brown et al., 1996.)

b. Grooming, yawning

Grooming forms an important part of the behavioral repertoire of almost all animals. In addition to cleaning the skin and removing parasites, grooming is a response to stress, unfamiliar surroundings, and can be evoked by central administration of several neuropeptides, especially those evoked by stress: CRH, ACTH, VP, and to a lesser extent, OT.

Both electrical stimulation of the PVN and infusion of OT into this area increase self-grooming behavior in the rat, suggesting that electrical stimulation may induce grooming by activation of the oxytocinergic systems originating from the PVN (Vanerp et al.,

1995). Central OT plays a physiologically relevant role in activating grooming behavior, especially genital grooming, which increases around parturition and copulation, when OT levels rise (Pedersen et al., 1988).

Yawning, a response evoked by several neuropeptides when centrally administered, is also induced by OT injections into the PVN (Melis and Argiolas, 1995).

c. Male social behavior

Male rats, administered OT centrally, demonstrate increased social behavior (nonsexual) with other rats, both male and female; they spend less time investigating younger male rats, have higher levels of anogenital sniffing of females, and more self-grooming (Witt, 1995).

d. Cognition

OT has intrinsic behavioral properties of an opposite nature to those of VP, that is, OT may be an amnesic neuropeptide, affecting both consolidation and retrieval of memory (Bohus et al., 1993).

11.2.8 Clinical Implications of Oxytocin

Physiological doses (2 to 5 mU/minute), rather than pharmacological doses (10 to 422 mU/minute) of OT are recommended to induce or augment uterine contractions sufficiently strong to dilate the cervix and expel the infant. This low dose prevents most of the potentially serious effects to the mother and fetus. However, this low dosage is effective only at term, when the uterus is highly sensitive to OT owing to the absence of progesterone and the increased number of OT receptors. The effectiveness of OT is enhanced by the concomitant stimulation of prostaglandins by this peptide. Because OT is normally secreted in spurts or pulses during labor, it is also more effective to administer exogenous OT in a pulsatile manner (Dawood, 1995).

There is only one report of an increase in female sexual behavior due to OT administration, modulated by steroids (Anderson-Hunt and Dennerstein, 1995). After an extensive search of the literature, these authors report a dearth of controlled studies in women and suggest that more research is needed to clarify the role of OT in human reproductive behaviors, including its "aphrodisiac" effect in women. Other reported effects of OT in humans include the induction of analgesia in low back pain involving the endogenous opiate system and suggestions that some forms of obsessive-compulsive behavior are related to OT dysfunction. OT may have an anxiolytic action in humans, and therefore may have therapeutic value in human depressive illness, panic attacks, and social phobias, as well as in deficits in social bonding.

In drug addicts, narcotic-analgesic drugs inhibit sexual behavior and cause impotence, perhaps by opioid inhibition of central OT transmission. There may be some involvement with OT systems since OT inhibits the development of opiate tolerance, dependence, and self-administration. Early childhood autism, similarly, may be linked to excessively high levels of brain opiates, perhaps due to elevated brain OT.

The biosynthesis of OT appears to be changed in acquired immunodeficiency syndrome (AIDS) patients, as indicated by a 40% reduction in the total number of OT neurons in the PVN (Guldenaar and Swaab, 1995), and a similar reduction of OT neurons in the PVN in Parkinson's disease (Purba et al., 1994). This suggests that there may be a correlation between loss of OT neurons and certain neurodegenerative diseases.

11.3 Vasopressin

11.3.1 Vasopressinergic Systems

There are several neuroanatomical and functional vasopressinergic systems. The HNS is the classical neuroendocrine route for the peripheral antidiuretic and pressor effects of VP. As discussed in section 11.1.3, the major sources of OT and VP are the magnocellular neurons of the SON and PVN which project mainly into the posterior pituitary to release VP and VP-neurophysin into the peripheral circulation. However, many parvocellular neurons secrete VP, which permits VP to exert important central actions.

Parvocellular VP neurons project to the brainstem and spinal cord, probably to control autonomic functions. Parvocellular neurons in the PVN that produce VP regulate pituitary functions via axons that project to the ME. Some parvocellular neurons in the PVN project to various brain areas, forming terminal VP-containing synapses. Other prominent VP-containing cell groups are in the SCN, the bed nucleus of the stria terminalis (BNST), and the medial amygdaloid nucleus, which project to several limbic structures, such as the lateral septum, ventral hippocampus, and the habenular area, regions considered to be involved in behavioral and physiological regulation of reproductive events, and in behavioral learning and memory. The central amygdaloid nucleus is also innervated by VP fibers from the BNST and contains a rich density of VP receptors, and consequently is a principal structure for mediating the effects of VP on cognition. Both immunocytochemistry and in situ hybridization show that the level of VP expression in these areas is greater in males than in females and is dependent upon testosterone (De Vries et al., 1994). This diverse origin and widespread distribution of VP fibers forms the anatomical basis for the numerous CNS functions regulated by VP (Buijs, 1987).

Additional extrahypothalamic-neurohypophyseal sources of VP include the pineal gland, the anterior pituitary, testis, pancreas, adrenal, ovary, and placenta. With the exception of the testis, in which VP has a paracrine antireproductive function, the function (if any) of VP in these tissues is unclear.

11.3.2 The Vasopressin Gene

11.3.2.1 Mutations of the Vasopressin Gene

The structural organization of the VP gene was discussed in section 11.1.4. The best-known mutation of the VP gene involves a single base deletion in the second exon of neurophysin II. In the *Brattleboro rat*, an animal model of this defect, an autosomal recessive defect is involved. If this mutation is homozygous, the animals completely lack both VP and neurophysin II and suffer from inherited diabetes insipidus, characterized by primary polyuria and polydipsia. In the human, in contrast, it is an autosomal dominant trait, and the disease is often late in onset, occurring in children between 2 and 6 years of age. The defective gene results in degeneration of magnocellular VP cells in the hypothalamus and their projections to the neurohypophysis. The magnocellular OT cells remain intact.

11.3.2.2 Regulation of the Vasopressin Gene

The VP gene is differently regulated in neurons of the HNS from neurons in the SCN or the BNST. Expression of the VP gene in nuclei of the HNS is finely adjusted to the peripheral requirements of VP. Osmotic stimuli, such as hypertonicity or salt loading, result in increased plasma VP levels and a marked rise in VP mRNA of the PVN and SON. The VP mRNA of the SCN is not affected by osmotic challenge.

Interestingly, testosterone increases VP immunoreactivity in the BNST, a sexually dimorphic structure, but has no effect on VP in the PVN, SON, or SCN.

There is a diurnal variation in the VP content of the SCN, a biological clock that generates daily rhythms in hormone secretion and behavior. VP levels in the SCN are highest in the day, around 5 P.M., and lowest at night, but there is no such diurnal rhythm in the PVN and SON (Burbach et al., 1988).

11.3.3 Synthesis, Storage, Release, and Inactivation

11.3.3.1 Synthesis and Storage

VP is synthesized as an N-terminal part of the larger VP-neurophysin precursor, *propressorphysin*, which includes an additional neurophysin and a C-terminal glycopeptide (Schmale et al., 1987). The peptide hormone remains intact in the precursor until proteolytic processing occurs in the secretory granules. The main products in the HNS are VP, neurophysin II, and CPP, of which only VP has been shown to have a hormonal effect.

In Brattleboro rats, the mutation results in a preprohormone that cannot be folded, processed, or properly degraded and which eventually destroys VP neurons. The C-terminus of the VP-neurophysin precursor is completely altered and the mutant protein is retained in the endoplasmic reticulum as its queer shape prevents normal intracellular transport (Schmale et al., 1993). A comparison between the human and Brattleboro rat precursor synthesis from gene to protein is shown in figure 11.15.

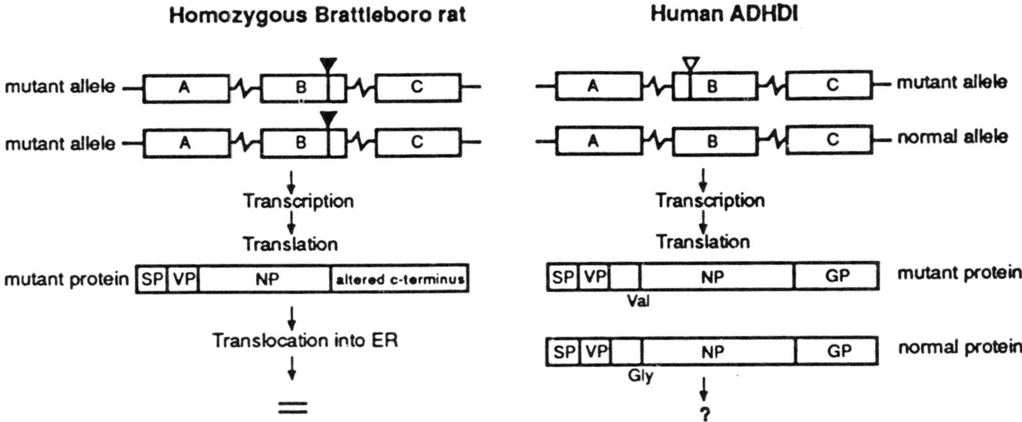

Figure 11.15
Schematic of vasopressin (VP) and neurophysin (NP) precursor synthesis from gene to protein in hereditary diabetes insipidus in homozygous Brattleboro rats and in human autosomal dominant hypothalamic diabetes insipidus (ADHDI). The boxes A, B, and C represent the three exons of the VP-NP gene. The solid arrowheads mark the site of nucleotide deletion in both the VP-NP gene alleles of the homozygous Brattleboro rat. The open arrowhead denotes the Gly 17-to-Val mutation in one VP-NP gene allele of a human family. SP, signal peptide; GP, C-terminal glycopeptide. (From Schmale et al., 1993.)

11.3.3.2 Release

a. Plasma hypertonicity and hypovolemia of the extracellular fluid

These are the classical stimuli for VP release. The release of VP into the circulation is due to the combined effect of excitatory and inhibitory inputs to the magnocellular cells of the SON and PVN. The scope of neural input to the neurosecretory cells in the PVN and SON may be of considerable integrative significance. Kiss et al. (1983) calculate that 2800 axon terminals are associated with a single neurosecretory cell in the PVN. The relationship between AP activity and hormone secretion is well established and the characteristic phasic pattern of magnocellular VP-secreting neurons is distinct from those secreting OT (see figure 2.10). This is not the final stage of VP secretion since presynaptic modulation of VP release from axon terminals occurs in the neurohypophysis, mediated by DA-containing fibers from the arcuate nucleus (D. A. Carter and Lightman, 1985).

b. Direct microdialysis with hypertonic solutions

This causes the release of both VP and OT within the hypothalamic nuclear region. Systemic osmotic stimuli elicit increases in intranuclear peptide release which are delayed and long-lasting, occurring over a 2.5-hour period. In contrast, plasma peptide levels peak at 30 minutes after the stimulus, indicating that increased plasma sodium elicits an increase in VP and OT into the extracellular space of the SON. The different patterns of peptide release in plasma and brain indicate that there may be independently regulated release into the different compartments (Ludwig et al., 1994)

c. Site of the osmoreceptors

Although Verney in 1947 postulated osmoreceptors in the hypothalamus, there is still no consensus as to their site, within or outside the CNS. There is very likely an osmoreceptor in the SON that mediates osmotic processing (Andersson, 1971) and there may be additional osmotic receptors within the CNS, for example, in the circumventricular organs (McKinley, 1985; Thrasher, 1985), and in the periphery, especially the hepatic portal vascular bed (Haberich, 1968). The importance of volume receptors in the vascular system was first stressed by Gauer (1968). Most probably, they are all implicated and interact to varying degrees, with a synergistic interaction between osmotic and volemic factors likely.

d. Thirst

One has to consider the many other mechanisms that regulate water balance and extracellular volume, including water intake, temperature, and water loss, to realize the complexity of VP regulation (figure 11.16). There is a linear relationship between thirst, plasma osmolality, and plasma VP. When the plasma osmolality approaches the threshold for thirst or VP secretion, the rate of water intake or excretion is rapidly corrected to protect from further change. The perception of thirst is satisfied by rapid drinking (especially of cold water), even before sufficient water can have been absorbed to correct the plasma osmolality; tongue, esophageal and gastric receptors are involved. Complete slaking of thirst, however, depends on the correction of plasma osmolality.

The remarkable water intake of patients with diabetes insipidus is an excellent example of the extremes to which physiological mechanisms can be pushed to maintain water homeostasis. Urine volume in such patients may reach 12 L/day in contrast to the normal 1 to 3 L, and to compensate, the patient will drink frequently, both night and day, to an extent that seriously interferes with normal living. Replacement with VP relieves the frequent urination and thirst, an

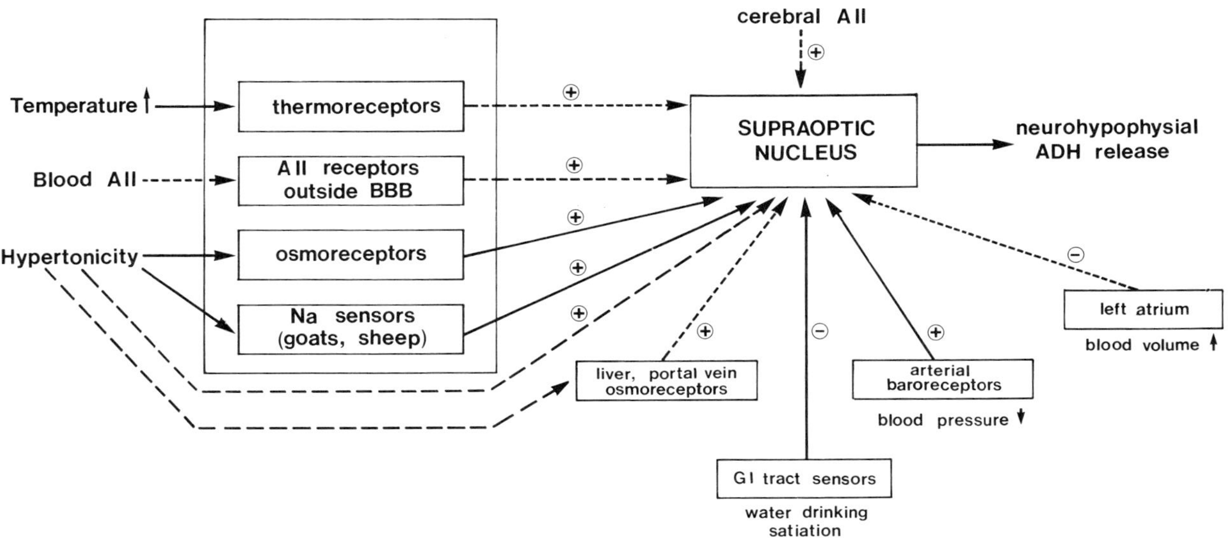

Figure 11.16
A summary of factors which may influence vasopressin (ADH) release in mammals. Solid lines indicate those factors and pathways likely to be physiologically significant in regulating vasopressin secretion; interrupted lines denote pathways of a more speculative nature which need further confirmation. ATII, angiotensin II; BBB, blood-brain barrier; GI, gastrointestinal. (From McKinley, 1985.)

action which typifies the antidiuretic action of VP, sometimes called ADH.

e. *Cardiovascular reflexes*

These form the major nonosmotic pathways for VP release. The loss of blood volume resulting from sustained hemorrhage results in electrophysiological responses and VP secretion analogous to those evoked by osmotic stimulation. Arterial pressure receptors in the carotid sinus and arch of the aorta act as high-pressure baroreceptors, whereas receptors in the right atrium act as low-pressure volume receptors. There is some debate about the significance of the atrial receptors in primates (McKinley, 1985).

If the neurosecretory cells of the SON and PVN are not themselves the osmoreceptors, they must receive neural inputs with the relevant information. *Afferent input* comes from the mid- and hindbrain, and from the anterior wall of the third ventricle, all of which receive information associated with osmolality or plasma volume. The ninth and tenth cranial nerves, with nerve endings in the walls of the atria and aortic arch, synapse in the nucleus of the tractus solitarius, from which noradrenergic fibers project to dendrites of the magnocellular neurons.

The efferent pathway for the cardiovascular reflexes consists of projections from the parvocellular neurons of the PVN (PVN autonomic neurons) to several

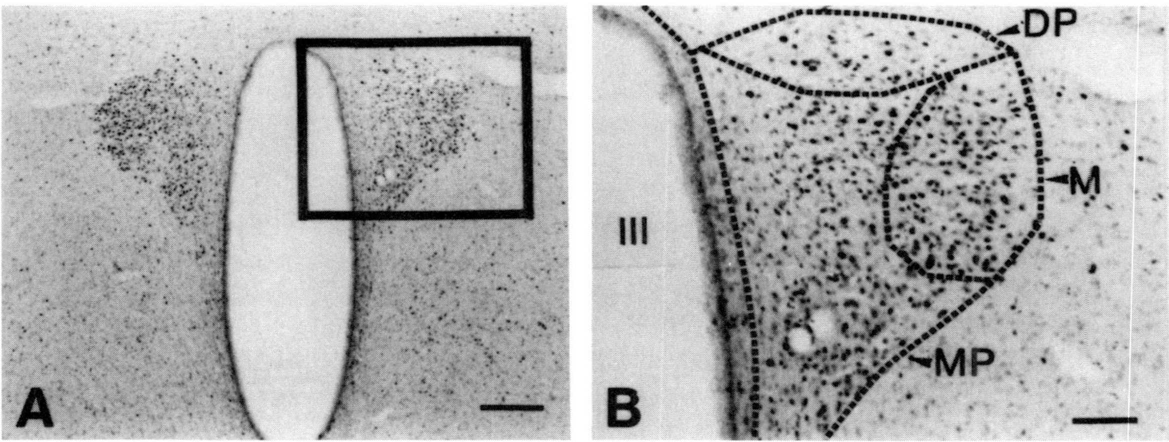

Figure 11.17
Coronal section of the paraventricular nucleus of the hypothalamus showing *fos* in cell nuclei after hemorrhage. Area in rectangle depicted in A is shown at higher magnification in B. Section has been counterstained with cresyl violet. Bars are 300 μm in A and 100 μm in B. III, third ventricle; MP, medial parvocellular; DP, dorsal parvocellular; M, magnocellular. (From Badoer, 1996.)

areas in the CNS involved in cardiovascular function. These areas include the nucleus of the solitary tract, the medulla, and the intermediolateral cell column of the thoracolumbar spinal cord. Some of these long projections to sympathetic preganglionic motor neurons in the spinal cord are important mediators of reflexes induced by changes in blood volume. Using the protein *fos* as a marker of neuronal activity, it is possible to investigate the effects of cardiovascular stimuli such as hemorrhage on neurons in the PVN in conscious animals. Badoer (1996) showed that in such animals, not only are the magnocellular neurons of the PVN activated but a good number of the PVN parvocellular neurons show heavy accumulation (figure 11.17). Sympathetic cardiac control is intensified by CRH and OT, probably by inhibiting vagal output.

AT II is a possible participant in the regulation of VP secretion. Hypovolemia results in increased renin production by the kidneys and the subsequent formation of AT I and AT II. Circulating AT II may stimulate VP release from the neurohypophysis. This inference is based on the observation that AT II, administered ICV, increases neurohypophyseal VP release into the peripheral circulation. This central AT II action is mediated by AT 1A receptors in the dorsal and medial parvocellular parts of the PVN, in some magnocellular PVN neurons, but not in VP-producing neurons in either the PVN or SON. Thus the stimulation of VP neurons must be indirect or via an unknown type of AT receptor (Lenkei et al., 1995). Whether AT II has a physiological role in VP release is debatable.

Interleukin-1 β, administered centrally, markedly increases VP release (Landgraf et al., 1995), suggesting that VP might oppose the central effects of the cytokine, including those on thermoregulation and behavior, and identifying another link between the neuroendocrine and immune systems, as discussed in chapter 8.

Estrogen causes exocytosis of granules from both the dendrites and cell bodies of the magnocellular neurons, with exocytosis from the dendrites predominating. Exocytosis occurs from both OT- and VP-producing magnocellular cells, but no secretory granules were exocytosed from the posterior pituitary. This is a rapid, direct action that excludes a genomic action and is not dependent on external calcium (Wang et al., 1995).

11.3.3.3 Inactivation

The removal of VP and OT from the circulation is mainly through renal and hepatic clearances, aided by inactivation in the small intestine. In the kidney, both filtration and peritubular metabolism are involved. Clearance of VP by the fetus is especially interesting as the VP excreted in the urine in the amniotic sac is recirculated in the fetus as it swallows the amniotic fluid. The VP is then absorbed from the gastrointestinal tract, apparently still biologically active (Claybaugh and Uyehara, 1993). Degradation of VP and OT also occurs in brain areas, but to a lesser extent. There are four major proteolytic enzymes that cleave VP: the tail portion is cleaved by a serine protease, which cleaves between positions 7 and 8, and by a carboxypeptidase, which cleaves between positions 8 and 9. The disulfide bond in the ring portion of VP is cleaved by a thiol:protein disulfide oxidoreductase, and an aminopeptidase cleaves the ring between positions 1 and 2. The different metabolites that result from these cleavages may have some biological activity.

11.3.4 Vasopressin Receptors and Second Messengers

At least three receptors for VP have been described: V1a, V1b, and V2, each of which is coupled to G proteins. The V1a receptor is found in many tissues, including brain, pituitary, liver, blood vessels, and kidney. Most VP binding sites in the CNS are of the V1a type and are present in several discrete regions, that is, the suprachiasmatic, the sigmoid, and the arcuate nuclei, but they are also diffusely distributed in the lateral hypothalamic and dorsochiasmatic areas, the anterior central amygdala, the mesencephalic central gray, and the choroid plexus. In general, VP receptors are concentrated in small areas of high receptor density and then decrease gradually from a frontal to a caudal direction (de Kloet et al., 1990).

The V1b receptor is localized in the anterior pituitary where it modulates the secretion of ACTH, but it is also found in many brain regions, as well as in a number of peripheral tissues (Lolait et al., 1995). Both V1a and V1b receptors act via phosphotidylinositol hydrolysis and mobilization of intracellular Ca^{2+}.

In the kidney, VP receptors are coupled to adenylate cyclase and cAMP and are classified as V2 receptors. VP receptors recognize OT but with a much lower affinity than VP.

Amphibians have two types of vasotocin receptors, V1 and V2, homologous to the vascular and hepatic $V1_{1a}$ and the renal V2 vasopressin receptors of mammals. The V2 renal subtype is necessary for the reabsorption of tubular water from the kidney, and the skin-bladder subtype is required for reabsorption from the skin and urinary bladder. A shorter version of vasotocin (vasotocinyl-Gly-Lys-Arg) *is hydrin* (vasotocinyl-Gly) which is active on skin and urinary bladder, but is devoid of antidiuretic action in the rat and frog, in contrast to vasotocin. Thus anuran amphibians appear to have developed two hydro-osmotic peptides, vasotocin and hydrin, derived from a single precursor through differental processing, and, on the other hand, two corresponding receptors in kidney and skin for internal and external water recovery (Rouille et al., 1995).

11.3.5 Vasopressin as a Neurotransmitter and Neuromodulator

VP may act as a neurohormone, neurotransmitter, or neuromodulator. As discussed in section 11.3.1, anatomical studies have shown that VP is contained in synaptic-like axon terminals in an extensive extrahypothalamic VP fiber network. VP, applied by iontophoresis, is a potent excitatory agent on the electrical activity of certain neurons in the SCN (Joels, 1987). This subpopulation of peptide-sensitive neurons possesses V1-type receptors and may contribute to the circadian cycle of electrical activity characteristic of the SCN.

In general, VP excites extrahypothalamic regions of the CNS that can be regarded as target sites for the peptide on the basis of immunocytochemistry, receptor binding, and behavioral studies. In almost all intracellular studies, VP depolarizes the membrane potential (figure 11.18). In the hippocampus, VP potentiates the effects of NE. In the lateral septum, VP may act as a neurotransmitter or neuromodulator, increasing the spontaneous activity of about 35% of neurons in this region, but also enhancing glutamate-evoked activity of these neurons. The long-term effects of VP on glutamate-induced excitation in septal and hippocampal neurons, and the maintenance of long-term potentiation in septal slices after fimbria fornix stimulation, provide a physiological basis for the understanding of the long-term memory effects of VP (van den Hoof et al., 1989).

11.3.6 Physiological Functions of Vasopressin

11.3.6.1 Renal Functions

VP, or ADH, has several functions in the kidney, most of which result in the conservation of water. These functions include modulation of solute and water transport, vasoconstriction, stimulation of prostaglandin synthesis, inhibition of renin release, and mitogenic effects. Each of these functions is mediated by either the V1 or V2 receptor subtype. Figure 11.19 illustrates some of the VP-responsive sites in the mammalian nephron. At the level of the glomerulus, VP causes a decrease in glomerular ultrafiltration rate, contraction of the glomerular mesangial cells, and prostaglandin production. These actions regulate glomerular filtration. VP also reduces blood flow in the vasa recta via a V1 receptor. In the thick ascending loop of Henle, VP stimulates Na^+, K^+, Cl^- transport. The most important action of VP is the reabsorption of water in the cortical collecting tubule, reducing tubule fluid flow from approximately 20% to 5% of the glomerular filtration rate. This is mediated by the V2 receptor, coupled to adenylate cyclase.

In the medullary interstitium there appears to be a mechanism for feedback modulation of V2 response through the concomitant occupancy of the V1 receptor on a neighboring cell, with the resulting production of prostaglandins. These, in turn, acting in a paracrine manner, modulate the V2 response to VP (Margolis et al., 1988).

11.3.6.2 Control of Pituitary ACTH Secretion

While VP is not the physiological CRH, it is involved in the regulation of ACTH secretion. Most studies indicate that VP enhances ACTH secretion, partly by potentiating responsiveness to CRH and perhaps by actually increasing CRH release. Most VP is produced in the magnocellular neurons and travels via axons to

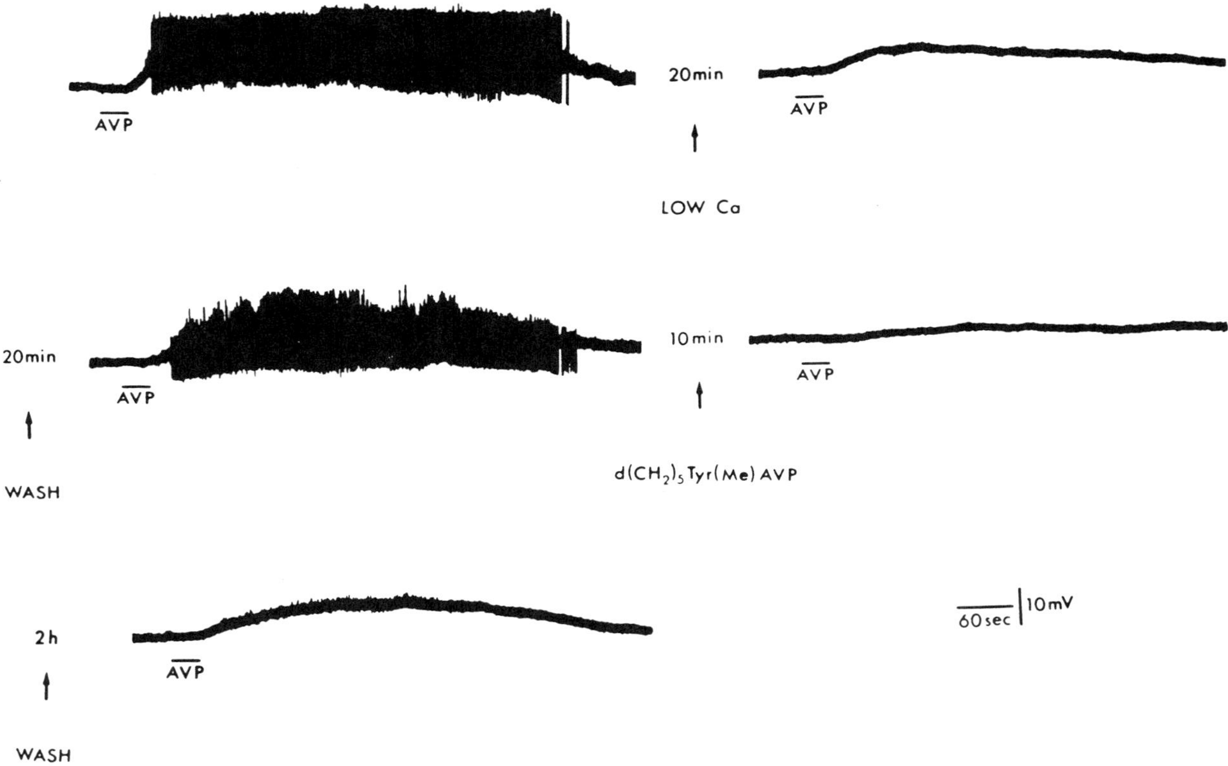

Figure 11.18
(Top left) Depolarization of the membrane of a lateral horn cell of the rat induced by 0.1 μM vasopressin (AVP). (Top right) In a low Ca^{2+}, high Mg^{2+} solution, the VP-evoked depolarization is markedly smaller. (Middle row) Application of the VP antagonist $d(CH_2)_5$ [Tyr(Me)^2] AVP (10^{-6} for 10 minutes) strongly blocks the effect of a subsequent application of AVP. (Bottom row) The peptide effect returns only partially after washout of the antagonist. (From Ma and Dun, 1985.)

the neurohypophysis, where it is released for peripheral functions. However, there are two and possibly three distinct pathways from the PVN to the ME that are involved in the regulation of ACTH secretion (figure 11.20). CRH and VP are the major neuropeptides in all three projections to the ME. One pathway involves CRH produced in the parvocellular neurons; a second group of parvocellular neurons produces both CRH and VP, and a third group of PVN magnocellular neurons produces VP. CRH and VP in the ME are delivered via the portal system to the anterior pituitary where they synergistically increase ACTH secretion. Details of these pathways are given by Antoni (1993). Additionally, as was discussed in chapter 9, the vascular route between the anterior and posterior pituitary can deliver VP directly to the corticotrophs and, via retrograde circulation through

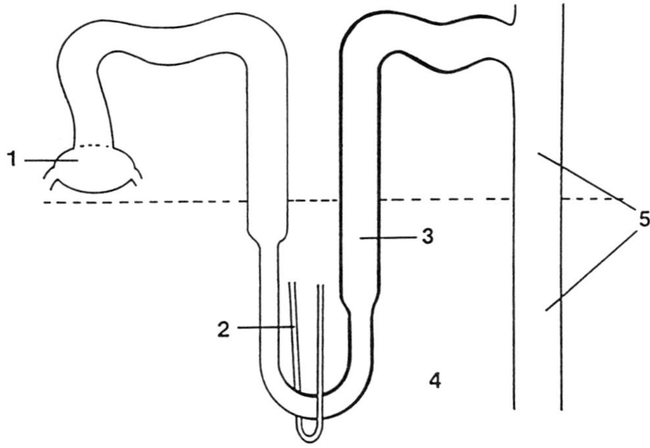

1	GLOMERULUS — mesangial contraction, PG elaboration, growth	V_1
2	VASA RECTA — medullary blood flow	V_1
3	MTALH — electrolyte transport, growth	V_2
4	MEDULLARY INTERSTITIUM — PG elaboration	V_1
5	CCT and MCT — water and solute transport, ? PG elaboration	V_2, ? V_1

Figure 11.19
Vasopressin (VP)-responsive sites and actions in the mammalian nephron. For each of the major recognized VP-responsive sites the corresponding functions and likely receptor subtype is given. An additional function not shown is modulation of renin release. MTALH, medullary thick ascending loop of Henle; PG, prostaglandin; CCT, cortical collecting tubule; MCT, medullary collecting tubule. (From Margolis et al., 1988.)

the hypothalamic-hypophysial portal system, back to the hypothalamus.

Whereas both VP and ACTH, released by stress, stimulate the neuroendocrine system, they have different and important actions on the motor and autonomic nervous systems (figure 11.21). CRH increases locomotor activity; VP depresses it. VP stimulates the parasympathetic system to result in passive coping with the stress; CRH activates the sympathetic nervous system to permit active coping (Bohus, 1993)

11.3.6.3 Cardiovascular Functions

Activation of the PVN increases blood pressure, heart rate, renal nerve activity, and plasma renin activity. Reciprocal connections between the PVN and brainstem autonomic centers, together with the direct innervation of sympathetic preganglionic fibers by PVN neurons, results in shared information and regulation of the physiological and behavioral cardiovascular responses to stress. The parasympathetic nervous system is also involved in conditioned emotional responses. The well-known "heart-stopping" response to stress (bradycardia) is controlled by the parasympathetic nervous system via the vagal nerves. This response is absent in Brattleboro rats but can be evoked by administration of VP. Vagal activity is facilitated by VP, NE, and DA.

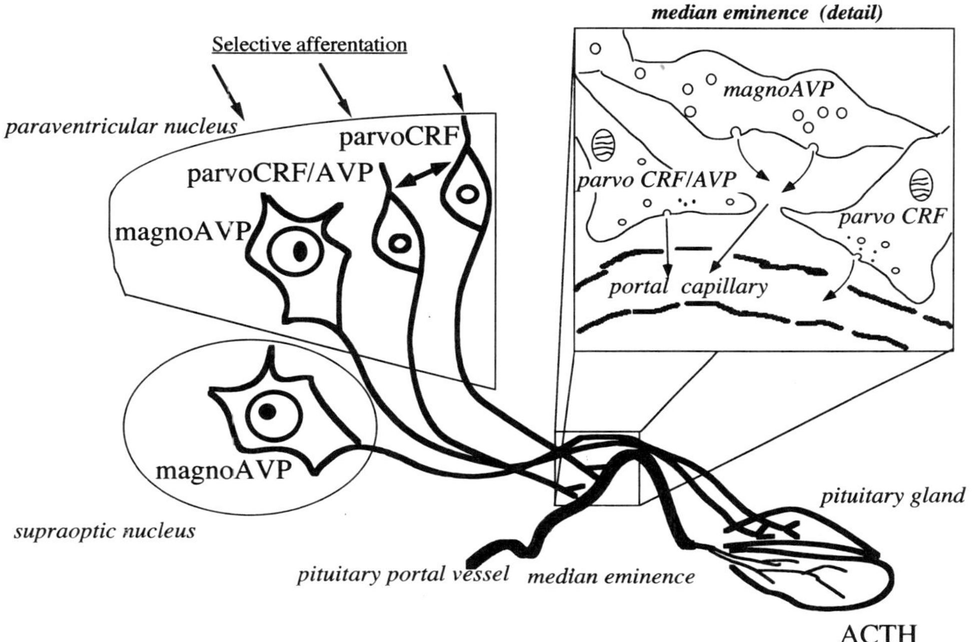

Figure 11.20
Scheme of the current concept of hypothalamic control of anterior pituitary ACTH secretion by multiple hypophysiotropic pathways to the median eminence. The double-headed arrow indicates that parvocellular corticotropin-releasing hormone and vasopressin (parvocell CRH/AVP) and CRH neurons may constitute a single functional entity. (From Antoni, 1993.)

11.3.7 *Behavioral Effects of Vasopressin*

11.3.7.1 Cognition, Memory, and Retrieval

More than 30 years ago the surprising discovery was made that neurohypophyseal hormones are involved in cognitive processes (De Wied, 1965). Removal of the neurohypophysis impairs the maintenance of an avoidance behavior, a deficit that can be restored by the administration of VP. As VP administration to normal rats prolongs the avoidance behavior, VP is considered to affect long-term memory processes, improving both the consolidation and retrieval of memory. VP reverses induced memory loss, including amnesia resulting from high dosages of epinephrine. OT, on the other hand, has opposite, amnesic effects (Bohus et al., 1978, 1993). Brattleboro rats, homozygous for hereditary diabetes insipidus and lacking endogenous VP, have serious retention deficits which can be corrected by VP. The mechanism(s) of these mnemonic effects are complex and many other factors are involved, including peripheral hormones, such as epinephrine and the gonadal steroids.

The amygdala is considered a site for the modulation of memory storage by hormones and neurotransmitters, a function that is dependent upon NE innervation. The vasopressinergic system involving

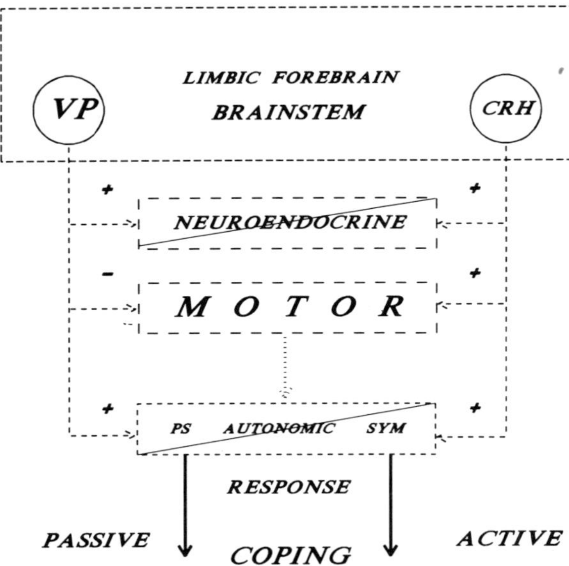

Figure 11.21
Differential effects of vasopressin (VP) and corticotropin-releasing hormone (CRH) neuronal systems in passive or active coping with environmental challenge. PS, parasympathetic mediation; SYM, sympathetic mediation. (From Bohus, 1993.)

the amygdala seems to be sexually dimorphic and regulated by testosterone (De Vries et al., 1985), and the antiamnesic effects of VP are seen in males but not in females (figure 11.22).

In contrast to the peripheral actions of VP, central functions of VP do not always require the full nonapeptide structure. VP 1–8 (des-glyNH_2) (DGLVP), a metabolite of VP found in the plasma but not in the brain, has most of the behavioral activities of VP but lacks its pressor and antidiuretic actions (De Wied, 1983). The main metabolites of VP and OT in the brain are formed after the cleavage of the Cys^1–Cys^6 bond and in a structure-activity study it was found that the presence of a glycinamide residue favors retrieval processes, whereas its absence encourages consolidation processes (De Wied et al., 1987). This is an excellent example of the neuropeptide concept, demonstrating that biologically active molecules, with specific functional differences, can be formed from the parent neuropeptide.

11.3.7.2 Drug Tolerance, Analgesia, and Temperature Regulation

VP and DGLVP facilitate the development of tolerance to morphine and ethanol, and high doses of VP systemically administered, have an antinociceptive effect in rats which can be blocked by a VP antagonist. VP has an antipyretic or fever-reducing effect, probably mediated by a receptor different from that moderating learning and memory effects. VP is also implicated in hibernation and VP injected into the lateral septum during hibernation disrupts this process.

11.3.7.3 Social Behaviors

Endogenous VP in the dorsal and ventral hippocampus and in the dorsal septal region plays a physiological role in social recognition and memory, as determined by the time spent by older rats in social investigation of young male rats (Greidanus and Maigret, 1996). Flank-marking in hamsters, a stereotyped behavior consisting of grooming and wetting of the flanks, is elicited by central administration of VP.

In the monogamous prairie vole, selective aggression and partner preference in males, two critical features of pair bonding, are dependent on central VP (Winslow et al., 1993). VP in the prairie vole brain is sexually dimorphic and important for paternal behavior Mating activates central VP pathways in the monogamous species, but OT and not VP is increased in CSF in polygamous rodents, such as the rat. This

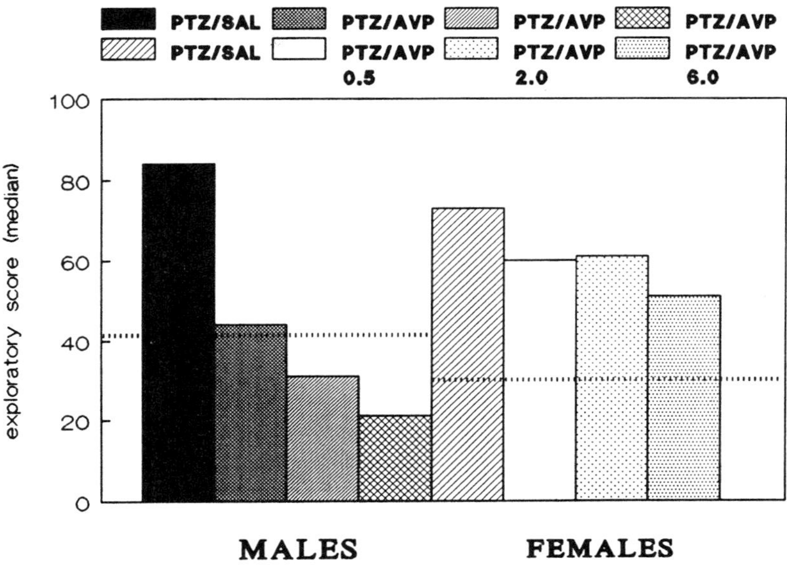

Figure 11.22
Sex dependence of the reversal of pentylenetetrazol (PTZ)-induced amnesia for exploration of a novel environment by arginine vasopressin (AVP) in male and female rats. PTZ was administered intraperitoneally immediately after the first exposure to the field. Exploratory scores represent the number of floor units entered on the second day. Broken lines show the behavior of nonamnesic controls (PTZ treatment six h after the first exposure). Six animals per group. (From Bohus et al., 1993.)

correlates with the specific difference in the distribution of VP and OT forebrain receptors in the monogamous vs. polygamous species.

11.3.8 Clinical Implications of Vasopressin

Since animal studies suggest that VP enhances memory processes, some clinical trials have attempted to evaluate the potential of VP in the treatment of human memory disorders. While these clinical trials are difficult to evaluate, as there are many sources of difference in patient groups, duration of treatment, necesary dosage, and so on, there does seem to be some improvement in patients with mild deficits, but not in those with profound brain degeneration (Jolles, 1987).

In healthy volunteers (Beckwith et al., 1984), and in diabetes insipidus patients (Van Ree et al., 1985), memory was reported to have been improved by VP treatment. Intranasal application of VP produced better results in healthy men than did i.v. administration (Pietrowsky et al., 1996).

While the total number of VP neurons in the SON and PVN remain unaltered throughout life, their size increases considerably in the age group of 80 to 100 years. The number of VP neurons in the human SCN, on the other hand, is markedly reduced during senescence, an effect more marked in patients with senile dementia of the Alzheimer's type (Swaab et al., 1987). There does not seem to be much hope for improvement of these conditions by administration of exogenous VP.

11.4 Summary

OT and VP are members of a family of highly related nonapeptides found throughout the vertebrate and invertebrate kingdoms. They are synthesized in the hypothalamus and stored in nerve terminals in the posterior pituitary. OT and VP are coded by two different genes and the OT and VP genes are similarly organized, reflecting their common evolutionary origin. In all mammals, both genes are close together on the same chromosome and they are oriented in opposite transcriptional directions. There are three encoding exons separated by two introns. Various amino acid substitutions, mostly in positions 3 and 8, account for the differences between the neuropeptides of this large and ancient family. They all have the same ring structure formed by a disulfide bridge between cysteine residues 1 and 6. Both OT and VP are expressed in specific groups of magnocellular neurons in the SON and PVN, but they are not colocalized, since the OT and VP genes are not expressed in the same cell. Collateral axons of the magnocellular neurons are widely dispersed throughout the CNS, permitting OT and VP to act as neuromodulators or neurotransmitters, important regulators of cardiovascular responses to stressful or osmotic stimuli. Local release of VP and OT may enable them to act in a paracrine or autocrine manner on neighboring cells.

Neurophysins, small acidic proteins about 10 times the length of VP or OT, form noncovalent complexes with the hormones: neurophysin I with OT, neurophysin II with VP. Neurophysins are stored within the secretory granules bound together with their respective neuropeptides and may ensure proper configuration of OT and VP for exposure to processing enzymes and excision of the neurophysin. The secretory granules are transported down the axons of the OT- and VP-containing magnocellular neurons to terminate in the posterior pituitary, close to fenestrated capillaries. They then enter the bloodstream to act as hormones.

11.4.1 Oxytocin

The *OT gene* is regulated by a composite of multiple interacting enhancers and repressors. Expression of the OT gene is controlled by several physiological conditions, such as development, puberty, stages of the female cycle, thyroid hormone levels, and variations in plasma osmolarity. Estrogens are strong inducers of uterine OT gene expression when primed by progesterone, but subsequent progesterone withdrawal is then required for full expression of hypothalamic OT. Uterine OT mRNA rises sharply in the late stages of pregnancy, but the uterus is protected from premature contractions by endogenous opioid inhibition until parturition, at which time OT is reflexly released from magnocellular neurons. Hypothalamic OT mRNA increases during lactation, chiefly due to activation of PVN neurons following suckling stimulation of nerve endings in the nipples, but also through local release of OT acting on autoreceptors. During lactation PRL acts directly on hypothalamic OT cells to increase OT mRNA. Maternal behavior provides a positive feedback to increase central OT release. In males, OT modulates tetosterone production and assists sperm transport. In both sexes, OT secretion is circadian in most mammals.

There is considerable variation in the distribution of *OT receptors* in different species. In the rat, OT receptors are present in the olfactory system, basal ganglia, limbic system, thalamus, ventromedial hypothalamus, some cortical regions, the brainstem, and spinal cord. OT receptors bind VP as well as OT with high affinity, but their distribution is very different from that of VP receptors. Peripheral OT receptors are coupled to inositol phosphates and they are regulated differently in various brain areas and during different physiological conditions associated with mating and sexual behavior. Both receptor number and affinity are increased by mating and pregnancy. In males, estrogen and testosterone act synergistically to regulate OT binding in the ventromedial hypothalamus. OT receptors are present in many peripheral tissues.

OT increases *uterine contractility* at parturition, contraction of the mammillary myoepithelial cells for *milk ejection*, and facilitates the spinal *nociceptive flexor reflex*. Through its projections to cortical, brainstem, and spinal neurons, and to opioid systems, as well as through local effects on neighboring parvocellular neurons, OT may influence cardiovascular and endocrine responses to stressful and osmotic stimuli, and affect the pain threshold.

OT is involved in a variety of *sexual and social behaviors* in avian and reptilian species, in which vasotocin is the active nonapeptide, as well as in mammals. In mammals, OT facilitates all aspects of reproductive behavior, including female receptivity, maternal behavior, and male mounting. OT acts on neurons in the CNS that control such behaviors: in the VMN in the female and PVN in the male. The olfactory bulb is another site of OT induction of maternal behavior. The female behaviors are dependent upon estrogen priming but OT may have a more direct effect on the alleviation of the distress of young separated from their mothers. In males OT is a potent activator of penile erection, and shortens ejaculation latency and the postejaculation interval.

In the mongamous prairie vole, which forms pair bonds after mating, OT is secreted during mating and is essential to pair bonding. In males VP is the essential "bonding hormone." Female mutant mice, lacking an immediate early gene *fos*B, are completely deficient in maternal behavior and all their neonates die. The defect is a specific disturbance in the olfactory pathway to the hypothalamus. *Nonsexual behaviors*, such as grooming, cognition, and yawning are affected by OT in both sexes.

11.4.2 Vasopressin

The main pathway for OT and VP to reach the systemic circulation is through the hypothalamic-neurohypophyseal system, by which axons from the magnocellular neurons in the PVN and SON pass through the infundibulum to reach the posterior pituitary. Central effects of VP are routed mainly through projections from recurrent axon collaterals of the magnocellular neurons, and through projections of parvocellular neurons from the PVN and many other brain regions.

A well-known *mutation of the VP gene* involves a single base deletion in the neurophysin encoding exon B. If this mutation is homozygous, as it is in the Brattleboro rat, the animal lacks VP and neurophysin II and suffers from inherited diabetes insipidus, characterized by polyuria and polydipsia. The defective gene results in the degeneration of the magnocellular VP cells in the hypothalamus while leaving the OT cells intact. An abnormal preprohormone is coded which cannot be processed to VP. *Expression* of the VP gene in neurons of the HNA is finely regulated by osmotic stimuli, hypertonicity causing a marked increase in hypothalamic VP mRNA and plasma

VP. The VP mRNA of parvocellular neurons, such as those in the SCN, is not affected by osmotic stimulation, but these neurons have a diurnal rhythm which is absent from the PVN and SON.

Plasma hypertonicity and a *reduction in blood volume* are the classic stimuli for *VP release*. Release of VP into the circulation is due to a balance of excitatory and inhibitory neural inputs to the magnocellular neurons of the PVN and SON, which results in the phasic secretion of VP by these excited cells. The release of VP accumulating in the nerve terminals in the posterior pituitary is presynaptically modulated by DA. Osmoreceptors and volume receptors for VP release probably exist but have not been definitively located. Thirst and the perception of thirst are potent regulators of VP release, and patients with diabetes insipidus, lacking VP, drink enormous quantities of water to compensate for the large volumes of water they excrete in their urine.

Nonosmotic stimuli, such as loss of blood volume, reach the PVN and SON from high-pressure baroreceptors in the carotid sinus and arch of the aorta. Receptors in the right atrium respond to low-pressure changes. The afferent pathway is via the ninth and tenth cranial nerves which synapse in the nucleus of the tractus solitarius, from which dendrites project to the magnocellular neurons. The efferent pathway for the cardiovascular reflexes consists of projections from the parvocellular neurons in the PVN to CNS centers controlling autonomic functions. AT II may be involved in the regulation of VP secretion, as may interleukin-1 β. Most ciculating VP is inactivated by the kidney and liver, and to a lesser extent by the small intestine. Central VP is degraded in the brain.

There are two types of *VP receptors*, the V1 receptor and the V2 receptor. Most CNS receptors are V1 receptors and are coupled to the phosphatidylinositol pathway. The pituitary V1 receptor differs somewhat and is classified as a $V1_b$ receptor. Peripherally, VP receptors include the hepatic and vascular $V1_a$ receptors. Kidney receptors are of the V2 type and utilize adenylate cyclase and cAMP as the second-messenger pathway. VP receptors recognize OT with much lower affinity than VP. Amphibians have two types of vasotocin receptors, V1 and V2, analogous to the mammalian vascular and hepatic $V1_a$ receptor and V2 kidney receptor, respectively.

VP actions are of great physiological importance. VP may act as a *neurohormone* in the kidney and vasculature; as a *neurotransmitter* in the CNS exciting extrahypothalamic neurons, especially in the SCN; and as a *neuromodulator* potentiating the effects of NE and glutamate in the brain. VP potentiates the action of CRH in stimulating the release of ACTH.

The *renal functions* of VP involve modulation of water and ion transport, vasoconstriction, stimulation of prostaglandin synthesis, and the regulation of the glomerular ultrafiltration rate. VP causes the reabsorption of water in the renal collecting tubule, acting through the V2 receptor. All these actions, and several others, result in *conservation of water*. The *cardiovascular effects* of VP include increase in heart rate, blood pressure, and plasma renin activity, accomplished through VP release from PVN axons terminating in brainstem autonomic centers and on sympathetic preganglionic fibers.

Behavioral effects of VP include improvement of long-term memory: animals lacking VP have serious retention deficits which can be corrected by VP administration. VP facilitates the development of tolerance to morphine and has antinociceptive and antipyretic actions. Endogenous VP plays a role in social recognition in rodents, and in aggression and partner preference in monogamous male voles.

Chapter 12 discusses the neuropeptides derived from the large prohormone, pro-opiomelanocortin (POMC). POMC gives rise to ACTH, MSH, β-lipotropin, β-endorphin, and a series of small fragments of varying known and unknown potencies. In addition to the classical endocrine functions of ACTH, this neuropeptide has developmental, regulatory, behavioral, and regenerative effects on the central and peripheral nervous systems, actions that will be described in some detail.

Anterior Pituitary Neuropeptides I. The POMC-Derived Neuropeptides: ACTH, MSH, β-LPH, β-EP

12

This chapter discusses the anterior pituitary neuropeptides derived from the prohormone pro-opiomelanocortin (POMC): ACTH, MSH. Detailed discussion of the receptors and functions of β-lipotropin and β-endorphin are included in chapter 14. The glycoprotein and growth hormone families of anterior pituitary neuropeptides are examined in chapter 13.

The anterior pituitary hormones, while named after their first identified endocrine effects on target organs, have numerous effects on other tissues, including the brain and the resulting behavior patterns. In the classical endocrine pathway, the anterior pituitary hormones ACTH, FSH and LH, and TSH are regulated by potent negative feedback loops from their target organ (adrenal cortex, gonads, thyroid) secretions, as well as through control by hypothalamic regulatory hormones. The glycoprotein hormones GH and PRL do not evoke endocrine secretion and are basically controlled by the hypothalamic mechanisms that were discussed in depth in chapter 10.

12.1 Development of the Pituitary Gland and Its Cell Types

The anterior pituitary develops from a section of somatic ectoderm, the hypophysial placode, which gives rise to Rathke's pouch. The anterior wall of Rathke's pouch gives rise to the anterior pituitary, the posterior wall produces the intermediate lobe of the pituitary, and the posterior, neural lobe of the pituitary is formed from an evagination of the floor of the hypothalamus. Figure 12.1 illustrates the development of the rat pituitary, from embryonic day 9 (e9). The front end of the neural plate grows in an anterior direction, accompanied by an elongation of the future hypophyseal area. The oropharyngeal membrane disintergrates to permit an opening between the mouth and foregut. The future hypothalamic area is formed from the expanded front end of the notochord (see figure 12.1, top row).

The next important stage involves the differentiation of the hypophyseal placode, which is a thickening of the ventral ridge ectoderm, seen at e11 in figure 12.1. On the next day, e12, the infundibulum evaginates from the base of the hypothalamic portion, and Rathke's pouch is clearly seen. At e13, anterior lobe stem cells appear in the anteroventral region of Rathke's pouch. What is especially interesting about figure 12.1 is that it illustrates the clear spatiotemporal pattern of development of the different anterior pituitary cell types and their genes. A glycoprotein subunit (GSU) common to the gonadotropins and TSH is expressed throughout the hypophyseal placode by e11. The TSH gene is expressed first on e14 in one group of anterior lobe cells, followed by cells expressing POMC in the more posterior region of this lobe (Swanson, 1993).

Several transcription factors, especially Pit-1, are essential trophic factors in pituitary development through their regulation of particular hormone genes. Pit-1 binds to the promoter regions of the GH, PRL, and TSH genes, controlling their pituitary-specific expression. Pit-1 is also required for the normal development and proliferation of the lactotrophs and sommatotrophs (Nelson et al., 1988).

The five phenotypically distinct cell types appear in the anterior pituitary in the following temporal sequence: corticotrophs, thyrotrophs, gonadotrophs, somatotrophs, and lactotrophs. Whereas these five distinct cell types, secreting six adenohypophyseal hormones, can be distinguished by techniques such

Figure 12.1
Overview of pituitary development based on schematic sagittal sections through rat embryos, starting on embryonic day 9 (e9) at the neural plate stage. The pro-opiomelanocortin (POMC) gene displays an especially interesting pattern of expression: it first appears in the basal hypothalamus on e13 (*), then in the anterior lobe on e14, and finally in the intermediate lobe on e15 (not shown). By e17, a definite spatial organization of cell types has formed. See text for more details. alr, anterolateral ridge; ALstm, anterior lobe stem cell area; anp, anterior neuropore; CF, cephalic flexure; EC, ectoderm; EN, endoderm; FB, forebrain vesicle; FG, foregut vesicle; FG, foregut; fpl, floor plate; GH, growth hormone; GSV, glycoprotein subunit; ha, hypophyseal region; HB, hindbrain vesicle; hp, hypophyseal placode; HY, hypothalamus; IL, intermediate lobe; ir, infundibular recess of third ventricle; LH/FSH, luteinizing hormone–follicle-stimulating hormone; M, mouth; MA, maxillary process; MB, midbrain vesicle; ME, neurohemal zone of median eminence; nch, notochord; NPLdi, neural plate, diencephalic part; och, optic chiasm; opm, oropharygeal membrane; P, pontine neuroepithelium; PL, posterior lobe; PRL, prolactin; prpl, prochordal plate (of notochord); RP, Rathke's pouch; S, Seessel's pouch; sph, sphenoid cartilage; stm, stem cell area; vr, ventral ridge; V3, third ventricle. (From Swanson, 1993.)

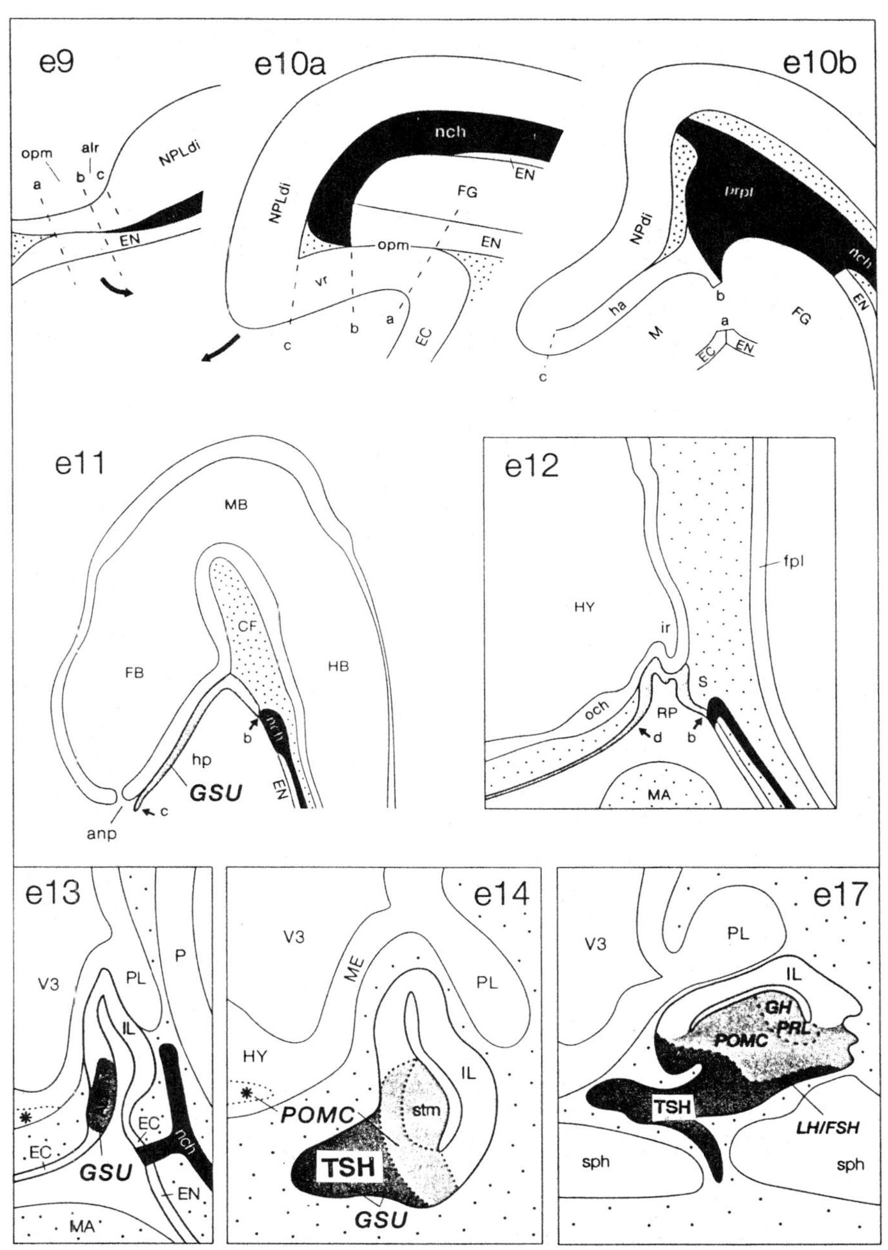
e9
opm
alr
a
b
c
NPLdi
EN
e10a
nch
EN
FG
NPLdi
opm
EN
vr
c
b
a
EC
e10b
brpl
NPdi
nch
EN
b
ha
M
FG
a
EC
EN
c
e11
MB
CF
FB
HB
b
nch
hp
GSU
EN
c
anp
e12
fpl
HY
ir
S
och
RP
d
b
MA
e13
V3
PL
P
IL
EC
EC
nch
GSU
EN
MA
e14
V3
ME
PL
HY
IL
POMC
stm
TSH
GSU
e17
V3
PL
IL
GH
PRL
POMC
TSH
LH/FSH
sph
sph

as immunocytochemistry, electron microscopy, immunoelectron microscopy, and in situ hybridization, it is likely that methodologies still to be developed may identify other important cell types.

12.2 Adrenocorticotropic Hormone, Melanocyte-Stimulating Hormone, β-Lipotropin, and β-Endorphin

12.2.1 Historical Significance

The many effects of pituitary hormones were clearly demonstrated by their removal through hypophysectomy (removal of the hypophysis or pituitary gland). It was noted that, in the rat, hypophysectomy resulted in an abrupt cessation of growth, and atrophy of the adrenals, thyroid, and gonads, changes that could be reversed by the administration of crude pituitary extracts (Smith, 1930). The fascinating story of the early research on anterior pituitary hormones, and the scientists who developed the field of endocrinology, is provided by Greep (1974).

The involvement of the pituitary gland in color change was known early in the twentieth century, first through experiments on larval amphibians (tadpoles), which became pale following removal of the pituitary. Implantation of pituitaries, or administration of pituitary extracts, restored the pigmentation to the melanocytes (P. E. Smith, 1916). MSH was first isolated from porcine pituitary by T. H. Lee and Lerner (1956) and named after its most obvious action, melanin dispersal (figure 12.2). Its effects on *behavior* and its *neurotrophic actions* on nerve development and regeneration did not become known until almost 25 years later (see section 12.2.9.3).

Clinically, Harvey Cushing (1909) introduced the concepts of hyper- and hypopituitarism: excess pituitary secretion leading to bilateral adrenal hyperplasia (Cushing's disease), or in other cases of pituitary tumors, gigantism and acromegaly; hyposecretion resulted in dwarfism. The isolation of the specific pituitary hormones responsible, ACTH and GH, came much later.

In the early 1950s crude extracts of the pituitary were shown to have adrenocorticotropic properties and ACTH 1–39 was the first pituitary polypeptide to be isolated and sequenced (Li et al., 1955). Subsequently, a higher-molecular-weight form of ACTH was detected: this was "big ACTH" (240 to 250 amino acids), the precursor of the linear 39–amino acid ACTH (Yalow and Berson, 1973). In one year three separate groups of investigators (Mains et al., 1977; Roberts and Herbert, 1977; and Nakanishi et al., 1977) discovered that the high-molecular-weight form of ACTH contained the sequences of ACTH 1–39, β-MSH, and β-lipotropin. β-lipotropin, a 91–amino acid sequence, in turn, contains the sequences of β-endorphin (β-lipotropin 61–91) and β-MSH (ACTH 1–16 or 1–22, depending on the species. Accordingly, this large precursor was named *pro-opiomelanocortin* to incorporate all three moieties. Figure 12.3A is a simplified diagram showing the pairs of basic residues at which POMC is cleaved into its major products, whereas figure 12.3B indicates the products of POMC processing in more detail. See also figures 3.9 and 3.10.

Pituitary extracts have been known for decades to have fat-mobilizing activity. β-Lipotropin was isolated from the pituitary in 1964 and named for its lipolytic action, which is, however, rather weak. Its physiological role as the precursor of β-MSH and β-endorphin is far more consequential. β-Endorphin, a neuropeptide derived from β-lipotropin, is an endogenous opiate with analgesic and euphoric properties, first isolated by Li and Chung (1976).

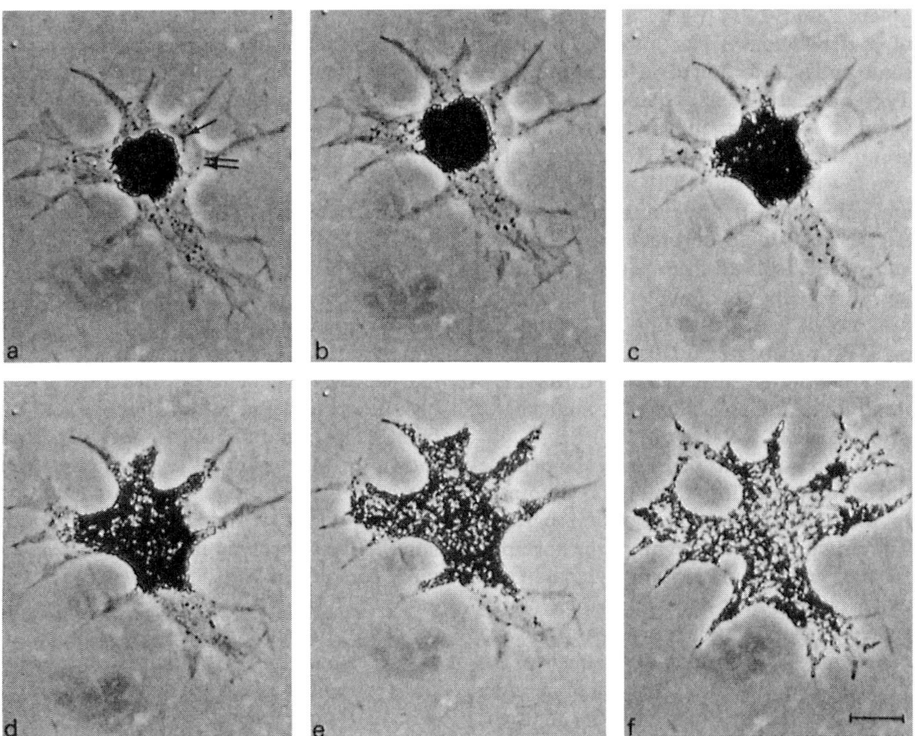

Figure 12.2
Melanin dispersion response of a 10-day cultured melanophore to 100 pg/mL α-melanocyte–stimulating hormone (α-MSH). a, Before addition of α-MSH. b, c, d, e, and f, At 2, 6, 10, 15, and 84 minutes after addition of α-MSH. Double arrows indicate the nucleus; single arrows indicate the nucleolus. (From Seldenrijk et al., 1979.)

12.2.2 Phyologenetic Distribution and Structure of POMC-Derived Neuropeptides

Most vertebrate species possess both anterior and intermediate lobes, including amphibians, reptiles, and fish, as well as most mammals. Birds, and many mammals (humans, the higher apes, elephants, mantees, whales, dolphins, and the armadillo) have little or no intermediate lobe. Adult humans do not have an intermediate lobe, although it is present in fetal life and capable of producing α-MSH (Kastin et al., 1968).

12.2.2.1 Pro-opiomelanocortin

POMC proteins, mRNAs, and genes have been highly conserved. Human and *Xenopus laevis* (the South African clawed frog) genes and their corresponding mRNAs are remarkably similar (Civelli et al., 1982). The POMC gene structure has been virtually unchanged in 350 million years of vertebrate evolution. However, *X. laevis* has two POMC genes, both of which are active (Martens, 1988).

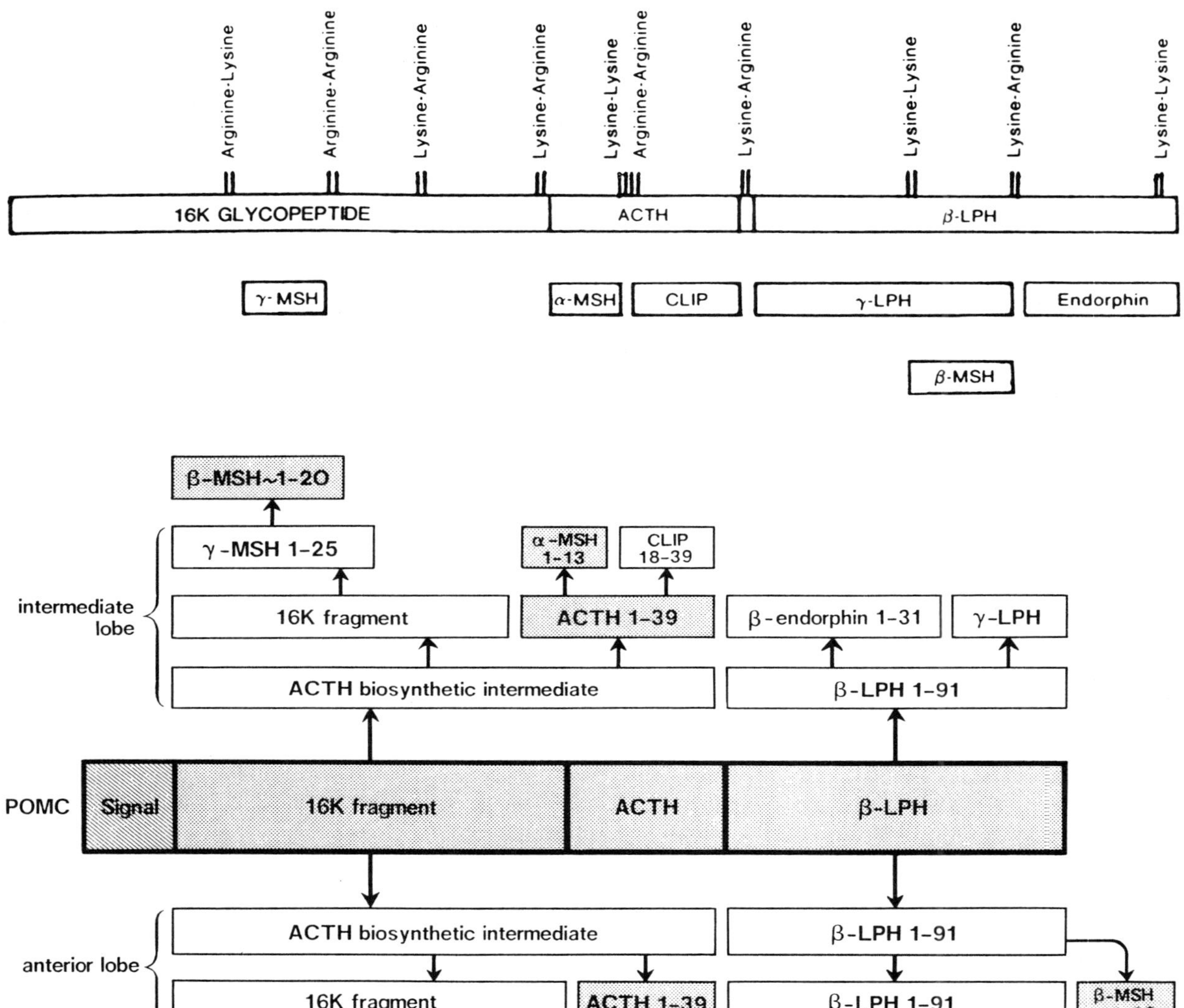

Figure 12.3
(Top) Diagrammatic representation of human pro-opiomelanocortin structure showing the pairs of basic residues. ACTH, adrenocorticotropic hormone; β-LPH, β-lipotropin; MSH, melanocyte-stimulating hormone; CLIP, corticotropin-like intermediate lobe peptide. (From Loh et al., 1988.) (Bottom) Tissue-specific processing of pro-opiomelanocortin (POMC).

Table 12.1
Sequences of POMC-derived neuropeptides[a]

The Melanocortins

ACTH 1–39

H-*Ser^{1}-Tyr-Ser-Met^{4}-Glu-His-Phe^{7}-Arg-Trp-Gly-Lys-Pro-Val^{13}*-Gly-Lys-Lys^{16}-Arg-Arg-Pro-Val-Lys -Val-Tyr-Pro^{24}-Asn-Gly-Ala-Glu-Asp-Glu-Ser-Ala -Glu-Ala-Phe-Pro-Leu-Glu-Phe^{39}-OH

α-MSH (ACTH 1–13)

Ser^{1}-Tyr-Ser-Met^{4}-Glu-His-Phe^{7}-Arg-Trp-Gly-Lys-Pro-Val^{13}-NH_2

β-MSH

H-Asp^{1}-Glu-Gly-Pro-Tyr-Lys-*Met^{7}-Glu-His-Phe^{10}-Arg-Trp-Gly*-Ser-Pro-Pro-Lys-Asp-OH

The Endorphins

β-Endorphin (1–31)

H-*Tyr^{1}-Gly-Gly-Phe-Met-Thr^{6}-Ser-Glu-Lys^{9}-Ser-Gln-Thr -Pro-Leu-Val-Thr^{16}*-Leu^{17}-Phe-Lys-Asn-Ala-Ile-Ile-Lys-Asn-Ala-Try-Lys-Lys-Gly-Glu^{31}-OH

α-Endorphin (β-endorphin 1–16)

H-*Tyr^{1}-Gly-Gly-Phe-Met-Thr^{6}-Ser-Glu-Lys^{9}-Ser-Gln-Thr-Pro-Leu-Val-Thr^{16}*

γ-Endorphin (β-endorphin 1–17)

H-*Tyr^{1}-Gly-Gly-Phe-Met-Thr^{6}-Ser-Glu-Lys^{9}-Ser -Gln-Thr-Pro-Leu-Val-Thr-Leu^{17}*

POMC, pro-opiomelanocortin; ACTH, adrenocorticotropic hormone; MSH, melanocyte-stimulating hormone.
[a] Common amino acid sequences are in italics.

12.2.2.2 Adrenocorticotropic Hormone

Similarly, the structure of the ACTH molecule has been highly conserved. Its entire biological activity is contained within ACTH 1–39, the natural product of POMC processing. Cleavage yields the sequence ACTH-MSH 1–13, but although many shorter ACTH fragments, especially the heptapeptide sequence ACTH 4–10 common to ACTH and MSH (table 12.1), have potent neurotrophic and behavioral effects, evidence is only now accumulating to show that they are also physiologically produced. Brain membranes form active fragments in vitro from large peptides and immunocytochemical studies have demonstrated the presence of ACTH 4–10 in the CNS during development and regeneration (Lee et al., 1994; Antonawich et al., 1994).

12.2.2.3 Melanocyte-Stimulating Hormone

MSH is included in this chapter on anterior pituitary hormones because it is produced by melanotrophs in the anterior pituitary of those species that lack an intermediate lobe. However, most research has been done on the intermediate lobe of the rat. Three distinct forms of MSH have been isolated and purified, α-, β-, and γ-MSH (see table 12.1). All three MSH sequences occur in the intermediate lobe precursor. They are structurally related, possessing a common heptapeptide core Met-Glu-His-Phe-Arg-Trp-Gly, which has inherent melanotropic activity, and this sequence also forms the midportion of β-lipotropin, suggesting that this segment is essential to bioactivity.

α-MSH has been identified in many species and shown to be highly conserved. The amino acid sequence of α-MSH is the same in all mammals, with an acetylated N-terminus and an amidated C-terminus, indicating that there is an "ancestral" POMC N-acetylating mechanism that has generally persisted throughout mammalian evolution (Dores et al., 1993). Amphibians secrete an α-MSH identical to the mammalian hormone, but teleost fish produce two forms of MSH, one of which is identical to mammalian α-MSH, except that it is not acetylated at the N-terminus. The other MSH is a 15–amino acid molecule, 13 residues of which are identical to mammalian ACTH 1–15 (Kawauchi et al., 1988). α-MSH is not produced in measurable amounts in adult human pituitaries, although there may be some produced by other brain areas. The human fetal intermediate lobe, however, may play a meaningful role in development because it produces significant amounts of α-MSH (Swaab et al., 1977).

β-MSH, on the other hand, shows extensive species heterogeneity, the length and amino acid composition varying considerably. β-MSH does not seem to be a significant secretion of the human pituitary; rather it is identified as a fragment of β-lipotropin, artificially formed during tissue extraction. *γ-MSH*, which is present in mammals and elasmobranchs but not in teleosts, has very little melanotropic activity. The glycosylated precursor of γ-MSH was originally termed the 16K segment of POMC.

12.2.2.4 β-Lipotropin and β-Endorphin

β-Lipotropin, a 91–amino acid peptide incorporated within the POMC precursor, is itself a precursor to a variety of peptides, including β-MSH and β-endorphin. The primary structure of *β-endorphin* (β-lipotropin 61–91) has also been highly conserved during evolution. In all species tested, it consists of 31 amino acids, with very little substitution. There are several forms of endorphins, α, β, and γ, each of which contains a sequence of β-endorphin 1–16. The structures of the POMC-derived neuropeptides are presented in table 12.1, with the common amino acid sequences in italics.

12.2.3 *Anatomical Distribution*

POMC is found in the cell bodies of the arcuate nucleus and in fibers that project from these cells to extrahypothalamic structures, including the nucleus accumbens, reticular formation, periaqueductal gray, and the medial amygdala. POMC arcuate neurons are larger than other arcuate neurons, being 10 to 15 μm in diameter with conspicuous dendrites, and are probably the main source of extrapituitary ACTH and MSH. The POMC arcuate neurons are anatomically distinct from those containing enkephalin or other known neuroactive substances (Chronwall, 1985). A second group of POMC neurons is located in the nucleus of the tractus solitarius of the caudal medulla. These neurons produce mainly α-MSH, CLIP, and β-endorphin, very little ACTH and β-lipotropin. POMC is present in spinal motor neurons. In addition to localization in the CNS, POMC is present in many other tissues, including the gut and pancreas (Krieger et al., 1980; Larson, 1977), and in lymphocytes, macrophages, and spleen (Lolait et al., 1986). POMC is also expressed in the testis, ovary, adrenal medulla, placenta, lung, skin, and heart.

ACTH 1–39, α-MSH *and* β-lipotropin are present in the anterior pituitary corticotrophs (figure 12.4) The corticotrophs form about 10% to 15% of adenohypophyseal cells and contain a large, irregular unstained perinuclear body, of unknown function and appropriately named the enigmatic body. Another characteristic marker of the corticotrophs is the presence of bands of filaments (type 1) in the perinuclear region. There is no sex difference in the morphology of the corticotrophs but they increase in size and

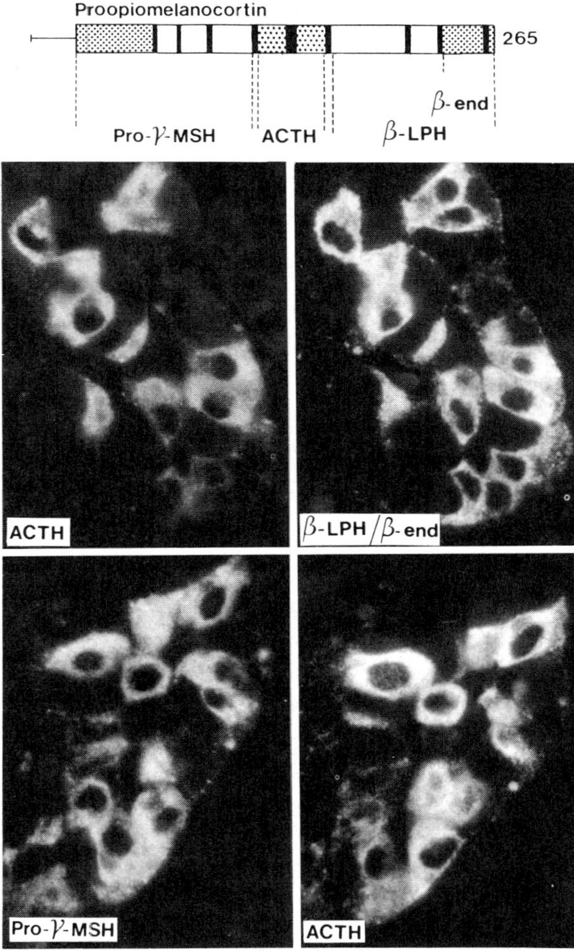

Figure 12.4
Coexistence of pro-opiomelanocortin-derived peptides in the porcine anterior pituitary. (Top) Immunofluorescence staining for ACTH and β-lipotropin (β-LPH) and β-endorphin (β-end) immunoreactants in a pair of consecutive semithin sections. (Below) Another pair of sections was stained for pro-γ-melanocyte-stimulating hormone (Pro-γ-MSH) and ACTH, respectively. The antigenic sequences recognized by the various antisera are indicated by dotted areas in the precursor structure represented by the bar at the top of the figure. (From Sundler et al., 1985.)

number in Cushing's disease, reflecting their overactivity in response to the lack of adrenal corticosteroid negative feedback. Some corticotrophs are also found in the intermediate lobe.

The melanotrophs in the intermediate lobe are granular cells with a well-developed rough endoplasmic reticulum and secretory granules. These cells contain MSH and the various peptide derivatives of POMC. α-MSH is found in many brain areas, with the highest levels in the hypothalamus and pineal gland: lower concentrations are found in the thalamus, brainstem, cerebrum, and cortex. Most hypothalamic α-MSH is in neurons of the arcuate nucleus, and nerve fibers from their perikarya project through the hypothalamus, thalamus and midbrain, amygdala, and telencephalon (for more details, see Eberle, 1988). Dopaminergic neurons that project to the intermediate lobe have their cell bodies in the anterior part of the arcuate nucleus and form an important inhibitory route for the control of the secretory activity of the intermediate lobe.

In animals such as amphibians and anurans, in which MSH is an important regulator of skin color change, the number and size of the secretory granules in the skin melanocytes vary according to adaptation to a light or dark background. MSH is also present in mammalian skin, including human skin, and human melanocytes express MSH receptors, but how MSH contributes to the regulation of skin pigmentation in humans is unknown (Thody et al., 1993). α-MSH is also present in immune cells (Smith et al., 1992) and may play a role in inflammatory reactions of the skin (Luger et al., 1997).

Extrapituitary sources of the POMC-derived neuropeptides include many hypothalamic nuclei, the pituitary stalk, and the median eminence (O'Donohue and Dorsa, 1982; Kiss et al., 1985) with lesser amounts in the amygdala, mesencephalon, and septum. α-MSH is also found in the meninges, choroid plexus, and ependyma following injection of ^{125}I-labeled MSH into the carotid artery. Immunoreactive α-MSH is present in the spinal motor neurons of immature but not adult mice (Haynes and Smith, 1985).

12.2.4 *Gene Expression, Regulation, and Processing of POMC*

POMC-expressing cells in the pituitary form a model neuroendocrine system of multihormonal interactions. The organization of the POMC gene, its regulation by CRH, and the gonadal steroids, and its processing were introduced in chapter 3, section 3.3.2 and 3.3.3. More detailed information is appropriate here.

12.2.4.1 The POMC Gene

In the pituitary, the product of transcription of the POMC gene is a 6.5 polyadenylated RNA containing three exons and two introns (see figure 3.11). When the introns are removed, the mature pituitary mRNA is 1200 bases long and the nucleic acid sequences which code for the POMC prohormone are within the second and third exons of the mRNA. The POMC 5′ flank contains multiple copies of at least three types of regulatory elements.

POMC gene expression varies in different types of tissues, and different species, both in the size of the mRNA and in its regulation. CRH is the only physiological ACTH-releasing factor known to increase POMC gene expression in the corticotrophs. CRH stimulation of POMC gene expression depends mainly on cAMP, but Ca^{2+} is also involved. The POMC gene in spinal motor neurons is upregulated following injury to the motor neurons; unilateral sciatic nerve section increases POMC mRNA in both the ipsilateral and contralateral ventral horns (Hughes and Smith, 1994).

12.2.4.2 Tissue-Specific Processing of POMC

The reader is referred to chapter 3 in which POMC was used as an example of neuropeptide processing, including tissue-specific processing, which was discussed there in some detail.

The POMC prohormone gives rise to a variety of neuropeptides, the type depending upon the degree to which the prohormone is processed, which in turn is dependent upon the specific enzymes present in that tissue. In the anterior lobe, POMC is processed by corticotrophs mainly to ACTH 1–39, β-lipotropin, and β-endorphin. In the intermediate lobe, POMC is processed further by melanotrophs to smaller peptides such as α-MSH, β-MSH, γ-lipotropin, CLIP, and β-endorphin (see figure 3.9). In addition to producing ACTH 1–39, the most powerful endogenous stimulus to adrenocortical secretion, several forms of MSH can be generated: α-MSH and β-MSH, both MSHs which do *not* stimulate the adrenal cortex; γ-MSH, which *can* stimulate the adrenal cortex to secrete corticoids but which has little melanotropic activity; CLIP, which may have insulinotropic properties and some activity on slow wave sleep; β-lipotropin and γ-lipotropin, which have lipolytic actions; and β-endorphin (β-lipotropin 61–91), the potent opiate neuropeptide. As humans lack an intermediate lobe, there is very little α-MSH in human blood. Nor does much β-lipotropin get processed into β-MSH; consequently β-lipotropin and ACTH are the predominant melanocortins in humans, whereas α-MSH is predominant in most other species.

Further processing by several enzymes results in glycosylation, phosphorylation, and the formation of amidated and acetylated biologically active neuropeptides. Completion of intermediate lobe peptides involves N-terminal acetylation of α-MSH, β-endorphin, and related peptides. N-terminal acetylation increases the melanotropic activity of α-MSH more than 10 times, reduces the corticotropic activity of ACTH approximately 10 times, and completely destroys the opiate activity of β-endorphin (Smyth et al., 1979). Since β-endorphin is released concomitantly with α-MSH, acetylation of the neuropeptides may be an important way to regulate their biological activity (O'Donohue and Dorsa, 1982).

β-LPH is processed in the pituitary gland to a 31–amino acid peptide β-endorphin (β-lipotropin 61–91) and several other related peptides that are formed by special proteolysis in the C-terminal region of its peptide chain. The main shortened forms are β-endorphin 1–27, and small amounts of α-endorphin (β-endorphin 1–16), and γ-endorphin (β-endorphin 1–17), as shown in table 12.1. β-Endorphin is the most potent analgesic: on a molar basis its potency is from 50 to 100 times greater than that of morphine. The analgesic action of β-endorphin is reversed by naloxone, an opiate antagonist, indicating that its actions are mediated at opiate receptors. N-acetylation removes all analgesic activity from β-endorphin.

The degree of proteolysis of β-lipotropin varies considerably in the anterior and intermediate lobes. In the latter, extensive proteolysis produces at least six β-endorphin–related peptides, only one of which shows high opiate activity: in the anterior lobe the predominant form is the amidated β-endorphin 1–31 form.

12.2.5 Regulation of POMC-Derived Neuropeptides

In what ratio are the POMC peptides secreted by the corticotrophs and melanotrophs? In general, the relative proportions in which the neuropeptides are secreted are the same as those in which they are present in the cell. This, in turn, reflects the differential tissue processing of POMC, which results in a greater concentration of MSH peptides in the melanotrophs of the intermediate lobe than in the corticotrophs of the anterior lobe. As the various POMC-derived peptides are stored together in secretory granules, they are consequently released together. However, this does not seem to hold true for the ratio of β-endorphin and ACTH peptides released from the anterior lobe. This may vary between 1 and 3, depending on the stress stimulus.

12.2.5.1 Regulation of Corticotroph Secretion

a. Corticotropin-releasing hormone

CRH is the primary positive regulator of ACTH secretion by the anterior pituitary. Regulation of secretion is distinct from regulation of transcription since both the neuropeptides CRH and VP, as well as KCl depolarization, increase ACTH secretion, but only CRH increases POMC transcription in anterior pituitary corticotrophs, a cAMP- and protein kinase–dependent mechanism. Much of our information on the synthesis and processing of POMC comes from ACTH-producing tumor cell lines, such as the AtT-20 cells. Peptide secretion from these cells is stimulated by CRH and inhibited by glucocorticoids. However, care must be taken when interpreting these results since the control of the tumor cells may differ fundamentally from that of normal pituitary cells. In the intact organism, the circadian rhythm in basal ACTH secretion is driven by the SCN activating the CRH-secreting neurons in the PVN.

b. Other neuropeptides and neurotransmitters

Whereas CRH is the most important physiological stimulus to POMC-derived peptide secretion, many other peptides and transmitters may act *synergistically* with CRH. These include VP, AT II, VIP, peptide histidine isoleucine (PHI), GHRH, NE, and epinephrine, all of which increase intracellular cAMP levels and consequently ACTH and MSH secretion (Levin and Roberts, 1991). Corticotrophs have been shown to have specific receptors for CRH, VP, AT II, and catecholamines, and receptors for PHI and GHRH probably also exist.

The role of VP as a stimulus to ACTH release was discussed in chapter 11, the consensus being that VP is a potent amplifier of CRH action but is relatively weak as an independent stimulus. However, experiments using an antiserum to VP show a marked attenuation of the stress-induced ACTH release, implying a more robust role for VP in stress-induced ACTH secretion (Tilders et al., 1985). The other secretogogues have additive or potentiating powers. The ACTH-releasing activity of AT II is to potentiate the action of CRH on ACTH release. The action of the other peptides also appears to be additive to that of CRH. The stimulating activity of epinephrine is probably indirect, through the release of CRH from the hypothalamus. Serotonergic neurons synapse on CRH neurons in the PVN and activate 5-HT_{2A} and 5-HT_{2C} receptors to increase ACTH secretion (Rittenhouse et al., 1994). Figure 12.5 illustrates some of

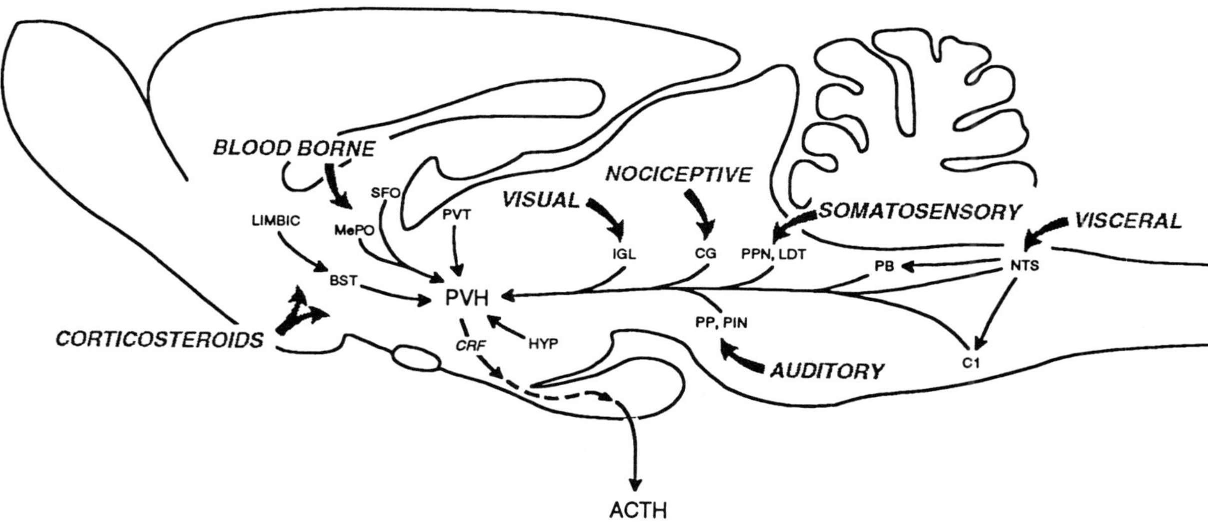

Figure 12.5
Suggested afferent routes for neural and hormonal modification of ACTH secretion. Schematic drawing of a midsagittal section through the rat brain showing the major afferent pathways that may influence corticotropin-releasing hormone (CRH) secretion in the paraventricular nucleus (PVN), and consequently ACTH secretion. Also shown are the types of information that these pathways may convey. BST, bed nucleus of the stria terminalis; C1, C1 adrenergic cell group; CG, central gray; HYP, hypothalamus; IGL, intergeniculate leaflet; LIMBIC, limbic system; LDT, laterodorsal tegmental nucleus; MePO, median preoptic nucleus; NTS nucleus of the solitary tract; PB, parabranchial nucleus; PIN, posterior intralaminar nucleus; PP, peripeduncuar nucleus; PPN, pedunculopontine nucleus; PVT, paraventricular nucleus of the thalamus; SFO, subfornical organ. (From Sawchenko et al., 1993.)

the many positive neural and endocrine influences on ACTH secretion, all acting through the PVN and CRH secretion.

c. *Inhibition of POMC secretion*

POMC secretion is inhibited mainly through a long-loop glucocorticoid negative feedback action on the hypothalamic secretion of CRH (see chapter 10, section 10.1.2.4), rather than on the corticotrophs directly. Both the secretion and release of ACTH are blocked by adrenal glucocorticoids. This feedback by corticosterone is through association with a high-affinity, type I corticosterone receptor. As these receptors are concentrated in the hippocampus and lateral septum, it is likely that interneurons are involved in transmitting the signal to the PVN. In vivo, dexamethasone, a synthetic glucocorticoid, is less effective than corticosterone in the inhibition of ACTH, and aldosterone, an adrenal mineralocorticoid, is even less active. The hypothalamic neuropeptide somatostatin is a potent inhibitor of ACTH release from AtT-20 cells but whether this is a physiological role for somatostatin is uncertain.

12.2.5.2 Regulation of Melanotroph Secretion

a. *Release of MSH*

α-MSH occurs in different molecular forms in the intermediate lobe, the most prevalent of which is the *N*, *O*-diacetyl form. In contrast, in the anterior lobe the nonacetylated α-MSH molecule is the predominant form. CRH appears to be the neuropeptide that stimulates the secretory activity of intermediate lobe cells, but its affinity and intrinsic activity are much lower than on the corticotrophs. Interestingly, the physiological control of corticotrophs and melanotrophs differs under stressful conditions. For the corticotrophs, CRH remains the main factor mediating ACTH release during stress. In contrast, epinephrine, possibly derived from the adrenal medulla, appears to be the stimulus to the release of α-MSH and β-endorphin from the melanotrophs but not from the corticotrophs of the anterior pituitary (Berkenbosch et al., 1983).

b. *Inhibition of MSH release*

Dopamine is the most important *inhibiting influence* on the secretion of MSH from the melanotrophs, acting through D_2 receptors coupled to adenylate cyclase. Lesions of the arcuate nucleus destroy the pathway of the DA fibers to the intermediate lobe and cause a rapid rise in circulating α-MSH and β-endorphin. Similarly, treatment with DA agonists, such as bromocriptine or apomorphine, inhibits the secretion of POMC-derived peptides via D_2 receptor stimulation. GABA and NPY also inhibit α-MSH release. The inhibitory action on MSH secretion of the putative MSH release inhibiting factor (MIF), a tail fragment of OT (Pro-Leu-Gly-NH_2), has not been convincingly demonstrated.

c. *Synthesis and release of α-MSH in amphibians*

Regulation of MSH synthesis and release in amphibians is an exceedingly complex procedure, for these lower vertebrates alter the color of their skin by changing the distribution of melanin and other pigments in the chromatophores of the integument. α-MSH is directly involved in the rapid change from concentration to dispersal of melanin granules. The multiple factors that regulate the synthesis and release of α-MSH from the melanotroph cells in the intermediate lobe include light, and the neuropeptides CRH, TRH, and *melanostatin*, a 36-amino acid peptide that is the amphibian counterpart of NPY (Valentijn et al., 1994). Other factors involved include melanin-concentrating hormone (MCH, see below), as well as the transmitters DA, GABA, and ACh. The changes in α-MSH secretion closely parallel changes in POMC mRNA and POMC synthesis (Loh et al., 1988). Similar to mammalian regulation, amphibian α-MSH release is inhibited by DA. The multihormonal control of MSH secretion in submammalian vertebrates is reviewed by Tonon et al. (1988).

d. Melanin-concentrating hormone

This neuropeptide, not POMC derived, has antagonistic effects to MSH. MCH is found in both the hypothalamus and pituitary of teleost fish, and in the lateral hypothalamus and sub–zona incerta areas but not in the pituitary of the mammalian brain. In rodents, the extrahypothalamic distribution of MCH fibers throughout the brain is extensive, with projections to the cerebral cortex, inferior colliculus, midbrain tegmentum, and the spinal cord (Knigge et al., 1996).

Salmonid MCH is a cyclic 19–amino acid peptide with one sulfide bridge and its amino acid sequence is

H-Asp-Thr-Met-Arg-Cys^5-Met-Val-Gly-Arg-
Val^{10}-Tyr-Arg-Pro-Cys-Trp^{15}-Glu-Val-OH

Mouse, rat, and human MCH are identical, and they differ from salmonid MCH by only a 2–amino acid N-terminal extension, and 4–amino acid substitutions, 1 within the Cys-Cys ring

In fish, MCH can rapidly reverse the melanin dispersal action of MSH and several analogs have been synthesized to determine the possible structural basis for its opposing action (Hadley et al., 1987). Although the physiological action of MCH in mammals is uncertain (Kawauchi, 1988), MCH and other neuropeptides derived from the same precursor may participate in multiple functions in the mammalian CNS, modulating behavior and the perception of sensory function (Baker, 1994) and influencing learning and memory, in directions opposite to that of MSH (McBride et al., 1994).

Some suggested functions of MCH derive from the areas of the mammalian brain in which MCH is most concentrated (lateral hypothalamus and zona incerta). This topography may permit extrapyramidal motor circuits to integrate appropriate motor behavior with hypothalamic visceral activity (Knigge et al., 1996). Similarly, these MCH-rich areas are regions involved in the regulation of feeding and MCH may have a role in the control of food intake (see chapter 16, section 4.2.4).

12.2.6 Structure-Activity Studies of the Melanocortins

As discussed in earlier chapters, ACTH 1–39 and its shorter peptide fragments, including α-MSH, are known as the *melanocortins*. Immunocytochemical studies localize ACTH 1–39 and ACTH 11–24 in the hypothalamus, thalamus, amygdala, and periaqueductal gray. The neurotrophic fragment ACTH 4–10 has a far more restricted distribution, being limited to processes in the septal area and the perimeter of the third ventricle, including the ME. ACTH 4–10 is also present in the ventral horn of the spinal cord (S. J. Lee et al., 1994).

12.2.6.1 Functional Tests

The relative effectiveness of these neuropeptides depends on the specific function for which they are being tested. In tests on skin darkening in amphibians or anurans, α-MSH is 10 to 100 times more potent than ACTH and 2 to 10 times more potent than β-MSH, depending on the species tested (Eberle, 1988). When the behavioral effects of ACTH and MSH compounds are compared, ACTH appears to be the most effective of the melanocortins inasmuch as 1 μg of ACTH 1–24, injected icv, can cause the rat to groom for more than 55 minutes of the hour following the injection

(Dunn, 1988). In tests based on the neurotrophic attributes of the melanocortins, α-MSH is the most potent (see section 12.2.9.3). However, if the assay is for stimulation of the adrenal cortex, only ACTH has corticotropic qualities, although β-lipotropin has weakly corticotropic properties in very high dosages.

12.2.6.2 The Specificity of the Message

Whereas ACTH 1–39 is the naturally occurring neuropeptide processed from POMC, ACTH 1–24 has the full biological activity of the 39–amino acid molecule, possessing both corticotropic and neurotrophic characteristics. The sequence ACTH 25–39 apparently conveys improved binding qualities of the ligand to its receptor. Stepwise shortening of ACTH 1–24 from the C-terminal to ACTH 1–13 (α-MSH) eliminates most of the in vivo corticotropic qualities (Greven and de Wied, 1973), thus permitting the investigation of the neurotrophic properties of the neuropeptide fragments without the complications of any evoked adrenal corticoids.

The message within the various short melanocortin fragments differs according to what is being measured. In behavioral tests the trisubstituted ACTH 4–9 analog Org 2766, which has lost almost all endocrine effects, is very active on avoidance behavior (see section 12.2.9.4), increasing passive avoidance by a factor of 1000 compared to ACTH 4–10. As is seen with many neuropeptides, tested on many different parameters, such as development, regeneration or behavior, low dosages (50 to 200 ng SC) facilitate, whereas high dosages (500 and 1000 ng SC) inhibit. Of particular interest is that substitution of the D-Phe^7 isomer of ACTH 4–10 has opposite effects on behavior to the L-isomer, but loses all activity when tested on electrophysiological parameters improved by the D-form of the peptide. Specific amino acid residues within the ACTH fragments and analogs display selectivity for different melanocortin receptors, a discrimination that can be correlated with their differential effects on discrete behavioral responses (Adan et al., 1994).

In studies on peripheral nerve regeneration, a detailed structure-activity investigation by Bijlsma et al. (1981) showed α-MSH to be more effective than Org 2766, which is more active than ACTH 4–10, the smallest fragment with neurotrophic properties. The ACTH 4–10 analog BIM 22015 has weaker neurotrophic properties but possesses myotrophic characteristics (Strand et al., 1993b). A more recent structure-activity study shows that α-MSH, desacetyl-α-MSH, and Org 2766 are equally effective when tested in the foot-withdrawal reflex, whereas ACTH 7–16 is without effect and ACTH 11–13 inhibits this response (Van der Zee et al., 1991). Figure 12.6 shows the amino acid sequences of the most biologically active ACTH peptides.

12.2.7 ACTH and MSH Receptors and Second Messengers

12.2.7.1 Localization of Binding Sites

Localization in the brain and spinal cord has become more specific and quantitative with the development of a radiolabeled MSH tracer [^{125}I]N- Leu^4, D-Phe^7-α-MSH (*NDP-MSH). Binding intensity is highest in the septal area, septohypothalamic nucleus, the bed nucleus of the stria terminalis, and the medial preoptic area. Moderate binding is seen in hypothalamic structures, including the median eminence, and the ventromedial, dorsomedial, arcuate, and paraventricular nuclei. All these binding sites recognize ACTH, α-MSH, and *NDP-MSH (Tatro, 1990). The presence of melanocortin receptors (MCRs) in the ME, a circumventricular organ lacking a BBB, may indicate a

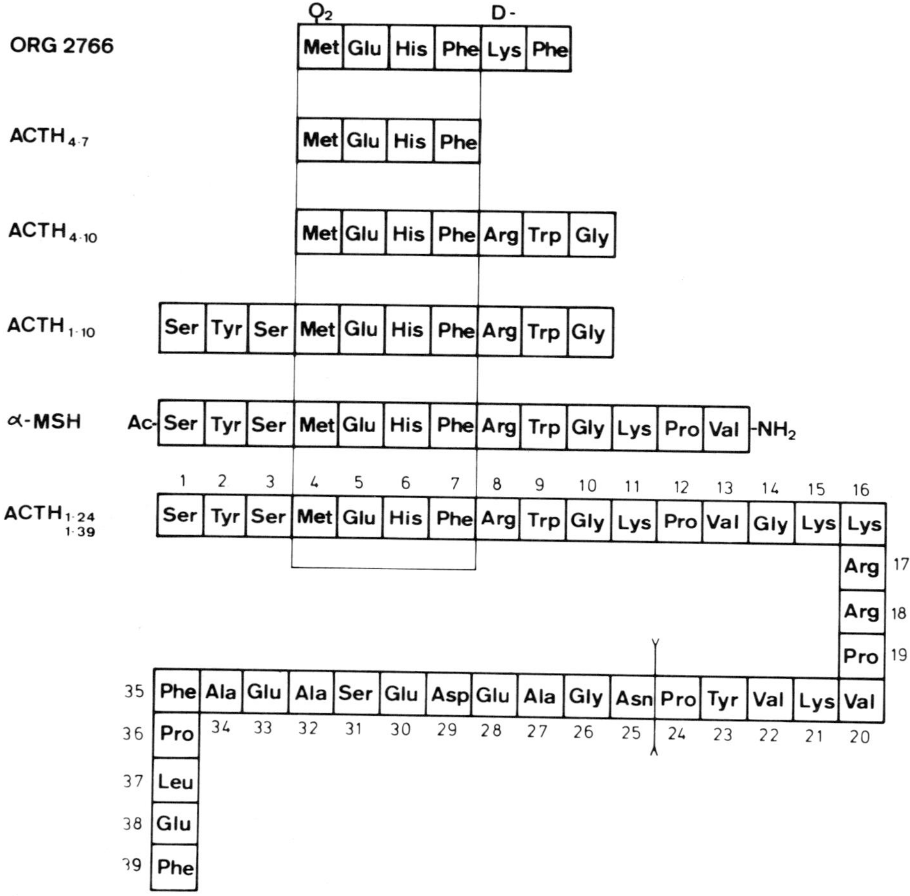

Figure 12.6
Primary structure of some of the adrenocorticotropic (ACTH)- and melanocyte-stimulating hormone (MSH)–related peptides discussed in the text. (From Flohr and Lüneborg, 1989.)

route which peripherally administered melanocortins use to exert their demonstrable effects on the CNS (Banks and Kastin, 1988).

Binding sites for the shorter melanocortin sequences, such as ACTH 4–10 and the potent neurotrophic ACTH 4–9 analog Org 2766, have been localized to limited regions of the septum and preoptic areas, hypothalamus, and hippocampus (Rees et al., 1980). Although there is no direct evidence to date that ACTH is processed physiologically to ACTH 4–10, highly specific immunoreactivity to ACTH 4–10 has been demonstrated in the rat brain during development, and in the spinal cord following peripheral nerve crush (Lee et al., 1994). This binding is not seen in normal adults, confirming the experimental observations that the melanocortins function in specific "time windows"—during development, in the presence of metabolically deranged systems such as diabetes, muscular dystrophy, neuropathy, and nerve regeneration—but are inactive or superfluous during normal adult nerve maintenance (Strand et al., 1989). There is an interesting pattern of regional and time-specific appearance of MCRs in the CNS in early postnatal life (Lichtensteiger et al., 1996), supporting the concept of "time windows" of effectiveness in different tissues during development.

12.2.7.2 Identification of Melanocortin Receptors

As the varied potencies of the melanocortins indicate, they must act through different receptor types. An exciting new development is the cloning, pharmacological distinction, and localization of five types of MCRs. These MCRs form a unique subfamily of G protein–coupled receptors, which are highly homologous to each other and activate cAMP. Some of their novel features are their very small size (297 to 360 amino acids), and the absence of several amino acid residues present in most G protein–coupled receptors, which may account for a tertiary structure that differs from most of the other G protein–coupled receptors (Cone et al., 1993) (figure 12.7). Surprisingly, MCRs appear to be more closely related to the cannabinoid receptor than to other neuropeptide receptors.

It has long been recognized that ACTH and ACTH fragments have effects on behavior independent of their adrenocortical stimulating activity—in fact, the ACTH fragments, including MSH, do not stimulate the adrenal cortex. These remarkable differences can now be explained on the basis of the differential distribution and affinity of MCRs.

Five MCRs have been cloned so far: MC1-R, MC2-R, MC3-R, MC4-R, and MC5-R (Chhajlani et al., 1993; Gantz et al., 1993; 1994; Mountjoy et al., 1992; Mountjoy et al., 1994; Roselli-Rehfuss et al., 1993). The structure of the MCRs is described concisely in a review by Adan and Gispen (1997). *MC1-R*, the MSH receptor, is specifically expressed in *melanocytes* and *melanoma cells*, and to a limited extent in testis and CNS. *MC2-R* is an ACTH receptor and localized in the *adrenal cortex*. The adrenal receptor is selectively activated by ACTH, which activates all MCRs, whereas the other MCRs recognize various forms of MSH with different degrees of ligand selectivity. MC1-R and MC2-R are generally absent in brain.

MC3-R, MC4-R, and MC5-R are the three *neural receptors*. The existence of multiple, pharmacologically distinct classes of MCRs in *brain* can be demonstrated using the highly potent, synthetic radiolabeled α-MSH analog, Nle^4,D-Phe^7-α-MSH (Tatro and Entwistle 1993; Adan et al., 1994). *MC3-R* is predominantly expressed in the limbic system and in regions of the hypothalamus and is activated almost equally by ACTH 1–39, α-MSH, γ_1, γ_2, and γ_3, MSH, and by β-MSH. Although MC3-Rs are potently activated

MSH RECEPTOR

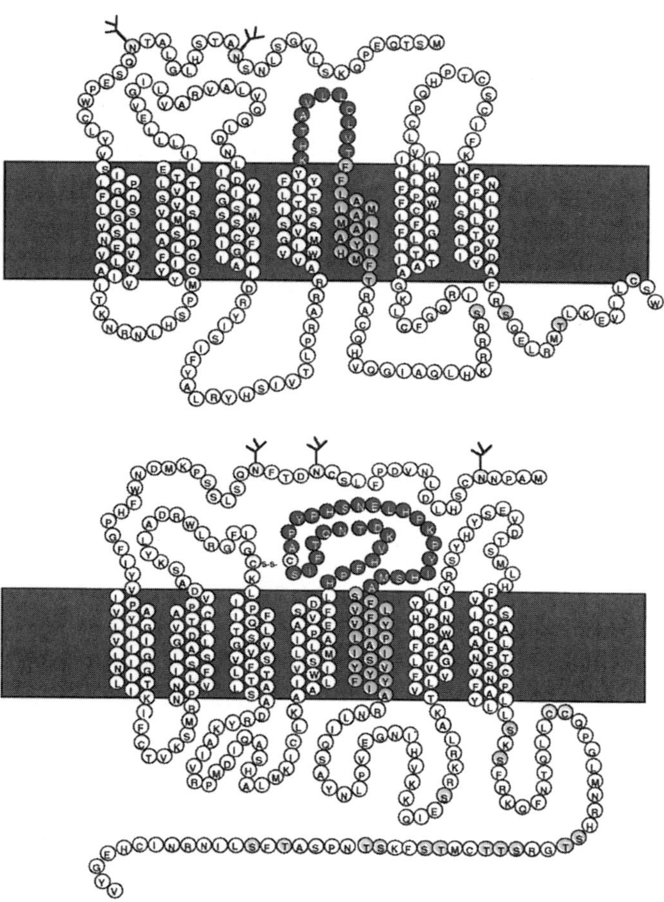

BOMBESIN RECEPTOR

Figure 12.7
Predicted structure of the human melanocyte-stimulating hormone (MSH) receptor and, for comparison, the bombesin receptor. Putative glycosylation sites are indicated with a branched structure, and putative phosphorylation sites are shaded. The small second extracellular loop and the small fifth transmembrane domains are also shaded for comparison with the bombesin receptor. The conserved cysteines and putative disulfide bond formed between the first and second extracellular loops are indicated in the bombesin receptor, but are absent in the MSH receptor. (From Cone et al., 1993.)

by γ-MSH peptides, these peptides do not affect MSH (MC1-R) or ACTH (MC2-R) receptors. γ-MSH lacks melanotropic activity and has been reported to induce opiate-like withdrawal symptoms (Van Ree et al., 1981) but its physiological function is not known (Roselli-Rehfuss et al., 1993). The MC3-R has a tenfold higher affinity for the ACTH peptides than the MC4-R (Schioth et al., 1997a).

The *MC4-R* is widely expressed and is found in practically every brain region, including the cortex, hypothalamus, brainstem, and spinal cord. MC4-R mRNA is found extensively in the PVN, suggesting a role in the central control of pituitary function (Mountjoy et al., 1994), perhaps through a negative feedback mechanism utilizing MSH. MC4-R is activated equally by ACTH 1–39 and α-MSH. ACTH 4–10 is a poor activator of both MC3 and MC4 receptors but does activate them when present in concentrations greater than 10^{-7} M, especially in those areas associated with the behavioral effects of the melanocortins (Gantz et al., 1993; Mountjoy et al., 1994).

The *MC5-R* is expressed in brain as well as in many peripheral tissues, including skin, adrenal gland, adipose tissue, skeletal muscle, and lymphoid tissue (Barrett et al., 1994; Chhajlani et al., 1993; Gantz et al, 1994; Griffon et al., 1994). Immunoreactive binding sites for ACTH and β-endorphin are present in skeletal muscle fibers of developing and diseased mice (Smith and Hughes, 1994), but these receptors have not as yet been identified or cloned. Their existence, however, helps to explain the effectiveness of melanocortins in peripheral nerve development and regeneration (see section 12.2.9.3). The expression of MC5-R in lymphoid organs could explain the anti-inflammatory action of the melanocortins. These data are summarized in table 12.2. MC5-R binds α-MSH, ACTH, β-MSH, the γ-MSHs and ACTH 4–10, β-endorphin, and CLIP (Labbe et al., 1994). Tatro and Entwistle (1994) point out that the existence of multiple, pharmacologically distinct classes of melanocortin receptors in the brain should provide a basis for the pharmacological targeting of central melanocortin receptors, with subsequent clinical implications.

Schwann cells (Dyer et al., 1993a) and skeletal muscle cells (M. E. Smith and Hughes, 1993) have receptors for α-MSH which may account for the neuroregenerative effects of α-MSH on peripheral nerve and denervated muscle (see section 12.2.9.3). No specific receptor has been found so far that responds to Org 2766, which has powerful effects on behavioral and regenerative processes. Dyer et al. (1993b) suggest that Org 2766 may act indirectly on NGF receptors on Schwann cells to evoke the release of neurotrophic factors that aid peripheral nerve regeneration. Similarly, there do not seem to be MCRs in dopaminergic systems in the brain, despite considerable evidence for melanocortins acting on DA systems (Antonawich et al., 1993, 1994; Wolterink et al., 1990). It is likely that there are still more MCRs to be identified.

12.2.7.3 Second Messengers

The second messenger system for the MCRs is primarily through adenylate cyclase and the resultant production of cAMP in a dose-dependent manner. Figure 12.8 shows the increase in cAMP in dorsal root ganglion cells elicited by increased concentrations of either α-MSH or Org 2766. Figure 12.8 also demonstrates the rather consistent effect seen with the administration of most neuropeptides—an inverted U-shaped curve as concentrations increase beyond an optimum. Melanocortin activity is dependent on extracellular Ca^{2+} and the MCRs appear to be a unique calcium-requiring receptor family (Salomon, 1990).

Table 12.2
Melanocortin receptors (MC-R) and their putative effects

Receptor Type	Main Tissue	Effect
MC1-R (MSH-R)	Melanocytes	Melanin dispersal
	Melanoma cells	
MC2-R (ACTH-R)	Adrenal cortex	Glucocorticoid secretion
MC3-R	Limbic system, arcuate nucleus	Behavior, neuroendocrine effects?
MC4-R	Cortex	Central control of pituitary?
	Periaqueductal gray	Grooming
	Hypothalamus	Autonomic effects
	Brain stem	
	Spinal cord	
MC5-R	Skin	Paracrine effects?
	Adrenals	
	Skeletal muscle	Neuromuscular function?
	Lymphoid organs	Anti-inflammatory actions?
	Gonads, uterus	Reproductive functions?
	Brain	

MSH, melanocyte-stimulating hormone; ACTH, adrenocorticotropic hormone.

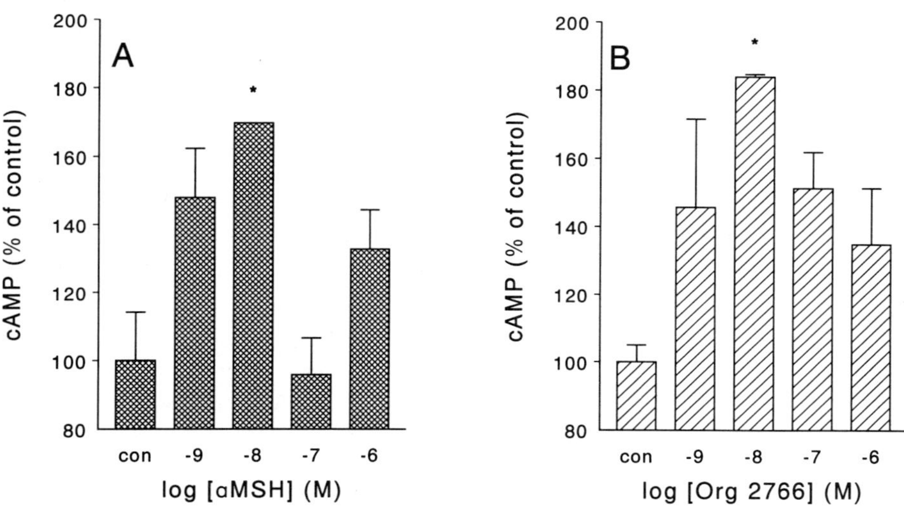

Figure 12.8
Effect of increasing concentrations of (A) α-melanocyte–stimulating hormone (α-MSH) or (B) Org 2766 (ACTH 4–9 analog) on cAMP production in dorsal root ganglia. Values are depicted as mean ±SEM of one representative experiment. $^*P < .05$. (From Hol et al., 1994.)

ACTH may also activate the phosphatidylinositol system through an involvement of the phosphoprotein B-50 (Gispen et al., 1983). A detailed discussion of signal transduction systems linked to the melanocortins is in Hol et al. (1994).

12.2.8 ACTH and MSH as Neurotransmitters and Neuromodulators

ACTH and its peptide fragments may be involved in *central neurotransmission*. Early studies by Torda and Wolff (1952) indicated that ACh synthesis is increased by ACTH and diminished by hypophysectomy. ACTH 1–39 stimulates the uptake of ^{14}C-choline by *brain* synaptosomes in vitro and also accelerates choline release, a Ca^{2+}-dependent process. Stimulation of choline uptake by ACTH 1–39 appears to be region-specific (figure 12.9), being apparent in synaptosomes from the hippocampus, parietal cortex, medulla-pons, olfactory tracts, and hypothalamus. Choline uptake is inhibited by ACTH in the anterior thalamus and cerebellum. Brain ACh metabolism is also enhanced by the ACTH 4–9 analog Ebiratide (Hoe 427), which differs from Org 2766 in that it has an additional octylamide side chain at the C-terminus, improving its resistance to enzymatic degradation (Wiemer et al., 1988). Figure 12.9 shows that ACTH-stimulated choline uptake is also augmented by the addition of epinephrine to the incubation medium.

ACTH or MSH peptides also interact with monoaminergic transmitter systems of the brain, influencing the activity of the regulatory enzymes, and thus neurotransmitter synthesis, release, and turnover. This topic is extensively reviewed by De Graan et al. (1990).

In the spinal cord, α-MSH acts directly as a neurotransmitter (Krivoy and Guillemin, 1961), and depolarization causes release of α-MSH from synaptosomes

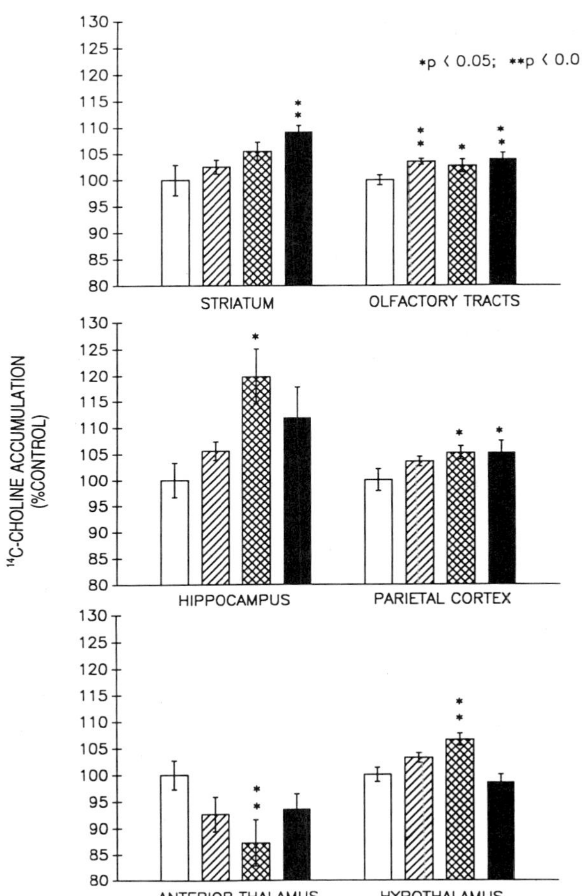

Figure 12.9
Effects of ACTH 1–39 and α-methyl-norepinephrine on ^{14}C-choline accumulation by synaptosomes from different brain areas. Open bars represent control; diagonal stripe, ACTH 0.1 μg/mL; cross-hatched, ACTH 1.0 μg/mL; black bars represent α-methyl-norepinephrine (10^{-6}M). $^{*}P < .05$; $^{**}P < .01$. (From Veals, 1979.)

and from hypothalamic slices, a Ca^{2+}-dependent process characteristic of neurotransmitters. Other evidence for MSH as a potential neurotransmitter is its ability to stimulate secretion by the lacrimal gland, which is also stimulated by epinephrine and ACh (Leiba et al., 1990). Binding of *NDP-MSH to lacrimal gland slices is dependent on Ca^{2+}, but establishment of MSH as a transmitter in the lacrimal gland awaits evidence that MSH is released from nerves innervating this structure. In general, however, the melanocortins are more likely to be neuromodulators, lending firm support to a concept of an integrated function of neuropeptides and neurotransmitters.

12.2.9 Functions of ACTH and MSH

12.2.9.1 Corticotropic Actions of ACTH

ACTH 1–39 and ACTH 1–24 possess full corticotropic and neurotrophic activity, but the corticotropic activity resides in the sequence ACTH 11–24. ACTH stimulation of MC2-Rs in the adrenal cortex, especially in the zona fasciculata, result in the secretion of the glucocorticoids cortisol and corticosterone.

12.2.9.2 Pigmentary Actions of MSH

The MSH neuropeptides bind with varying degrees of effectiveness to the MC1-Rs found mainly on melanocytes and melanoma cells, to affect the distribution of melanin. The importance of this action is mainly protective color change in lower vertebrates. In higher vertebrates, MSH has taken on a wide variety of other functions, some of which are described below.

12.2.9.3 Melanocortins as Neurotrophic Factors

The first demonstrated neurotrophic activity of fragments such as ACTH 1–10, ACTH 4–10, and ACTH 4–7 were changes in the CNS that involve behavior, attention, and learning (see review by De Wied and Jolles, 1982). A peripheral neurotrophic effect of the melanocortins was initially shown by Strand and Kung (1980) who demonstrated that ACTH could affect peripheral nerve regeneration. Considerable additional evidence for the neurotrophic activity is outlined below

a. CNS effects of ACTH and MSH during development

POMC and its derived melanocortin peptides are present within the fetal rat CNS as early as gestation day 12, suggesting an organizational role for these neuropeptides, which may be indirectly exerted through the evocation of corticosteroids. However, administration of the smaller melanocortins, which do not target the adrenal cortex, also have lasting effects. Endogenous MSH has a major role in early development: it is present in the fetal brain early in gestation and, in the rat, increases until the day of birth (Thody et al., 1979). It has an important physiological role at this time, stimulating fetal growth and brain development and acting as a signal for the initiation of parturition (Swaab et al., 1977). In the human fetus, which produces α-MSH, the fetal adrenal cortex is responsive to α-MSH and not to ACTH; consequently α-MSH may act as a signal for adrenocorticoid production during gestation (Kastin et al., 1968).

Learning and social behaviors α-MSH or Org 2766 administered to neonatal rats increases social interaction and improves the learning of a difficult task in young adulthood (Beckwith et al., 1977; Champney et al., 1976). Interestingly, these effects are sex-dependent, as improvement in learning is seen only in males, while the social behavior changes are especially evident in adult female rats treated neonatally with

MSH. This sexually dimorphic sensitivity to neonatal MSH exposure is probably due to a difference in neurocircuitry organized by the gonadal steroids during the initial period of the sexual differentiation of the brain.

Acceleration of maturation Additional evidence for a role for melanocortins in development is shown by the acccelerated eye opening of infant rats treated perinatally with α-MSH, an indication of maturation of neuronal circuitries (Van der Helm-Hylkema and de Wied 1976; Segarra et al. 1991). Similarly, neonatal ACTH 4–10 or Org 2766 administration accelerates the maturation of the developing neuromuscular system (figure 12.10A and B), an effect involving central as well as peripheral motor systems. These changes are morphological, electrophysiological, and functional (Frischer and Strand, 1988; Rose and Strand, 1988; Saint-Come et al., 1982). Figure 12.11 shows the increased complexity of the neuromuscular junction of neonatal muscle following treatment with ACTH 4–10.

Effects on brain monoamines Whereas a direct response to ACTH and MSH peptides can be seen in developing 5-HT neurons in culture (Azmitia and de Kloet, 1987), in the intact organism the 5-HT and catecholamine systems are greatly influenced by corticosteroids released via ACTH action on the adrenal cortex. Since the monoamines act as important regulatory signals for their own development, as well as for the maturation of many other neural systems (Lauder, 1990; Whitaker-Azmitia, 1991), increases in their concentrations during this sensitive period could alter the growth and maturation of numerous central circuitries. Thus, exposure to increased ACTH during development could result in widespread pertubations in the adult brain, influenced by the combined actions of the peptide, the corticosteroids, and the monoamines. The lasting effects of neonatal ACTH and MSH peptide exposure strongly suggest an organizational role for these peptides on the neurocircuitry regulating many behaviors, including the sexual, as discussed below.

Sexual behavior Sexual behavior in adults is markedly affected by perinatal administration of ACTH. Serotonergic neuronal pathways that subserve motor behaviors, such as female and male sexual reflexes, are affected by the melanocortins, which appear to act as trophic factors during development, increasing 5-HT neurite outgrowth and fiber density. Prenatal exposure to ACTH 1–24 results in distinct changes in 5-HT (see figure 9.5) and DA innervation of the brain, changes that persist in the medial preoptic area in adulthood (Alves et al., 1993; Segarra et al., 1991). These anatomical changes are accompanied by severe depression of sexual activity in males (figure 12.12), and to a lesser extent, in females (Alves et al., 1993).

b. Regenerative and neuroprotective effects of melanocortins

Peripheral effects Strand and Kung (1980) were the first to show that ACTH promotes the regeneration of crushed sciatic nerve, assessed by an accelerated return of sensory and motor function in adrenalectomized rats. That this is truly a peptidergic function was made clear when the noncorticotropic melanocortins and their analogs were shown to be as effective as the large molecule in improving peripheral nerve regeneration and neuromuscular performance (Bijlsma et al., 1981; Dekker et al., 1987; Saint-Come and Strand, 1985, 1988; Verhaagen et al., 1987a). Early axonal sprouting, formation of a greater number

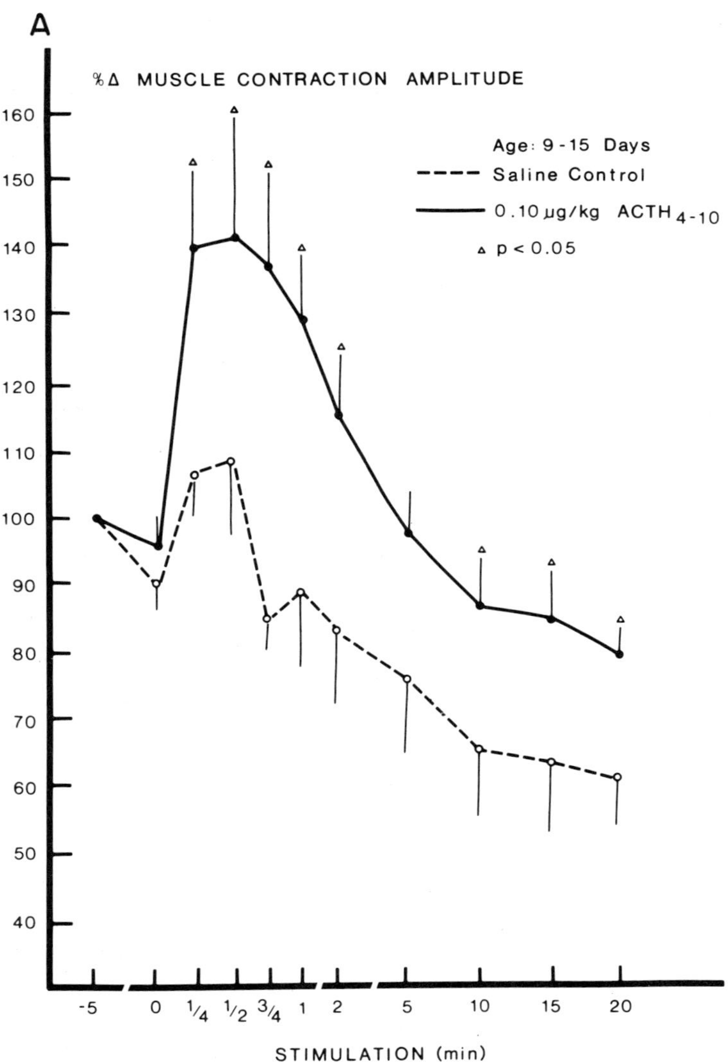

Figure 12.10
Time-sensitive effects of ACTH 4–10 during neuromuscular development. (A) Administration of ACTH 4–10 (0.1 μg/kg intraperitoneally) 30 minutes before continuous nerve stimulation of the extensor digitorum longus muscle increases muscle contraction strength in 9 to 15-day-old neonates. The peptide also evokes treppe (initial increase in contraction amplitude), characteristic of mature but not immature muscle. (B) Similar treatment of 21 to 25-day-old rats has no effect on muscle strength or treppe. (From C. M. Smith and Strand, 1981.)

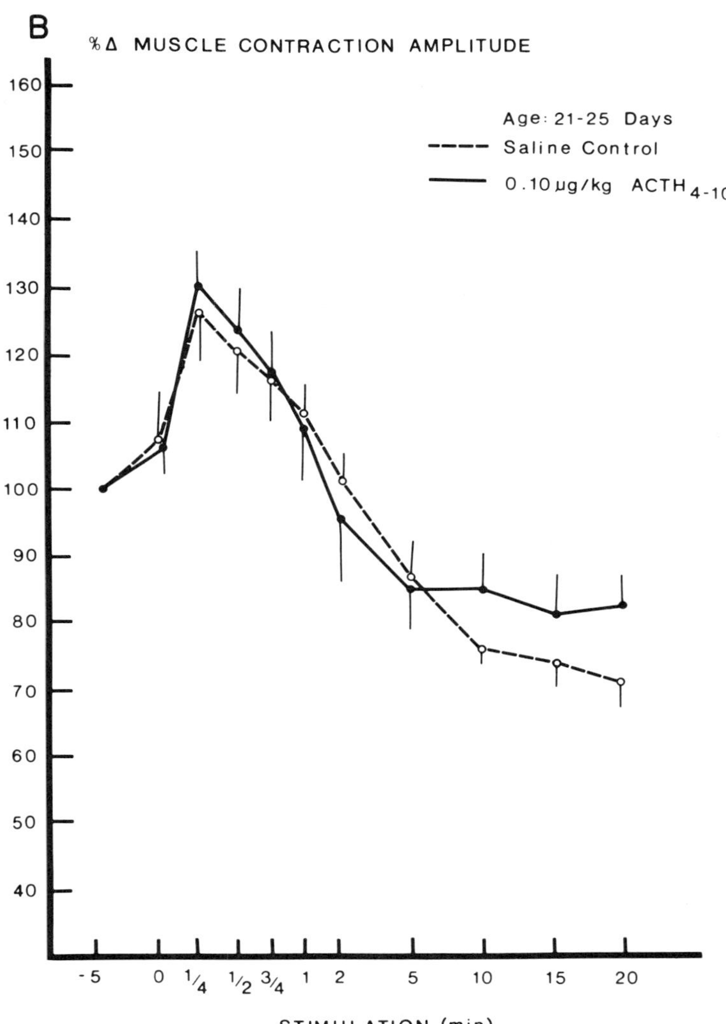

Figure 12.10 (continued)

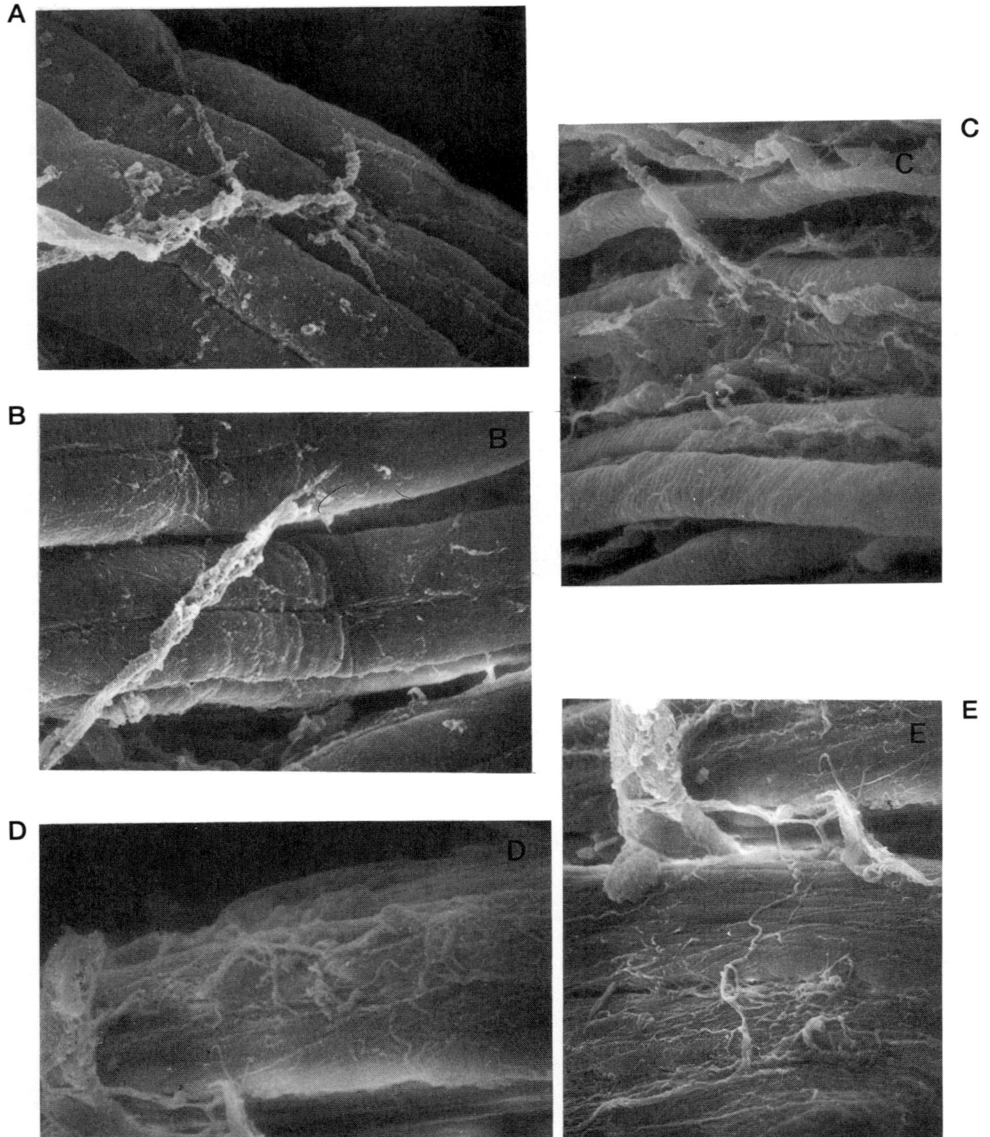

Figure 12.11
Scanning electron micrographs of endplate regions from the extensor digitorum longus muscles of 15-day-old rats. (A) Saline-treated neonate. The nerve can be seen branching into narrow terminals along the muscle fiber. X3420. (B) Org 2766-treated (10 μg/kg) neonate. There is a marked reduction in nerve terminal branching X3610. (C) ACTH 4–10–treated (10 μg/kg) neonate showing extensive nerve terminal branching. X2000 (D) Org 2766–treated (0.01 μg/kg) neonate, with extensive arborization of nerve terminals. X5000. (E) Higher magnification of D showing the extensive nerve terminal branching. This figure demonstrates that the more potent *Org 2766 is inhibitory* at a dosage which for *ACTH 4–10 facilitates* nerve terminal branching. When the dosage of Org 2766 is reduced considerably, it too becomes stimulatory. (From Frischer and Strand, 1988.)

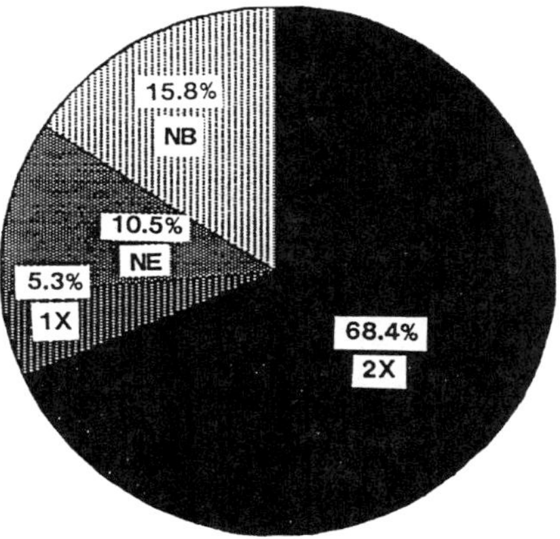

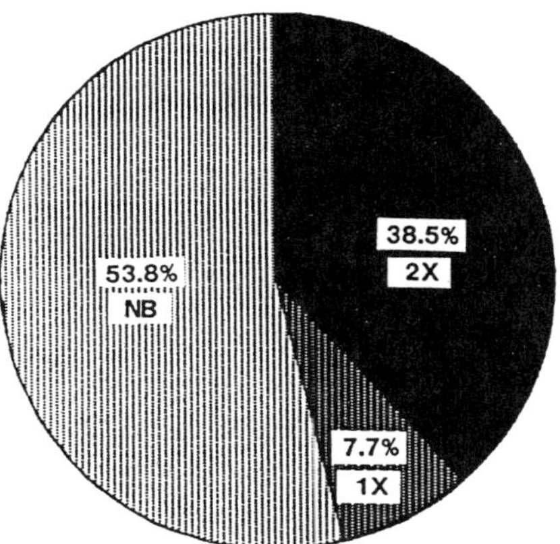

Figure 12.12
Overall sexual behavior displayed by sexually experienced male rats treated prenatally with saline or ACTH 1–24 (500 μg/kg twice daily intraperitoneally to pregnant females, gestation days 14 to 21). 2X, percent males that completed at least two ejaculatory series; 1X, percent males that completed only one ejaculatory series per trial; NE, percent males that did not complete one ejaculatory series; NB, percent males that did not mount. Kolmogorov-Smirnov test: $P < .05$. (From Segarra et al., 1991.)

Table 12.3
Melanocortin (10 μg/48 hours) effects on endplate parameters of extensor digitorum longus muscle 15 days after sciatic nerve crush

Parameters	Saline	ACTH 4–10	α-MSH
Nerve terminal branching (μm)	257 ± 4	337 ± 13***	370 ± 18***
Perimeter (μm)	232 ± 6	235 ± 6	256 ± 5**
Area (μm^2)	3501 ± 200	3573 ± 189	4092 ± 153*

From Strand et al. (1993b).
ACTH, adrenocorticotropic hormone; MSH, melanocyte-stimulating hormone.
Mean ± SEM. $^*P < .05$; $^{**}P < .01$; $^{***}P < .001$ vs. crush and saline.

of small motor units, and a more highly complex reinnervation site (table 12.3 and figure 12.13), have been suggested as the basis for enhanced melanocortin-mediated recovery from a nerve lesion. The mechanisms suggested include changes in B-50 (Van der Zee et al., 1989) and the evocation of a naturally occurring ACTH-MSH peptide signal by nerve damage (Bär et al., 1990). This suggestion is supported by the demonstration that the relatively low levels of ACTH 4–10 present in the adult spinal cord are markedly increased following unilateral peroneal nerve crush. This increase is restricted to distinct populations of ventral horn motor neurons in the lower lumbar region, where the cell bodies of this nerve originate (figure 12.14). Of considerable interest is the observation that, whereas motor neuron loss is severe on the side of the nerve injury in the saline-treated rats, there is considerable rescue of motor neurons, in *both* ventral horns, in animals treated with ACTH 4–10, which perhaps facilitates the expression of the naturally occuring neuropeptide (Lee et al., 1994). This implies that the melanocortins may excite a

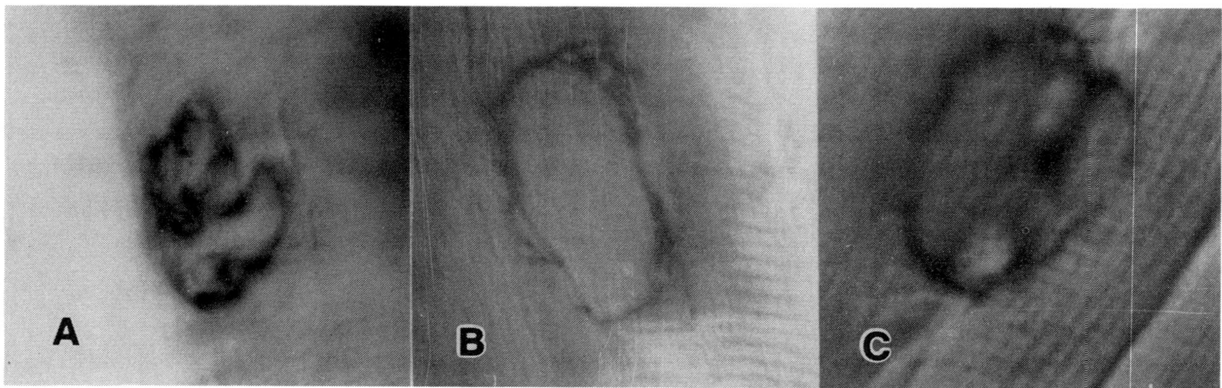

Figure 12.13
Light micrographs of silver-cholinesterase–stained endplates at the denervated extensor digitorum longus muscle. (A) α-Melanocyte-stimulating hormone–treated. (B) Saline–treated. (C) ACTH 4–10–treated. Increased density and complex branching are clearly evident in the peptide-treated endplates. (A and C). The saline-treated sample, (B) reveals an open, simple endplate interior. (From Strand et al., 1988.)

neuroprotective, as well as a regenerative, outcome following nerve damage.

The concept of neuroprotection is further supported by the observation that the melanocortins are most beneficial when administered directly following nerve damage, or simultaneously with neurotoxic chemotherapy (Antonawich et al., 1994; De Koning et al., 1988; Duckers et al., 1994; Gerritsen van der Hoop et al., 1990; Hamers et al., 1993; S. J. Lee et al., 1994; Verhaagen et al., 1987b). The plasticity of neuropeptide content and their receptors is not restricted to the melanocortins, as several other neuropeptides, both stimulatory and inhibitory, are altered by axotomy (Hökfelt et al., 1994).

Central effects Melanocortins also influence functional recovery of damaged central neurons, although this ameliorative action is probably a neuroprotective rather than a regenerative one, as shown by studies on lesioned dopaminergic systems, and lesions of the fimbria fornix (Antonawich et al., 1993; Atella et al., 1992; Hannigan and Isaacson, 1985; Pitsikas et al., 1990; Spruijt et al., 1990; Wolterink et al., 1990). The location of the central lesion and the peptide dosage, as well as the dosage regimen, are important determining factors. Generally, studies examining motor functional recovery have more consistently demonstrated a beneficial role for the melanocortins and their analogs than assays involving cognitive behavior, such as learning. Functional recovery from central lesions may involve compensatory events within the disturbed system (Lüneburg and Flohr, 1988). This has been suggested for recovery from septal, hippocampal, neocortical, parafascicular, and vestibular lesions. For a more detailed discussion of this mechanism, see Strand et al. (1993a).

In vitro experiments have demonstrated a direct trophic effect of melanocortins on cultured primary

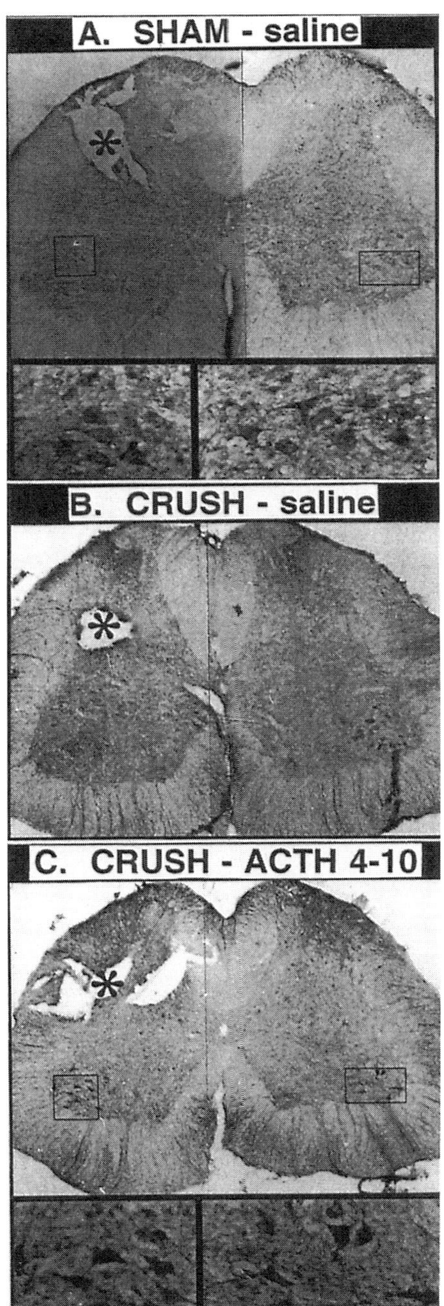

sensory and motor neurons (S. J. Lee et al., 1991; Van der Neut et al., 1992, Strand et al., 1993b). CNS neurons in tissue culture exposed to ACTH and MSH peptides survive better and increase neurite outgrowth and protein synthesis. Again, a differential response to specific melanocortins is found: midbrain serotonergic neurons mature more rapidly with ACTH fragments but not with α-MSH (Azmitia and de Kloet, 1987). On the other hand, spinal cord slices respond to α-MSH by an increase in B-50 expression and greater neurite outgrowth, but ACTH 4–10 and Org 2766 are ineffective in this system (Van der Neut et al., 1992). Dissociated mixed spinal cord cells respond well to all the melanocortins, including their analogs, even in the absence of NGF, which may indicate that interaction between cell types plays a role in the effectiveness of the neuropeptides (Strand et al., 1993c).

The molecular and biochemical events which occur during the regenerative response of the mature nervous system to trauma, may closely mimic those processes that occurred previously during development. ACTH 4–10-like immunoreactivity is widespread in the CNS only during postnatal development, to disappear in the mature adult, and then to reappear fol-

Figure 12.14
ACTH 4–10-like immunoreactivity (ACTH 4–10-IR) in lumbar spinal cord sections of the rat. (A) Sham-crushed sections show slight ACTH 4–10 distribution throughout the cord. (B) Following nerve crush and saline treatment, ACTH 4–10-IR is localized to the motor neurons contralateral to the lesion. There is a severe loss of motor neurons on the injured side of the cord. (C) Following treatment with ACTH 4–10, starting on the day of nerve crush, motor neuron number is retained on both sides of the cord, and both sides show ACTH 4–10-IR. Asterisk indicates the side of the lesion or sham crush. (Adapted from S. J. Lee et al., 1994.)

lowing lesions in the nigrostriatal system or in ventral horn motor neurons following peroneal nerve crush (S. J. Lee et al., 1994; Antonawich et al. 1993). Despite the inspiring advances in our knowledge of the melanocortin receptors and their interactions with signal transduction systems, the mechanisms by which the ACTH and MSH peptides exert their undeniable protective and trophic actions remain unclear. What is known is that the specificity of the message in the melanocortin sequences is very marked: slight variations may permit them to modulate many diverse physiological systems and be sensitive to tissue, stage of development, maturation, and regeneration, as well as sex. Unraveling these interactions will certainly be the focus of future research involving these important regulatory neuropeptides.

12.2.9.4 Melanocortins and Behavior in Adults

a. Learning, memory, and attention

These functions are affected by the melanocortins. There is an enormous literature on this subject, which has been comprehensively reviewed (Beckwith and Kastin, 1988; De Wied and Jolles, 1982; De Wied and Wolterink, 1989; Sandman and O'Halloran, 1988). Many of these effects are best demonstrated in hypophysectomized rats in which there are deficits in learning. Administration of ACTH 1–24, 1–10, or 4–10 restores the rate of active avoidance acquisition, when a stimulus signals impending punishment.

In intact rats, ACTH peptides also delay the extinction of acquired responses, whether the responses are reinforced originally by punishment or by reward. Similarly, ACTH peptides facilitate the acquisition and retention of passive avoidance behavior, such as the bar-press avoidance of an electric shock, with low dosages enhancing retention of the response and high dosages having the reverse effect. In both active and passive avoidance behavior, the structural requirements of the ACTH fragments for specific behavioral responses are surprisingly different, a phenomenon which may be explained by the specificity and distribution of MCRs. Substitution of D-Phe^7 in the ACTH 1–10 or ACTH 4–10 structure reverses the effects of these compounds on active avoidance behavior (Bohus and de Wied, 1966).

ACTH and its related peptides also delay extinction of the rewarding effect of brain self-stimulation in rats and facilitate sexual motivation. ACTH may cause either facilitation or inhibition, depending upon dosage and the complexity of the task. These results have been interpreted as an effect on learning, attention enhancement, or motivation, independent of adrenal steroids (De Wied 1969, 1976; Sandman and Kastin, 1977).

The most potent effects of α-MSH on learning are its enhancement of visually learned behaviors and the reversal of a visual discrimination, effects again related to the specific conditions of training. In a study of cyclic and linear analogs of α-MSH on retrieval of memory, three of the cyclic analogs and three of the linear analogs improved retrieval, while one linear analog antagonized the effect. An analog with D-Phe^7 substitution and α-MSH itself had no effect, demonstrating that structural modifications of α-MSH alter its potency in learning and memory situations (Beckwith et al., 1989).

ACTH and MSH effects on memory storage are time-dependent and short-lived, and may involve ACTH release of NE (Gold and Delanoy, 1981), an interesting indication of stress-evoked hormones cooperating in a time-dependent phenomenon essential to survival. This view is strengthened by the changes in heart rate and electrocardiographic recordings that accompany neuropeptide-induced behavioral changes.

b. Immobility response

The species-specific, stereotypal dorsal immobility response, which may mimic that of the prey carried by a predator, is inhibited by ACTH 4–10 and ACTH 7–16, but potentiated by the D-Phe^7 analogs of these fragments. γ-MSH 1–12, an opiate antagonist, attenuates the immobility response. A similar immobility behavior, known as behavioral depression, follows kindling, a widely used model for epilepsy, evoked by repeated, subconvulsive electrical stimulation of the amygdala and other brain regions. Immobility following hippocampal kindling is reduced by many of the D-substituted ACTH fragments but not the L-fragments (Bohus et al., 1986).

c. Grooming, yawning, stretching, and penile erection

Intracerebroventricular injection of ACTH 1–24 evokes remarkable, nonlearned behaviors which are not seen after peripheral administration of the peptides but can be elicited by either ACTH or α-MSH in adrenalectomized animals (Ferrari, 1958). These behaviors include excessive grooming, yawning, stretching, and penile erection in young male rats (Bertolini et al., 1975). The brain regions sensitive to the yawning and stretching syndome are the hypothalamic areas lining the third ventricle and a septal-hippocampal-cholinergic pathway has been implicated for its evocation.

Birds and small mammals display enhanced grooming behavior in response to stressful or novel environmental stimuli, which also activate the HPA axis. Since excessive grooming can also be elicited in hypophysectomized rats, the pituitary cannot be directly involved in the response to i.c.v. administration of ACTH. The site of ACTH-evoked excessive grooming is the periaqueductal gray.and it is mediated by the MC4 receptor (Adan et al., 1994).

d. Social behavior

ACTH and its fragments induce long-lasting muricidal behavior in 52% of young male rats, an aggressive response spontaneously induced by adrenalectomy, which is characterized by high levels of endogenous ACTH (Miachon et al., 1995). ACTH has an anxiogenic effect in an animal model of anxiety, possibly modulating serotonergic pathways in the midbrain and hypothalamus. ACTH 1–24, ACTH 4–10, Org 2766, and α-MSH all decrease social interaction and exploratory behavior in male rats, without reducing motor activity. However, the effects of these peptides vary with the conditions of the test (File and Vellucci, 1978).

e. Melanocortins and feeding behavior

The MC4 receptor may play a role in the regulation of fat, glugagon, and insulin. Knockout mice lacking the MC4-R are hyperphagic, obese, and develop hyperinsulinemia and hyperglycemia. Melanocortinergic neurons exert a tonic inhibition of feeding behavior and the MC4-R and MSH are necessary for the biological response to leptin, a hormone produced by adipocytes which allows the body to maintain constant stores of fat (Fan et al., 1997). This is discussed in more detail in chapter 16, section 16.4.2.

f. Cognitive tests in humans

Beckwith (1988) comprehensively summarizes the complex results of cognitive tests on the effects of α-MSH, ACTH 4–10, and Org 2766 in healthy young adults, healthy and cognitively impaired elderly adults, and on clinical populations. In general, ACTH analogs maintain alertness during long-term performance but have no direct effect on learning or memory. It appears that α-MSH may have a mildly beneficial effect on some aspects of visual recall, and ACTH 4–10 may be of some benefit to severely retarded adults. In both animal and humans, *attention* with its corresponding positive effects on the processing of information before it enters memory, appears to be a crucial element in the effects of MSH (Kastin et al., 1971; Sandman et al., 1972). Both ACTH 4–10 and Org 2766 have mild euphoric effects and may therefore be involved with positive reinforcement.

The reported effects are conflicting, due perhaps to the differences in the tests used to assess learning and memory. The discrepancies in the results may be due to variations in dosage, sex, age, the choice of tasks, and the complexity of the phenomena studied. Better tests need to be devised to extend the neurotrophic effects of the melanocortins in animals to learning and memory in humans.

12.2.9.5 Various Central and Peripheral Effects of Melanocortins

a. Autonomic responses

I.v. injections of ACTH, ACTH 4–10, or α-MSH cause pressor and cardioaccelerator effects, the tachycardia probably being due to increased sympathetic influences (Bohus et al., 1993). These changes are also seen during passive avoidance, suggesting that ACTH and MSH peptides act centrally to affect autonomic responses.

b. Inflammation and immunity

α-MSH and its C-terminal tripeptide 11–13 (Lys-Pro-Val) inhibit inflammation when administered systemically, effects that are mediated by pathways involving both central and peripheral sites of action (Macaluso et al., 1994). Administration of ACTH suppresses several immune functions, not only through glucocorticoids but by acting directly on ACTH receptors on lymphocytes and monocytes (Johnson et al., 1982), lending credence to the concept of a close association between stress and immune responses, as discussed in chapter 8.

c. Analgesia

ACTH and α-MSH antagonize the analgesic effects of opiates, including β-endorphin, possibly via opiate receptors, yet stress-induced sedation and hypokinesia, which are not mediated through opiate systems, are facilitated by ACTH 4–10 (Wolterink and Van Ree, 1988).

d. Locomotion

In general, motor activity is not affected by the melanocortins in the intact adult rat, but is dramatically increased by ACTH administration to neonates (figure 12.15). However, very high doses of ACTH 1–24 depress, and low dosages stimulate, motor activity of the rat in an open field, responses that may involve the opiate system (Amir et al., 1980). α-MSH potentiates the motor effects of L-DOPA in mice, and decreases audiogenic seizures (Plotnikoff and Kastin, 1976).

e. Fever

ACTH and MSH peptides have antipyretic effects and α-MSH is one of the most potent endogenous antipyretic agents, able to inhibit IL-1–induced fever. Endotoxin administration increases the levels of circulating α-MSH, which in turn, alleviates the resulting fever (Martin and Lipton, 1990).

f. Anticonvulsive effects

The melanocortins counteract convulsive seizures induced by various experimental means, with varying degrees of effectiveness. The smaller peptides, ACTH 4–10, the ACTH 4–9 analog Org 2766, and the

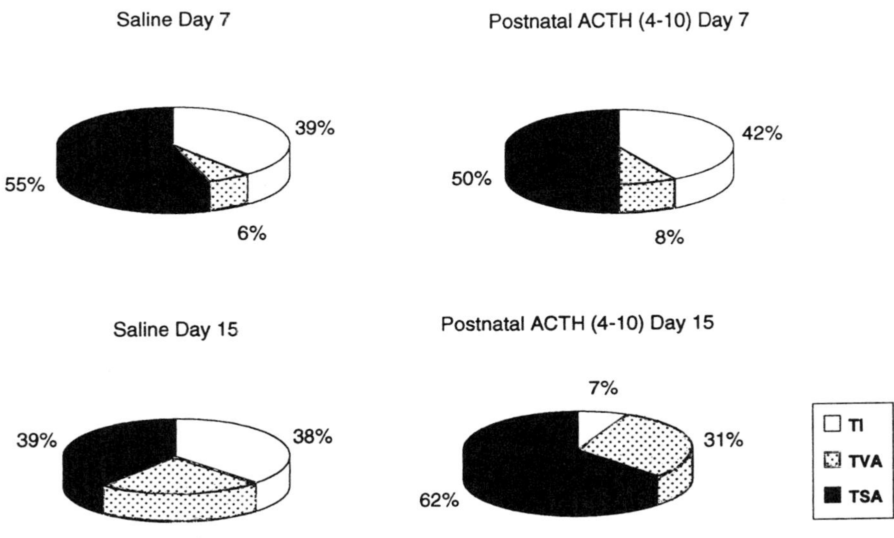

Figure 12.15
Postnatal administration of ACTH 4–10 increases active behavior in neonates. Both total very active behavior (TVA) and total slight activity (TSA) are increased in 15-day-old rat pups by melanocortin treatment (10 μg/kg subcutaneously daily from day of birth to day prior to the experiment). This effect is not seen at 7 days of age. There is a marked decrease in total inactivity (TI) in peptide-treated 15-day-old rats. (From Rose et al., 1988.)

ACTH 4–9 analog BIM 22015, reduce the severity of the convulsions, whereas ACTH 1–39 and ACTH 1–24 are inactive (Croiset and de Wied, 1992; Calvet et al., 1992)

g. Electrophysiological effects

Krivoy and Guillemin (1961) first demonstrated that β-MSH, but not ACTH 1–24, increases spinal motor neuron excitability. Increased neuronal excitability has been demonstrated in many areas of the CNS following administration of α-MSH, β-MSH, or ACTH, and in some cases by ACTH 4–10. Alterations in the electrical activity of the brain, including cortical evoked potentials, and EEG activity of the preoptic and hypothalamic areas and the hippocampus, indicate that ACTH 4–10 and α-MSH increase the state of arousal in the limbic-midbrain system, permitting the animal to respond more rapidly and effectively to stress (De Wied and Jolles, 1982). The ACTH and MSH peptides also increase neuromuscular efficiency during recovery from peripheral nerve damage, increasing the proportion of small motor units (figure 12.16), and thus, presumably, improving the fine control of muscles. These peptides also increase muscle contraction strength, action potential amplitude, and decrease fatigue, actions that involve spinal motor neurons and perhaps higher motor centers (see reviews by Strand et al., 1989, 1993a).

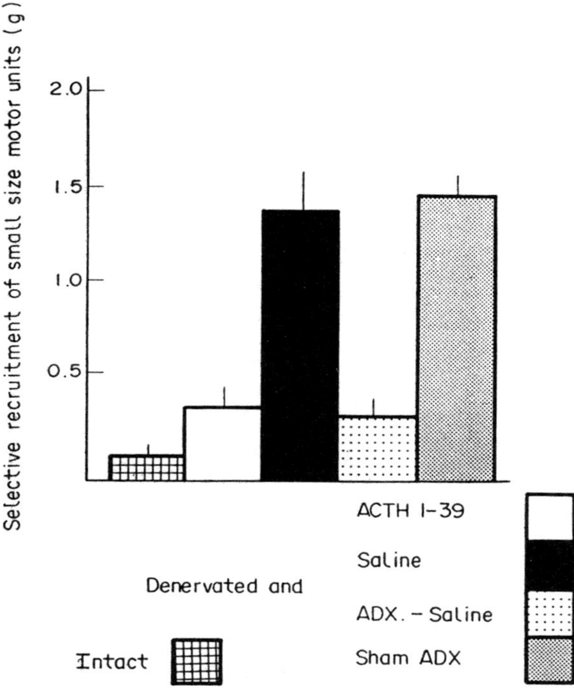

Figure 12.16
The mean size of motor units responding to continuous stimulation (1 Hz for 1 minute) was larger in denervated vs. intact rats ($P < .05$). Treatment with adrenocorticotropin (ACTH) reduced motor unit size vs. saline controls ($P < .05$). Adrenalectomized (ADX) saline-treated rats, with high endogenous ACTH levels also had smaller contracting motor units than saline-treated or sham-ADX, saline-treated animals ($P < .05$). Bar: Standard error of the mean. Six rats per group. (From Saint-Come et al., 1985.)

12.2.10 Clinical Implications of POMC-Derived Neuropeptides

In patients with *pituitary deficiency of ACTH,* a potentially life-threatening situation, particularly in stress, the administration of cortisone is usually preferred to that of ACTH itself, since ACTH deficiency does not usually lead to complete mineralocorticoid (aldosterone) deficiency. This is unlike those suffering from adrenal insufficiency (Addison's disease), which may be due to adrenal failure or to pituitary ACTH dysfunction, who require both glucocorticoids and mineralocorticoids as replacement therapy, with increased amounts necessary during stress. Disturbances of adrenal function due to hypothalamic lesions occur relatively rarely.

Cushing's disease, characterized by an *excess of ACTH secretion,* may be caused by a pituitary adenoma, an adrenal adenoma, or by an ACTH-secreting carcinoma of the lung or thyroid. If the hypersecretion is due to a pituitary tumor, the various therapies used include transsphenoidal microsurgery to remove the pituitary, pituitary irradiation, or the administration of ACTH-suppressive drugs, such as cyproheptadine or bromocriptine. Plasma β-lipotropin immunoreactivity is usually high in patients with Cushing's disease, but plasma α-MSH is usually not measurable as melanotrophs are not regulated by adrenocorticoids. However, due to the high levels of ACTH, which contains the core melanotropic sequence, increased pigmentation is often seen.

The use of MSH and the ACTH and MSH peptide fragments has been more limited clinically, although there is extensive evidence from animal models that the melanocortins accelerate recovery from nerve trauma, ameliorate many neuropathies, and may be helpful in alleviating convulsive seizures. These animal models include peripheral nerve lesions, diabetic neuropathy, cisplatin-induced sensory neuropathy, experimental allergic neuritis, motor neuropathy resembling that of motor neuron disease, and motor neuropathy in the wobbler mouse. Most of this very interesting work has been done by Gispen and his colleagues and is reviewed by Gispen et al. (1994).

Clinical trials involving the administration of Org 2766 to prevent the development of neuropathy in women with ovarian cancer treated with the chemotherapeutic drug cisplatin have been reported. Signs of neurotoxicity as assessed by the vibration perception threshold (a measurement of sensory nerve function which is specifically affected by cisplatin neurotoxicity) were decreased in the peptide-treated women (Gerritsen van der Hoop et al., 1990). Similar positive results were obtained in a small pilot study of patients with atrophy of spinal motor neurons (progressive spinal muscular atrophy), carpal tunnel syndrome, and multiple sclerosis: treatment with ACTH 4–10 significantly increased muscle action potentials indirectly evoked through nerve stimulation (Strand et al., 1977). Diseases primarily of myogenic origin, such as muscular dystrophy, did not respond to the neuropeptide. The possibilities for treatment of neuropathies and nerve trauma are encouraging, although considerable clinical studies are still required. Evidence from animal studies indicates that neuropeptides may have therapeutic implications in memory disorders, mental retardation, pain, depression, impotence, obesity, fever, and insomnia (Kastin et al., 1987)

12.3 Summary

ACTH 1–39 was the first pituitary peptide to be isolated and sequenced. This achievement was followed by the discovery of a large precursor molecule that contains the sequences of ACTH 1–39, β-MSH (ACTH 1–16 or 1–22) and β-lipotropin (ACTH 61–91). The precursor was named pro-opiomelanocortin (POMC) to indicate its embodiment of the three moieties. POMC gene structure, mRNAs, and proteins have been highly conserved, as has been the structure of ACTH. The entire biological activity of ACTH is contained within ACTH 1–39, which is also cleaved biologically to ACTH 1–13 (α-MSH). POMC gives rise to three forms of MSH, α-, β-, and γ-MSH each of which contains a common heptapeptide core that is essential to biological activity. β-Lipotropin is a precursor of β-MSH and β-endorphin.

POMC is found in cell bodies of the arcuate nucleus and their projections to extrahypothalamic structures, and in the nucleus of the tractus solitarius, and in spinal motor neurons. Outside the CNS, POMC is found in the gut and pancreas, lymphocytes, macrophages, and spleen, as well as in the gonads, adrenal medulla, and lung. *POMC gene expression* varies in different types of tissues and species and is increased by CRH. Processing of POMC is tissue-specific. In the anterior lobe POMC is processed by corticotrophs mainly to ACTH 1–39, β-lipotropin, and β-endorphin. In the intermediate lobe POMC is processed further to small peptides such as α-MSH, β-MSH, γ-lipotropin, CLIP, and and several β-endorphin–related peptides. β-Lipotropin and ACTH are the predominant melanocortins in humans, whereas MSH is predominant in most other species. In the intermediate lobe, N-acetylation increases the potency of α-MSH but reduces the corticotropic activity of ACTH and completely destroys the opiate activity of β-endorphin. β-Lipotropin is processed in the pituitary gland to β-endorphin (β-lipotropin 61–91). POMC expression in spinal motor neurons is upregulated by peripheral nerve section.

The pituitary corticotrophs contain ACTH 1–39, α-MSH, and β-lipotropin, and some corticotrophs are present in the intermediate lobe. Most hypothalamic α-MSH is in the arcuate nucleus, the neurons of which send projections to many other brain regions. In animals with an intermediate lobe, MSH is present in the melanotrophs of that structure. MSH is found in low concentrations in several peripheral organs.

Regulation of corticotroph secretion is primarily through CRH, which increases POMC transcription in the corticotrophs. Other neuropeptides, especially VP, may act synergistically with CRH and neurotransmitters such as epinephrine and 5-HT are also involved. POMC secretion is inhibited through a long-loop glucocorticoid feedback on CRH secretion. CRH stimulates the *melanotrophs* of the intermediate lobe to secrete MSH. The secretory activity of the melanotrophs is inhibited by DA acting through D_2 receptors coupled to adenylate cyclase. In amphibians, the regulation of MSH synthesis and release is complex as MSH is directly involved in movement of melanin and other pigments in skin color changes. Light; CRH; TRH, and melanostatin, an amphibian counterpart of NPY; MCH; and several neurotransmitters are all implicated. MCH has effects that are antagonistic to MSH in lower vertebrates, but its effects in mammals, perhaps modulating behavior and the perception of sensory function are uncertain.

The *functional efficacy* of the melanocortins depends on the peptide and the function being tested. Many shorter synthetic fragments of ACTH, and their synthetic analogs, have potent neurotrophic and behavioral effects. In skin darkening in amphibians, α-MSH is 10 to 100 times more potent than ACTH, and 2 to 10 times more potent than β-MSH. Similarly, α-MSH is more potent than ACTH as a neurotrophic agent. In behavioral tests, however, ACTH is the more effective melanocortin. Only ACTH 1–39 and ACTH 1–24 have corticotropic and neurotrophic effects, since shortening of ACTH 1–24 eliminates most of the corticotropic properties. In tests of peripheral nerve regeneration, ACTH 4–10 is the shortest fragment with neurotrophic properties, but α-MSH, ACTH 4–10, and ACTH 4–9 analogs are more potent than ACTH 4–10.

MCRs have recently been identified with the aid of a radiolabeled MSH tracer. They are most concentrated in the septal area, the bed nucleus of the stria terminalis, and the medial preoptic area. More moderate binding is found in hypothalamic nuclei and the ME. Binding of the ACTH fragments is limited to regions of the septum, preoptic areas, hypothalamus, and hippocampus in adults. ACTH 4–10 binding is seen in developing brain and in the spinal cord following peripheral nerve injury, but not in normal adults, supporting the concept that melanocortins are active during specific “time windows” of development and regeneration.

Five different MCRs have been cloned, pharmacologically distinguished, and localized. The MSH receptor MC1-R is specifically expressed in melanocytes and is distinct from the ACTH receptor, MC2-R, which is restricted to the adrenal cortex. MC3-R is found in the limbic system and hypothalamus and is activated by γ-MSH peptides which do not affect the other MCRs. MC4-R is found in almost all brain regions, especially the PVN, and in the spinal cord. MC5-R is expressed in brain and many peripheral tissues, including skeletal muscle and lymphoid organs. The melanocortins use adenylate cyclase and cAMP as the second-messenger system, but may also activate the phoshatidylinositol system through involvement of the phosphoprotein B-50.

ACTH and MSH peptides act as *neurotransmitters* and *neuromodulators*, increasing ACh synthesis and release. They interact with brain monamine transmitters, depolarize spinal motor neurons, and increase neuronal excitability in many areas of the CNS. They increase the state of arousal and improve the efficiency of the motor system.

The most obvious *function of ACTH* is to stimulate the secretion of glucocorticoids by the adrenal cortex, that of *MSH* to affect color change by regulating the distribution of melanin. However, the melanocortins have many other functions. Their neurotrophic effects can be demonstrated during development, in adulthood, and in regeneration. POMC and its derived melanocortins are present in the fetal rat CNS early in gestation, and endogenous MSH has a major role in early development, stimulating fetal growth and brain development and perhaps acting as a signal for the initiation of parturition. MSH, ACTH 4–10, and the ACTH 4–9 analog Org 2766 accelerate the maturation of central neuronal circuitries and of the developing neuromuscular system. Perinatal administration of ACTH negatively influences subsequent sexual behavior, changes that correspond to changes in the monoaminergic innervation of the brain, including the POA. MSH administered to neonates increases social interaction and improves learning in young adulthood, a sexually dimorphic response.

In *adults*, the melanocortins affect *learning, memory, and attention*, effects best shown in hypophysectomized animals. There is a high degree of specificity of the structural fragments of ACTH for the particular behavior studied, probably due to the specificity and distribution of the MCRs. The nonlearned *immobility response* is inhibited by ACTH 4–10 and ACTH 7–16, but potentiated by the D-Phe^7 analogs of these fragments. Icv. injection of ACTH 1–24 causes excessive grooming, yawning, and penile erection; the excessive grooming is mediated by the MC4-R. Additional behavioral responses induced by the melanocortins include muricidal behavior in young male rats, and anxiogenic effects. In humans, cognitive tests indicate that ACTH analogs maintain alertness, but have no direct effect on learning or memory.

ACTH and MSH peptides act centrally to affect autonomic responses, causing pressor and cardioaccelerator effects. They are involved in inflammation and immunity and antagonize the analgesic effects of opiates, including β-endorphin. High doses of ACTH depress, and low doses stimulate, motor activity, perhaps through involvement of the opiate systems. The small ACTH fragments counteract convulsive seizures, but ACTH 1–39 and 1–24 are ineffective.

The melanocortins promote the regeneration of peripheral nerves, improving neuromuscular performance by accelerating axonal sprouting, the formation of more small motor units, and a more highly complex reinnervation site. Suggested mechanisms include changes in B-50 and the evocation of endogenous ACTH and MSH resulting from nerve injury. Experiments indicate that the melanocortins may provide a neuroprotective as well as regenerative effect following nerve damage, both in the brain and spinal cord.

The ACTH and MSH neuropeptides have a direct trophic effect on sensory and motor neurons in culture with differential responses to specific melanocortins indicated. Midbrain serotonergic neurons mature more rapidly with ACTH fragments but do not respond to α-MSH. Spinal cord slices respond to α-MSH but not to the ACTH fragments, and dissociated mixed spinal cord cells respond well to all the melanocortins.

Chapter 13 continues with the pituitary neuropeptides: the glycoproteins FSH, LH, and TSH, the growth hormone-prolactin family, GH, PRL, and placental lactogen. A novel neuropeptide, secretoneurin, which was first discovered in the pituitary, but is also widely distributed throughout the nervous system, is included in this chapter.

Anterior Pituitary Neuropeptides II. The Glycoprotein and Growth Hormone Families; Secretoneurin

13

13.1 Pituitary Glycoprotein Hormones

13.1.1 Glycoprotein Structure

All vertebrates synthesize three different glycoprotein hormones: follicle-stimulating hormone (FSH), luteinizing hormone (LH), and thyroid-stimulating hormone (TSH). The glycoproteins are heterodimers formed by a noncovalent association between an α subunit, common to all glycoprotein hormones, and a unique β subunit, encoded by a discrete β subunit gene (figure 13.1). It is the β subunits that confer the biological specificity for the glycoprotein receptors in the target organs. Neither subunit is active individually. FSH, LH, TSH, and chorionic gonadotropin (CG) each possess 92 amino acids in their α subunits, but have 118, 121, 112, and 145 amino acids, respectively, in their β subunits. The biosynthesis of LH, FSH, and TSH is regulated at all levels of the classical pathways for peptides.

Chorionic gonadotropin, as its name implies, is secreted by the placenta and has best been characterized in humans and equids (horses, donkeys, zebras). It belongs to the same family of hormones as the pituitary gonadotropins. Human chorionic gonadotropin (hCG) is composed of α and β subunits: the α subunits are identical to those of LH and FSH, whereas the β subunits give it its distinctive biological characteristic, which is to maintain the corpus luteum during pregnancy.

Both the α and β subunits are *glycosylated* and there is considerable heterogeneity in the composition of the sugars in the different hormones and under different physiological circumstances. The sugars may be either *N*-linked chains attached to Asp residues or *O*-linked attached to Ser or Thr residues. The addition of sugar chains to the subunits occurs cotranslationally with cleavage of the signal peptide as the subunits enter the RER. The sugar chain is critical for triggering receptor signaling in the target tissue.

13.1.2 Gene Structure and Expression

Each subunit is coded by a different gene and the genes for the α and β subunits are on different chromosomes. The human *α subunit gene* spans about 9.4 kb, is 4 amino acids shorter than in other species (92 in humans, 96 in other species) (Nagaya and Jameson, 1994), and is stabilized by five disulfide bonds. All α subunit genes contain four exons and three introns, with the coding sequences present in exons 2, 3, and 4. A single gene encodes this subunit in all species studied. The transcriptional start is identical in pituitary gonadotrophs and thyrotrophs but tissue-specific processing and multihormonal control of the α gene result in the specificity of the neuropeptide hormone produced. Based on the information that the α gene is regulated by cAMP at the transcriptional level, a cAMP regulatory element (see figure 13.1) has been identified in the α gene promoter, the

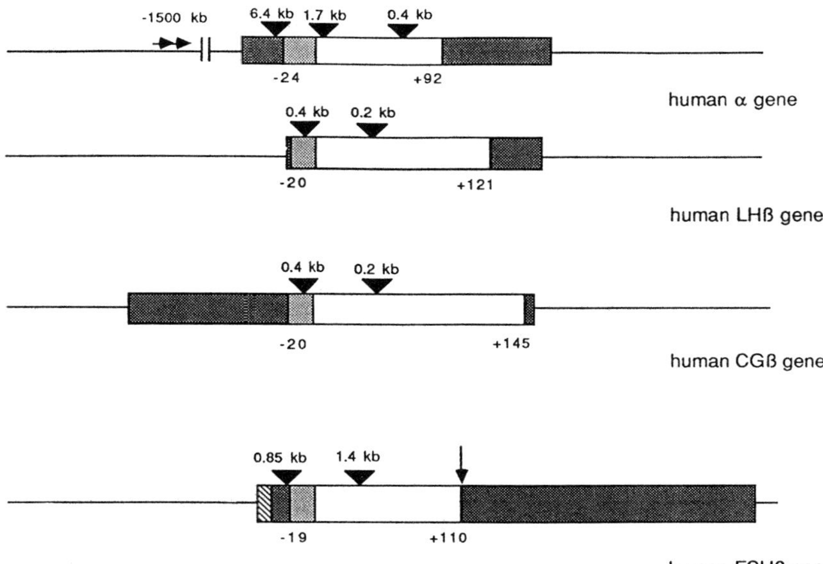

Figure 13.1
Structure of the human gonadotropin genes, α, luteinizing hormone–β (LHβ), chorionic gonadotropin–β (CGβ), and follicle-stimulating hormone–β (FSHβ). Untranslated regions are shown by dark-shaded areas. Signal peptides and mature apoproteins are represented by stippled and unshaded regions, respectively. Solid triangles demonstrate the positions of introns. Intron sizes are marked above these triangles. Numbers below each diagram signify amino acids' position with respect to the first amino acid of the mature apoprotein. The pair of horizontal arrows in the diagram of the α gene denote the position of the directly repeated cAMP regulatory element. In the diagram of the FSHβ gene, the hatched region represents the extended 5′-untranslated region produced by alternative splicing that occurs in 35% of transcripts. The solid arrow indicates a polyadenylation site utilized by 20% of transcripts. (From Gharib et al., 1990.)

DNA sequences responsible for controlling the expression of the genes (Jameson et al., 1986).

There are differences in the number of exons, their length, and the transcriptional start sites of the β subunits in different species, details of which may be found in the article by Nagaya and Jameson (1994). Like the α subunit, the β subunit possesses several (six) disulfide bonds, predicting that the two subunits are tightly coiled. The β subunit of ovine LH consists of 120 amino acids and has many primary amino acid sequences in common with the 96 amino acids of the ovine LH α subunit. The α subunit of TSH is produced in excess of the α subunits so that the synthesis of the β subunit is rate-limiting in the production of TSH.

13.2 The Gonadotropins

13.2.1 Anatomical Distribution of the Gonadotrophs

The gonadotrophs of the anterior pituitary are unusual in that they produce both LH and FSH, as has been convincingly shown by antibodies against the specific β subunit of each hormone. These cells are scattered throughout the glandular parenchyma, and to a more limited extent, also in the pars tuberalis, and represent about 14% of the cell population in both male and female adult rats. There is a strange state of functional heterogeneity in the various sizes of the gonadotrophs and the secretory granules may contain both gonadotropins, or LH and FSH may be found in separate granules.

13.2.2 Differential Regulation of Luteinizing Hormone and Follicle-Stimulating Hormone

Hypothalamic control of FSH and LH, and the role of the gonadal steroids in the negative and positive feedback loops was discussed in chapter 10, section 10.1.3.6.7 and 8. In addition, the gonadal peptides, inhibin, activin, and follistatin, are involved in an intricate feedback mechanism (figure 13.2).

13.2.2.1 Expression of Gonadotropin Subunit mRNA

LH mRNA and FSH mRNA, indicators of gonadotropin synthesis, are regulated differentially during the 4-day estrous cycle in rats. During late proestrus, both LH β mRNA and FSH β mRNA increase rapidly. In transgenic male mice, expression of the FSH β subunit gene is suppressed by testosterone at the level of the pituitary (Kumar and Low, 1995). An interesting observation that supports the significance of the pulsatile release of GnRH, discussed in chapter 10, is that continuous GnRH stimulates only α subunit mRNA synthesis and that pulsatile GnRH is required to stimulate the LH β gene (Shupnik and Fallest, 1994).

Using unit gravity sedimentation techniques to separate the gonadotrophs, Denef et al. (1980) found that most cells, regardless of size, contain both FSH and LH, but that some cells have only FSH or LH.

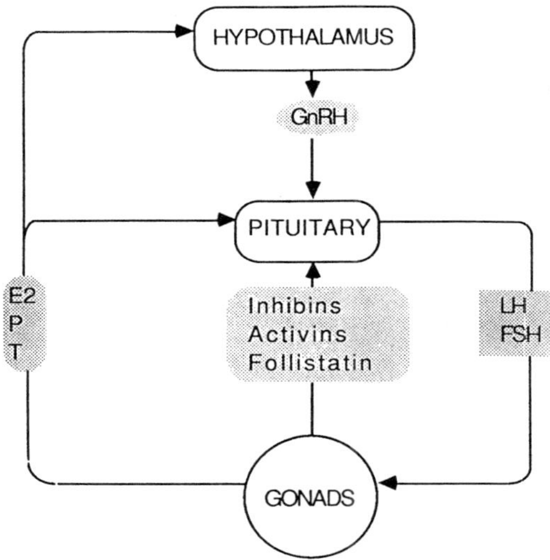

Figure 13.2
Hypothalamo-pituitary-gonadal axis. The hypothalamic neuropeptide gonadotropin-releasing hormone (GnRH) is released in a pulsatile fashion into the portal circulation and interacts with receptors on gonadotroph cells in the pituitary. The gonadotrophs secrete luteinizing hormone (LH) and follicle-stimulating hormone (FSH) which stimulate steroidogenesis in the gonad. The sex steroids estradiol (E_2), progesterone (P), and testosterone (T) have effects on LH and FSH biosynthesis and secretion that may be mediated at the hypothalamus, the pituitary, or both. Additionally, the gonad produces inhibins, activins, and follistatin. These gonadal peptides affect the synthesis and secretion of FSH and LH by the pituitary. See text for details. (From Gharib et al., 1990.)

Depending on the age and sex of the animal, and the size of the gonadotrophs, the release of either FSH or LH is favored. Whether this is causative or merely a correlation is still to be determined.

13.2.2.2 External Signals to the Gonadotrophs

Patterns of neuronal excitation and hormonal environment are important variables that influence the differential regulation that determines the release of

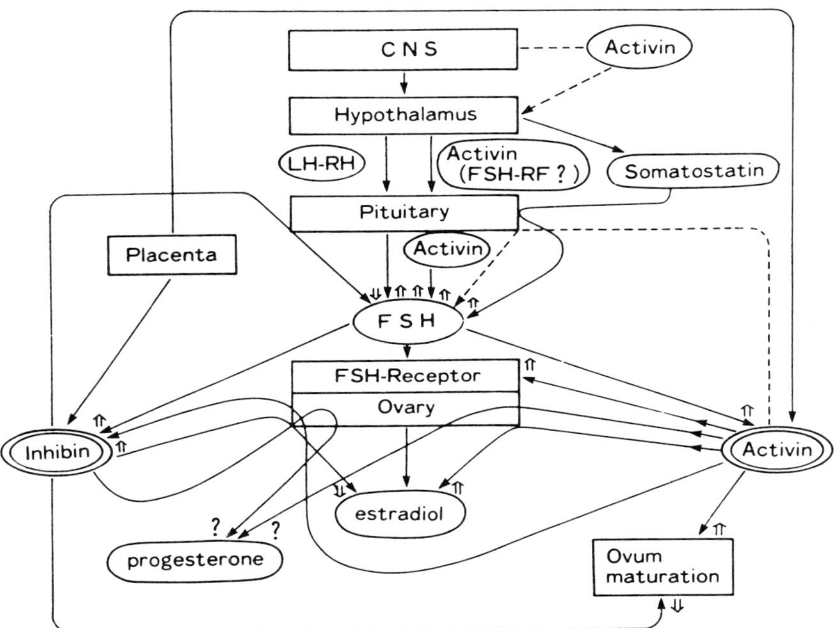

Figure 13.3
Mode and site of action of inhibin and activin in reproduction. Closed arrows show sites of action of inhibin or activin. Open upward arrows show stimulatory effects. Open downward arrows show inhibitory effects. LH-RH, luteinizing hormone–releasing hormone; FSH-RF, follicle-stimulating hormone–releasing factor (From Igarashi et al., 1993.)

FSH or LH. High pulse frequency favors LH, as does steroid feedback, but gonadal peptide feedback regulates FSH. However, little is known about the specific intracellular pathways that select one gonadotropin over the other.

13.2.2.3 Regulation of FSH by Inhibin, Follistatin, and Activin

Whereas GnRH and the *gonadal steroids* (testosterone in the male and estrogen and progesterone in the female) are the dominant factors regulating FSH secretion, the importance of the *gonadal peptides* is becoming increasingly evident. The inhibitory peptides are inhibin and follistatin; activin stimulates FSH secretion (figure 13.3).

Inhibin, produced by the granulosa cells of the ovarian follicles and the Sertoli cells of the testis, suppresses pituitary FSH but not LH. This forms a closed-loop endocrine feedback system in which FSH stimulates inhibin formation by the ovary, and inhibin in turn represses FSH synthesis by the anterior pituitary gonadotrophs (Burger, 1989). Inhibin is a peptide consisting of two subunits, the 18-kD α unit and the 14-kD β unit, linked by disulfide bonds. Each subunit is encoded by a different mRNA species. There are slight species differences in the α subunit but almost no differences in the β subunit, indicating a high degree of conservation in this molecule (Ying, 1988).

Follistatin, or FSH-suppressing protein, is a polypeptide glycoprotein produced in the pituitary that bears no structural similarity to the gonadal peptides. Its main action is to suppress pituitary basal FSH secretion in a dose-dependent manner and it counteracts the effects of activin, acting in an autocrine manner. It has similar but lesser effects on LH.

Activin is formed from two β subunits of inhibin and has biological activities opposite to those of inhibins. Activin stimulates both the synthesis and release of FSH from the pituitary, but induces no change in LH, although it may increase the number of LHRH receptors (Braden and Conn, 1992). If activin and inhibin are added to the same culture medium, their actions are competitive and the final released amount of FSH depends on their reciprocal doses. On a molar basis, the inhibitory action of inhibin is more potent than the stimulatory action of activin (Igarashi et al., 1993). Activin is present in the interstitial cells of the testis and ovary, and is also secreted by the gonadotrophs, acting in a positive autocrine fashion to increase FSH secretion.

13.2.3 Synthesis and Secretion of Luteinizing Hormone and Follicle-Stimulating Hormone

The biosynthesis of LH and FSH is complex, consisting of the classical pathway of transcription and translation, and proceding through extensive post-translational modifications, especially the addition of oligosaccharides. It is regulated at all these levels. The LH β promoter contains binding sites for the estrogen receptor, the cAMP response element binding factor, and a nuclear steroidogenic factor-1 (SF-1).

In the *male*, there is only one pattern of pituitary LH secretion, that is, the basal, episodic discharge. In contrast, there are two basal forms of discharge in the *female*, consisting of a sharp rise followed by a rapid decay in plasma LH levels approximately once each hour during most of the estrous cycle. Then there is an abrupt preovulatory LH rise on the afternoon of proestrus, which lasts for several hours, and upon which ovulation is dependent (see figures 10.15 and 10.16). FSH secretion is pulsatile but the pulses are much more variable in amplitude and frequency than the LH pulses. Similar hormonal changes are seen during the menstrual cycle (figure 13.4).

Chronic stress, or the administration of ACTH, delays sexual maturation in rats through an inhibition of LH secretion, an effect that is dependent upon the adrenal steroids (Mann et al., 1982).

13.2.4 Functions of Luteinizing Hormone and Follicle-Stimulating Hormone

LH has been much more extensively studied than FSH, mainly because of the earlier development of a sensitive radioimmunoassay for LH. LH stimulates steroidogenesis, ovulation, and corpora lutea formation in the female, acting on granulosa and luteal cells in the ovary. In the male, LH stimulates testosterone production by the Leydig cells of the testis, an action that is dependent on FSH induction of Leydig cell LH receptors. LH stimulates spermatogenesis indirectly through its effects on testosterone production.

13.2.4.1 LH Effects on Steroidogenesis

In the *testis*, steroid biosynthesis occurs in the Leydig cells, which are the only testicular cells to have LH receptors. LH stimulates the transport of cholesterol from lipid droplets within the cytoplasm to the inner

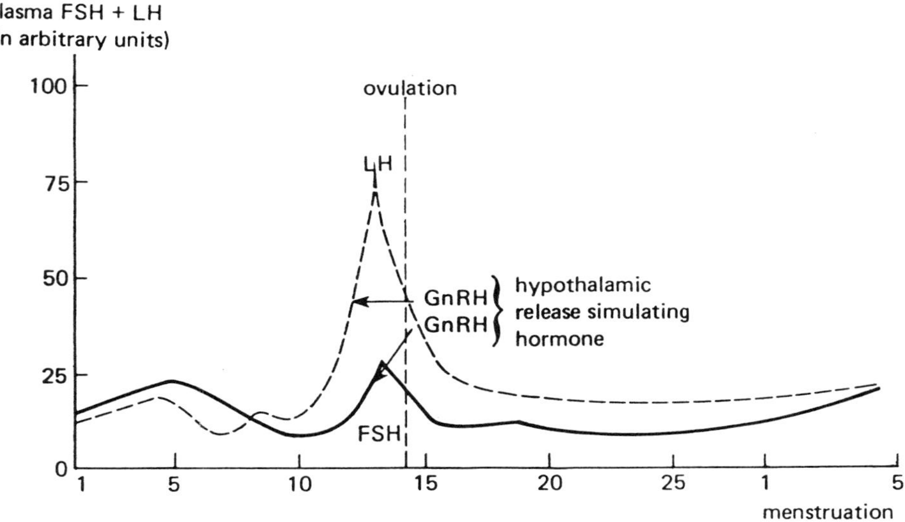

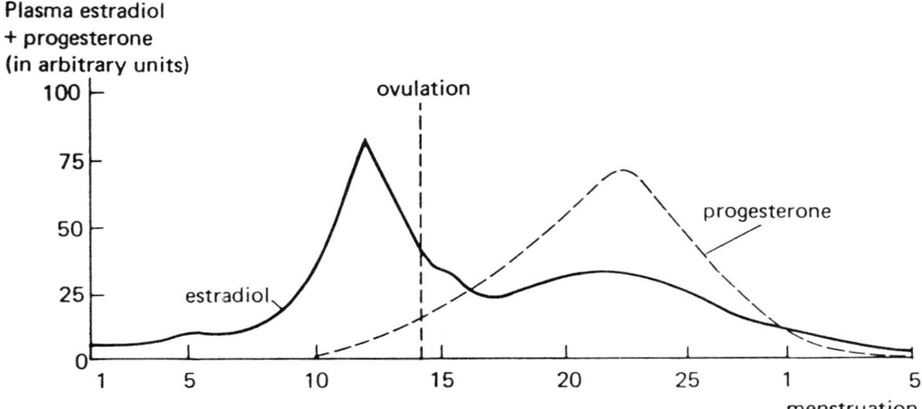

Figure 13.4
Gonadotropin (follicle-stimulating hormone and luteinizing hormone) and ovarian hormones during the menstrual cycle. During the early phase of the cycle, FSH and LH levels rise. Estradiol from the ovary reaches a peak the day before the LH surge, which causes ovulation 24 hours later. In the second, luteal phase of the cycle, estradiol levels decline whereas progesterone levels rise. All gonadotropin and ovarian steroid levels diminish prior to menstruation. GnRH, gonadotropin-releasing hormone.

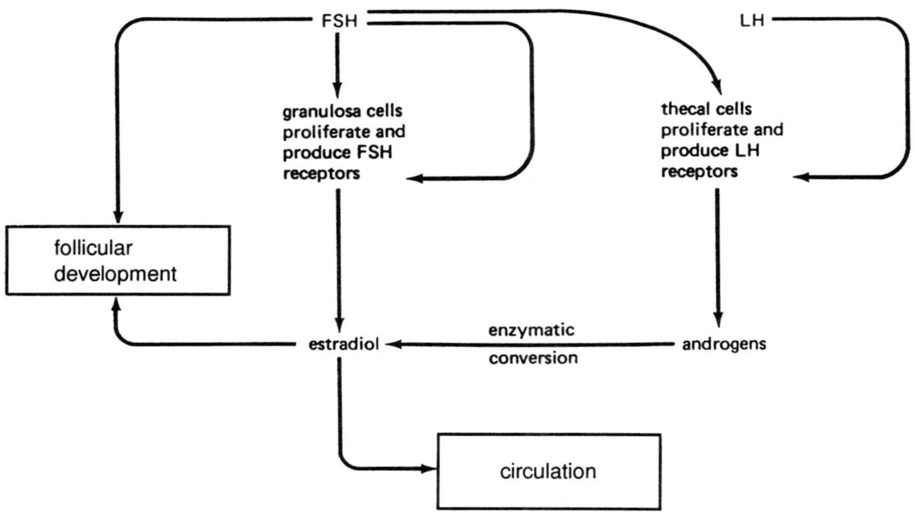

Figure 13.5
The two-cell, two-gonadotropin concept of gonadal steroidogenesis and the synergistic action of follicle-stimulating hormone (FSH) luteinizing hormone (LH), and estradiol necessary for the development of the ovarian follicle. As levels of FSH increase in the first part of the estrous or menstrual cycle, there is an increase in the number of granulosa cells and in their FSH receptors. This enhances the response of the granulosa cells to FSH and large amounts of estradiol are secreted into the circulation and into the antrum of the follicle. FSH also stimulates thecal cell growth and development of thecal LH receptors. LH stimulates the thecal cells to secrete androgens, which diffuse into the follicular granulosa cells where they are converted to estradiol. Estradiol and FSH together regulate follicular development.

mitochondrial membrane, resulting in increased pregnenolone production. Pregnenolone is then transferred to the microsomes to complete the synthesis of androgens.

In the *ovary*, the thecal and the granulosa cells are the major steroid-producing cells. In most species the thecal cells function primarily to produce androgens, and estrogens to a lesser degree, whereas granulosa cells convert androgens produced by the thecal cells and aromatize them to estrogens (figure 13.5). Following luteinization, the process by which granulosa cells differentiate into the luteal cells of the corpus luteum under the influence of LH, the biosynthetic pathway of the granulosa cells is changed so that steroid synthesis is switched from estrogen to progesterone.

13.2.4.2 FSH Effects on the Ovary and Steroidogenesis

FSH binding accelerates early follicular development. This response of the granulosa cells of the follicles is not due to changes in FSH receptor numbers but rather to an increase in the stimulatory G protein of the adenylate cyclase system, and an increased responsiveness to cAMP (Richards and Hedin, 1988). FSH stimulates steroidogenesis and the maturation of the ovum, These are slowly developing phenomena which require relatively constant stimulation. FSH is cleared by the liver much more slowly than is LH, permitting it to have a plasma half-life of from 100 to 250 minutes, considerably longer than the 30-minute half-life of LH.

13.2.4.3 The Two-Cell Type, Two-Gonadotropin Concept

This concept describing cellular cooperation in follicular estrogen and progesterone biosynthesis involves both thecal and granulosa cells, as well as both FSH and LH. The thecal cells are stimulated by LH to produce androgens, which diffuse into the granulosa cells where they are used for estrogen biosynthesis under the influence of FSH. FSH binding sites are exclusively located on granulosa cells. LH binding sites are found initially on thecal cells and only later in the cycle are they found on the granulosa cells, as the process of luteinization commences (see figure 13.5). Progesterone biosynthesis occurs in the granulosa cells initially in response to FSH stimulation, but this is later amplified by LH after the LH receptors have differentiated.

13.2.4.4 FSH Effects on the Testis

In the male, the primary function of FSH is the differentiation of the Sertoli cells in the testis and the maturation of the gametes. The internal environment of the seminiferous tubules is controlled by the Sertoli cells, which are regulated by many hormonal and cellular factors. FSH affects several aspects of Sertoli cell metabolism. The hormone markedly alters energy-yielding reactions, such as phosphorylase activity, leading to glycogen breakdown and energy production, processes essential to the high energy demands of the gametes. FSH also increases Sertoli cell secretion of a Leydig cell stimulatory factor which affects testosterone production by these cells. There is a synergistic action of FSH and LH in men: both are needed to induce quantitatively normal spermatogenesis and inhibin secretion (Bremner and Matsumoto, 1990).

13.2.5 Gonadotropin Receptors and Second Messengers

13.2.5.1 LH Receptors and Second Messengers

The LH receptor is an integral membrane protein with one or more components, found in granulosa, luteal, and Leydig cells. It is activated by LH and, via G proteins, utilizes the adenylate cyclase system and cAMP to regulate the biosynthesis of steroid hormones in gonadal cells. LH acts to stimulate steroidogenesis by directly or indirectly influencing several processes involved in the mobilization, transport, and metabolism of cholesterol, the precursor of the steroids. These pathways are described in detail by Gore-Langton and Armstrong (1988).

13.2.5.2 FSH Receptors and Second Messengers

The FSH receptor, like the LH receptor, is a membrane-bound glycoprotein of approximately 146,000 molecular weight, found chiefly on the granulosa cells of the ovary and the Sertoli cells of the testis. The receptor may be multimeric, containing several subunits. The FSH receptor is probably complexed with G proteins and adenylate cyclase, acting via the cAMP-dependent protein kinase pathway. The interaction of FSH with its receptors is influenced by Ca^{2+}, Mg^{2+}, or Mn^{2+} and inhibited by Co^{2+} or Ni^{2+}, which changes receptor affinity (Reichert and Dattatreyamurty, 1989).

13.2.6 Behavioral Effects of the Gonadotropins

Estrogen is required for lordosis and its behavioral actions are facilitated by progesterone. To the extent that the gonadotropins regulate the gonadal steroids, FSH and LH have indirect behavioral effects. GnRH, on the other hand, facilitates lordosis by acting directly on midbrain neurons, primed with estrogen (Sakuma and Pfaff, 1980).

13.2.7 Clinical Implications of the Gonadotropins

Gonadotropin deficiency is usually managed by gonadal steroid replacement therapy. In *men* the criteria of successful therapy include the maintenance of beard growth, libido, and potency. Administration of excessive amounts of androgens may cause edema, gynecomastia, disturbing sexual drive, nightmares, and acne. Long-standing gonadal insufficiency may take many months before a positive outcome is attained.

In *women*, sex hormone replacement therapy consists of a combination of estradiol and progesterone, which restores the menstrual cycle and reverses the atrophy of the breasts and uterus. This type of hormone replacement therapy is also extensively used in postmenopausal women to reduce circulatory changes (hot flashes), vaginal atrophy, and psychological depression. Estrogen is also believed to provide a neuroprotective action in aging women and perhaps reduce the incidence of Alzheimer's disease.

In cases of infertility due to gonadotropin failure, high doses of an estrogen antagonist (clomiphene) are administered to induce ovulation. Many patients so treated respond with superovulation and multiple fetuses. If clomiphene therapy is unsuccessful, pulsatile administration of GnRH is often attempted, as described in chapter 10. An additional option is the administration of human menopausal gonadotropin (rich in FSH-like gonadotropins) followed by daily injections of hCG, which has LH-like effects (Martin and Reichlin, 1987).

Gonadotropin hypersecretion may cause precocious puberty. The gonadotropin secretion in these children is actually normal but premature, and the best treatment appears to be superagonist GnRH therapy, although there are conflicting opinions about its safety. The superagonist suppresses gonadotropins and sex steroids, reverses sexual maturation, and slows growth rates (Mansfield et al., 1983). Gonadotropin-secreting tumors are fairly rare, develop late in life, and are usually treated by partial surgical removal and x-ray therapy.

13.3 Thyroid-Stimulating Hormone (Thyrotropin)

TSH activity is present in the pituitary glands of all vertebrates studied. Its effects on amphibian metamorphosis following hypophysectomy were dramatically demonstrated by P. E. Smith (1916) (see also chapter 12, section 12.2). The most important function of TSH is control of thyroid gland function, and consequently the secretion of the thyroid hormones thyroxine (T_4) and triiodothyronine (T_3), which influence almost all physiological processes, including early growth and development, reproduction, metabolism, and behavior.

13.3.1 The Importance of Pit-1 in Thyrotroph Development

The development of the thyrotrophs, the TSH-producing cells of the anterior pituitary, is dependent upon the presence of the *Pit-1 transcription factor*. Pit-1 is a pituitary-specific factor which binds to sites within the TSH promoters to activate them. Pit-1 may participate in the physiological regulation of TSH by hypothalamic factors, through increasing the cAMP responsiveness of the promoters (Baringa et al., 1985). In various mouse mutants in which Pit-1 loses its ability to bind DNA, the offspring have very small pituitaries which completely lack GH, PRL, and TSH cells but have normal numbers of corticotrophs and gonadotrophs, indicating that a functional Pit-1 is essential to the growth and development of the somatotrophs, lactotrophs and thyrotrophs (Castrillo et al., 1991). The expression of these three genes can be modulated by changes in the hormonal environment and it is thought that some of these effects may be mediated by Pit-1.

13.3.2 Gene Structure

The gene for the α subunit of TSH encodes a single polypeptide chain of 96 amino acids containing two N-linked carbohydrate groups, in common with the α subunit of the other glycoprotein hormones, LH, FSH, and hCG. The gene is located on the short arm of chromosome 6 and possesses four exons and three introns. The gene for the TSH β subunit encodes a polypeptide chain of 110 amino acids containing one N-linked sugar (Shupnik et al., 1989). This gene is located on the long arm of chromosome 1 and consists of three exons and two introns. Arg is essential to the dimerization of the two subunits.

13.3.3 Glycosylation

The correct subunit conformation is critically dependent upon normal glycosylation. Magner (1990) suggests that TSH may be a prototype of a new class of physiologically essential glycoproteins whose biological functions depend on proper oligosaccharide structures. During translation, the oligosaccharides protect the TSH subunits from intracellular breakdown. In a study of site-directed mutagenesis, when the glycosylation sequence of the TSH β subunit was deleted, TSH synthesis decreased by 90% (Lash et al., 1992). Even more significantly, the structures of the oligosaccharides may be regulated by endocrine factors during TSH biosynthesis, resulting in different forms of TSH being secreted under different physiological and pathological conditions.

13.3.4 Regulation of Thyroid-Stimulating Hormone and the Triiodothyronine Receptor

13.3.4.1 Negative Feedback by Thyroid Hormone

The hypothalamic regulation of TSH by thyrotropin-releasing hormone (TRH) was discussed in chapter 10. TRH not only stimulates TSH biosynthesis and secretion but also regulates the post-translational glycosylation steps in TSH processing (Jackson, 1994). However, TSH secretion is primarily regulated by negative feedback from circulating *thyroid hormone* and the set-point of the thyroid hormone–LTSH interaction is determined by input from the hypothalamus.

The T_3 receptor has been identified in liver and kidney cells as a nuclear receptor, the product of the *c-erb-A* gene, part of a gene superfamily that includes related oncogenes and steroid receptor genes, but other hormones, such as steroids, do not bind to the thyroid hormone receptor.

There are several isoforms of the thyroid hormone receptors (TR) on pituitary thyrotrophs, all of which contain a C-terminal T_3 binding domain and an N-terminal DNA binding domain (Lechan et al., 1994). The most potent thyroid hormone is T_3, which is derived from the precursor hormone T_4 (figure 13.6). The two thyroid hormones receptors that bind T_3 are the TRα and TRβ_2 receptors, which are encoded by two separate thyroid hormone receptor genes,

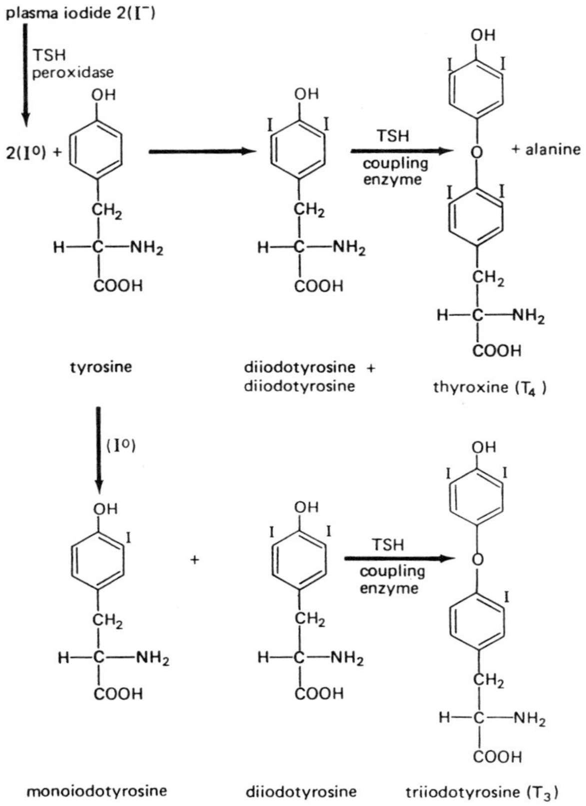

Figure 13.6
The synthesis of thyroid hormones. Before the iodide can be incorporated, it must be oxidized (I°) by a peroxidase system of enzymes, which is under the influence of thyroid-stimulating hormone (TSH).

TRβ_2 on chromosome 3 and TRα on chromosome 17 (Evans, 1988). The TRβ_2 isoform, a protein of 514 amino acids, is found in the anterior pituitary and both the TRβ_2 and the TRα isoforms coexist in TRH neurons in the hypothalamus. This permits T_3 to regulate TSH at both the hypothalamic and pituitary levels.

Serotonin participates in the physiological control of TSH secretion by increasing TRH secretion or facilitating the pituitary TSH response to TRH (Silva and Nunes, 1996). The *endogenous opiates* also stimulate TSH secretion, predominantly during the nocturnal TSH surge in humans (Samuels et al., 1994).

13.3.4.2 Inhibitors of TSH Secretion

Stress is a potent inhibitor of TSH secretion in humans and many other species. This involves both the CNS and the modulatory effects of other stress-evoked hormones, such as ACTH and corticosteroids. Both dopamine and somatostatin inhibit TSH secretion through direct effects on the pituitary thyrotroph. It is also possible that GABA inhibits TSH secretion.

13.3.4.3 Acute Cold

Acute exposure to cold evokes a rapid release of TSH in the rat and the human infant, but is absent in the adult human. This appears to be a neuroendocrine reflex involving hypothalamic TRH release. In the rat, chronic exposure to cold elevates plasma levels of TSH and free thyroid hormones, which remain high during 5 days of cold stress, whereas plasma ACTH levels return to normal after the first day. This indicates that cold stress activates the HPA system briefly, as does any stress, but that prolonged cold stress specifically targets the hypothalamo-pituitary-thyroid axis as a means of maintaining body temperature (Fukuhara et al., 1996).

13.3.5 TSH Stimulation of Thyroid Hormone Synthesis, Storage, Release, and Recycling

TSH binds to thyroid follicular cell membranes, activating the adenylate cyclase system and increasing cAMP levels. TSH increases the amount and the activity of the RER and the Golgi apparatus, the synthetic elements of the thyroid follicle. TSH stimulation increases pinocytotic activity at the apical follicular membrane, resulting in the engulfing of the colloidal protein *thyroglobulin* by phagocytosis into the follicle cells to be used as the substrate for the synthesis of the thyroid hormones. In the absence of TSH, the columnar cells of the follicle become flattened and colloid accumulates in the swollen lumen (goiter).

TSH also stimulates the *incorporation of iodide* into thyroglobulin for tyrosine iodination and the subsequent synthesis of the thyroid hormones T_4 and T_3. The follicular cells trap iodide and transport it across an electrical gradient across the cell to the luminal surface where it is converted by a peroxidase to an oxidized species of iodine (I°). I° is then incorporated into tyrosine groups of thyroglobulin. The first product is monoiodotyrosine (MIT), followed by diiodotyrosine (DIT). Two molecules of MIT condense to form T_4, a synthesis that is speeded up by TSH. The most active thyroid hormone, T_3, is probably formed by the coupling of one molecule of MIT and one of DIT, or by the loss of iodine from T_4 (see figure 13.6).

The hormone-containing thyroglobulin contains about 18 molecules of T_4 for every T_3 molecule. In this form, the thyroid hormones may be stored in the follicles for several months. Thyroglobulin is usually broken down to its constituent T_3 and T_4 components, as well as to other iodinated compounds, by a proteolytic enzyme. The hormones are released into the circulation, whereas the thyroglobulin remains in the follicles to be recycled. This reaction, like all the others involving the synthesis and release of thryoid hormones, is stimulated by TSH. The second messenger is cAMP and cAMP has the same effect as TSH stimulation.

An immunoglobulin secreted by lymphocytes, *long-acting thyroid stimulator (LATS)*, is present in the plasma of hyperthyroid persons but not in normal persons. It seems to stimulate the thyroid in a manner similar to that of TSH (through cAMP), but its action is much longer lasting. It is not known whether it is the cause or result of hyperthyroidism.

13.3.6 Pulsatile and Circadian Secretion of Thyroid-Stimulating Hormone

TSH is secreted in a pulsatile manner. In humans, TSH pulse frequency is approximately nine per 24-hour period, increasing slightly in hypothyroid patients to 11 per 24-hour period. The rat has a much higher peak frequency, about 60 per 24 hours and increasing to about 10 times that frequency in hypothyroid rats (Bruhn et al., 1992). There is also a circadian rhythm for TSH secretion. In humans, TSH rises in the evening to reach a peak between 11 P.M. and 4 A.M. It drops to its lowest point around 11 A.M. (Salvador et al., 1988). In the nocturnal rat, TSH peaks between 10 A.M. and 2 P.M., with lowest levels at 6 A.M.

13.3.7 Clinical Implications of Thyroid-Stimulating Hormone

TSH is not used clinically, but the availability of TRH for clinical studies has resulted in its extensive use in humans. Apart from its therapeutic use, the administration of TRH yields important information about the negative feedback control of TSH through the hypothalamo-pituitary-thyroid axis and assists in the diagnosis of the dysfunctional state. Most TSH-deficient patients are treated with synthetic L-thyroxine.

13.3.7.1 Hypothyroidism

Insufficient production of the thyroid hormones may be hypothalamic, pituitary, or thyroid in origin. It may be a failure to convert T_4 to T_3, the biologically active hormone, or a genetic failure in the development of the thyroid hormone receptors. Hypothyroidism may also be the result of antibodies against thyroid hormone receptors, or due to a lack of iodine in the diet. If hypothyroidism occurs in utero, or in early postnatal life, cretinism may result, with characteristic mental and growth retardation. In *adults*, hypothyroidism is characterized by low basal metabolic rate, decreased cardiac output, low body temperature, lethargy, mental depression, weight gain, and edema of the face and eyelids. Many of these symptoms are related to decreased activity of the sympathoadrenal system.

13.3.7.2 Hyperthyroidism

Hyperthyroidism may also be hypothalamic, pituitary, or thyroid in origin. As might be expected from the negative feedback control of the pituitary-thyroid axis, patients with hyperthyroidism do not respond to TRH injection since the high levels of thyroid hormone inhibit the secretion of TSH. Hyperthyroidism is characterized by elevated basal metabolism, increased cardiac output, increased body temperature, and many other manifestations of increased sympathoadrenal activity. Antithyroid drugs that inhibit the formation of thyroid hormones include inhibitors of iodide transport, the thionamides, sulfonamides, and the sulfonylureas. Tumors secreting TRH, TSH, or thyroid hormones may be removed surgically or by irradiation.

13.3.7.3 Psychological Disturbances

Patients with abnormally elevated or depressed thyroid function, whatever the initial cause, often show disturbances in cognition and behavior. There is a correlation between a blunted TSH response to TRH in patients with clinical depression, and a small number of depressed patients show improvement with TRH (Kastin et al., 1972).

13.3.7.4 Muscle Diseases

Myogenesis, muscle growth, and differentiation are influenced by thyroid hormone levels. Thyroid hormone may have a direct effect on the expression of some muscle genes: in cardiac muscle it has been clearly demonstrated that DNA sequences required for thyroid hormone induction are present in the 5′ flanking sequence of the α-myosin heavy chain gene (Gustafson et al., 1987). There is an association between immune-mediated thyroid disorders and acquired myasthenia gravis in hypothyroid humans and in dogs.

13.4 The Growth Hormone Family

Growth hormone not only promotes growth but is an important anabolic hormone, stimulating protein synthesis, glyconeogenesis, and lipolysis. *Prolactin* was named after its lactogenic action in rabbits and pigeons, but PRL has no lactogenic activity in humans. It does, however, have a mammotropic effect, stimulating cell proliferation in the mammary glands and milk secretion (Walker et al., 1991). There is considerable overlap in the range of functions affected by GH and PRL. Both influence growth and development, osmoregulation, reproduction, lipid metabolism, and adrenal steroidogenesis, but the effects may vary in intensity and between species. GH induces growth in invertebrates as well as vertebrates and, in mammals, postnatal growth is dependent on GH. While *placental lactogen* (*PL*) is produced by the placenta and not the pituitary, it is closely related to the GH family and is therefore included in this discussion.

13.4.1 Evolution of the Growth Hormone and Prolactin Family

The two branches of the GH and PRL family of neuropeptides diverged prior to the evolution of vertebrates. The *chorionic somatomammotropins* of primates also show close homology to GH and probably diverged from GH during primate evolution. Similarly, the PLs bear a strong sequence homology to PRL. The analogous protein in fish has sequences intermediate between GH and PRL and is termed *somatolactin*.

Both GH and PRL are found in all vertebrate groups except the subphylum Agnatha (e.g., lamprey) and there is strong evidence that the GH/PRL gene duplication occurred approximately 430 million years ago from the ancestral proto–GH-PRL (Niall, 1982; Miller and Eberhardt, 1983). It is also possible that gene duplication occurred even earlier (perhaps 700 to 800 million years ago), prior to the separation of the vertebrates and the ancestors of the molluscs and arthropods, since putative GH and PRL analogs have been found in arthropods and molluscs, and even in some protozoa. The duplication of the primordial gene probably gave rise to two separate precursors, one for the GH and PL genes, and the other for the PRL gene. The GH-PL and PRL genes then segregated onto two different chromosomes, since the human GH-PL genes exist in multiple copies on chromosome 17, whereas the human PRL gene is a single copy on chromosome 6 (Owerbach et al., 1980). Following divergence of these precursor genes, distinct regulatory sequences were introduced, permitting the differential regulation of the three hormones.

All mammalian GH and PL genes are structurally similar, having five exons and four introns, and they share 91% to 99% sequence identity throughout their coding regions. Of the 66 kb in the human PL-GH cluster, 21% of the sequence consists of 48 copies of the 300-bp repetitive *Alu* sequence (E. Y. Chen et al., 1989). The human PL-GH locus probably evolved in three steps, involving large sequence duplications that preferentially begin and end with *Alu* elements (figure 13.7). Primate GH has several differences from other mammalian GHs. Humans and the rhesus monkey have five GH genes. Specific mutations in primate GH permitted it to rapidly acquire PRL activity, which may be advantageous in widening the scope of GH action.

13.4.2 Structures of Growth Hormone, Prolactin, and Placental Lactogen

Human GH is a single-chain polypeptide of 191 amino acids, with two disulfide bonds between Cys^{53} and Cys^{165}, and between Cys^{182} and Cys^{189}. Human PL is very similar to GH with the same number of disulfide bonds and amino acids, most of which are identical. Human PRL, with a molecular mass of 23 kD, has 199 amino acids and a third disulfide bond between Cys^{4} and Cys^{11}. Although the PRL molecule is encoded by a single gene, it is structurally heterogeneous due to post-translational modifications.

13.4.3 Growth Hormone and Prolactin Receptors

The GH and PRL receptors belong to the *hematopoietic superfamily*, which includes receptors for erythropoietin, the interleukins, the interferons, and several white blood cell–stimulating factors. These

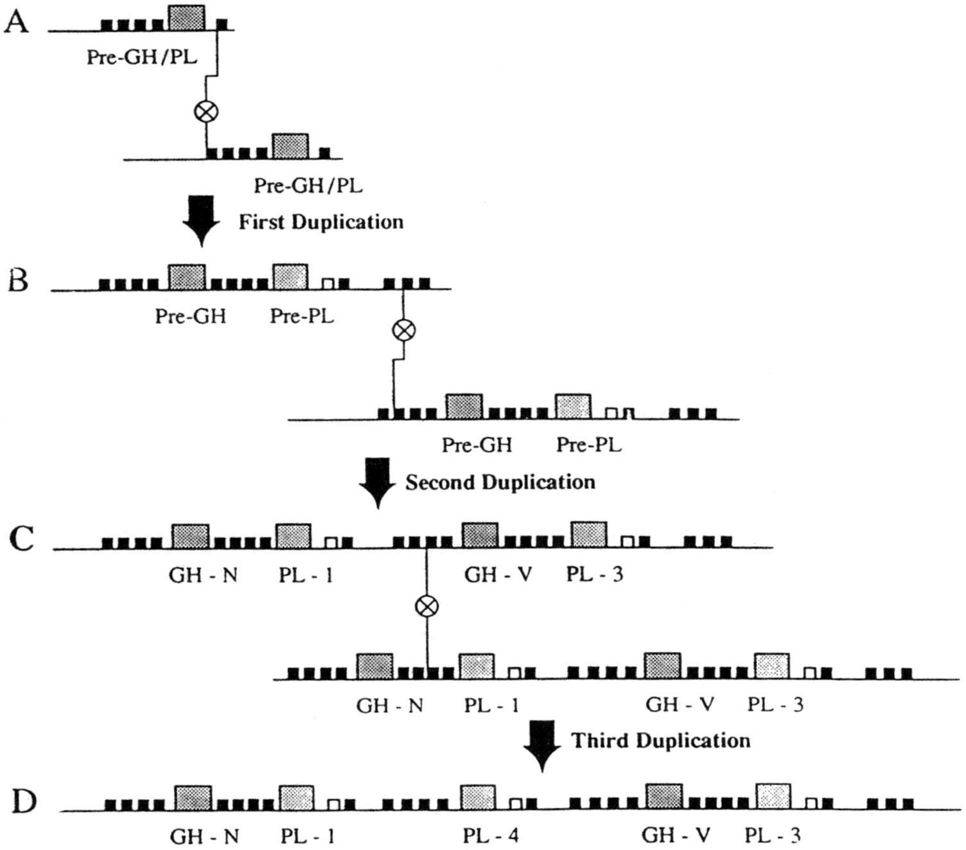

Figure 13.7
Schematic diagram of the evolution of the human growth hormone–placental lactogen (GH/PL) gene family. Gene sequences are indicated by stippled boxes; Alu sequences by solid boxes, and partial alu sequences by open boxes. The last indicate differences between the 3′ ends of the PL and GH genes. The present gene family is believed to have originated from a single ancestral gene by three duplications and nonreciprocal crossover events. (From Hirt et al., 1987).

receptors are all glycoproteins with an extracellular N-terminus and a single transmembrane domain. The tertiary structure of most of these hormones is organized as four antiparallel α helices. The signal transduction systems used by GH are still largely unknown but PRL activates tyrosine kinase, leading to phosphorylation of transcription factors known as signal transducer and activator of transcription.

13.4.3.1 The GH Receptor

GH molecules *circulate* in both the bound and free forms. The bound hormones form a complex with large and small serum *binding proteins*. The smaller protein, with a higher affinity, is identical to the extracellular domain of the GH receptor. One GH molecule binds two GH receptors and although the two binding sites on GH are distinct they differ only in one residue (Asn-19). GH rapidly causes dimerization of the receptor which initiates signal transduction (Cunningham et al., 1991). These events, starting from the release of GH from the pituitary, are summarized in figure 13.8.

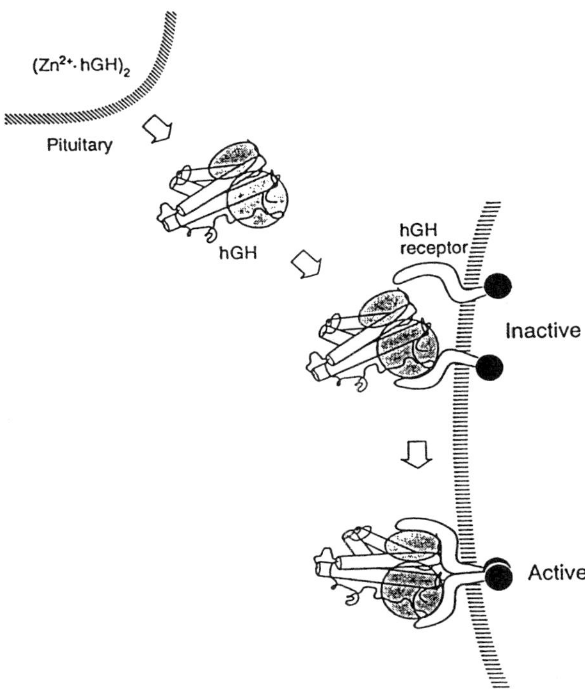

Figure 13.8
Summary of molecular endocrinology of human growth hormone (hGH). hGH is released as a $(Zn^{2+}\text{-hGH})_2$ complex from the pituitary. On dilution in the circulation, the dimer dissociates into a monomeric form, in which it is available to bind via site I to the hGH receptor. The membrane-bound hGH then complexes with a second receptor molecule using site II on hGH and binding determinants on the first receptor. Receptor dimerization by GH initiates signal transduction. (From Wells et al., 1993.)

Because GH lacks specific target sites but instead affects most tissues, which respond with different biological reactions, the GH receptors are heterogeneous in structure and may have different signal transduction mechanisms, none of which have been positively identified to date. The GH receptor is a single-chain polypeptide of approximately 638 amino acids, deviating somewhat in different species. The size of the native GH receptor is probably 120 kD, but it varies with tissue-specific modifications and possible dimerization.

The *extracellular domain* is extensively *N*-glycosylated at Asp residues, and the NH_2 portion consists of three disulfide loops linking six cysteines, which are highly conserved across species. The *intracellular domain* is essential to signal transduction and may be subdivided into subdomains responsible for distinct GH actions. The proximal portion is responsible for the proliferative actions of GH: only the 54 amino acids adjacent to the membrane are needed for proliferative action, and this region includes a conserved, proline-rich box common to all the receptors in this group that have proliferative functions. This includes the PRL receptor. Residues 249 to 381 are necessary for the metabolic effects of GH and residues 436 to 620 are involved in transcriptional events.

In mammals, the liver possesses the highest concentration of GH receptors but GH receptors are also found in many other tissues, including adipose tissue, lymphatic and immune cells, pancreas, intestine, lungs, heart, kidney, brain, cartilage, skeletal muscle, corpus luteum, and testis. The GH receptor is rapidly internalized following binding with GH and most GH receptors are found associated with intracellular membranes and organelles.

a. *Regulation of the GH Receptor*

A markedly reduced number of GH receptors and reduced GH secretion are found in different conditions of growth failure, as occurs in chronic renal failure or fasting. The rise in estrogen levels in puberty increases GH receptor number in the liver of female rats, and the receptor number doubles or triples during pregnancy. GH induces an upregulation of both GH and PRL receptors.

13.4.3.2 The PRL Receptor

The classic PRL receptor is a glycosylated protein with a molecular weight of approximately 41 kD and may exist as a higher-molecular-weight dimer. It consists of a 210–amino acid extracellular domain, a single 24–amino acid transmembrane region, and a short 57–amino acid cytosolic domain. There are five extracellular cysteines, four of which are close to the N-terminal region, with the fifth near the transmembrane domain. Three different forms of the PRL receptor are generated by the alternative splicing of a single gene and the many diverse effects of PRL are attributed to the heterogeneity of the PRL molecule and its receptors. One of these is a larger variant of the PRL receptor, with a longer cytosolic domain (358 amino acids) which has been cloned from rabbit mammary glands (Edery et al., 1989).

Binding sites for PRL are widely distributed in mammalian tissue, including the mammary gland, ovary, uterus and placenta, the testis, epididymis, seminal vesicle, and prostate. The liver, pancreas, intestine, kidney, lymphatic tissue, and immune cells, brain, and eye also contain PRL receptors. The long form of the PRL receptor is present in mammary gland (Edery et al., 1989), hypothalamic DA neurons (Arbogast and Voogt, 1997), in the PVN, SON, medial preoptic area, and in the arcuate and ventromedial nuclei, regions that support maternal behavior (Bakowska and Morrell, 1997). Although PRL receptors are absent from adult olfactory bulb, they are abundant in the olfactory system of the fetal and neonatal rat, implicating a novel role for PRL in the regulation of neonatal behavior and maternal-infant interactions (Freemark et al., 1996).

A soluble form of the PRL and GH receptor has been found in milk (Postel-Vinay et al., 1991). Primate GH is also lactogenic and binds to both GH and PRL receptors. Following binding of PRL to its receptor, the complex is rapidly internalized (Kelly et al., 1994), which accounts for the high concentration of PRL receptors in intracellular membranes and organelles. In a manner suggestive of the GH receptor, the aggregation of two or more PRL receptors appears to be needed to evoke a response.

Regulation of the PRL receptor varies according to the target organ and physiological state. Estradiol appears to regulate the short form of the hypothalamic PRL receptor but not the long form (Shamgochian et al., 1995). During pregnancy, PRL receptor number in the mammary gland is limited by high estrogen and progesterone levels, but PRL receptors increase markedly in number during lactation, following the steep fall in ovarian and placental steroids that occurs at parturition. Contact with pups induces the expression of PRL receptor mRNA in the choroid plexus of the brain of lactating rats, coincident with the expression of maternal behavior (Sugiyama et al., 1996). Some aspects of maternal behavior, such as crouching and licking, can be induced in male rats by contact with foster pups, and this behavior is associated with increased serum PRL and long-form PRL receptor mRNA (Sakaguchi et al., 1996). In the liver, PRL receptors are stimulated by estrogen, whereas in the prostate, PRL receptors are increased by testosterone and decreased by estrogen. PRL up-regulates its own receptors.

13.4.4 Differentiation of Somatotrophs and Lactotrophs

In most species, the GH-secreting cells, the somatotrophs, are the most numerous of the pituitary cell types and human GH may make up almost 50% of the cell population. The somatotrophs and lactotrophs appear after the other three anterior pituitary cell types—the somatotrophs appearing on day 16 of embryogenesis, whereas the lactotrophs are not evident until 4 to 10 days after birth. GH and PRL are usually found in discrete secretory granules, but some pituitary cells secrete both GH and PRL, some of which may be colocalized within the same granule (Frawley, et al., 1982, 1989). The specific expression of GH in somatotrophs and PRL in lactotrophs has been attributed to the short promoter in the 5′-flanking region of the GH and PRL genes. Pit-1 binds at specific sites of the GH and PRL genes, to activate the promoters via cAMP (see section 13.3.1) and may be involved in determining the expression of these genes and thus the final pathway leading to either GH or PRL production. There is a sexual dimorphism in the postpubertal expression of GH and PRL, with males having higher GH levels and females higher PRL levels, and it is probable that this is due to differential levels of Pit-1, and of Pit-1 mRNA expression in the somatotrophs and lactotropes of the two sexes (Gonzalez-parra et al., 1996).

13.4.5 Mammosomatotropes

Mammosomatotrophs are plurihormonal cells found in normal pituitaries and in pituitary tumors that secrete GH and PRL. Mammosomatotrophs possess receptors and secretory characteristics of both somatotrophs and lactotrophs, although they are more like the former. Mammosomatotrophs form a substantial percentage of pituitary cells, but their number varies considerably according to age, sex, and physiological state. They proliferate under the influence of estrogen, whereas testosterone has an inhibitory influence on mammosomatotroph generation. LHRH tips the balance in favor of PRL-secreting cells. Interesting evidence for a regulatory role for GHRH comes from transgenic mice expressing the GHRH gene: these animals develop a massive increase in the number of pituitary mammosomatotrophs (Asa et al., 1990). The apparently unlimited ability of these cells to differentiate into either somatotrophs or lactotrophs, depending on the hormonal environment, may indicate that they are either transitional cell types or that they represent a "stem" cell capable of transformation into either type.

13.5 Growth Hormone

13.5.1 Synthesis and Secretion of Growth Hormone

The number and size of the somatotrophs and their secretory granules vary during ontogeny, puberty, and the reproductive stage, and with age. These changes are not reflected in the basal level of circulating GH but they are accompanied by decreased frequency and reduced amplitude of episodic GH release. GH is *synthesized* in the somatotrophs as a pre-GH molecule of 217 amino acids. Subsequent cleavage yields the 191–amino acid neuropeptide hormone, with a molecular weight of 22 kD. A smaller 20-kD molecule is synthesized following alternative splicing. The amount of GH produced by the pituitary amounts to almost half the total content of neuropeptides in the anterior pituitary.

GH is *synthesized* in the somatotrophs as a pre-GH molecule of 217 amino acids. Subsequent cleavage yields the 191–amino acid neuropeptide hormone, with a molecular weight of 22 kD. A smaller 20-kD molecule is synthesized following alternative splicing. GH molecules circulate in both the bound and free forms. The binding of GH to serum binding protein and to its receptor are described in section 13.4.2.1.

13.5.2 Neural and Humoral Regulation of Growth Hormone

The regulation of GH secretion by GHRH and somatostatin was discussed in chapter 10. This chapter emphasizes regulation by peripheral hormones and growth factors such as the insulin-like growth factors (IGFs) (see section 13.5.2.3) acting at the level of gene transcription or the interaction between GHRH, somatostatin, and GH. Neural systems and their transmitters also play an important role in the regulation of GH.

15.5.2.1. Pulsatile Secretion of GH

In all mammalian species, including humans, GH is secreted in a pulsatile manner, which is dependent on sequential crucial events that regulate normal growth during infancy, puberty, and adolescence. The pattern is also influenced by age, sex, food intake, nutritional status, and physical activity. The diurnal pattern of GH secretion in young and old men is shown in figure 13.9.

The pulsatile pattern results from the interaction of the two opposing regulatory hypothalamic neurohormones, GHRH and somatostatin (see figure 10.17), both of which are necessary for pulsatile GH secretion, but the pattern is markedly affected by neural input. The adrenergic systems affect GH secretion in a complex manner. GH secretion is stimulated by α_2-adrenergic agonists but negatively modulated by α_1- and β-adrenergic agonists, which act on somatostatin, preventing its release. The cholinergic systems are also involved: ACh seems to inhibit hypothalamic release of somatostatin.

13.5.2.2 GH Regulates Its Own Pulsatile Secretion

Ultrashort-loop feedback is exerted by GH on pituitary somatotrophs, which have GH receptors. However, GH receptors are also found on lactotrophs and thyrotrophs and autoregulation could be mediated through paracrine factors, such as the IGFs produced by these cells (Harvey et al., 1993). *Short-loop feedback* occurs through GH involvement with reciprocal feedback actions on hypothalamic somatostatin and GHRH neurons. High levels of GH result in an increase in somatostatin mRNA and somatostatin levels, and a decrease in GHRH mRNA and GHRH secre-

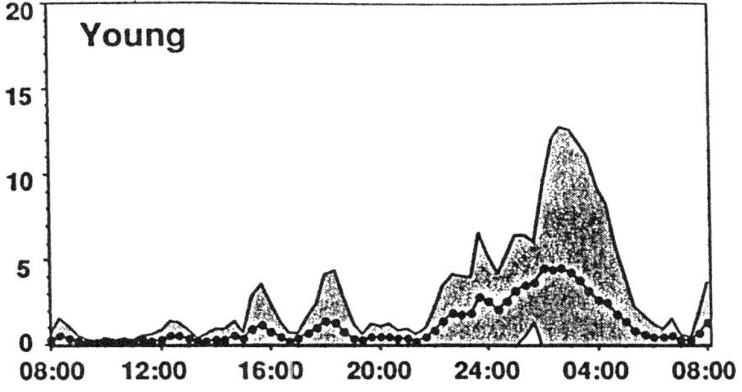

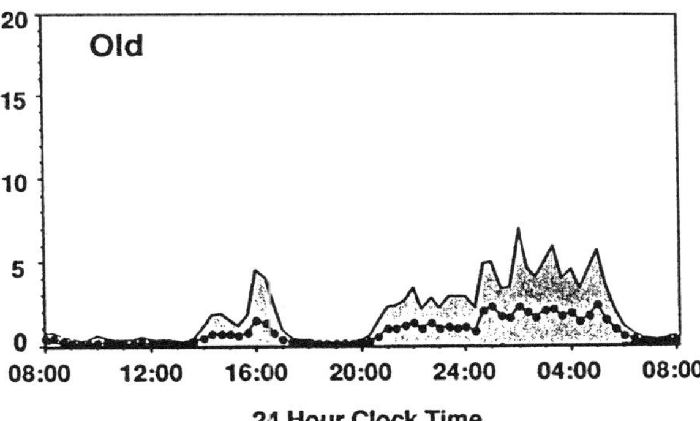

Figure 13.9
The normal diurnal pattern of growth hormone secretion in young (age 26 ± 4years) men and the reduced nocturnal peak amplitude in old (68 ± 6years) men, sampled at 20-minute intervals. (From Corpas et al., 1993.)

tion. A fall in GH has the opposite effects, that is, a decrease in somatostatin mRNA and somatostatin, accompanied by an increase in GHRH mRNA and GHRH secretion.

13.5.2.3 The Long-Loop Feedback via Peripheral Humoral Factors

This is a slower system and involves pathways mediated by peripheral endocrines and metabolites. Unlike other pituitary hormones, GH does not have a specific

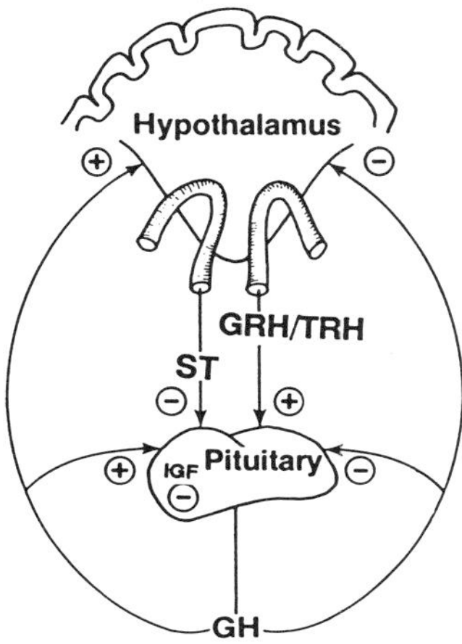

Figure 13.10
Autoregulation of growth hormone (GH) secretion. At hypothalamic sites, GH stimulates the release of somatostatin (ST) and inhibits the release of growth hormone–releasing hormone (GRH) and thyrotropin-releasing hormone (TRH). At pituitary sites, ST may inhibit GH synthesis and release directly, or indirectly through increased activity of insulin-like growth factors (IGF). (From Harvey, 1995.)

target organ that provides a specific secretion that acts as a feedback mechanism for GH. GH has widespread effects on the growth and metabolism of most tissues, and consequently there are central and peripheral sites at which GH acts to regulate its own secretion (figure 13.10). Some of these factors are depicted in figure 13.11. These include the following:

a. Insulin-Like Growth Factors

IGFs (formerly called somatomedins) are synthesized in the liver and other peripheral tissues in response to GH stimulation and act on both hypothalamic and pituitary receptors to inhibit GH secretion. IGF-I and IGF-II are structural homologs of the insulin A and B chains. The main IGF is IGF-I, which stimulates somatostatin synthesis and release, and directly inhibits

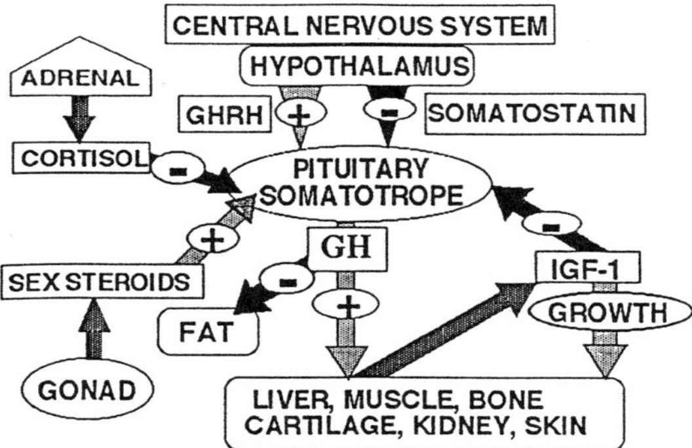

Figure 13.11
Physiological regulation of growth hormone (GH) and insulin-like growth factor–1 (IGF-1) secretion. The pituitary somatotroph (GH-secreting cell) is under dual stimulatory (GH-releasing hormone, GHRH) and inhibitory (somatostatin) control by the CNS, and negative feedback control by IGF-1. In addition, gonadal steroids exert a positive modulating effect at the pituitary level. GH stimulates IGF-1 production at various peripheral tissues. GH, acting primarily via locally released (paracrine) and secreted (endocrine) IGF-1, has stimulatory effects on growth and differentiation of a variety of tissues, and also promotes lipolysis and loss of body fat. (From Corpas et al., 1993.)

GHRH synthesis and release. IGF-I also acts on the pituitary to inhibit GH gene transcription and GH release, a topic discussed in detail in Harvey et al. (1995, pp. 163–148). IGFs are also synthesized in the pituitary in response to GH and directly inhibit basal GH release and the transcription of the GH gene. The mechanism may be via autocrine or paracrine effects, or both, on the somatotrophs, which have IGF receptors. The effects of GH on growth, including chondrogenesis, skeletal growth, and protein synthesis, are all mediated by IGF-I. The effects on carbohydrate and lipid metabolism, on the other hand, appear to be direct effects of GH on the target tissues.

b. Sex Steroids

There is a sexually dimorphic pattern of GH release, with males having higher but less frequent pulses than females. The "default" pattern of GH secretion is that of the female, and it is the exposure to androgen during the critical period of postnatal development (see chapter 9, section 9.5) that establishes the characteristics of the GH pulse in male rats. The sex steroids probably act directly on the expression of somatostatin and GHRH in the hypothalamus. In humans, the sex differences in the pattern on GH secretion are less evident: both estradiol and androgens increase the amplitude of the GH pulse. However, estrogens inhibit growth probably because of their depressive effect on liver production of IGFs.

c. Thyroid Hormones, Glucocorticoids, and Activin

The *thyroid hormones* and *corticosteroids* are key ingredients in the regulation of the hypothalamic-somatotroph axis. Both these hormones are active at the level of the pituitary, rather than of the hypothalamus. T_3 is an important positive regulator of the rat GH gene (Brent et al., 1989). It regulates transcription by the binding of its nuclear receptor to a *cis*-element thyroid hormone reponse element. Adrenocortical function is stimulated by GH, and glucocorticoids may provide a long-loop feedback secretion control. Glucocorticoids enhance GH gene transcription and increase GHRH receptor synthesis, but hypersecretion of glucocorticoids inhibits normal growth in all species studied. Activin produced by the gonadotrophs acts in a paracrine manner to decrease GH mRNA levels, and, by decreasing Pit-1 binding to the GH promoter, inhibits the action of the promoter and decreases somatotroph proliferation (Struthers et al., 1992).

d. Immune factors

GH has many stimulatory effects on immune function (reviewed in Harvey et al., 1995, pp. 407–413). Thymic factors and cytokines provide a long-loop reciprocal influence on GH secretion at both the hypothalamic and pituitary levels.

e. Metabolic Factors

As might be expected from the wide-ranging effects of GH on tissue metabolism, the products of carbohydrate and fat metabolism, in turn, provide another long-loop inhibitory mechanism controlling GH. The levels of glucose and free fatty acids are inversely related to GH levels, providing a fine day-to-day and hour-to-hour control of GH release that is correlated with the immediate metabolic state of the organism. A drop in blood glucose due to prolonged fasting, strenuous exercise, or hypersecretion of insulin rapidly raises GH levels (figure 13.12). Feeding causes a drop in plasma GH levels.

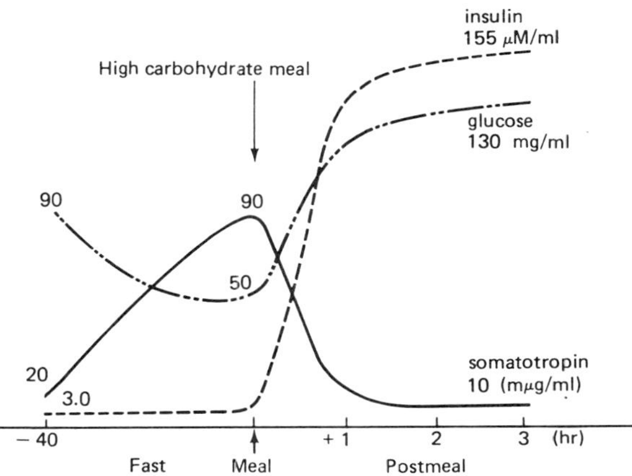

Figure 13.12
Low blood glucose levels induce a marked rise in growth hormone (GH, somatotropin) titers, whereas insulin levels are severely depressed. A meal rich in carbohydrates raises both blood glucose and insulin levels and GH levels fall. (From Roth et al., 1963.)

13.5.3 Actions of Growth Hormone

In normal mammals, including humans, GH causes an increase in body weight and height, skeletal growth, nitrogen retention (muscle growth), and, in rodents, increased tail length. GH increases protein, fat, and carbohydrate metabolism. Its effect on cartilage deposition forms the basis for the most widely used bioassay for GH: the tibia test, which measures the width of the cartilage plate of the tibia from a hypophysectomized rat or mouse as a response to GH. The skeletal response to GH is much greater if GH is administered in a pulsatile manner, rather than by continuous infusion.

Genetic dwarf models have been used extensively to study GH mechanisms. Transgenic mice expressing a mutant GH unable to cause GH receptor dimerization fail to grow (W. Y. Chen et al., 1991). The Ames dwarf mouse, the result of a spontaneous mutation in a colony of laboratory mice at the University of Iowa in Ames, grow to only one-third the size of normal mice but live at least a year longer. These mice lack not only GH but also TSH and PRL, complicating the interpretation of the role of GH and longevity. In addition, both spontaneous and transgenic dwarf mice lack somatostatin (Hurley et al., 1997).

Similarly, the Snell dwarf mouse, whether the spontaneous or transgenic mutant, lacks GH, PRL, TSH, and somatostatin. Administration of GH to this dwarf mouse increases growth rate and plasma concentrations of IGF-I, increases the tibial ossification center and the size of the metaphysis (growth zone adjacent to the epiphysis), and increases the number of capillaries in the metaphysis. GH also affects protein metabolism in these dwarf models, as shown by an increase in the rate of protein synthesis in muscle. In GH-deficient children receiving GH therapy, protein metabolism is markedly improved, as measured by an increase in the rate of whole-body protein synthesis, protein degradation, and protein accretion.

13.5.3.1 Effects on Other Peripheral Hormones

In addition to its effect on IGFs, already discussed, GH increases insulin and glucagon secretion. In the thyroid, GH appears to increase the conversion of T_4 to T_3, the active form of the hormone. GH may also stimulate the adrenal cortex in some species and has been reported to play a modulatory role in the actions of the gonadal steroids.

13.5.3.2 Effects on Sleep

The temporal relationship between the first few hours of sleep and the pulsatile secretion of GH is present in normal persons of both sexes from early childhood until late adulthood. In adults, most of the GH pulses during sleep coincide with slow wave sleep, and this secretion of GH is basically dependent on GHRH. Both GH and GHRH promote slow wave sleep, and as the secretion of GH decreases by two- to threefold in adults 30 to 40 years old, so does the amount of slow wave sleep. Further decrease in GH secretion occurs with aging, coincident with the characteristic insomnia of senescence (Vancauter and Plat, 1996).

13.5.4 Growth Hormone Secretion in Childhood and Adolescence

Prior to puberty, the gonadal steroids do not seem to be of importance in the regulation of human GH. Puberty, however, has dramatic effects on GH physiology. A characteristic feature is the *pubertal growth spurt*, which occurs in girls at an average age of 11 to 12 years, and in boys at 13 to 14 years. Endogenous GH levels rise during middle to late puberty, associated with marked increases in circulating gonadal steroids, and the sex hormones, together with GH, are the decisive factors regulating the pubertal growth spurt. Studies of children with deficiencies in either GH or hypoganadism, or a combination of these defects, show that both GH and the gonadal steroids are required for normal adolescent growth. However, in children with precocious puberty and GH deficiency, the sex steroids seem able to promote adolescent growth independent of GH secretion (Attie et al., 1990). The gonadal steroids also have a limiting effect on ultimate height gain, acting on skeletal maturation and the closure of the epiphysial plates, which occurs earlier in females than in males.

13.5.5 Clinical Implications of Growth Hormone

13.5.5.1 Hyposecretion of GH

a. Deficiencies in GH due to Hypothalamic or Pituitary Disorders

As discussed in chapter 10, section 10.1.4.9, patients lacking GH are often administered GHRH provided that the pituitary is responsive. The main disadvantage of GHRH administration is the requirement for frequent injections.

In childhood, severe GH deficiency leads to *dwarfism*, whereas lesser deficiencies result in various degrees of *growth failure*. Skeletal maturation is delayed and other organ systems are often affected. The GH deficiency may be of pituitary or hypothalamic origin. Hypothalamic or pituitary GH deficiency may be successfully treated with recombinant human GH. The use of recombinant human GH not only provides a practically unlimited supply of the hormone but it precludes the possibility of contamination of the natural pituitary hormone with viruses causing Creutzfeldt-Jakob disease. In *adults*, GH deficiency leads to muscle weakness, fatigue, and a general feeling of malaise. There is a relative increase in adipose tissue mass. GH administration is usually beneficial.

a. *Deficiency of GH due to Psychosocial Causes*

Failure of children to grow has sometimes been traced to an extremely stressful social environment, which is accompanied by a low level of GH. Adequate nutrition and removal of the child to an improved social environment rapidly lead to a reversal of the syndrome. GH administration may be of additional benefit (Boulton et al., 1992).

a. *Disorders in IGF Production*

Laron dwarfs, who lack hepatic GH receptors, or whose receptors are dysfunctional due to an autosomal recessive disorder (Daughaday and Trivedi, 1987), have normal or elevated serum concentrations of biologically active GH. However, GH is unable to stimulate hepatic production of IGF-I and consequently severe growth retardation results (Golde et al., 1980). This type of dwarfism responds dramatically to administration of IGF-I but not at all to GH. Similar low IGF-I levels are characteristic of adolescent African pygmies (Merrimee et al., 1990).

13.5.5.2 Hypersecretion of GH

If hypersecretion of GH occurs before the closing of the epiphyses, *gigantism* results. If it occurs after this event, *acromegaly*, with thickening of the skin and bones, especially the facial bones, is the outcome. In most cases, GH hypersecretion is due to a pituitary tumor and only very rarely to an elevated GHRH level. Destruction of the tumor by various types of irradiation or by surgical ablation may be followed, or supplanted, by the administration of bromocriptine (a DA agonist) or of potent, long-lasting somatostatin analogs.

13.5.5.3 Hypogonadism

The use of GH, in combination with the sex steroids, is the usual treatment of choice in children with disordered growth associated with hypogonadism. One of these syndromes is *Turner's syndrome*, a chromosomal deficiency (XO instead of XX) resulting in ovarian dysgenesis, short stature, and several other physiological abnormalities.

13.5.6 Agricultural Significance of Growth Hormone

GH enhances feed-to-gain efficiency (weight gained per unit of feed consumed) in pigs, sheep, cattle, and fish, in that order. Bovine GH (bGH) stimulates milk production in dairy cows, but the effect is markedly affected by the adequacy of the cow's diet. bGH consistently improves feed efficiency (milk produced/feed intake). There are no significant differences in the composition of the milk following bGH administration so that it is deemed safe for human consumption, and prolonged bGH treatment does not appear to affect the health of the animals. Consequently, the U.S. Food and Drug Administration approved the commercial use of GH in 1994 despite considerable consumer resistance (Harvey et al., 1995, pp. 407–413).

13.6 Prolactin

As discussed above, PRL and GH have similar actions on a wide variety of biological functions, several of which can be attributed to the growth-promoting effects of these neuropeptides. PRL, however, has special growth-promoting effects on the mammary gland, prostate, and seminal vesicles in mammals, the crop sac of pigeons and doves, the tail fin of larval anurans and urodeles, and the gills, nuptial, and cloacal pads of amphibians. In fish, PRL acts on the kidney and, in some species, the seminal vesicles. PRL is also a potent regulator of angiogenesis.

13.6.1 Synthesis and Secretion of Prolactin

The PRL and GH genes were discussed in section 13.4.1. PRL is synthesized in the lactotrophs by the usual process of protein synthesis. The PRL molecule consists of 198 amino acids with three disulfide bonds, two of which form small loops in both the N- and C-terminal ends of the molecule. The third bond links the amino acid residues 58 and 174 in a large internal loop which causes the entire molecule to fold over itself. This tertiary structure is essential to PRL's biological actions, which are lost when this disulfide bond is broken (Doneen et al., 1979).

Due to differences in post-translational modifications, such as proteolytic cleavage, glycosylation, and phosphorylation, PRL exists in several molecular variants, with different immunoreactivity and biological potency (Markoff et al., 1988; Andries et al., 1996). They may activate different receptors and this may account for the extremely diversified biological functions ascribed to PRL.

There are far fewer lactotrophs than somatatotropes, lactotrophs comprising 5% to 10% of the total anterior pituitary cell population, whereas the GH-producing cells are reported to make up almost half of the anterior pituitary cell population. This disparity is not surprising given the importance of GH throughout the life of both sexes; PRL is of less consequence except during pregnancy and lactation.

The lactotrophs are the last pituitary cell type to differentiate during embryonic life, probably owing to the combined influences of cell-specific transcriptional factors such as Pit-1 and an inhibitory control by DA neurons, either in the pituitary or from hypothalamic sources. They display several characteristics more akin to neurons than to endocrine cells, such as a high resting membrane potential (−50 to −70 mV) and spontaneous electrical activity. In addition, lactotrophs may be distinguished from other anterior pituitary cells by their remarkable heterogeneity, both in structure and in function. The lactotrophs vary in size and distribution, with the highest density in the region bordering the intermediate lobe; they also vary in responsiveness to stimulation by TRH. The number of lactotrophs fluctuates considerably with the physiological state, such as gestation and lactation.

13.6.2 Regulation of Prolactin

The tonic inhibition of PRL by hypothalamic DA, suckling-induced PRL release, and the role of α-MSH and estrogen in overcoming the tonic DA inhibition were discussed in chapter 10, section 10.2.2, and illustrated in figure 10.20. The extraordinary pleiotropic regulation of PRL secretion is examined by Martínez de la Escalera and Weiner (1992) and is supported by the long list of factors believed to be significant in the control of PRL secretion and release. The neuropeptides OT, TRH, and VIP are important modulators of PRL release but are not the primary prolactin releasing factors. Several other neuropeptides, including MSH, AT II, NPY, SP, galanin, endothelin, and PRL itself, may act as paracrine or autocrine agents to alter PRL release (Ben-Jonathan et al., 1991). Numerous neurotransmitters are also implicated in PRL release: 5-HT and histamine (Jorgensen et al., 1996), GABA (Reyroldan et al., 1997), nicotine (a cholinergic agonist) (Shieh and Pan, 1997), and glutamate and NO (Aguilar et al., 1997). The list continues with opiates (Blackford et al., 1992), glucocorticoids (Wiedermann et al., 1995), melatonin (Juszczak and Stempniak, 1997), and ethanol (Subramanian, 1997). Many of these agents may also act at the hypothalamic level to affect DA release.

13.6.3 Actions of Prolactin

The many and diverse actions of PRL on different tissues and in different species are summarized below and depicted in figure 13.13. Much of the comparative data is taken from Ensor (1978).

13.6.3.1 Reproduction

In teleost fish, PRL acts synergistically with androgens to promote growth and secretion in the seminal vesicles. In amphibians and reptiles, there is no reliable indication of a reproductive function for PRL. In birds, PRL has an antigonadal action, blocking testicular growth but only in nonmigratory species. It is in mammals that PRL assumes a vital function in reproductive events.

a. Mammary gland

In preganancy PRL is essential to mammary gland development through cell proliferation, but this action is dependent upon the synergistic action of ovarian and adrenal steroids, together with insulin (Shiu and

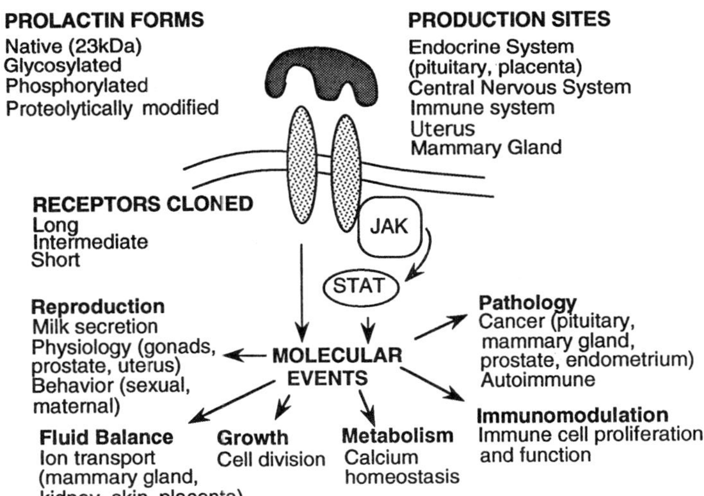

Figure 13.13
Functional diversity of prolactin (PRL) actions and molecular heterogeneity of PRL and its receptor. Molecular variants of PRL produced by different cell types activate a heterogeneous population of receptors in target cell membranes. Receptor signaling mechanisms include activation of tyrosine kinases of the Janus family (JAK), leading to phosphorylation of transcription factors known as signal transducer and activator of transcription (STAT). PRL exerts actions on reproduction, fluid balance, growth, metabolism, and immune functions, as well as angiogenesis. (From Clapp and Martínez de la Escalera, 1997.)

Friesen, 1980). Although circulating levels of PRL increase toward the end of pregnancy, lactation does not begin until parturition, when there is a sharp decrease in the ovarian and placental steroids which inhibit milk protein synthesis by PRL (Kleinberg et al., 1983). PRL stimulation of milk protein synthesis requires the concomitant presence of glucocorticoids and insulin.

b. Ovary

PRL has been called a "luteotrophic" hormone in rodents and some other species since low levels of PRL stimulate luteal function, assisting in the luteinization of granulosa cells, and maintaining their ability to synthesize progesterone, most probably indirectly through the inhibition of pituitary LH secretion. PRL also may induce and maintain LH receptors on luteal cells during late gestation. In contrast, the high levels of PRL characteristic of lactation and hyperprolactinemia inhibit progesterone production by immature ovarian follicles and prevent ovulation (Gibori and Richards, 1978). This accounts, at least in part, for the contraceptive effect of suckling, provided suckling is maintained on an almost continuous basis (McNeilly, 1979).

c. Testis and accessory sex organs

Low levels of PRL act synergistically with LH to augment testosterone production by the Leydig cells, but high concentrations diminish this response. PRL appears to be involved in prostate gland growth, stimulating cell proliferation of normal, hyperplastic, and malignant prostatic cells in culture (Syms et al., 1985).

13.6.3.2 Electrolyte Balance

PRL regulates salt balance in teleost fish, stimulating renal tubular reabsorption and the glomerular filtration rate, and decreasing water reabsorption from the urinary bladder. In addition to these actions on the kidney and bladder, PRL inhibits active ion efflux from the gills and causes the secretion of an impermable mucous coat over the skin of the fish. The ability of PRL to stimulate secretion of "crop milk" of pigeons and doves is the basis for the international bioassay standard for determining the specific activity of PRL preparations. PRL receptors are present on the crop sacs of pigeons and the involvement of prostaglandins in PRL action is likely. The evidence for PRL action in osmoregulatory processes in mammals is less striking. PRL facilitates Na^+ reabsorption by the distal convoluted tubules of the kidney and activates Na^+, K^+-ATPase in the mammary gland and amnion (Horrobin, 1981).

13.6.3.3 Adrenal Secretion

PRL acts synergistically with ACTH to promote glucocorticoid, aldosterone, and androgen secretion by the adrenal cortex in vitro, an observation that may be physiologically significant since glucocorticoids act synergistically with PRL to promote mammary gland development and lactation (Shiu and Friesen, 1980).

13.6.3.4 Hepatic Factors

The growth-promoting action of PRL is seen in its ability to stimulate hepatic mitosis in vitro and to stimulate the liver to release a factor (*synlactin*) that may mediate many of the biological actions of PRL, in a manner reminiscent of the stimulation of IGFs by GH (Mick and Nicoll, 1985).

13.6.3.5 Angiogenesis

The N-terminal 16-kD fragment, but not the larger 23-kD PRL, is a potent inhibitor of angiogenesis, the formation of new capillary blood vessels. In addition, endothelial cells contain a unique receptor for PRL fragments that differs structurally and functionally from the classic PRL receptor. Adding to the complexity of PRL regulation of the formation of capillaries is the role of two placental proteins, proliferin and proliferin-related protein, which are members of the PRL hormone family. Proliferin stimulates angiogenesis, whereas proliferin-related protein inhibits it. These regulatory actions of angiogenesis are clearly reviewed by Clapp and de la Escalera (1997).

13.6.3.6 Immunological Functions

PRL is an important growth factor for lymphocytes and restores immunocompetence in rodents and humans. PRL receptors are found in all immune cell types and PRL is also produced and secreted by lymphocytes so that both pituitary PRL and locally produced PRL contribute to immunoregulation (Yu-Lee, 1997).

13.6.3.7 Behavioral Effects

PRL induces *parental behavior* in cichlid fish, amphibia, and birds, and may be involved in fish and bird migration. Prolactin-induced migration in some birds is accompanied by increased restlessness and food consumption. There is debatable evidence for a role for PRL in *maternal behavior in mammals*: if PRL is involved it probably plays a subsidiary role to estrogen and OT, and PL may also play a role. Supporting a more significant role for PRL in maternal behavior are experiments with male rats in which maternal behavior (crouching and licking) can be triggered and maintained by PRL administration, when the males are kept in contact with pups. This is accompanied by elevated serum PRL levels and brain PRL receptor mRNA in the adult males (Sakaguchi et al., 1996). In a different type of experiment, penile erectile function was suppressed by excess PRL secreted by three additional anterior pituitaries transplanted under the kidney capsule: plasma PRL levels were significantly raised (Sato et al., 1997). In similar experiments that evoked hyperprolactinemia, rats demonstrated a number of behavioral changes, including excessive grooming, enhancement of drug-induced stereotypy, facilitated acquisition of active avoidance behavior, and decreased responsiveness to electrical footshock (Drago et al., 1982, 1986).

Lactation in mammals is accompanied by a striking hyperphagia and markedly elevated levels of PRL, an adaptation of obvious survival importance. The increased food intake can be elicited by central administration of PRL (Sauve and Woodside, 1996).

13.6.4 Clinical Implications of Prolactin

No human or animal model of a genetic defect of the PRL receptor has as yet been reported. Nor have there been any reports of a disease resulting from PRL deficiency. However, *hypersecretion of PRL* in women results in the hyperprolactemia-galactorrhea-amenorrhea syndrome, and loss of sexual activity. The hypersecretion may result from a pituitary tumor secreting PRL or from the loss of the tonic hypothalamic inhibition of PRL secretion. Not all patients with high PRL levels develop galactorrhea (milk secretion) so it is likely that other hormones are necessary for its development. The amenorrhea may be due to the inhibitory influence of PRL on pituitary gonadotropin secretion. Surgical removal of the tumor restores normal ovarian function and the menses.

PRL is a growth and differentiation factor for the mammary gland and may be a causative factor in mammary cancer in rodents and perhaps in humans. For microadenomas secreting high levels of PRL, medical treatment with a DA agonist such as bromocriptine or pergolide, is preferable to surgery.

Vascular-associated diseases, including rheumatoid arthritis, an autoimmune disease associated with angiogenesis, and certain ocular diseases associated with pathological angiogenesis, theoretically could benefit from the administration of inhibitory PRL fragments.

PRL-secreting tumors are much less frequent in men than in women and the accompanying symptoms include disturbances in the visual field and headache due to pressure from the encroaching tumor, decreased libido and potency, low testosterone levels, and azoospermia or oligospermia. Depending on the size of the tumor, treatment is surgical or medical.

Drugs or hormones that deplete or block the central monoaminergic neurons may induce hyperprolactemia by removing the normal inhibitory influence of DA neurons. Many of these drugs are commonly used clinically, for example, haloperidol, chlorpromazine, sex steroids, and opiates.

13.7 Secretoneurin

Secretoneurin is a recently identified novel peptide of 33 amino acids that was first described in frog brain (Vaudry and Conlon, 1991), then isolated from the pituitary gland (Fischer-Colbrie et al., 1995). However, it is widely expressed throughout the nervous system, including the sympathetic nervous system and the retina, and is found in many endocrine tissues, especially the adrenal medulla, so that like so many other neuropeptides it cannot always be easily classified according to its source. Its distribution is generally in phylogenetically older forebrain structures and it is highly conserved from frog to human, with more than 90% homology between birds and mammals (Fischer-Colbrie et al., 1995). The structure of human secretoneurin is

Thr-Asn-Glu-Ile-Val-Glu-Glu-Gln-Tyr-Thr-Pro-Gln-Ser-Leu-Ala-Thr-Leu-Glu-Ser-Val-Phe-Gln-Glu-Leu-Gly-Lys-Leu-Thr-Gly-Pro-Asn^{31}-Asn-Gln

The structure of rat secretoneurin differs from human only at position 31, where Ser substitutes for Asn.

In the spinal cord, secretoneurin is co-localized in sensory fibers with tachykinins, having a similar distribution to that of SP. Tissue levels of both substances are depleted in the dorsal horn after systemic capsaicin treatment. In the brain, secretoneurin is found in the extended amygdala (which links the hypothalamic limbic and striatal pallidal functions) from the nucleus accumbens to the central and medial amygdala. Some hippocampal pathways are strongly immunoreactive for secretoneurin. Secretoneurin is present very early in brain development and its distribution is found as early as embryonic day 16 in the rat. By postnatal day 15 the distribution of secretoneurin in the brain is essentially the same as in the adult (figures 13.14 and 13.15) and the processing enzymes necessary for the production of secretoneurin from its prohormone secretogranin II are developed before embryonic day 14 (Saria et al., 1997).

Secretoneurin is formed by endoproteolytic cleavage by prohormone convertases PC1 and PC2, from a large precursor *secretogranin II*, one of the proteins of the *secretogranin-chromogranin family* (Vaudry and Conlon, 1991). These proteins have been detected in the large, dense-core vesicles of neurons and endocrine cells, and have been analyzed using immunocytochemistry, immunoblot, reversed phase high-performance liquid chromatography (HPLC), high-performance gel filtration, and radioimmunoassay. Most of brain secretogranin undergoes post-translational processing, and secretoneurin represents secretogranin II amino acids 156–186 (Kirchmair et al., 1993).

There are only two clearly demonstrated actions of secretoneurin as yet. Secretoneurin displays a potent and specific chemotactic activity towards monocytes but not to other blood cells (Reinish et al., 1993) and

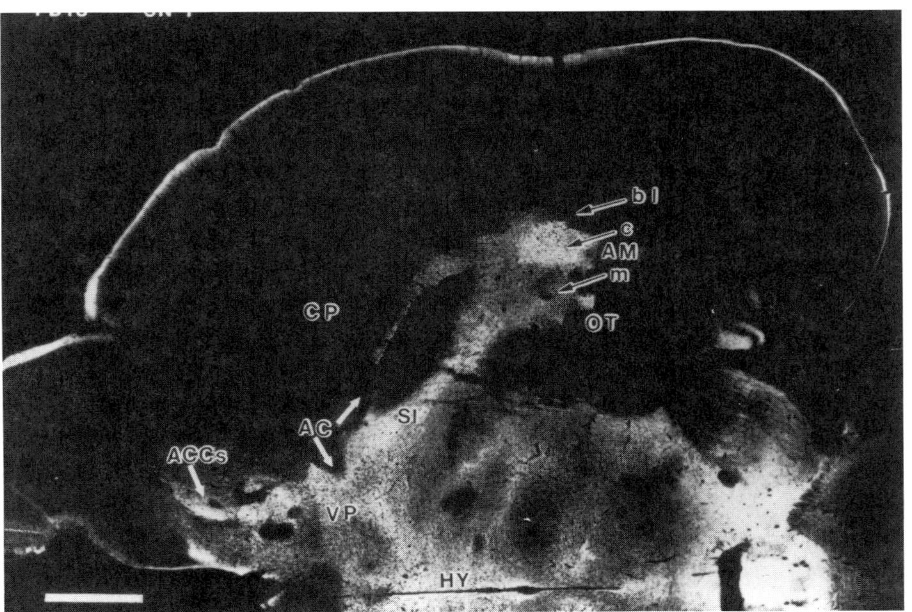

Figure 13.14
Illustration of a horizontal section of postnatal day (PD) 15 rat ventral forebrain using secretoneurin (SN)-immunostained slides as negatives; therefore, SN-immunoreactive (IR) structures appear white. By PD 15 the pattern of SN-IR is similar to that of the adult rat brain. SN-IR is apparent in the medial or shell portion of nucleus accumbens (ACCs) and the ventral extension of the striatopallidum (VP). The SN-IR continues into the bed nucleus of the stria terminalis, which lies in a dorsal plane (not shown here). Also, note SN-IR extending laterally from the anterior hypothalamus (HY) and overlapping the ACCs and VP. From these forebrain regions SN-IR extends caudad through the substantia innominata (SI) to the amygdaloid nucleus (AM). Note the intense SN-IR in the medial and central A < (Amm, Amc), while relatively less SN-IR is apparent in lateral and basal lateral AM (Ambl). Little SN-IR is evident in the caudate-putamen (CP) at PD 15. OT, optic tract. Bar = 1 mm. (From Saria et al., 1997.)

it has been shown that there are specific high-affinity binding sites for secretoneurin on monocytes. Secondly, secretoneurin induces DA release in the striatum of the rat brain (Saria et al., 1993). It is possible that secretoneurin has a part in water homeostasis since secretogranin mRNA is specifically upregulated in osmotically stimulated rats in hypothalamic areas involved in osmoregulation, such as the PVN and SON.

13.8 Summary

FSH, LH, and TSH are glycoproteins synthesized by all vertebrates .The other member of this family is CG, which is produced by the placenta and restricted to primates and horses. The specificity of these heterodimeric glycoproteins resides in the β subunit, whereas the α subunit is common to all the

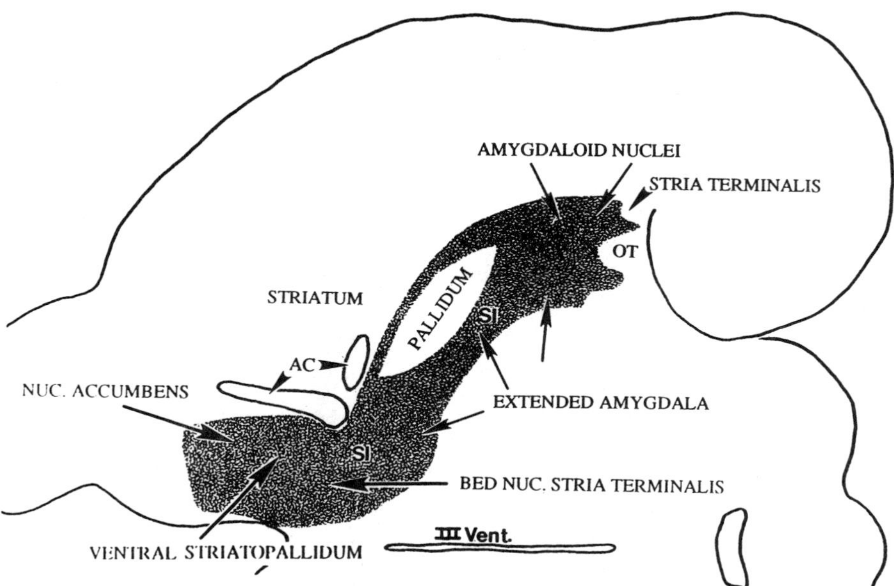

Figure 13.15
Schematic representation of intense secretoneurin-immunoreactive labeling (derived from figure 13.13) of the extended amygdala and ventral striatopallidum (shaded area). AC, shell portion of the nucleus accumbens; OT, optic tract. (From Saria et al., 1997.)

glycoproteins. Both subunits are glycosylated and the sugar chain triggers receptor signaling in the target organ. Each subunit is coded by different genes on different chromosomes.

A single gene encodes all α subunits but tissue-specific processing and multihormonal control results in the specificity of the resulting neuropeptide. The α gene is regulated by cAMP. There are several differences in the structure of the β genes in different species, including the number of exons, their lengths, and the transcriptional start sites. FSH, LH, TSH, and CG, each possess 92 amino acids in their α subunits, but have 118, 121, 112, and 145 amino acids, respectively, in their β subunits. The biosynthesis of LH, FSH, and TSH is regulated at all levels of the classical pathways for peptides.

FSH and LH *gonadotrophs* are scattered throughout the glandular parenchyma of the anterior pituitary, constituting about 14% of the cell population. They produce both LH and FSH. The differential regulation of hypothalamic control of LH and FSH has been discussed in chapter 10. The expression of mRNA for LH and FSH β subunits is increased in late proestrus. Continuous GnRH stimulates only α subunit mRNA and pulsatile GnRH is required for stimulation of the LH β gene. FSH secretion is inhibited by the gonadal peptides *inhibin* and *follistatin. Activin*, formed from two β subunits of inhibin, is produced by the gonads and the pituitary gonadotrophs and stimulates the synthesis and release of pituitary FSH without affecting LH. Both the *LH receptor* and the *FSH receptor* are membrane-bound glycoproteins complexed with G proteins and adenylate cyclase, acting via the cAMP-dependent protein kinase pathway.

In the male there is only a basal, episodic LH discharge, whereas the female has two forms of basal discharge. During most of the estrous and menstrual cycles, there is a sharp peak, then fall in LH each hour. An abrupt preovulatory rise lasts for several hours and is essential to ovulation. FSH pulses are more variable. LH stimulates the synthesis of androgens in the Leydig cells of the testis and the synthesis of progesterone by the corpus luteum. In the ovary FSH accelerates follicular development, steroidogenesis, and ovum maturation. The two gonadotropins cooperate in the biosynthesis of estrogen and progesterone involving both thecal and granulosa cells. In the testis, FSH promotes differentiation of the Sertoli cells and the maturation of the gametes. Both FSH and LH are required for normal spermatogenesis. FSH and LH have indirect behavioral effects due to their regulatory actions on gonadal steroids.

TSH is present in the pituitary gland of all vertebrates and through its influence on thyroid hormone production, is essential to almost all physiological processes, including early growth and development, reproduction, metabolism, and behavior. The *thyrotrophs* of the pituitary are dependent on the *Pit-1 transcription factor*, which activates the TSH promoter. Pit-1 is also essential to the normal growth and development of the somatotrophs and lactotrophs but not to the gonadotrophs. The correct subunit conformation of the TSH β subunit is dependent on normal glycosylation: deletion of its glycosylation sequence almost completely abolishes TSH synthesis. TSH secretion is *regulated* by TRH (see chapter 10) and by negative feedback from circulating thyroid hormones, the most potent of which is T_3. TSH is secreted in a pulsatile manner, about nine pulses per 24 hours in humans, with a circadian rhythm that reaches a peak between 11 P.M. and 4 A.M. In rodents the pulse frequency is much higher and TSH levels peak between 10 A.M and 2 P.M.

The T_3 receptor has been identified in liver and kidney cells as a nuclear receptor, the product of the *c-erb-A* gene, part of a gene superfamily that includes related oncogenes and steroid receptor genes, but other hormones, such as steroids, do not bind to the thyroid hormone receptor. There are several isoforms of thyroid hormone receptors, the TRα and TRβ_2 receptors, which are encoded by different genes. As these receptors are present in the hypothalamus and the pituitary, T_3 regulates TSH at both levels. Both 5-HT and the opiates stimulate TSH secretion, which is inhibited by stress and the stress-evoked hormones, and by DA and somatostatin. Cold stress, however, increases TSH through TRH release via a neuroendocrine reflex, and is an important component of the maintenance of body temperature.

TSH stimulates *thyroid hormone* synthesis, storage, release, and recycling, increasing cAMP levels, and causing the engulfing of thyroglobulin into the thyroid follicles for use as a substrate for thyroid hormone synthesis. TSH stimulates the incorporation of iodide into thyroglobulin for the synthesis of T_3 and T_4. The hormones may be stored in this manner, then released by proteolysis into the circulation as needed.

GH and PRL gene duplication may have occurred prior to the evolution of vertebrates, giving rise to two separate precursors, one for the GH-PL gene and the other for the PRL gene, which are present on different chromosomes. The introduction of distinct regulatory sequences, permitted the differential regulation of the three hormones. Mammalian GH and

PRL genes are structurally similar, but primate GH has several important differences from mammalian GH, and specific mutations in primate GH have resulted in GH acquiring PRL activity. Thus there is considerable overlap in the functions affected by GH and PRL. Both affect growth and development, osmoregulation, reproduction, lipid metabolism, and adrenal steroidogenesis, but their potencies vary in different species.

The *GH and PRL receptors* belong to the hematopoietic superfamily, all glycoproteins with an extracellular N-terminus and a single transmembrane domain. They are arranged as four antiparallel α helices. *GH receptors* are heterogeneous and may have different signal transduction systems, none of which have been positively identified as yet. Circulating GH may be free or bound to serum binding proteins, the smaller of which is identical to the extracellular domain of the GH receptor. Binding of GH to the receptor rapidly causes its dimerization which initiates signal transduction. In mammals, the liver has the highest concentration of GH receptors, which are rapidly internalized after binding with GH. *PRL receptors* exist in three forms, and their binding sites are widely distributed in mammalian tissue. Following binding to PRL, the receptor is rapidly internalized. Primate GH is also lactogenic and binds to PRL receptors. PRL receptors increase considerably in number during lactation, following the steep fall in ovarian and placental steroids that occurs at parturition. PRL receptor numbers are influenced by gonadal steroids, and upregulated by PRL itself.

The *somatotrophs*, GH-producing cells, are the most numerous cell type of the anterior pituitary and appear later than the FSH-, LH-, and TSH-producing cells. The *lactotrophs* (PRL-producing) only appear a few days after birth. GH and PRL may be found colocalized or in separate secretory granules. Pit-1 may be responsible for the expression of the GH and PRL genes and thus the final pathway leading to either GH or PRL production. The higher levels of GH in males, and the higher levels of PRL in females may be due to differential Pit-1 levels in the somatotrophs and lactotrophs of the two sexes. The *mammosomatotrophs*, which secrete both GH and PRL, are found in normal pituitaries and in pituitary tumors, and proliferate under the influence of estrogen but are inhibited by testosterone. GnRH increases the number of these cells.

GH is a 191–amino acid neuropeptide and a smaller GH molecule is also synthesized after alternative splicing. GH secretion is *pulsatile*, affected by crucial events that affect growth during infancy, puberty, and adolescence. Age, sex, nutritional status, and physical activity are important influences on GH secretion. Males have higher but less frequent pulses than females. The pulsatile pattern is due to the balance between the stimulatory effect of GnRH and the inhibitory effect of somatostatin, modified by adrenergic and cholinergic inputs. In addition, GH regulates its own production by somatotrophs which have GH receptors, and GH has reciprocal feedback interactions with hypothalamic GnRH and somatostatin, high levels of GH increasing somatostatin levels, and decreasing GHRH levels. A fall in GH has the reverse effects. Both GH and GHRH promote slow wave sleep and there is a temporal relationship between sleep and pulsatile secretion of GH.

GH has no specific target organ to produce a long-loop feedback mechanism, but there are several peripheral response mechanisms that *regulate GH. IGFs* synthesized in the liver and other peripheral organs, as well as in the pituitary, act on both hypothalamic and pituitary receptors to inhibit GH secretion. The *effects of GH* on growth include increased body weight and height; skeletal growth; muscle growth; protein, fat and carbohydrate metabolism; and cartilage deposition. The actions of GH on growth are mediated by IGF-I, whereas GH has a direct effect on carbohydrate and lipid metabolism. The pubertal growth spurt and normal adolescent growth require both an increase in GH and *sex steroids*. T_3 is an important positive regulator of the GH gene and *glucocorticoids* increase GH gene transcription and GHRH receptor synthesis. However, hypersecretion of glucocorticoids provides a long-loop negative feedback on GH, inhibiting growth. *Thymic factors* and *cytokines* form another long-loop reciprocal influence on GH, which, in turn, has many stimulatory effects on immune function. *Metabolic factors*, such as glucose and free fatty acids, produced as a result of GH actions on carbohydrate and lipid metabolism, provide fine control over GH release.

PRL is synthesized in the pituitary lactotrophs. It is a large molecule of 198 amino acids with three disulfide bonds, the third of which forms a looped tertiary structure essential to biological activity. There are several molecular PRL variants with different biological activities as well as three PRL receptors. The lactotrophs are far fewer in number than the somatotrophs and appear later in embryonic life, are highly heterogeneous both in their structure and function, and their number varies during gestation and lactation. They are remarkable in their similarity to neurons in their electrophysiological characteristics.

PRL release is tonically inhibited by hypothalamic DA, and the role of α-MSH, estrogen, and suckling in overcoming this inhibition was discussed in chapter 10, section 10.2.2.2. Several other neuropeptides may act in the pituitary as autocrine or paracrine agents to alter PRL release, or they may act at the hypothalamic level to affect DA release, or they may do both. There is a nocturnal rise in PRL associated with sleep and there is also a circadian rhythm of PRL secretion which is greater in women than in men, being associated with the follicular and luteal phase of the cycle.

In addition to its general growth-promoting actions, PRL has *specific effects* on the growth of the crop sac of pigeons and doves, the tail fin of larval anurans and urodeles, and the gills, nuptial, and cloacal pads of amphibians. In fish, PRL acts on the kidney, and in some species, the seminal vesicles. But it is in mammals that PRL assumes its vital role in *reproduction*. PRL, together with ovarian and adrenal steroids and insulin, provides the stimulus to mammary gland development in pregnancy. Lactation only occurs after parturition when there is a sharp decline in the ovarian and placental steroids that inhibit milk protein synthesis. PRL stimulation of milk synthesis requires the synergistic action of glucocorticoids and insulin. The high levels of PRL during suckling inhibit progesterone production by ovarian follicles and prevent ovulation. In males, PRL acts synergistically with LH to increase testosterone production, but high PRL levels have an inhibiting effect. PRL may be involved in normal and malignant growth of prostate cells, and in the regulation of angiogenesis. PRL is associated with *behavioral effects* in fish, amphibians, birds, and mammals.

Secretoneurin is a 33–amino acid peptide first isolated from the pituitary, but it is widely distributed in the CNS and in many endocrine glands. Secretoneurin is formed from a large precursor molecule, secretogranin II, and is colocalized in sensory fibers with tachykinins with a distribution similar to that of SP. Secretoneurin has a potent and specific chemotactic activity toward monocytes and induces DA release in the striatum. It may be involved in water homeostasis.

Chapter 14 continues the examination of β-endorphin, one of the neuropeptides derived from POMC and β-lipotropin. The endorphins form one of the three endogenous opiate families, the other members being the enkephalins and dynorphins. The structural and functional characteristics of these three important families are compared.

Endogenous Opiate Neuropeptides: Endorphins, Enkephalins, Dynorphins, Tyr-MIF-1, and Nociceptin

14

14.1 Historical Background

Opium has been used as a drug at least since classical Greek times for its analgesic and euphoric qualities. The word *opium* is derived from the Greek for poppy juice and the opium alkaloid was isolated from poppies in 1803 and named morphine after *Morpheus*, the Greek god of dreams. In 1680 the English physician Thomas Sydenham wrote, "Among the remedies which it has pleased Almighty God to give man to relieve his sufferings, none is so universal and efficacious as opium." This encomium has since been tempered by our awareness of the toxicity and addictiveness of opiates, but no other class of drugs has as powerful an analgesic action. Consequently, the search continues for synthetic analogs which have the analgesic qualities without the addictive properties of the opiates. Although this task has not been successful, many useful compounds structurally related to morphine have been synthesized. One of these that is extensively used clinically is *methadone*, a morphine substitute developed for pain relief but which is useful for detoxification and maintenance of the heroin addict.

The discovery of endogenous opiates, named *endorphins* by Eric Simon in 1975 (Simon and Hiller, 1978), and the more widely distributed *enkephalins*, was a process different from the discovery of most other biologically active molecules, for the receptors were identified before the ligands were. In the search for nonaddictive morphine analogs, it was found that the addictive and analgesic properties of morphine and its analogs were remarkably *stereospecific*. This was correctly interpreted as requiring an equally demanding stereospecificity of their receptors, which set off an active search for the highly specific opiate binding sites in the CNS and other tissues. In 1973, three laboratories independently reported the existence of stereospecific opiate binding sites in the brain (Pert and Snyder, 1973; Simon et al., 1973; Terenius, 1973). A search for endogenous ligands for these receptors ensued and several groups reported, almost at the same time, the existence of opiate activity in brain and pituitary gland (J. S. Hughes, 1975; Hughes et al., 1975; Teschenmacher et al., 1975). These stereospecific opiate receptors exist in all vertebrates and it is unlikely that the receptors have been conserved throughout evolution only to bind plant opiates. Opiates have also been demonstrated by immunocytochemical means in most invertebrates. Every aspect of the system is stereospecific, including synthesis, degradation, and receptors.

The opiate system interacts with other systems, including neurotransmitters and hormones, and is altered by many stressors. In addition to pain regulation and actions on behaviors such as reinforcement and reward, opiates are clearly involved with neuroendocrine regulation, being present in very high concentrations in the hypothalamus and intermediate and posterior pituitary. The endogenous opiates are widely and differentially distributed in the CNS and act as neuromodulators and neurotransmitters, exerting a profound influence on many physiological and pathological states, including cardiovascular and gastrointestinal functions. Opiates depress the respiratory system and may cause hyperglycemia and akinesia. As was discussed in chapter 8, there is an intimate communication system between the neuroendocrine system and the immune system, which produces both ACTH and endorphins, and which has receptors for opiates on lymphocytes (Smith and Blalock, 1981).

Opioid was the term originally used to refer only to endogenous compounds with morphine-like actions, but this distinction has gradually disappeared and the more encompassing term, *opiate*, is now more commonly used for all such compounds, endogenous or not (Olson et al., 1991).

14.2 Families and Distribution of the Endogenous Opiates

14.2.1 The Three Endogenous Opiate Gene Families

The major endogenous opiates are the *endorphins*, the *enkephalins*, and the *dynorphins*, which are coded for by three separate genes, all of which have been cloned. The *endorphins* arise from β-lipotropin, which is cleaved from POMC (see chapter 12, section 12.2). β-Lipotropin, in turn, serves as a prohormone for several fairly large amino acid fragments, α-, β- and γ-endorphin (see table 12.1). The precursor molecules for the endorphins, enkephalins, and dynorphins are shown in figure 14.1.

The two *enkephalins*, leu-enkephalin and met-enkephalin, are pentapeptides differing only at the C-terminal, possessing either leucine (leu-enkephalin: *Tyr-Gly-Gly-Phe-Leu*) or methionine (met-enkephalin: *Tyr-Gly-Gly-Phe-Met*). Both enkephalins are derived from a precursor molecule, *proenkephalin* (see figure 14.1).

The *dynorphins* are opiate peptides derived from a different precursor, *prodynorphin*, sometimes called proenkephalin B (see figure 14.1), which shows considerable amino acid sequence homology with proenkephalin. The possibility that the three genes may have the same evolutionary ancestor is based on the overall similarity of the genes, the similar size and position of their introns, and the clustering of six cystine residues near the N-terminals. The repeated nucleotide sequences within the individual genes suggest that each arose by duplication of a short primordial gene segment, perhaps as far back as *Tetrahymena*.

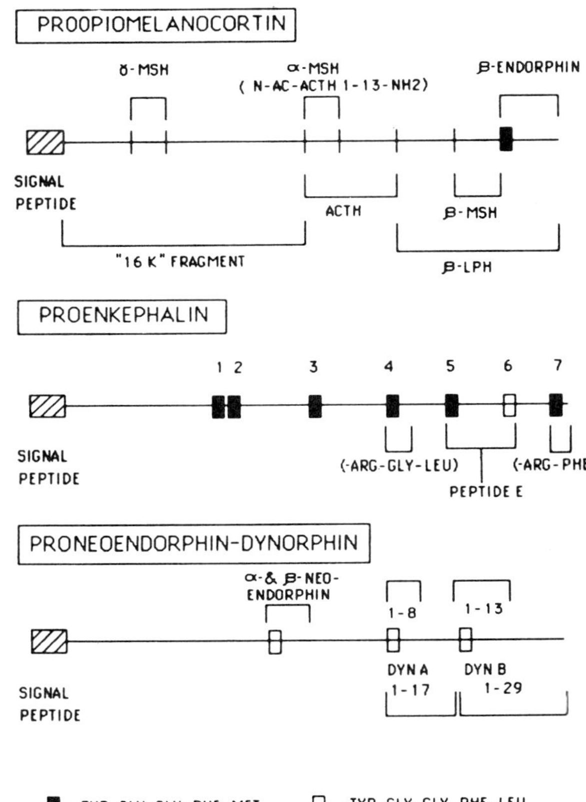

Figure 14.1
Schematic representation of the structure of the three opiate peptide precursors. Note that the opiate-active core sequence Tyr-Gly-Gly-Phe-Met (met-enkephalin) appears in both pro-opiomelanocortin and proenkephalin, whereas the opiate-active sequence Try-Gly-Gly-Phe-Leu (leu-enkephalin) is common to both proenkephalin and proneoendorphin-dynorphin (prodynorphin). α-MSH, α-melanocyte–stimulating hormone; β-LPH, β-lipotropin. (From Khachaturian et al., 1985.)

14.2.2 Differential Distribution of Opiate Neuropeptide Families

The three opiate neuropeptide families are differentially expressed throughout the CNS. The endorphins are found in all cells of the intermediate lobe and those anterior pituitary cells that contain ACTH. The enkephalins are present in the intermediate and posterior pituitary, but are absent from the anterior lobe. β-Endorphin and enkephalin are found in different neuronal systems within the brain, although some systems may overlap (figures 14.2 and 14.3). The enkephalin-containing neurons seem to be

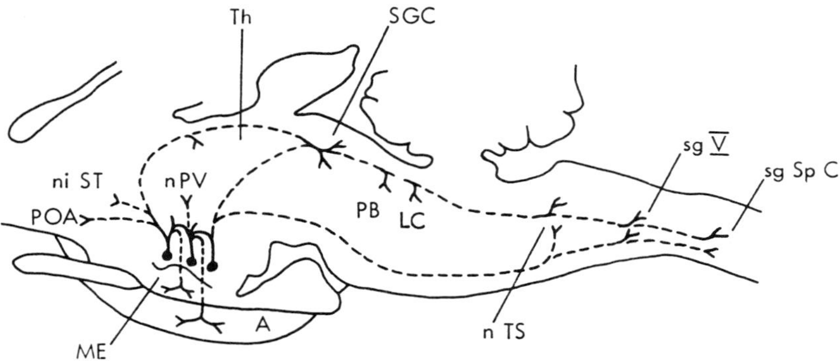

Figure 14.2
Sagittal view of the rat CNS showing the main possible projections of the β-endorphin–immunoreactive neurons, with cell bodies in the arcuate nucleus and medial basal hypothalamus. Projections are to the POA, anterior preoptic area; ni ST, nucleus of stria terminalis; nPV, paraventricular nucleus; Th, dorsomedial thalamus; ME, median eminence; SGC, periaqueductal gray; PB, nucleus parabrachialis; LC, locus ceruleus; n TS, nucleus of tractus solitarius; sg V, substantia gelatinosa of the spinal nucleus of the trigeminal nerve: sgSpC, substantia gelatinosa of the spinal cord; A, amygdala. (From Cuello, 1983.)

mostly short interneurons, although they also form projection systems (see figure 14.3). There are also considerable amounts of opiate peptides in peripheral tissues, especially in some endocrine glands. The distribution of the three types of opiates is considered in more detail in section 14.3.

14.2.3 Structural Similarities of Endogenous Opiates and Morphine

Figure 14.4 shows that the N-terminal Tyr^1 ring of met-enkephalin and leu-enkephalin corresponds to the A ring of morphine. Table 14.1 lists some endogenous opiate peptides, most of which show a structural homology in that the first four residues are identical. The N-terminal region of the molecule is constant and carries the "message" to the "address" (Schwyzer, 1977). The rest of the molecule varies, resulting in functional heterogeneity and the binding to different receptors.

14.2.4 The Tyr-MIF-1 Family

Four structurally related small peptides have been isolated from brain tissue, two of which, *Tyr-MIF-1* (Tyr-Pro-Leu-Gly-NH_2) and *Tyr-W-MIF-1* (Tyr-Pro-Trp-Gly-NH_2), bind to a Tyr-MIF-1 site and to a μ opiate site, whereas the third member of this family, *MIF-1* (Pro-Leu-Gly-NH_2), binds to neither site (Erchegyi et al., 1992; Hackler et al., 1993). The fourth member, *Tyr-K-MIF-1* (Tyr-Pro-Lys-Gly-NH_2), unlike many other peptides with Tyr-Pro at the N-terminal, does not bind to opiate receptors but only to its own site in brain tissue (Hackler et al., 1994).

Tyr-MIF-1 and Tyr-W-MIF-1 have opposite effects on opiate systems. Tyr-MIF-1 antagonizes both endogenous and exogenous opiate-induced analgesia and has been suggested to belong to an endogenous antiopiate system (Galina and Kastin, 1986). Tyr-MIF-1 also reacts with nonopiate systems, mainly the

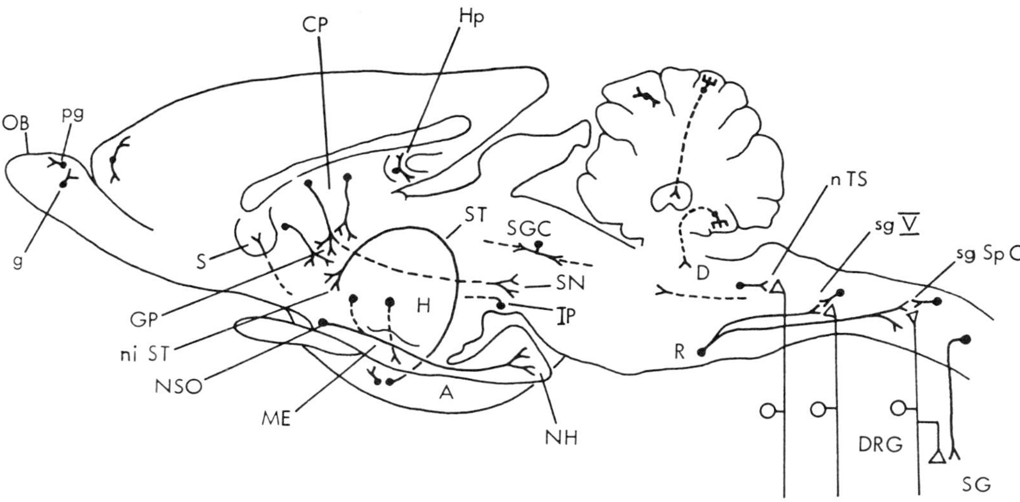

Figure 14.3
Sagittal view of the rat CNS showing the major neuronal systems containing enkephalin-immunoreactive neurons. The best-established systems are represented by solid lines; broken lines indicate less certain projections. The most conspicuous enkephalin-immunoreactive system is in the corpus striatum with cell bodies in the caudate putamen (CP) and fibers radiating to the globus pallidus (GP). This nucleus contains the richest concentration of enkephalin in the CNS. Enkephalin-immunoreactivity is found in many local circuit neurons, as indicated. Those present in areas of central projections of sensory neurons (cell bodies represented by open circles and nerve terminals as open triangles) are implicated in the processing of pain information. OB, olfactory bulb; S, septum; Hp, hippocampus; ni ST, nucleus of stria terminalis; ST, stria terminalis; NSO, supraoptic nucleus; ME, median eminence; NH, neurohypophysis; H, hypothalamus; A, amygdala; IP, nucleus interpeduncularis; SN, substantia nigra; SGC, periaqueductal gray; D, Deiters' nucleus; R, caudal nuclei of raphe system; n TS, nucleus of tractus solitarius; sg V, substantia gelatinosa of trigeminal nerve; Sg Sp C, substantia gelatinosa of spinal cord; DRG, dorsal root ganglia; SG, sympathetic ganglia. (From Cuello, 1983.)

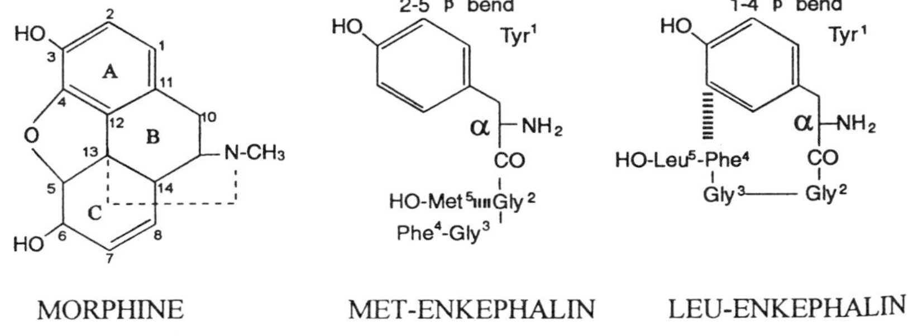

Figure 14.4
Comparison of structure of ± morphine with that of met-enkephalin and leu-enkephalin. The A ring of morphine corresponds to the N-terminal Tyr[1] ring of the enkephalins. (From Borsodi and Tóth, 1995.)

Table 14.1
Endogenous opiate peptides

Precursor	Opioid-Peptide	Structure	Selectivity
Pro-opiomelanocortin (POMC)	β-Endorphin	*Tyr-Gly-Gly-Phe-Met*-Thr-Ser-Gln-Thr-Pro-Leu-Val-Thr-Leu-Phe-Lys-Asn-Ala-Ile-Ile-Lys-Asn-Ala-Tyr-Lys-Lys-Gly-Glu	$\mu, \varepsilon > \delta \gg \kappa$
Proenkephalin A	[Leu[5]]Enkephalin	*Tyr-Gly-Gly-Phe-Leu*	$\delta > \mu \gg \kappa$
	[Met[5]]Enkephalin	*Tyr-Gly-Gly-Phe-Met*	$\mu \sim \delta \gg \kappa$
	[Met[5]]Enkephalin-Arg[6]-Phe[7]	*Tyr-Gly-Gly-Phe-Met*-Arg-Phe	κ_2
Prodynorphin (proenkephalin B)	Dynorphin A (1–17)	*Tyr-Gly-Gly-Phe-Leu*-Arg-Arg-Ile-Arg-Pro-Lys-Leu-Lys-Trp-Asp-Asn-Gly	$\kappa \gg \mu > \delta$
	Dynorphin A (1–13)	*Tyr-Gly-Gly-Phe-Leu*-Arg-Arg-Ile-Arg-Pro-Lys-Leu-Lys	$\kappa > \delta \sim \mu$
	Dynorphin A (1–8)	*Tyr-Gly-Gly-Phe-Leu*-Arg-Arg-Ile	$\kappa > \delta \sim \mu$
Others			
β-Casein derivatives	Morphiceptin	Tyr-Pro-Phe-Pro-NH_2	μ
	β-Casomorphin	Tyr-Pro-Phe-Pro-Gly-Pro-Ile	
α-Gliadin derivatives	Gliadorphin	Tyr-Pro-Gln-Pro-Gln-Pro-Phe	
Frog brain peptides			
Phyllomedusa sauvagei	Dermorphin	Tyr-D-Ala-Phe-Gly-Tyr-Pro-Ser-NH_2	μ
	Deltorphin	Tyr-D-Met-Phe-His-Leu-Met-Asp-NH_2	
Phyllomedusa bicolor	[D-Ala[2]]Deltorphin I	Tyr-D-Ala-Phe-Asp-Val-Val-Gly-NH_2	
	[D-Ala[2]]Deltorphin II	Tyr-D-Ala-Phe-Glu-Val-Val-Gly-NH_2	

From Borsodi and Toth (1995).
Tyr-Gly-Gly-Phe-Leu is the peptide sequence common to Leu-enkephalin and the dynorphins. The first 4 amino acids of the sequence are the same for Met-enkephalin. $\gg$, considerably greater than.

dopaminergic and GABAergic systems, and stimulates gastrointestinal motility. Tyr-MIF-1 and Tyr-W-MIF-1 bind to both μ_1 and μ_2 sites (Zadina et al., 1996), perhaps functioning as a mixed μ_1 receptor agonist and μ_2 receptor antagonist in the endogenous opiate system (Gergen et al., 1997). Tyr-W-MIF-1 inhibits electrically induced contractions of guinea pig ileum and produces profound analgesia after icv injection, effects that correspond to its binding to μ opiate receptors (Zadina et al., 1994a). Cyclization of Tyr-W-MIF-1 enhances analgesic activity by about 200-fold, with the duration of the analgesia comparable to that of morphine, as well as that of Tyr-D-Ala-Gly-N-MePhe-Gly-ol (DAMGO) one of the most effective analogs of enkephalin known (Zadina et al., 1994b).

Recently, from an ingenious study that generated 20 Tyr-W-MIF-1 derivatives, Zadina et al., (1996) isolated two new μ-selective peptide ligands from mammalian brain, named endomorphin-1 (Tyr-Pro-Trp-Phe-NH_2) and endomorphin-2 (Tyr-Pro-Phe-Phe-NH_2). These two peptides have the highest affinity and specificity for the μ opiate receptor found so far in the mammalian nervous system. They have potent μ-selectivity, including analgesia. Endomorphin-1–like immunoreactivity is present in several brain regions known to contain dense μ opiate receptors (thalamus, hypothalamus, cortex, and striatum). This discovery should provide important new molecular techniques for clarifying the endogenous opiate systems in the brain and spinal cord.

14.2.5 Nociceptin

Nociceptin, or orphanin FQ, is a newly discovered neuropeptide of 17 amino acids with an amino acid sequence resembling that of dynorphin:

Phe-Gly-Gly-Phe-Thr-Gly-Ala-Ala-Lys-Ser-Ala-Arg-Lys-Leu-Ala-Asn-Gln

Nociceptin is an endogenous ligand for the opiate receptor–like (ORL_1) receptor (Mollereau et al., 1996) but differs from the other opiate receptor agonists in that it does not possess the N-terminal tyrosine residue that is required for agonist activity at the μ, δ, and κ opiate receptors (Reinscheid et al., 1996).

Nociceptin induces hyperalgia when administered i.c.v. in mice. Nociceptin also inhibits electrically induced contractions of the mouse vas deferens, a nonopiate action as it is not blocked by opiate antagonists (Berzeteigurske et al., 1996). Similarly, the release of tachykinins from sensory nerves mediated by nociceptin is not affected by opiate antagonists (Giuliani and Maggi 1996).

14.3 Processing and Specific Distribution of Endogenous Opiates

14.3.1 β-Lipotropin and β-Endorphin

The tissue-specific processing of POMC and post-translational modifications, such as N-acetylation of the N-terminal tyrosine of β-endorphin, which inactivates this opiate, were discussed in chapter 12, section 12.2.4.2. β-Lipotropin, a 91–amino acid peptide cleaved proteolytically from POMC (see figures 3.10, and 12.3), contains several fragments with opiate activity. These are listed in table 14.2. Several of these fragments, most notably β-endorphin, are cleaved from β-lipotropin during physiological processing. The enkephalins have their own precursor molecules and processing enzymes, as discussed below.

Table 14.2
Fragments of β-lipotropin (1–91) with opiate activity

Amino Acid Sequence	Name of Fragment
60–65	Arginine-enkephalin
61–64	Methionine-enkephalin
61–76	α-Endorphin
61–91	β-Endorphin
61–77	γ-Endorphin

β-Endorphin, the 31–amino acid C-terminal peptide of β-lipotropin, is the predominant active opiate derived from β-lipotropin. β-Endorphin is localized in two cell groups in the brain: the arcuate nucleus of the hypothalamus and the nucleus tractus solitarius of the brain stem (Schafer et al., 1991). Processes of arcuate nucleus neurons project far to innervate forebrain regions, such as the medial preoptic area, the septum, the nucleus accumbens, the bed nucleus of the stria terminalis, and the periaqueductal gray. These processes also extend into midbrain and hindbrain regions. Neurons from the tractus solitarius send projections to the caudal brain stem and spinal cord (Tsou et al., 1986). β-Endorphin is densely localized in the anterior pituitary and the intermediate lobe. Whereas almost all the β-endorphin in the brain and anterior lobe is nonacetylated, in the intermediate lobe most β-endorphin is processed to yield the inactive acetylated form [*N*-acetyl] β-endorphin (1–26). The C-terminal tetrapeptide (β-endorphin 28–31) *melanotropic-potentiating factor*) has several biological actions in the nervous system and promotes glucose uptake in muscle (Evans and Smith, 1997).

14.3.2 Proenkephalin A

The precursor protein *proenkephalin* was first discovered in the adrenal gland, and its role in the biosynthesis of the enkephalins was clarified by Lewis et al. (1980). Proenkephalin contains one copy of leu-enkephalin, four copies of met-enkephalin, and one copy each of a met-enkephalin C-terminal–extended heptapeptide and octapeptide (see figure 14.1). These peptides are all separated by dibasic peptides, sites of proteolytic cleavage. Human brain proenkephalin contains 267 amino acids and is coded for by a gene with four exons and five introns, and a 24–amino acid N-terminal signal peptide.

Brain and adrenal proenkephalin appear to be identical, although there are differences in processing: in the brain the shorter pentapeptides predominate (met-enkephalin and leu-enkephalin), whereas in the adrenal medulla the longer, C-terminal–extended derivatives of met-enkephalin are more common. These larger molecules are metabolically more stable and thus have a longer half-life but, in general, the enkephalins are rapidly degraded by peptidases. However, their activity is retained and their half-life prolonged by the substitution of D-amino acids in position 2 or 5 of leu-enkephalin.

Proenkephalin-containing neurons are much more widely distributed in the brain than POMC-containing neurons (see figures 14.2 and 14.3). Enkephalinergic neurons form both local circuits and long projection tracts. Proenkephalin is found in the cerebral cortex, basal ganglia, and limbic system, several basal telencephalic structures such as the nucleus accumbens, the bed nucleus of the stria terminalis, and the amygdala. Proenkephalin is also present in the hypothalamus and thalamus, the spinal cord, and the anterior and posterior pituitary. In addition, it is found in various peripheral tissues such as the adrenal medulla and reproductive system (Schafer et al., 1991).

14.3.3 Prodynorphin (Proenkephalin B)

Prodynorphin is a 30-kD presursor molecule which is processed to produce several peptides structurally related to leu-enkephalin. Prodynorphin contains three sequences of leu-enkephalin and several opiate peptides, all of which are C-terminal extensions of leu-enkephalin (see figure 14.1). These include α- and β-neoendorphin, dynorphin A (1–17), dynorphin A (1–8), and dynorphin B (1–29), sometimes called leumorphin. The products of prodynorphin may vary with tissue-specific processing, yielding first peptides selective for one type of receptor (dynorphin 1–17 and α-neo-endorphin, which prefer κ receptors) and then, by subsequent processing, the δ-specific leu-enkephalin. Tissue-specific processing may cause cleavages not only at dibasic sites but also at some single arginine sites, so that the product of post-translational processing depends on the specific enzymes present in the tissue.

Dynorphin is a heptadecapeptide of considerable potency (Goldstein et al., 1981), but its physiological role is uncertain. It has been reported to be an important mediator of electroacupuncture (Han and Xi, 1984). The primary amino acid structure of dynorphin A (1–17) is

Tyr-Gly-Gly-Phe-Leu-Arg-Arg-Ile-Arg-Pro-
Lys-Leu-Lys-Trp-Asp-Asn-Gly.

It can be seen from the amino acid residues shown in italic that dynorphin contains leu-enkephalin as its N-terminal sequence.

Prodynorphin is widely distributed throughout the brain. Like the proenkephalins, the precursor for the dynorphins is found in local and long-tract projections, often in parallel with the proenkephalin systems. There are many similarities in distribution to that of proenkephalin, but there are also differences. The ventral pallidum is densely innervated by dynorphin cells and fibers, whereas the globus pallidus is enriched with enkephalins. In the magnocellular neurons of the hypothalamus, dynorphin is coexpressed with VP, with which it is coreleased in response to dehydration (S. J. Watson et al., 1982).

14.3.4 Circulating Opiate Neuropeptides

Immunoreactive opiates are present in the CSF and in the peripheral circulation. During stress, ACTH and its related peptides are released simultaneously from the anterior pituitary. In the human, most of the β-lipotropin is secreted into the circulation intact so that circulating levels of the endorphins are very low. However, variations in endorphin levels in CSF can be correlated with different types of pain (Almay et al., 1978). Met-enkephalin is present in the circulation and in the adrenal vein in high concentrations, but its release does not appear to be controlled by stress.

14.3.5 Nociceptin

Nociceptin is processed from a larger precursor, prepronociceptin, and the complete coding sequences for the gene encoding the precursor have been identified. The overall structure and organization of the gene are highly conserved in mouse, rat, and human and are markedly similar to those of the endogenous opiate peptides, suggesting that the four genes belong to the same family. The human prepronociceptin gene is located on human chromosome 8p and is chiefly transcribed in the brain and spinal cord. In the mouse CNS, nociceptin mRNA is highly expressed in discrete neuronal sites with a pattern distinct from that of the opiate peptides.

In the short time since its discovery, many physiological properties of nociceptin have been reported. These include central control of water balance; regulation of arterial blood pressure; hyperanalgesia when injected i.c.v, but analgesia when administered into the spinal cord; ataxia; loss of the righting reflex and the spinal nociceptive flexor reflex; and inhibition of mouse vas deferens contractions. None of these actions are affected by opiate antagonists. Electrophysiological studies show that nociceptin applied microiontophoretically to CNS nociceptive neurons has an inhibitory modulatory effect on N-methyl-D-aspartate (NMDA)–evoked responses from these neurons (X. M. Wang et al., 1996) and appears to act presynaptically to inhibit the release of the neurotransmitter GABA in periaqueductal gray neurons (Vaughan et al., 1997).

14.4 Opiate Receptors

14.4.1 Opiate Antagonists and Agonists

Opiate antagonists bind to opiate receptors with high affinity but are unable to trigger the subsequent events, such as analgesia. They are invaluable pharmacological tools for identifying receptor types. Some substances, like *naloxone*, bind to opiate receptors as a pure antagonist without any apparent agonist activity: other substances have mixed antagonist and agonist

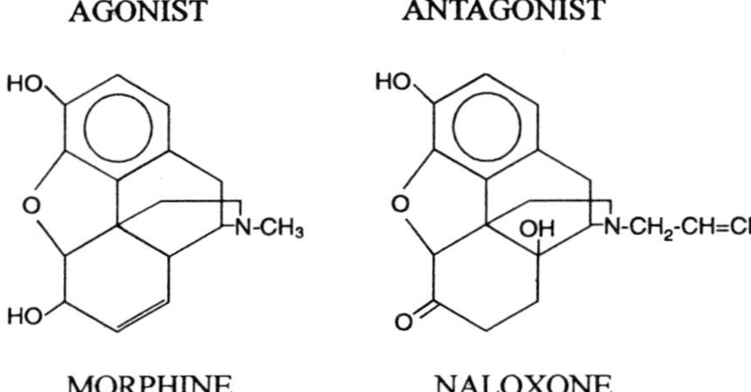

Figure 14.5
Chemical structure of the classical opiate ligands, morphine and its antagonist, naloxone. (From Borsodi and Tóth, 1995.)

actions depending on the dosage, the species, and the test situation (Brady, 1993). Naloxone is, chemically, *N*-allylnoroxymorphone, and has become indispensable for determining the selectivity of opiate agonist action: minute amounts of naloxone can prevent or reverse the effects of morphine. *Nalorphine* is another morphine antagonist that selectively antagonizes the respiratory depression induced by opiates, but morphine and naloxone remain the standards against which opiate activity and opiate antagonism are measured. Various morphine analogs have been synthesized, one of the most potent being *etorphine*, which is 1000 times as potent as morphine. Figure 14.5 shows the chemical structure of the classical opiate ligands, morphine and naloxone.

14.4.2 *Distribution of Opiate Receptors*

14.4.2.1 Receptor Autoradiography

Early binding studies of opiate ligands to brain membranes showed marked variations in the number of receptors in different regions of rat brain (Pert and Snyder, 1973). The binding is highest in the striatum, lowest in the cerebellum, with moderate levels in other brain regions. The phylogenetically newer structures in primates, such as the diencephalon and telencephalon, but also the older limbic system, have the highest number of opiate binding sites (Atweh and Kuhar, 1983) and they are most frequently found in association with three major systems: the *sensory*, *limbic*, and *neuroendocrine systems*.

In *sensory systems*, opiate receptors are concentrated on afferent pathways in the dorsal horn of the spinal cord, and in the substantia gelatinosa of the cord and medulla. These are important structures for transmission of pain and temperature to the CNS and are major sites of analgesic action of opiates. Local application of opiates to the substantia gelatinosa specifically blocks the transmission of nociceptive stimuli. The periaqueductal gray of the midbrain and thalamus are significant areas for pain control. The enkephalin and endorphin pathways exert a descending inhibitory influence on the transmission of nociceptive impulses in the spinal cord. Electrical stimulation of the periaqueductal gray elicits considerable analgesia.

In the *limbic system* the high concentration of opiate receptors is associated with the effects of opiates on mood and behavior. However, there are considerable differences in the distribution of opiate receptors in rodent and primate brains. In the rodent forebrain the highest concentrations are in the cortical layers of the amygdala and basal ganglia, whereas in the primate amygdala the receptors are uniformly distributed.

In *neuroendocrine systems*, the high concentration of endogenous opiates and opiate receptors in the hypothalamus suggests that they may be important in neuroendocrine regulation. There are few opiate receptors in the anterior pituitary, which has β-endorphin but little or no enkephalin, but the posterior pituitary is rich in opiate receptors, enkephalin, and dynorphin.

14.4.2.2 Immunohistochemical Localization of Specific Opiate Receptors and mRNAs

The recent cloning of the three opiate receptor types, σ, δ, and κ, has allowed the specific localization of each type, with a precision not permitted by autoradiographic methods. This is possible through the use of specific antibodies for each receptor type combined with immunohistochemical techniques. For example, determination of the immunohistochemical distribution of the κ receptor–like protein uses antibodies generated to the C-terminal 42 amino acids of the cloned receptor, a region of the receptor that has little homology to the μ and σ receptors (Mansour et al., 1996). In situ hybridization techniques can be used to visualize the receptor mRNAs and thus the cells that synthesize the receptors. One of the most interesting findings from these techniques is that there is not always a correlation between the expression of a receptor mRNA and a binding site for that receptor; in these instances it seems that the receptors are synthesized in one region and transported to another, where they are incorporated into the presynaptic membrane (figure 14.6).

14.4.2.3 Opiate Receptors in Pain Pathways

Opiates regulate the ascending and descending pain pathways to produce analgesia. There are two main ascending pain pathways, the first being the *neospinothalamic tract*, which projects to the thalamus and then to the somatosensory cortex for the perception of primary pain. The second pain pathway, the *paleospinothalamic tract*, projects to the periaqueductal gray in the reticular formation, then to the thalamus, and finally, diffusely, to the limbic and subcortical areas involved in secondary or subjective pain, accounting for the highly subjective and individual perception of pain (Besson and Chaouch, 1987). Intracerebral injection of the opiates in these areas induces an intense analgesia that is specifically blocked by naloxone, a μ receptor antagonist, but not by δ or κ antagonists.

In the ascending pathways, all three types of receptors modulate primary sensory transmission and are localized in the dorsal root ganglia, spinal cord, and spinal trigeminal nucleus. At the thalamic level, however, the μ and κ receptors predominate. In the descending pain pathway, it is again the μ and κ receptors that are found at higher levels, such as the periaqueductal gray and raphe nuclei, whereas all three opiate receptor types are present in the reticular nuclei (Mansour et al., 1995).

14.4.3 Classification of Receptors by Function

On the basis of neurophysiological and behavioral tests, at least four types of opiate receptors were postulated, three of which were named for the prototype drugs used with which the receptors bind: mu (μ) for *m*orphine, kappa (κ) for *k*etocyclazocine, and *s*igma (σ) for SKF 10047 (*N*-allylnormetazocine) respectively. σ Binding sites seem to overlap with binding sites for the nonopiate drug of abuse, phencyclidine (angel dust) and for antipsychotics such as haloperidol, and as their reactions are not reversed by naloxone, their classification as opiate receptors is dubious (Simon and Hiller, 1994).

The third, confirmed opiate receptor type is the delta (δ) receptor, so named because it is the predominant receptor in the vas *d*eferens. The μ, δ, and κ receptors are the most important for the action of the endogenous opiates and all three receptor types have been cloned (Reisine and Bell, 1993). The μ, δ, and κ receptors are homologous to each other at both the nucleic acid and amino acid levels, and their transmembrane loops and intracellular loops are highly conserved. In general, the μ and δ receptors bind enkephalins and endorphins and the κ receptors potently

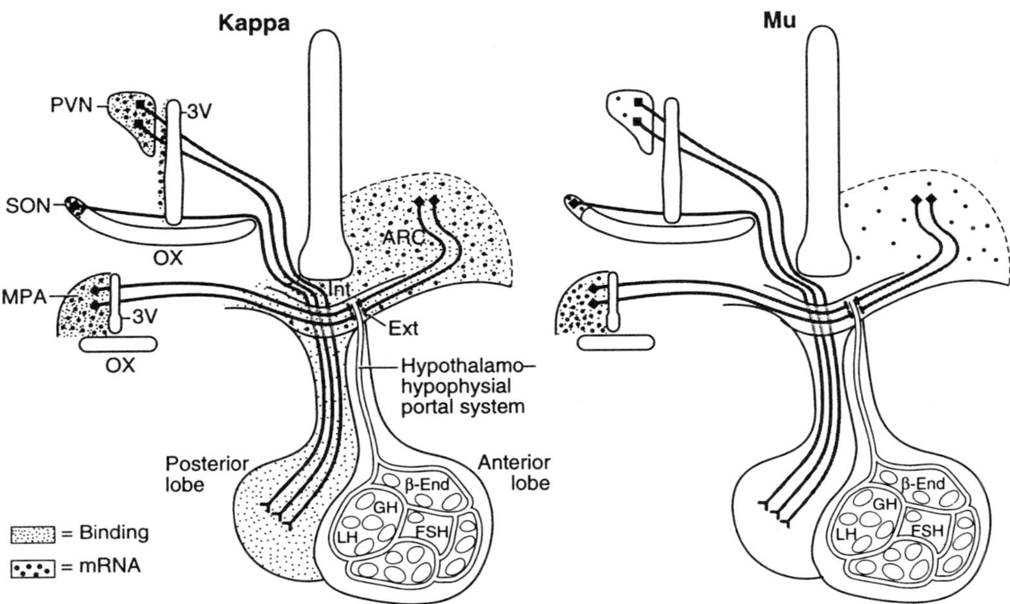

Figure 14.6
Schematic representation of the μ and κ receptor mRNA and binding distributions in the hypothalamus and pituitary. κ Receptors and mRNA are present in the paraventricular (PVN) and supraoptic nuclei (SON) of the hypothalamus. κ Receptor agonists, such as dynorphin, inhibit the release of vasopressin and oxytocin from these magnocellular nuclei. The posterior lobe contains only the κ receptors and not their mRNA, indicating that the receptors are probably synthesized in the PVN and SON, then *transported to the neural lobe.* κ Receptor binding and mRNA are also localized in the medial preoptic area (MPA) and arcuate nucleus (ARC) where κ agonists can affect the release of anterior pituitary hormones. The MPA also has high levels of μ receptors and their mRNA, indicating a route for the inhibitory effects of μ agonists on the release of luteinizing hormone–releasing hormone. There are comparatively few cells that express receptor mRNA in the PVN, SON, or ARC. 3V, third ventricle; Ext, external layer of median eminence; Int, internal layer of median eminence; OX optic chiasm; β-End, β-endorphin; GH, growth hormone; FSH; follicle-stimulating hormone. Fine stippling represents distribution of receptor autoradiographic grains produced by μ, δ, or κ receptor ligands in the hypothalamic-pituitary axis. Black dots symbolize the distribution of cells expressing the receptor mRNA. (From Mansour et al., 1995.)

Table 14.3
Tentative classification of opiate receptor subtypes and their actions

Receptor	Analgesia	Other
μ		
μ_1	Supraspinal	Prolactin release Feeding Brain acetylcholine release
μ_2	Spinal	Respiratory depression Gastrointestinal transit Brain dopamine turnover Feeding Guinea pig ileum bioassay Most cardiovascular effects
κ		
κ_1	Spinal	Diuresis Feeding
κ_2	Unknown	
κ_3	Supraspinal	
δ		Mouse vas deferens bioassay
δ_1	Supraspinal	
δ_2	Spinal and supraspinal	

From Pasternak et al. (1988).

bind dynorphin. The opiates can react with more than one receptor but usually with different affinities and potencies. There are several subtypes of each receptor type, but these subtypes are established on pharmacological evidence, and as yet no subtype has been cloned. It is also possible that subtypes may be based on post-translational alterations. Table 14.3 lists the opiate receptors, their subtypes, and major physiological functions.

Bioassays of the potency of the different opiate peptides demonstrate that morphine reacts preferentially with the μ receptor, inhibiting contractions of the guinea pig ileum, whereas the enkephalins inhibit the contractions of the mouse vas deferens through their reactions with δ receptors. These are simple, widely used tests that permit the ranking of relative agonist and antagonist potencies of many compounds. The test involves inducing twitches by a series of single electrical stimuli which, in the guinea pig ileum, can be inhibited in a dose-dependent manner by morphine and dynorphin. The inhibitory action of these opiates is blocked by naloxone. In the mouse vas deferens it is the enkephalins that inhibit muscle contractions, an action that is also blocked by naloxone. β-Endorphin is equally effective in both tissues. Figure 14.7 shows the original recordings made by J. S. Hughes (1975) of the depressant effect of crude brain extract on vas deferens contractions. The antinociceptive properties of the opiates are tested in rodents by the hot-plate method for the mouse, and the tail-flick response in the rat.

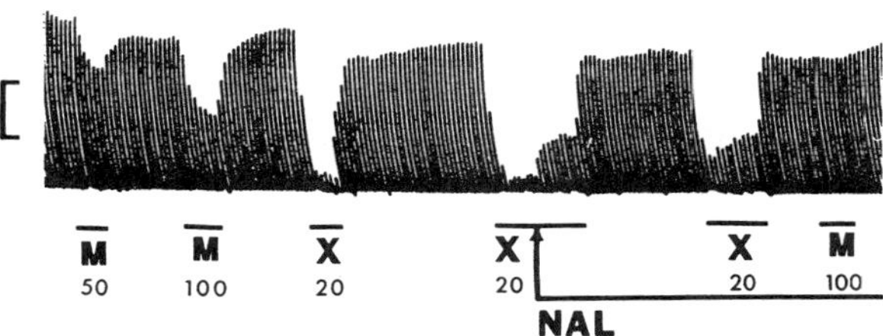

Figure 14.7
Effect of crude extract from pig brain on neurally evoked contractions of mouse vas deferens. Addition of this extract (X 20) caused a decrease in the contraction amplitude greater than that produced by the administration of morphine (M 50 and 100 ng). Concurrent administration of naloxone (NAL, 60nM) partially antagonized the effect of the extract. Naloxone itself had no effect on contractions of the vas deferens. Vertical calibration 100 mg. (From J. S. Hughes, 1975.)

14.4.4 *Classification of Receptors by Gene Family*

The cloning of the opiate receptor cDNAs and genes has shown that, based on gene structure and amino acid sequence homologies, opiate receptors can be classified as one gene family (Evans et al., 1992; Uhl et al., 1994; J. B. Wang et al., 1993; Yasuda et al., 1993). The three opiate receptor genes are located on different chromosomes in the human genome. They are very similar in extron and intron organization and may have been derived from a single ancestor gene (J. B. Wang et al., 1994). Interestingly, there is a high degree of amino acid sequence similarity between the μ and somatostatin receptors, raising the possibility that some ligands may be able to bind both receptors (Pelton et al., 1985). Opiate receptors are members of the G protein–coupled receptors containing seven transmembrane domains and share approximately 60% to 67% amino acid sequence similarity, chiefly in the transmembrane spanning regions and intracellular loops. Differences occur mainly in the amino acid sequences in the N- and C-termini, the fourth transmembrane region, and in the second and third extracellular loops. Selectivity for ligands and differential sensitivity to agonists and antagonists may depend on these variations. For example, the second extracellular loop and the C-terminal portion of the κ receptor are involved in binding dynorphin and can differentiate between peptide and nonpeptide ligands (Reisine et al., 1994). However, peptide agonists may rely on different domains of the same receptor to distinguish between μ and δ receptors and μ and κ receptors (B. Watson et al., 1996).

14.4.4.1 μ Receptors

These receptors display high affinity for morphine and lesser affinities for enkephalin. The human μ receptor is encoded by a single gene of more than 50 kb containing introns separating several functional receptor domains and is localized to chromosome 6q25 (J. B. Wang et al., 1994). The μ receptors are widely distributed in the brain and spinal cord, mainly postsynaptically but occasionally presynaptically (Ding et al., 1996). High levels of mRNA for μ receptors are found in the thalamus, striatum, locus ceruleus, and the nucleus of the solitary tract; lesser amounts are distributed throughout the brain and spinal cord. For excellent detailed maps of the distribution of the three opiate receptor types, see Mansour et al. (1995). The μ receptors are involved in the processing of sensory information.

14.4.4.2 δ Receptors

The δ receptors have high affinity for enkephalin peptides and micromolar affinities for morphine. There may be an enkephalin-preferring δ receptor subtype. The human δ receptor is encoded by an intron-containing gene located on chromosome 1p34 (Evans et al., 1992). The δ receptors are more limited in their distribution to sensory brain areas than the μ receptors, being restricted to olfactory-related areas such as the olfactory bulb, the olfactory tubercle, and the amygdala (Mansour et al., 1987). The δ receptors are highly concentrated in the cortex, striatum, and lateral reticular area, implying that they may be involved in the integration of sensorimotor information.

14.4.4.3 κ Receptors

The κ Receptors display high affinity for dynorphin peptides. Human κ receptors are encoded by an intron-containing gene on chromosome 8. The κ receptors represent approximately 10% of the total opiate binding sites in the rat brain and are found in high concentrations in the nucleus accumbens, substantia nigra, ventral tegmental area, and the nucleus of the solitary tract. The κ receptors are the predominant receptor type in the hypothalamus and are also present in the neural and intermediate lobes of the pituitary (Mansour et al., 1995, 1996). The κ receptors are involved in important functions such as antinociception, fluid homeostasis, hormonal regulation, nigrostriatal function, and the control of visceral responses. They are believed to be involved with the processing of sensory information but to a much lesser extent than the μ receptors.

14.4.4.4 ORL_1 Receptors

The "orphan" opiate receptor–like or ORL_1 receptor, also a member of the G protein–coupled family of receptors, binds nociceptin as its natural ligand. The primary structure of the ORL_1 receptor is most closely related to that of opiate receptors, with about 60% homology, yet its pharmacological properties are not opiate as they are not affected by the opiate antagonists. The receptor activates the adenylate cyclase pathway, increases intracellular Ca^{2+} concentration, and increases the inwardly rectifying K^+ conductance. These changes account for the inhibitory actions of nociceptin in cells expressing ORL_1 and are not affected by naloxone (Vaughan and Christie, 1997b). Through the use of nociceptin analogs it has been shown that the highly basic, internal core of nociceptin may be essential to the affinity and activity of the ligand at the ORL_1 receptor (Butour et al., 1997). These studies, and several others, indicate that despite the similarity in structure of nociceptin and dynorphin, the latter is not a ligand for the ORL_1 receptor.

14.4.5 Correlation of Opiate Receptors with Neurotransmitters and the Hypothalamo-Pituitary-Adrenal Axis

The fine resolution obtained from immunohistochemical studies permits the correlation of the phenotype of the cell in which the opiate receptor is localized with the transmitters and neuropeptides it may regulate. The presence of the μ receptor in the cells of the locus ceruleus satisfactorily explains the inhibition of these neurons by μ receptor agonists which inhibit NE release. Localization of the μ and κ receptor–expressing cells in the medial preoptic area, the arcuate nucleus and the external layer of the median eminence are compatible with their roles in inhibiting the release of LH and increasing PRL, GH, POMC, and cortisone release. The localization of κ receptor mRNA in the PVN and SON suggests that these receptors may be involved in the inhibition of VP and OT release (Mansour et al., 1995). Opiates may regulate the melanocortin system, down-regulating the expression of POMC mRNA in the hypothalamus, as well as reducing the MC4 receptor RNA in the periaqueductal gray (Alvaro et al., 1997).

14.4.6 Opiate Second-Messenger Systems

Using cloned opiate receptors it has become possible to study the coupling of opiate receptors and signal transduction pathways in various cells, including frog oocytes. These studies confirm similar intrinsic properties for all three opiate receptors in modulating the activity of the three effector pathways, that is, adenylate cyclase and K^+ and Ca^{2+} channels. In some cases, a single receptor in the same cell may activate multiple effector pathways (Kaneko et al., 1994). The opiate receptors, when activated, act on adenylate cyclase to inhibit cAMP formation, decrease the conductance of voltage-gated Ca^{2+} channels, or activate inwardly rectifying K^+ channels. These changes are mediated by G_i or G_o proteins and result in inhibition of neuronal activity.

Although activation of opiate receptors generally inhibits neuronal excitability, opiates are frequently excitatory in vivo, probably due to disinhibition mechanisms. It has not been possible to show a direct coupling of opiate receptors to an excitatory system, such as the phosphoinositide cascade, although the μ opiate receptor seems to be able to couple to IP_3 turnover (Uhl et al., 1995). The cloned opiate receptors expressed on *Xenopus* (frog) oocytes mediate the oscillatory Cl^- current response by mobilizing Ca^{2+} from internal stores via inositol phosphate formation. Gi_i and G_o proteins are probably involved and may stimulate phospholipase C (Kaneko et al., 1994). Opiate second-messenger systems are reviewed by Kieffer (1995).

14.4.7 Conformational States of Opiate Receptors

Opiate receptors can exist in different conformational states which determine the degree of their agonist/antagonist binding affinities. One state, the *agonist state*, preferentially binds agonists. The other state, the *antagonist state*, preferentially binds antagonists. Na^+ in the incubation medium increases the affinity of antagonist binding while decreasing that of agonist binding (Simon and Hiller, 1988).

14.5 Actions of Opiates

14.5.1 General Actions

Opiates have two main direct effects on neurons. The first is an *inhibition of firing rate*, especially of neurons involved in the reception of nociceptive information. The opiates, morphine and the endogenous opiates, cause membrane hyperpolarization and reduce the amplitude of synaptic potentials. This inhibitory action can be shown in many brain areas. β-Endorphin and dynorphin inhibit most of the neurons in hypothalamic slices and this inhibition can be blocked by receptor-appropriate antagonists (Lin and Pan, 1994). Dynorphin decreases excitatory transmission from the dentate granule cells of the hippocampus, potentially counteracting the excitation involved in epilepsy or long-term potentiation, an effect mediated by κ receptors (Drake et al., 1994). Many other brain regions are inhibited by opiate administration; a comprehensive review of opiate effects can be found in the yearly review of endogenous opiates by Olson et al. in the journal *Peptides*. In some cases the opiate peptides act as *neurotransmitters* and are found in nerve terminals from which they are released by depolarization in a Ca^{2+}-dependent manner (Henderson et al., 1978; Iverson et al., 1978).

The second effect is the *inhibition of neurotransmitter release*. This is the basis for the bioassays in isolated peripheral systems, such as the mouse vas deferens and the guinea pig ileum, initially worked out by Kosterlitz and his colleagues (Lord et al., 1977). All three major types of receptors inhibit the contractions of mouse vas deferens, with δ agonists producing the strongest suppression (Cohen et al., 1994). The opiates also inhibit transmitter release in the CNS, a topic reviewed by Cox and Baizman (1982); the transmitters affected include epinephrine, dopamine, acetylcholine and substance P. In these examples, the opiate peptides are acting as *neuromodulators*.

14.5.2 Analgesic Effects

Pain is a composite of sensory, cognitive and affective phenomena and the control of pain by the endogenous opiates peptides is extremely complex. In experimental animals the central and peripheral administration of some enkephalin analogs, and the central administration of β-endorphin, produce analgesia to a variety of nociceptive stimuli (Frederickson, 1984). It is interesting that pain is the only basic sensation affected by the opiates; touch and proprioception are not affected.

In addition to the qualitative differences between the actions of the opiates, the predominant type of opiate receptor involved depends largely on the quality of the nociceptive stimulus, be it chemical, mechanical, electrical, or thermal. For example, an analgesic response to thermonociceptive stimuli involves μ and δ agonists, but not κ receptors. On the other hand, when visceral pain is tested, it is the μ and κ agonists that relieve pain, but not the κ agonists (Schmauss and Yaksh, 1984).

14.5.2.1 Central Analgesic Actions

Enkephalins

The enkephalins are important in pain regulation at spinal and supraspinal levels. Met-enkephalin released from the adrenal medulla in response to stress modulates the antinociception that accompanies stress. Antibodies against met-enkephalin partially diminish electroacupuncture-induced analgesia at both the level of the midbrain and spinal cord (Han and Terenius, 1982). An enkephalin analog, FK 33-824, has potent analgesic activity and highly selective μ receptor activity against experimental pain in humans (Roby et al., 1983).

β-Endorphin

In animal experiments, repeated administration of β-endorphin produces tolerance, and sudden withdrawal results in the signs characteristic of morphine withdrawal (Oyama et al., 1980). Microinjections of antibodies to β-endorphin into the periaqueductal gray decrease the analgesia elicited by electroacupuncture, but there is no effective action by β-endorphin on basal nociceptive thresholds.

In humans, β-endorphin produces long-lasting analgesia in cancer or obstetrical patients, when administered intraventricularly, intrathecally, or epidurally, but i.v. administration is ineffective. Endogenous endorphin levels contribute to the individual pain threshold and tolerance level. High levels of CSF endorphins in postoperative patients correspond well with their need for opiate analgesics, their greater pain tolerance, and higher pain thresholds (Clement-Jones and Rees, 1982).

Physical exercise is one of the most potent stimuli for β-endorphin release, and the perception of post-exercise pain is believed to be due to the increased β-endorphin levels in plasma. In rats, aerobic exercise increases CSF β-endorphin and may alter brain dynorphin and enkephalin systems, affecting post-exercise blood pressure and the pain threshold. These effects are elicited by stimulation of nerve endings in the ergoreceptors of the contracting muscles and appear to be mediated by different opiate receptors (Hoffmann et al., 1996).

Similarly, the steep rise in plasma β-endorphin during the last stages of *pregnancy and during delivery* accompany an elevation of the pain threshold in pregnant women. These opiate levels return to normal shortly after delivery, suggesting that they are activated by the stress of parturition. The normal increase in endorphins in maternal and fetal blood may alleviate the pain and trauma of parturition for both mother and infant. β-Endorphin levels also rise sharply in the distressed fetus suffering from anoxia or acidosis (Abboud, 1988).

14.5.2.2 Peripheral Analgesia and Regeneration After Injury

The peripheral analgesic actions of the enkephalins can be demonstrated after s.c. injection into rat paws sensitized with prostaglandin E_2 (Nakasawa et al.,

1985), and β-endorphin receptors, present on mice muscle fiber membranes, increase in density in pathological conditions (diabetic) (Evans and Smith, 1996). Animal models of nerve injury show many changes in neuropeptide content of the spinal cord after peripheral nerve injury (Zhang et al., 1993): β-Endorphin levels rise in the ventral horns, an increase that remains for more than 7 days (S. Hughes and Smith, 1994). Damage to the spinal cord is exacerbated by dynorphin and recovery promoted by antiserum to dynorphin. The comparative physiology of the peripheral actions of the opiates is discussed by Stefano (1989).

14.5.3 Neuroendocrine Effects

Morphine causes lactation in rats by sharply increasing the secretion of *prolactin*. The endogenous opiates have a similar effect, acting on hypothalamic neurons rather than on anterior pituitary cells, lowering DA release into the hypophyseal portal blood. In this model, β-endorphin is far more potent than dynorphin or the two enkephalins, a result perhaps of the greater resistance of β-endorphin to enzymatic degradation. As these effects are prevented by naloxone, it is presumed that that opiate receptors are involved (Meites, 1984). The endogenous opiates do not seem to be implicated in PRL release in humans.

Growth hormone secretion is stimulated by morphine and by the endogenous opiates, with the response being due to an inhibition of somatostatin release as well as to increased GHRH release (Chichara et al., 1978). Opiates do not seem to be important modulators of GH secretion in humans.

Gonadotropin release in rodents is inhibited by morphine and the endogenous opiates, with the action being on hypothalamic neurons, mediated by monoaminergic neurons: NE and epinephrine have direct excitatory effects on LHRH neurons (Ramirez et al., 1984). β-Endorphin is primarily involved in the frequency-modulated release of LHRH, an inhibitory action that is sex steroid–dependent. Naloxone causes a prompt rise in gonadotropins and increases the frequency of spontaneous LH pulsatile secretion. Similar results are seen in humans.

Thyroid-stimulating hormone (TSH, thyrotropin) secretion is inhibited by opiates, most probably through suppression of TRH. In humans, the administration of morphine, methadone, or the metenkephalin analog D-Ala^2, MePhe^4, Met-(O)^5-ol (DAMME, FK33-824, Sandoz) elevates circulating TSH and potentiates the TSH response to TRH (Grossman et al., 1981), a small effect that does not indicate any vital control of TSH by opiates in humans.

ACTH and corticosterone secretion in rodents is affected by opiates in a manner that depends on the duration of the opiate administration. Acute administration of a variety of opiate agonists increases ACTH and corticosterone secretion, but long-term administration suppresses the HPA system. The inhibition is most likely at the hypothalamic level. In humans, the opiates tonically suppress the HPA axis probably through δ or κ receptors on pituitary corticotrophs, although there may be some hypothalamic involvement (Delitala, 1991).

Vasopressin and *oxytocin* are regulated by opiates through an enkephalin pathway from the SON and PVN to the neurohypophysis, and by β-endorphin neurons projecting from the arcuate nucleus and from the anterior pituitary gland. In addition, the VP and OT neurons themselves contain opiate peptides which are *colocalized* in the neurosecretory granules and released upon depolarization. OT and met-enkephalin are colocalized, and VP is colocalized with dynorphin (S. J. Watson et al., 1982). Figure 14.6 represents the distribution of κ receptor binding and mRNA in the hypothalamus and pituitary; the presence of these receptors and their mRNA in the PVN and SON suggests that the κ receptors are synthesized in these nuclei and respond to κ agonists by inhibiting VP and OT release from the posterior pituitary. The presence of κ receptors, but not their mRNA, in the posterior lobe suggests that these receptors are transported from the PVN and SON to presynaptic terminals in the posterior lobe.

The preponderance of evidence suggests that *opiates inhibit VP release.* The endogenous opiates may act in a paracrine manner upon opiate receptors on OT and VP nerve terminals or on pituicytes, or may constitute a feedback inhibitory loop on SON and PVN neurons. The data are somewhat conflicting for humans but, in general, the opiates appear to modulate some aspects of VP secretion, probably through the δ or κ receptors, with dynorphin being the endogenous ligand (Delitala, 1991).

OT release in animals is inhibited by opiates: morphine and its derivatives inhibit suckling-induced and ACh-mediated OT release. Endogenous opiates may modulate OT release during parturition in an inhibitory manner (Leng et al., 1985). In humans, it appears that OT secretion is regulated in much the same way as VP secretion.

The conflicting and unclear effects of opiates in humans arise from the difficulty of administering opiates to humans; consequently many studies are performed on heroin addicts or chronic methadone users, who may have other severe physiological disturbances.

14.5.4 Electrophysiological Effects

All three main opiate types shorten the Ca^{2+} component of the action potentials of sensory neurons in culture, by inhibiting Ca^{2+} entry. All three major opiate receptor agonists also hyperpolarize the resting potential by opening K^+ channels (Tallent et al., 1994).

The endogenous opiate system is involved in some *electroencephalographic (EEG)* changes. In drug abusers, morphine-induced changes in the EEG are associated with the positive subjective effects of morphine (Phillips et al., 1994). Of interest to ice cream lovers is the report that there is an increase in EEG activity in the right hemisphere in response to painful stimuli on days when ice cream lovers are not allowed to eat this delicacy. The increase in EEG activity occurs in the left hemisphere on days when they are given ice cream. The investigators interpret this as a differential cortical control mediated by the endogenous opiates for pleasurable and painful stimuli (Krahn et al., 1994).

As might be expected from the sedating action of the opiates, they increase both shallow and deep slow wave sleep. On a spinal level, opiates increase the threshold for spinal motor reflexes; dynorphin reduces dorsal root evoked potentials and has a biphasic effect on ventral root potentials (Ristic and Isaac, 1994).

14.5.5 Food and Water Intake

In general, opiate agonists stimulate feeding and the μ and κ antagonists suppress it, but the δ antagonists have variable effects. I.c.v administration of β-endorphin or dynorphin increases food intake, a process that is reduced by naloxone, and genetically obese rodents stop eating when treated with opiate antagonists (Margules et al., 1978). The opiate system is probably involved in the overeating and weight gain associated with the administration of NPY since these changes are blocked by naloxone (Lambert et al., 1994). The various antagonists have different effects on the differential intake of carbohydrates, fat, and protein, and total nutrients; the palatability of the diet, the species tested, and the route of administration of the antagonist all affect the results. Several areas of the brain are involved in opiate mediation of eating: the ventral striatum, nucleus accumbens, and the lateral hypothalamus. Electrical stimulation of the lateral hypothalamus induces eating that is modified by opiate agonists and antagonists, particularly involving the μ and κ receptors. (Papadouka and Carr, 1994). The opiate system also mediates a variety of behaviors needed for the acquisition of food, including foraging activity due to its stimulation of locomotion and its suppression of sexual activity.

Interestingly, eating changes the plasma levels of the endogenous opiates, such as β-endorphin, which is increased after an unappetizing meal but not after a highly palatable high-energy meal. Because opiates modulate eating, a link between the opiate system and eating disorders, such as bulimia and anorexia, has been investigated without much success, although the levels of β-endorphin are higher in the plasma and CNS of obese patients, and reduced in anorexic patients.

Opiate mediation of drinking is unclear as there are conflicting reports. Depending on dosage and the specific opiate involved, opiate agonists may increase, decrease, or have no effect on drinking. In general, opiate antagonists inhibit drinking. Morphine and other opiates have a strong antidiuretic effect due to release of antidiuretic hormone (VP), which will affect water balance and drinking.

14.5.6 Other Physiological Systems

The endogenous opiates influence cardiovascular and gastrointestinal functions, depress the respiratory system, and increase locomotor activity. The immune system is suppressed by chronic opiate administration. The opiate system seems to be involved in hypertension and may modulate some cardiovascular responses to extreme stress, but is probably not involved in mild stress. Morphine and the endogenous opiates, by inhibiting the motility of the gastrointestinal tract, cause constipation. The opiates, including β-endorphin, depress respiration, modulating both normal respiration and respiration under stress. The hyperlocomotion evoked by the opiates is not affected by antagonists, indicating that the endogenous opiate system is probably not involved in basic locomotor control, although there are several reports of the deleterious effect of dynorphin on motor function (Qu and Isaac, 1993). In many systems, opiates lower body temperature but there is significant species variation, and variation according to the conditions of the investigation.

14.5.7 Behavioral Effects

14.5.7.1 Reproductive Behavior

The endogenous opiates may be involved in sexual behavior since i.c.v administration of β-endorphin strongly inhibits lordosis in female rats and copulatory activity in male rats, both behaviors that are stimulated by naloxone. Enkephalinase inhibitors facilitate copulation and the enkephalins may be released before or during sex to stimulate ejaculation (Agmo et al., 1994).

14.5.7.2 Catatonia and Seizures

The major behavioral reponse to the i.c.v. injection of β-endorphin into rat brain is the dramatic development of *catatonia*, a state of prolonged muscular rigidity and immobility, similar to the catatonia seen in *schizophrenic* humans (Bloom et al., 1976). Similar neuroleptic-like effects are obtained with γ-type endorphins (De Wied, 1987). This stimulated intensive research into the metabolism of endorphins in schizophrenia but no conclusive evidence for any abnormal changes in endorphin levels has been found. The endogenous opiates with μ activity tend to induce convulsions, whereas the κ agonists have anticonvulsive action, implicating the endorphins in *epileptic seizures*.

14.5.7.3 Reward Behaviors

Opiates exert marked effects on *mood and motivation*. In humans they produce euphoria and drug-seeking behavior, and long-term administration causes tolerance and physical dependence. These drugs activate endogenous reward pathways, a process that is causal to the subsequent addiction. Koob and Bloom (1988) suggest the existence of a common reward pathway in which the nucleus accumbens receives input from the ventral tegmental area (source of the ascending mesolimbic DA system) and the limbic and olfactory cortices. Activation of opiate receptors in this circuitry is common to the rewarding effects of opiates, cocaine, and other psychostimulants, as well as alcohol. In particular, the mesolimbic DA system serves to integrate sensorimotor responses. There is a subtle balance between the opiate and DA systems in the control of the reward system: chronic inhibition of DA activity (either through a lesion or by administration of neuroleptics) dramatically increases the rewarding aspects of opiates (Stinus et al., 1986).

The *motivational effects* of opiates have been studied in experimental animal models, including self-administration, intracranial self-stimulation, and the conditioned place preference paradigm (Koob and Goeders, 1989). The results indicate that there is an endogenous, tonically active, μ receptor–mediated reward system, which when disrupted results in aversive states. Opiates are also important in positively motivated, rewarding situations for which β-endorphin seems to be of particular signicance (Herz, 1997). The opiates may affect *learning* and *memory*, as measured by classical avoidance tasks, but the result appears to be dependent on several variables, including dosage, species, age, and the specific paradigm being studied.

14.5.7.4 Tolerance and Dependence

The rapid development of tolerance and dependence, characteristic of exogenous opiates such as morphine, is also evoked by the repeated administration of the endogenous opiates. Tolerance is the loss of responsiveness to a drug, whereas dependence is shown by the abnormal physiological and behavioral symptoms that appear following drug withdrawal. These include diarrhea, weight loss, changes in body temperature and pupil dilation, changes in locomotion, "wet dog shakes," and teeth chattering. Place and taste aversion, decreased contact with others, and irritability are common. Detailed references may be found in the reviews by Olson et al. (1991, 1994, 1995).

There are several theories as to the mechanism of tolerance and dependence, one of which is the sensitization of the nucleus accumbens during the time of dependence, which then becomes the site of the aversive reactions of withdrawal (Koob et al., 1989). Repeated administration of opiate agonists reduces the number of opiate receptors and blocks receptor-effector coupling (Cox, 1994). Tolerance to opiates is also affected by DA, and OT blocks tolerance to morphine and the endogenous opiates (Sarnyai and Kovacs, 1994). Tolerance to morphine is prevented by MIF-1, which acts as an agonist in opiate-naive animals but as an antagonist in the tolerant state (Zadina et al., 1994b).

14.5.7.5 Interaction of Opiates with Alcohol

Alcoholism is one of the most widespread addictions, and like opiates, is characterized by tolerance and dependence. The withdrawal symptoms of alcohol and morphine have many symptoms in common. Chronic ethanol treatment affects opiate content, biosynthesis, and release. Alcohol causes the release of opiate peptides, especially β-endorphin, and studies in rats have shown that high doses of morphine reduce ethanol consumption but low doses of morphine increase it (Ulm et al., 1995). There are several different theories to explain this but they generally agree on an opiate imbalance that mediates the reinforcing effects of alcohol (Swift, 1995). Opiate antagonists, such as naltrexone and naloxone, are more effective than opiate agonists in reducing alcohol consumption in experimental animals and in humans (O'Malley, 1995).

14.5.7.6 Active Avoidance Behavior and Excessive Grooming

β-Endorphin, like ACTH 4–10, delays the extinction of active avoidance behavior, and α-endorphin (the N-terminal 16–amino acid peptide) is considerably more potent than the 31–amino acid parent molecule. In contrast, γ-endorphin (β-endorphin 1–17) accelerates extinction. β-Endorphin, given i.c.v., is a most potent stimulus for excessive grooming, an effect that can be blocked by naloxone. For a review of the structure and behavioral activity relationships of the endorphins and the ACTH and MSH neuropeptides, see de Wied (1979); Van Nispen and Van Wimersma Greidanus (1990).

14.6 Clinical Implications of Opiates and Opiate Antagonists

The clinical use of *morphine* and its derivatives for pain relief is invaluable. Its misuse by addicts leads to suffering, crime, and disease. Naloxone is a lifesaving drug in cases of opiate overdosage, the most critical effect of which is respiratory depression and consequent coma. *Naloxone* rapidly reverses these effects and restores the patient to almost normal breathing. The synthetic opiate, *methadone*, has been used successfully in the treatment of heroin addiction, when combined with proper dosage, slow induction, and on-site counseling. In heroin and alcohol addiction, a disruption of the endogenous opiate system occurs, especially of the HPA stress-responsive axis, which may contribute to the actual acquisition of drug-seeking behavior and addiction, persistence of addiction, and relapse to use of addictive drugs following restoration of the drug-free state (Kreek, 1996). The U.S. Food and Drug Administration has approved the clinical use of *naltrexone* for alcoholism (Nightingale, 1995). This opiate antagonist offers a new, safe, and effective medication for preventing relapse following detoxication. Naltrexone reduces the pleasurable effects of alcohol and enhances the effectiveness of psychosocial therapy (Volpicelli et al., 1995). Naltrexone is now widely used in the treatment of alcoholism, together with antidepressants and psychotherapy, since alcoholism is a complex disease, often with a genetic background.

Clinical use of the endorphins and enkephalins is still in its infancy, but the development of potent enkephalin analogs, which resist degradation and retain their analgesic properties without the accompanying addictive characteristics, shows much promise.

14.7 Summary

The endogenous opiates are involved in pain regulation, behaviors such as reinforcement and reward, and in neuroendocrine regulation. They are widely and differentially distributed in the CNS and exert a profound effect on many physiological systems, including the cardiovascular, gastrointestinal, respiratory, and immune systems.

The three endogenous opiate families are the endorphins, enkephalins, and dynorphins, which are coded for by three separate genes. The endorphins arise from β-lipotropin, which is cleaved from POMC, as explained in chapter 12. The enkephalins, all of which are pentapeptides, are derived from proenkephalin. The dynorphin precursor is prodynorphin. The three genes have a strong structural similarity and may have arisen from an extremely old gene.

The *endorphins* β-lipotropin, the 31–amino acid C-terminal peptide of β-lipotropin, is localized in the arcuate nucleus and the nucleus tractus solitarius of the brain stem and also in the anterior and intermediate lobes of the pituitary. In the brain and pituitary, β-endorphin is in its active, nonacetylated form in contrast to the acetylated, inactive β-endorphin of the intermediate lobe. Physical exercise is a potent stimulus to β-endorphin release, and β-endorphin levels rise steeply in the late stages of pregnancy and during delivery, increasing pain thresholds. β-Endorphin levels also increase in the distressed fetus. Repeated administration of β-endorphin produces tolerance, and sudden withdrawal results in signs and symptoms comparable to morphine withdrawal.

The *enkephalins* are pentapeptides with either Leu or Met at the C-terminal and have a structural similarity to morphine. They are derived from proenkephalin, which is found in the adrenal gland and reproductive system, and in the widely distributed enkephalinergic systems of the brain, including the hypothalamus, thalamus, and pituitary gland. The enkephalins are important in pain regulation at spinal and supraspinal levels and are involved in electroacupuncture-induced analgesia, but are rapidly degraded by peptidases in tissues and in the circulation.

The *dynorphins* are derived from prodynorphin, the products of which vary with the tissue in which it is processed. Prodynorphin is widely distributed throughout the brain, in local and long-tract projections, with some similarities to proenkephalin distribution.

Four tetrapeptides with opiate activity, Tyr-MIF-1, Tyr-W-MIF-1, MIF-1 and Tyr-K-MIF-1, have been isolated from human brain cortex. They vary in their binding specificities and may form endogenous opiate and antiopiate systems. A related tetrapeptide, endomorphin-1, has high selectivity for the μ opiate receptor.

Nociceptin has structural similarities to dynorphin and has pharmacological characteristics similar to those of the opiates, but its actions are not affected by opiate antagonists.

Opiate receptors are most concentrated in the diencephalon and telencephalon, frequently in association with the sensory, limbic, and neuroendocrine systems. In the sensory system, opiate receptors are concentrated in the dorsal horn of the spinal cord and the substantia gelatinosa of the cord and medulla. Local application of opiates to these areas blocks nociceptive transmission. Opiate receptors in the limbic system are associated with opiate effects on mood and behavior, and opiate receptors in the hypothalamus with neuroendocrine integration. The anterior pituitary has few opiate receptors, scant amounts of enkephalin, but has considerable amounts of β-endorphin. The posterior pituitary has many opiate receptors, and both enkephalin and dynorphin.

Opiate receptors form one gene family the most important of which are the μ, δ, and κ receptors. Morphine reacts preferentially with the μ receptor, the enkephalins and endorphins with the δ receptor, and dynorphin with the κ receptor. Opiate receptors are G protein–coupled with seven transmembrane domains and they inhibit adenylate cyclase in a guanosine triphosphate (GTP)–dependent manner, decrease Ca^{2+} conductance, and affect K^+ channels. The μ receptor couples to IP_3 turnover as well.

Opiate antagonists bind to opiate receptors with high affinity but do not trigger the subsequent physiological effects, such as analgesia. *Naloxone* binds to opiate receptors as a pure antagonist and is invaluable for the determination of opiate agonist activity, and as a blocker of opiate activity. Other morphine antagonists include nalorphine and naltrexone. Etorphine is a highly potent morphine *agonist*. The conformation of the opiate receptor determines its agonist or antagonist binding affinity. The presence of Na^+ increases the affinity for the antagonist and decreases the affinity for the agonist.

Opiates are powerful *analgesics*, modulating pain transmission at all levels of the ascending pain pathways. Opiates also act as *neuromodulators* to inhibit neurotransmitter release in the CNS and in isolated peripheral systems, an effect that is the basis of bioassays based on inhibition of the contractions of mouse vas deferens and guinea pig ileum. The endogenous opiates affect the *EEG* differentially for both pleasurable and painful stimuli, and have *sedative* effects. The opiates have important *neuroendocrine effects*, increasing the release of PRL, GHRH, and GH, and inhibiting the release of somatostatin, TRH, and TSH. The *HPA axis* is affected by the opiates, as is the release of VP and OT, but other opiates may increase VP release.

Other *physiological systems* are depressed by the opiates, including the cardiovascular, respiratory, gastrointestinal, and immune systems. In many species, opiates lower body temperature. The opiates have several effects on *behaviors* such as copulation and lordosis, convulsive activity, mood and motivation, and alcohol addiction.

In chapter 15, a new neuropeptide family appears, the tachykinins, of which substance P is the most familiar. Like so many other neuropeptides, the tachykinins were first discovered in the gut and then found to be widely distributed in the CNS and periphery.

Tachykinins: Substance P, Neurokinin A, and Neurokinin B

15

15.1 History

Tachykinins belong to an evolutionary conserved family of peptide neurotransmitters, in which, however, only the functionally important C-terminal sequence Phe-X-Gly-Leu-Met-NH_2 has been conserved. In this sequence X is an aromatic (Tyr or Phe) or hydrophobic residue (Val or Ile) (table 15.1). Tachykinins are found in invertebrates, lampreys, elasmobranchs, amphibians, and mammals (Waugh et al., 1995). The *nonmammalian tachykinins*, eleidosin, physalaemin, and kassinin, were identified as hypotensive, sialogenic, and spasmogenic agents in extracts of salivary glands of the octopus by Erspamer (1949) and the structure of eleidosin, the most potent of these agents, was established by Erspamer and Anastasi in 1962. Eleidosin was later shown to be similar in structure and action to the mammalian tachykinin, substance P.

Of the three important *mammalian tachykinin* peptides, *substance P (SP)* is an undecapeptide; *neurokinin A (NKA*, formerly substance K) and *neurokinin B (NKB*, formerly neuromedin K) are decapeptides (see table 15.1). *Kinins* form a group of endogenous peptides that cause vasodilation, increase vascular permeability, cause hypotension, and induce contraction of smooth muscle. The *tachykinins* (*tachys*, swift) evoke a sharp contraction of the smooth muscle of the gut, but their potencies differ considerably depending on the pharmacological model used. The three mammalian tachykinins are involved in different biological activities due to the several different types of tachykinin receptors.

Table 15.1
Amino acid sequences of mammalian and nonmammalian tachykinins

Peptide (equivalent nomenclature)	Abbreviation	Amino acid sequence[a]
Mammalian tachykinins (neurokinins)		
Substance P	SP	Arg-Pro-Lys-Pro-Gln-Gln-Phe-Phe-Gly-Leu-Met NH_2
Neurokinin A (substance K, neurokinin-α, neuromedin L)	NKA	His-Lys-Thr-Asp-Ser-Phe-Val-Gly-Leu-Met NH_2
Neurokinin B (neurokinin-β, neuromedin K)	NKB	Asp-Met-His-Asp-Phe-Phe-Val-Gly-Leu-Met NH_2
Nonmammalian tackykinins		
Eleidosin	ELE	Glu-Pro-Ser-Lys-Asp-Ala-Phe-Ile-Gly-Leu-Met NH_2
Physalaemin	PHY	Glu-Ala-Asp-Pro-Asn-Lys-Phe-Tyr-Gly-Leu-Met NH_2
Kassinin	KAS	Asp-Val-Pro-Lys-Ser-Asp-Gln-Phe-Val-Gly-Leu-Met NH_2

From Cuello (1987).
[a] The homologous sequences at the C-terminal end are indicated within boxes.

Substance P was the first member of this triad to be discovered. Euler and Gaddum (1931) isolated SP from extracts of intestine and from brain, as a substance that stimulated atropine-resistant contractions of rabbit ileum. It was one of many substances isolated by them at that time and because it was in *p*owdered form, they named it substance *P*. In view of its significant role in *p*ain transmission, its name is now more appropriate. SP was recognized as a sensory transmitter by Lembeck (1953), but little work was done until much later when SP was isolated and sequenced from bovine hypothalamus by Susan Leeman and her collaborators (Leeman and Hammerschlag, 1967; Chang and Leeman, 1970; Chang et al., 1971, Tregear et al., 1971).

It was not until the early 1980s that the other two mammalian tachykinins were discovered. NKA was the second tachykinin to be identified (Maggio et al., 1983) and sequenced (Kimura et al., 1983). Several differently named neurokinins were isolated by different investigators; their sequences subsequently showed them to be either the cationic peptide NKA or the anionic peptide NKB (Kimura et al., 1983; Kawanga et al., 1983; Hunter and Maggio, 1984) (figure 15.1). Since then the pace of investigation of the tachykinins has accelerated, aided immensely by the isolation and cloning of the genes that code for multiple tachykinins and their receptors, as well as by the availability of tachykinin agonists and antagonists.

15.2 General Functions of Tachykinins

Tachykinins are involved in a multitude of physiological processes due to their widespread distribution, centrally and peripherally. Tachykinins are found extensively in the periphery where they function as potential regulators of blood flow and vascular permeability, salivation, and micturition. Tachykinins are potent constrictors of smooth muscle and thus they are involved in the regulation of gastrointestinal motility and intestinal secretions, and are potent spasmogens of airway smooth muscle They function as pain transmitters from the periphery. Centrally, tachykinins act as neurotransmitters and neuromodulators in the brain and spinal cord, and SP regulates processes involving sensory perception in addition to pain (vision, olfaction, and audition). The tachykinins are inactivated by multiple peptidases in the tissues, especially by the airway epithelium (Maggi, 1995).

15.3 Anatomical Distribution of Tachykinins

15.3.1 In the Central Nervous System

SP is widely distributed thoughout the CNS. In the *brain*, SP is found in considerable amounts in the basal ganglia and nucleus accumbens; somewhat lesser levels are present in the cerebral cortex (Cooper et al., 1981). There is extensive evidence that SP interacts with nigrostriatal and various limbic nuclei DA neurons (M.S. Reid et al., 1990) and forebrain nuclei (Bannon et al., 1991). SP is found in important structures of the endogenous pain control system (midbrain periaqueductal gray, nucleus raphe magnus, and the nucleus reticularis gigantocellularis pars alpha) (Li et al., 1996). SP neurons are present in large numbers in the human posterior hypothalamus and in the basal forebrain (Chawla et al., 1997). The hypothalamic distribution indicates that SP may be widely involved in many hypothalamic functions, such as sexual behavior, pituitary hormone release, and water homeostasis.

All three tachykinins are found in most neurons in the corpus striatum, together with the opiate peptides enkephalin and dynorphin (Lucas and Harlan, 1995). NKB neurons are the predominant tachykinin in the anterior hypothalamus and are also present in the basal forebrain, indicating a distinct and complementary distribution from the SP neurons in these regions (Chawla et al., 1997). Whereas SP is found throughout the rat brain, NKB appears more in forebrain than in brainstem structures, suggesting that NKB may be involved in olfactory, gustatory, visceral, and neuroendocrine processing of information (Lucas et al., 1992).

In the *spinal cord* immunohistochemistry clearly shows SP to be located in a population of primary sensory neurons in dorsal root ganglia. The number of SP-containing neurons decreases markedly in lumbar dorsal root ganglia after peripheral axotomy (Barbut et al., 1981). SP is present in both central and peripheral neurons involved with *autonomic reflexes*. There is a marked difference in the distribution of the three tachykinin neuropeptides in the spinal cord (figure 15.2): SP and NKA are distributed in the same manner in the spinal cord, whereas NKB is limited to lamina II. SP and NKA are expressed by sensory neurons, but NKB is not expressed in detectable amounts in most peripheral tissues, nor is it found in sensory ganglia. mRNA for NKA is prominent in spinal cord laminae I and II and in the thoracic intermediolateral cell column, whereas the NKB precursor is prominent only in lamina III. Only preprotachykinin (PPT) mRNA is present in sensory neurons of the dorsal ganglia and in medullry raphe neurons which project to the spinal cord, indicating that spinal NKB is localized in interneurons or ascending pathways. See Helke et al. (1990) for a detailed description of the differential distribution of the NKA and NKB precursor mRNAs in the CNS.

15.3.2 In the Periphery

SP is found in substantial amounts in the myenteric and submucous nerve plexuses at all levels of the gut,

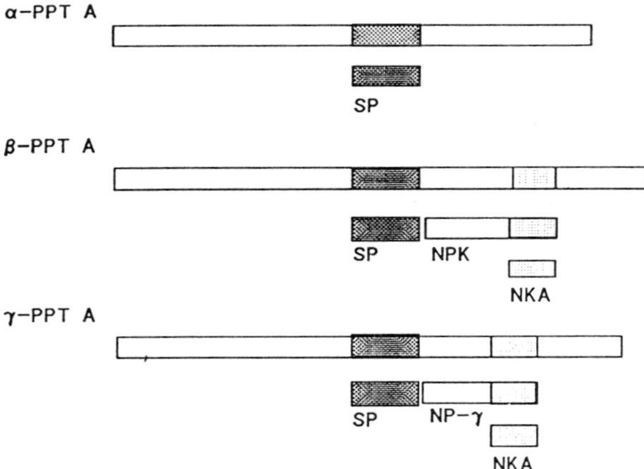

Figure 15.1
Structural relationships between the tachykinin precursors produced from the three preprotachykinin A (PPT A) mRNA species and the main biologically active products. Note that substance P (SP) is produced by processing of all three precursors. Neurokinin A (NKA) is produced from β- and γ-PPT-A. The N-terminally extended forms of NKA, that is, neuropeptide K (NPK) and neuropeptide-γ (NP-γ), are produced from β- and, γ-PPT-A, respectively. (From Dockray, 1994).

in rodents, dogs, and humans. Most SP-containing neurons in these plexuses are intrinsic in origin but some neurons are extrinsic and arise from the sensory ganglia (Costa et al., 1981). SP is also present in the pancreas and the salivary glands. A considerable proportion of circulating SP comes from the intestine. SP is also found in connective tissue, in taste buds, and in the lingual epithelium surrounding the taste buds, suggesting that SP may play a role in taste and oral pain. NKA-immunoreactive nerve fibers are localized around the secretory elements of the rat salivary glands (Virta et al., 1991). NKA is also found in the region of the gastroesophageal junction.

15.4 Co-Localization of Tachykinins

15.4.1 In the Brain

SP, NKA, and 5-HT are colocalized in neurons of the ventral medulla that project to the spinal cord. SP is colocalized differentially with other neuropeptides in the visceral afferent neurons of the vagus and glossopharygeal nerves located in the nodose and petrosal ganglia, respectively. For example, SP is contained in some, but not all neurons that contain calcitonin gene–related peptide (CGRP) (Helke et al., 1991). SP and other tachykinins coexist with ACh in neurons of the myenteric plexus; SP is colocalized with enkephalin in nerve fibers of the gut; and SP and 5-HT coexist in some nerve fibers of the myenteric plexus.

15.4.2 In the Spinal Cord

SP nerve terminals innervate the interomediolateral cell column of the thoracic spinal cord, where SP coexists with 5-HT, NKA, and TRH. However, despite their coexistence with SP, neither 5-HT nor TRH are involved in the regulation of SP release. SP, however, regulates the basal release of 5-HT acting through NK1 receptors, whereas NKA and TRH have no effect on 5-HT release (Yang et al., 1996).

15.4.3 In the Gastrointestinal Tract

SP and NKA are colocalized, mainly in the midcolon. It is probable that SP is colocalized with other neuropeptides in most of its nerve terminals, but if there is a pattern to the colocalization, it is by no means clear.

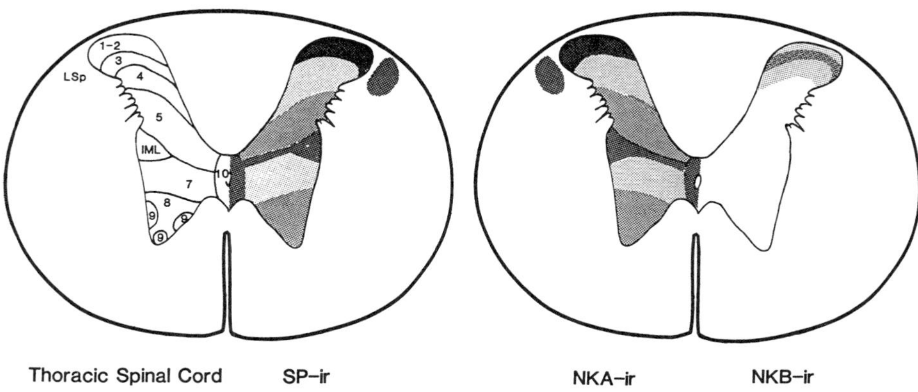

Figure 15.2
Schematic illustrations of the laminar divisions of the thoracic spinal cord in the rat (far left) and the distributions and relative intensities of substance P (SP), neurokinin A (NKA), and neurokinin B (NKB) immunoreactivity (ir) in fibers and terminals of the rat thoracic spinal cord. The pattern of SP and NKA distribution is the same: labeling is very dense in the dorsal horn, dense in the interomediolateral (IML) cell column, and moderate in the ventral horn. NKB labeling is moderately dense in lamina II but absent from almost all other cord areas. LSp, lateral spinal nucleus. (From Helke et al., 1991.)

15.5 Tachykinin Genes, Precursors, and Processing

There are two genes that encode mammalian preprotachykinins. The *preprotachykinin A (PPT-A)* gene encodes the precursor of several tachykinin neuropeptides, including SP and NKA. Neuropeptide K and neuropeptide-γ (NP-γ are N-terminally extended forms of NKA. *Differential* splicing results in three different PPT-A mRNAs (α, β, and γ). SP is encoded by all three PPT-A mRNAs, whereas NKA is produced by both β and γ PPT-A mRNA but not by α-PPT-A mRNA (Krause et al., 1987) (figure 15.1). NP-γ is a 21–amino acid peptide belonging to the tachykinin family and includes NKA in its terminal sequence.

The other gene encodes *PPT-B* which is the precursor of NKB. The gene contains two peptide sequences which are flanked by pairs of dibasic amino acids: the decapeptide NKB and a 30–amino acid nontachykinin peptide consisting of amino acids 50–79 of PPT-B (Lang and Sperk, 1995).

15.6 Expression and Regulation of the Preprotachykinin Gene

Peripheral autonomic ganglia are extensively used as a model for studying mechanisms of gene regulation and neurotransmitter action. Denervation of the ganglion considerably increases the PPT mRNA which encodes SP, as well as increasing SP itself, suggesting that the preganglionic nerve normally suppresses ganglionic SP production. The mechanisms that regulate SP and the conventional ganglionic transmitters (cholinergic and noradrenergic) are the same, that is, nerve impulse activity, but there appears to be *peptide-specific regulation* for different peptides colocalized in the same neurons because nerve impulse activity does not alter the level of NPY in the ganglion (Kessler and Freidin, 1991).

The expression of the PPT gene is developmentally and hormonally regulated in the *anterior pituitary*. Male anterior pituitaries contain more PPT mRNA than female pituitaries, but the exact hormonal control is uncertain. Testosterone may mediate this sex difference in tachykinins that appears at puberty, and estrogens may be an inhibiting factor in females, but the sex steroids appear to be mediating rather than decisive influences (Jonassen and Leeman, 1991). However, in contrast to mRNA levels of SP, reports on plasma, hypothalamic, and anterior pituitary levels of SP and NKA in male rats and in female rats during the estrous cycle and after ovariectomy show SP levels to be much lower in male rats and ovariectomized females, and also that intact females show wide fluctuations in SP and NKA content during the estrous cycle (Duval et al., 1996).

It has also been suggested that endogenous *nerve growth factor (NGF)* sensitizes both the peripheral nociceptors and the dorsal horn neurons responding to noxious stimuli (McMahon, 1996). NGF is elevated in inflamed tissues.

15.7 Tachykinin Receptors and Second Messengers

15.7.1 Types of Tachykinin Receptors

The mammalian tachykinins bind to specific receptors which are divided into three types: NK1, NK2, and NK3. All three tachykinin receptors have been cloned and contain seven membrane-spanning segments, indicating their inclusion in the G protein–linked receptor family, but they have different affinities and are distributed differently in various tissues. There is a 50% to 66% amino acid homology between the three rat receptor sequences.

Substance P is considered the natural ligand for NK1 receptors. NKA is the natural ligand for NK2 receptors, and NKB the ligand for NK3 receptors. However, NKA and NKB are fully effective agonists at the NK1 receptors, SP and NKB are equally effective agonists at NK2 receptors and, SP and NKA are fully effective agonists at NK3 receptors. It must be emphasized that the distribution and affinities of these receptors are species- and tissue-specific, and that there is considerable overlap of function. For example, NK1, NK2, and NK3 agonists can all cause contraction in guinea pig lung strips (Killingsworth and Shore, 1995). NP-γ has a higher affinity than NKA for central NK2 receptors and although NP-γ has a lower affinity for NK1 receptors, it nevertheless potently stimulates salivary secretion, which is mediated by NK1 activation. NP-γ is the most potent of the tachykinins in the control of water intake in the rat, acting as an antidipsogenic agent (Polidori et al., 1995).

The *genes coding* for the NK1, NK2, and NK3 receptors have been cloned, and a fourth receptor, which may be an NK4 receptor or an NK3 receptor subtype, has also been cloned. The gene for the NK1 receptor has been characterized. It is encoded by five exons dispersed over about 45,000 base pairs, which makes the NK1 recepter unusual among G protein–coupled receptors (Hershey et al., 1991). Only three members of this superfamily contain introns within the coding region of their genes: the NK1 receptor, the opsins, and the D_2 receptor.

15.7.2 Distribution of Tachykinin Receptors

The wide distribution of tachykinin receptors, as briefly outlined here, accounts for the highly diversified functions of this family of neuropeptides.

15.7.7.1 In the CNS

NK1 receptor sites are widely, but discretely distributed in the rat *brain*, especially in the olfactory bulb, the amygdalo-hippocampal area, some thalamic and hypothalamic nuclei, parts of the cerebellum, and the hypoglossal nucleus. There are quite important differences in the distribution of NK1 receptors in the mouse brain, as compared to that of the rat, which may be relevant since most behavioral studies have been performed in rats, whereas future experiments in transgenic animals over- or underexpressing the NK1 receptor will likely be performed in mice (Dam and Quirion, 1994).

There is a dense population of NK1 receptor–immunoreactive neurons in lamina I of the *spinal cord* at all levels, with the receptors covering almost all the dendritic and somatic surface of these neurons. Several distinct populations of NK1 receptors are located in laminae II to V, and in the neurons of the intermediolateral cell column (Brown et al., 1995). NK1 receptors are also present in *sympathetic ganglia*.

NK2 receptors are sparsely distributed in the CNS, found in low amounts in various regions including the striatum and spinal cord. *NK3 receptors* are strikingly prevalent in midcortical laminae throughout the cortex, in a pattern very different from that of the NK1 or NK2 receptors in the cortex. Many other brain regions show high densities of NK3 receptors: the SON, amygdalo-hippocampal area, medial habenula, and interpeduncular nucleus (Dam and Quirion, 1994). Many NK3 binding sites are in areas rich in DA neurons and this perhaps explains the modulatory effects of neurokinins on DA neurons in these regions.

15.7.2.2 In the Periphery

NK1 binding sites are present in the *respiratory tract*, but there are many species differences, as seen by the presence of NK1 receptors in rodent tracheal and bronchial smooth muscle but not in that of the human (Strigas and Burcher, 1993). NK2 binding sites, however, are found in both rodent and human airways, but no NK3 sites have been identified in the mammalian respiratory tract (Burcher et al., 1994). NK1 receptors are found on submucosal glands and epithelium, whereas the NK2 receptors are limited to smooth muscle, where they directly activate contraction.

The *gastrointestinal tract* of mammals is enriched with NK1, NK2, and NK3 receptors, chiefly on smooth muscle. In the human, NK1 receptors are present in gastrointestinal smooth muscle and also in the myenteric ganglia, epithelium, and lymph nodules. NK2 receptors are mainly found on the muscularis mucosae as well as on smooth muscle (Gates et al., 1988).

NK1 receptors are densely located in *salivary glands*, and are also found in the basolateral membranes of the the *taste buds*. NK1 receptors are present in *lymphoid tissue*. In the *skin*, NK1 receptors are predominant, as might be expected from the potent action of SP in causing plasma extravasation and cutaneous vasodilation. Similarly, NK1 receptors present in *joints* may explain the involvement of SP in inflammatory joint diseases. In the *urinary bladder*, contraction is mediated by NK2 receptors, but there are species differences. In the *reproductive tract*, NK1 receptors appear to predominate in the vas deferens, NK2 receptors in the uterine endometrium, myometrium, and blood vessels. All tachykinins cause contraction of *vascular smooth muscle* but there seems to be a different pattern of NK receptor distribution: NK1 receptors on rabbit jugular vein, NK2 receptors on rabbit pulmonary artery, and NK3 receptors on rat portal vein. These and other species and functional discrepancies are discussed by Burcher et al., (1994).

Table 15.2
Structure and properties of rat tachykinin receptors

	NK1 Receptor	NK2 Receptor	NK3 Receptor
Amino acid residues	407	452	390
Molecular weight	46,364	51,104	43,851
Core homology	66% to NKA 54% to NKB	55% to NKB	
Possible N-glycosylation sites	2	4	1
Possible phosphorylation sites:			
3rd loop	5	2	1
C-terminus	26	28	14
2nd messenger	IP_3-Ca^{2+}	IP_3-Ca^{2+}	IP_3-Ca^{2+}
Desensitization	+++	++	+
Expression sites:			
nervous system	+++	+	−++
peripheral tissues	+++	++	+++

Adapted from Ohkubo and Nakanishi (1991).
NKA, neurokinin A; NKB, neurokinin B; IP_3 inositol 1,4,5-triphosphate. + represents relative activity or numbers.

15.7.3 Tachykinin Second Messengers

The tachykinin receptor binding activates G(q), which in turn activates the phospholipase C cascade and the release of intracellular Ca^{2+} , as well as opening Ca^{2+} channels in the cell membrane. The development of selective agonists and antagonists for each receptor has revealed a striking interspecies and intraspecies heterogeneity among the tachykinin receptors (Otsuka et al., 1995). Most nonpeptide NK1 antagonists display a marked difference in affinity for rat vs. human NK1 receptors. Some of the properties and structures of tachykinin receptors are compared in table 15.2.

15.7.4 Specific Actions of Tachykinin Receptors

Analogs of the endogenous ligands show much greater selectivity than the natural ligands (about 1000-fold) for the different receptor subtypes. In addition, selective antagonists, which are either nonpeptides or modified peptides, for the receptor subtypes have been developed and have been of considerable help in distinguishing the actions of the tachykinin receptors.

15.7.4.1 Actions of NK1 Receptors

The actions of SP are mediated by the NK1 receptor which is is characterized by subnanomolar affinity for SP and 30 to 100nM affinity for other tachykinins, including NKB and *senktide*, a selective NK3 agonist (Huang et al., 1995). *Spantide I* (Leu^{11} SP) and *Spantide*

II ([D-NicLys[1],3-Pal[3],D-Cl_2Phe[5],D-Trp[7,9],Nle[11]] SP) are antagonists that are considered to be fairly specific for NK1 receptors (Maggi et al., 1991). The rank order of binding of the tachykinins to the NK1 receptor is SP > NKA > NKB (Regoli et al., 1987).

The NK1 receptors mediate actions on the cardiovascular system, plasma extravasation from blood vessels, and the regulation of sympathetic preganglionic neurons. NK1 receptors are pervasive in airway secretory processes, including mucus secretion and ion transport, as well as inflammatory actions in the airways (Lundberg, 1995). NK1 receptors are also found in canine and human small intestinal muscle (Mao et al., 1996). Grooming may involve NK1 receptors (Stoessl et al., 1995).

15.7.4.2 Actions of NK2 Receptors

NKA is the most potent agonist of the NK2 receptors. NK2 receptors contribute to the resting tone of the small intestine by depolarizing tonic neurons, and mediate contraction of the bronchus. This seems to be an exclusive action of the NK2 receptors, a concept supported by the finding that NKA fibers are located around intrinsic neurons of local ganglia and within the smooth muscle layer of the bronchus (Sheldrick et al., 1995). NKA receptors are involved in the spinal processing of nociceptive information in the normal and inflamed joint and in the maintenance of inflammation-evoked hyperexcitability of dorsal horn neurons (Neugebauer et al., 1996).

The C-terminal Ser and Thr phosphorylation sites in the NK2 receptor have a critical role in *desensitization*, in which the tissue becomes insensitive to further action of the peptide a few minutes after application. Removal of these phosphorylation sites results in a receptor that maintains activation of the signaling pathways (Alblas et al., 1995).

15.7.4.3 Actions of NK3 Receptors

These receptors mediate transmission in the ascending excitatory reflex pathway in the ileum and mediate intestinal contractions in the guinea pig in response to activation by NKB. NK3 receptors are also present in the endothelium of rat mesenteric arteries. Vasodilation induced by an NK3 agonist is mediated by the release of NO (Mizuta et al., 1995).

15.8 Tachykinins as Neurotransmitters and Neuromodulators

SP is a *neurotransmitter* in many terminals of primary sensory (afferent) fibers (Nicoll et al., 1980; Otsuka et al., 1982). Its main effect is a slow excitatory influence, producing a long-lasting depolarization, which is induced by suppression of the inwardly rectifying potassium conductance, mediated, not through the cAMP system, but through a G protein that is resistant to pertussis (Nakajima et al., 1991). The critical role of SP in increasing spinal cord excitability after activation of sensory afferents from skin and muscle is taken over by VIP following peripheral nerve section, when SP levels fall and VIP increases (Wiesenfeld-Hallin et al., 1991). This is a good example of a fail-safe procedure in which one neuropeptide can replace another in a pathological or injurious condition.

SP and NKA are also involved in motor pathways. SP is morphologically positioned to modulate the effects of neurotransmitters with which it is colocalized. SP is colocalized with 5-HT in raphe neurons descending to synapse on ventral horn motor neurons. 5-HT activates the stretch reflex through these motor neurons but also has an autoinhibitory action on its own release from raphe terminals. The coreleased SP prevents this autoinhibition, thereby maintaining the stretch reflex. In addition, SP con-

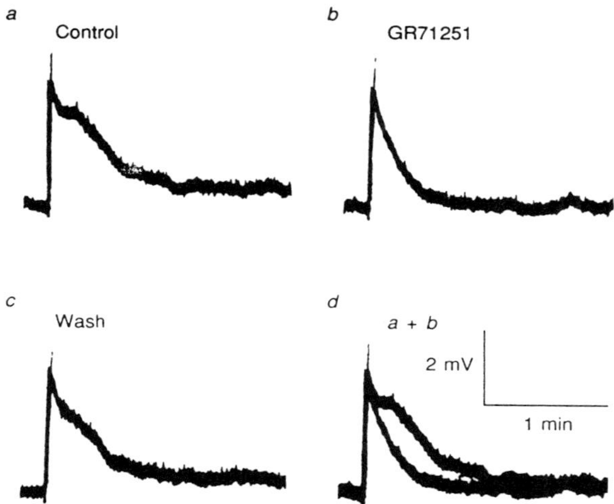

Figure 15.3
Intracellular recordings showing the effect of a neurokinin 1 (NK1) receptor antagonist GR71251 on the slow depolarization of motor neurons evoked by descending fibers in the neonatal rat spinal cord. Sample records from a single experiment. (a) Control response. (b) 12 minutes after adding the NK1 antagonist. (c) 20 minutes after washing out GR71251. (d) Superimposition of records in a and b. (From Kurihara et al., 1995.)

tained in serotoninergic terminals synapsing on motor neurons acts as a neurotransmitter mediating slow EPSPs evoked by descending fibers (figure 15.3). SP also facilitates the flexor reflex through increased spinal cord excitability. Both these actions of SP on reflex action can be blocked by pretreatment with the SP antagonist (spantide II) (figure 15.4).

Another example is specific *modulation of ACh action on Renshaw cells.* ACh released from ventral horn motor nerve collaterals stimulates Renshaw cells in the ventral horn, resulting in Renshaw cell inhibition of the ventral horn motor neurons. This inhibition is prevented by the coordinated release of the colocalized 5-HT and SP from the terminals of the raphe neurons. 5-HT inhibits Renshaw cell firing, whereas SP presynaptically blocks the release of ACh, which would otherwise stimulate the Renshaw cells (figure 15.5). SP alone has no effect on the excitation caused by muscarinic agonists or excitatory amino acids. SP acts as a *neuromodulator* in suprachiasmatic cells in vitro, modulating the response of 47% of the cells to excitatory amino acid agonists glutamate and *N*-methyl-D-aspartate (NMDA) (Piggins et al., 1995).

15.9 Specific Actions of Tachykinins

15.9.1 Axon Reflex

SP is present in sensory neurons in the dorsal ganglia and transported from these bipolar cells into their peripheral and central branches, to reach nerve terminals in peripheral tissues and in the dorsal horn of the spinal cord (Hökfelt et al., 1975). Some of the primary afferent nerves not only conduct impulses toward the CNS in an orthodromic direction but, through axon collaterals, conduct impulses back toward the periphery in an antidromic direction. Neuropeptides are released from the sensory nerve collaterals that terminate around blood vessels. This recurrent pathway forms the axon reflex. In addition, neuropeptides may be released from collaterals that form free nerve endings in the adjacent tissues (figure 15.6).

15.9.2 Inflammatory Response

SP is one of the best-known neurogenic mediators of immune hyperactivity, acting as a general inflammatory agent inducing the proliferation and activation of immune cells. Tachykinins trigger the adhesion of neutrophils and esosinophils to leaky venules, as well as plasma leakage caused by SP or capsaicin. The

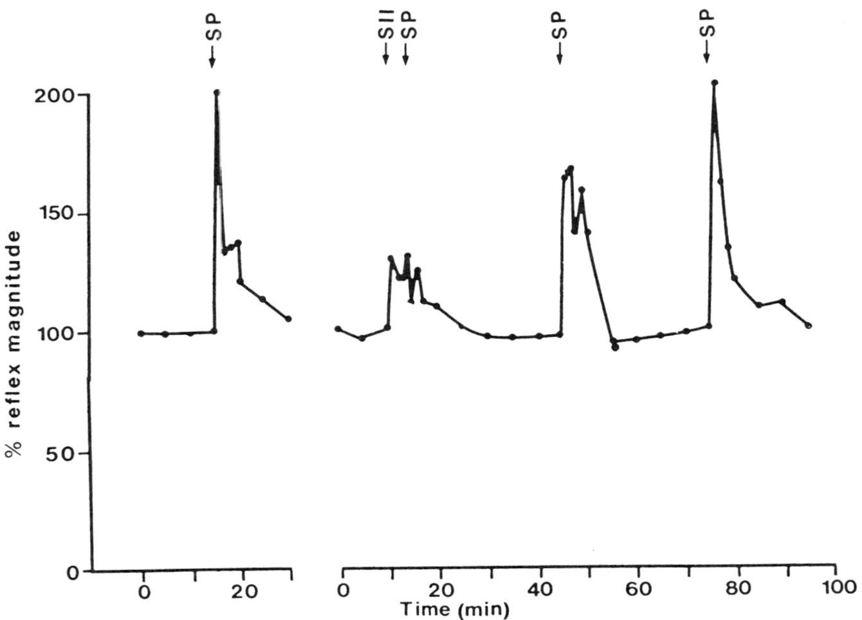

Figure 15.4
The antagonistic effect of intrathecal administration of the substance P (SP) antagonist spantide II on the facilitation of the flexor reflex by SP. The flexor reflex was recorded from the biceps femoris or semitendinosus muscle in decerebrate, spinalized, unanesthetized rats. The reflex was evoked continuously (1 minute) by single shocks to the sural nerve and was integrated. Baseline responses, defined as 100% reflex magnitude, were established for at least 20 minutes. The arrows indicate when the drugs were injected. The effect of a test dose of 10 ng SP is indicated on the left. Three micrograms of spantide II has a weak facilitatory action (slight agonist activity at low dosage) but almost totally antagonized the reflex facilitation by SP injected 3 minutes later. Thirty minutes after injection of spantide II, the response to SP was 70% of the control value, and after 55 minutes, the facilitation by SP returned to the control levels. (From Wiesenfeld-Hallin et al,. 1990.)

response of the immune cells is mediated through specific NK1 receptors (McCormack et al., 1996).

Injury to a muscle (inflammation or ischemia) or a joint (inflammation) sensitizes the peripheral nociceptors. Subsequent axon reflexes result in the release of the inflammatory neuropeptides (SP, NKA, and CGRP) which potentiate the *inflammatory response*. The secretion of these neuropeptides is affected by several tissue factors released by injury. These injury factors include the kinins (bradykinin and kallidin) and the prostaglandins.

Peripherally, the tachykinins SP and NKA act as potent vasodilators and increase vascular permeability, which accelerates the healing process by permitting chemotaxis of immune cells and plasma extravasation, a process known as *neurogenic inflammation*. This protective action is seen especially in the skin, eye, and respiratory tract (Holzer, 1988).

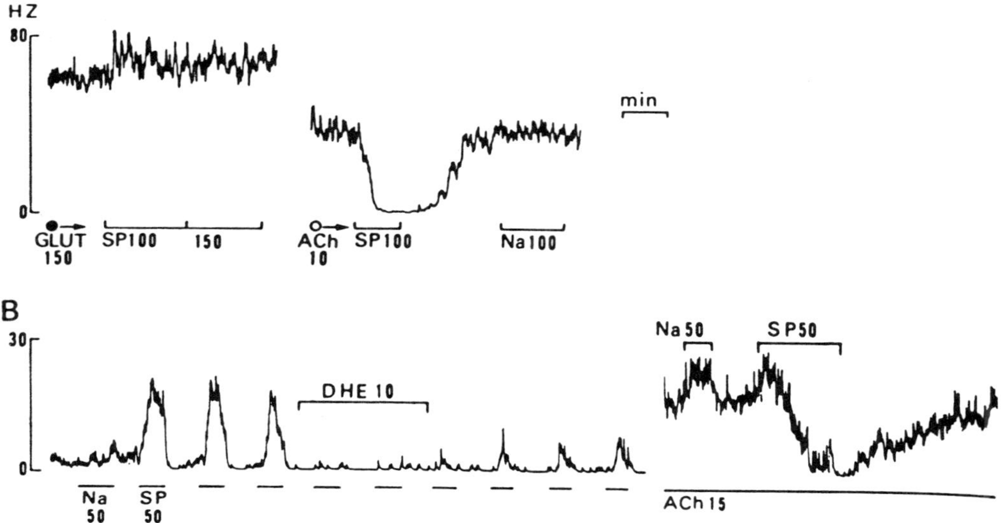

Figure 15.5
Microelectrophoretic application administration of substance P (SP) to two Renshaw cells, depicted by the top and bottom lines, respectively. (Top) SP had no effect on the excitation maintained by continuous administration of glutamic acid (GLUT), but abolished the firing evoked by acetylcholine (ACh). A current control affecting Na^+ had no effect. (Bottom) SP caused an excitation that was abolished by the simultaneous administration of dihydro-β-erythroidine (DHE), a cholinergic antagonist. The ordinate scale shows the frequency of firing (Hz). Microphoretic currents are expressed in nA. (From Ryall and Belcher, 1977.)

The *central release* of these neuropeptides sensitizes dorsal horn neurons, as seen by their increased background activity, increased receptive field size, and increased responsiveness to peripheral stimuli (Sluka, 1996). Centrally, the release of SP is presynaptically modulated by opiate peptides.

15.9.3 Pain

There is a complex neuronal network in the periphery and the spinal cord for the processing of nociceptive information. SP is distributed in nociceptive pathways and the nerve terminals of these pathways parallel the reactivity to met-enkephalin interneurons. Action potentials from small-diameter pain fibers in skin and some mucous membranes travel along primary sensory afferent neurons to release SP at their central nerve endings in the dorsal horn. Segmental interneurons containing *met-enkephalin* presynaptically inhibit the passage of this sensory information to secondary ascending sensory neurons, by reducing the release of SP. The acute administration of *capsaicin*, a neurotoxin contained in red peppers and hot chilies, causes the release of SP and thereby intense pain. Prolonged capsaicin administration depletes SP from nerve terminals, decreasing pain sensitivity.

SP exerts its effects via the NK1 receptor in the transmission of nociceptive messages at the level of

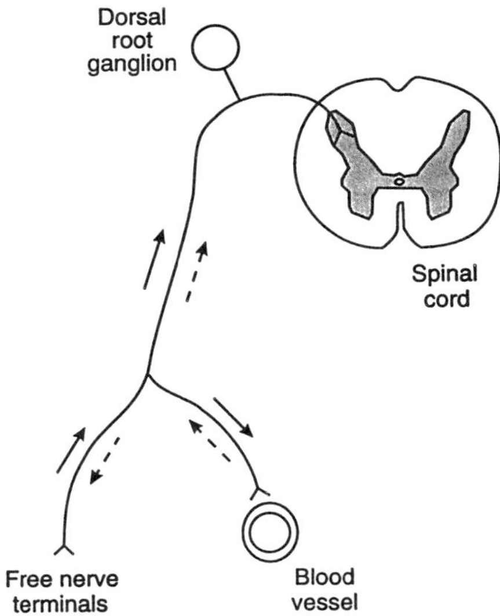

Figure 15.6
Release of neurotransmitters from the peripheral terminals of primary afferent sensory nerves by the axon reflex. Stimulation of free nerve endings sends action potentials (APs) to the dorsal root ganglia (arrows) and to the CNS. The APs may also invade nearby peripheral branches of the sensory nerves to be conducted peripherally (antidromically) to cause transmitter release from their terminals in blood vessels. Products of tissue injury may also evoke APs which invade the sensory branches antidromically (arrowheads) to release neurotransmitter or neuropeptide or both from their terminals. (From J. J. Reid et al., 1995.)

the spinal cord. Two different models of persistent pain, chronic inflammation of the hindpaw (which results in *increased SP levels*) and sciatic nerve section (which is associated with *decreased SP*), have been used to try to correlate levels of SP with changes in the NK1 receptors. Paradoxically, there is an increase in SP receptor immunoreactivity in both models, indicating that receptor upregulation of the receptor is not solely dependent upon the change in concentration of SP in the dorsal horn (Abbadie et al., 1996).

Recently, it has been shown that there are subpopulations of SP neurons in the spinal cord, some of which respond to mild noxious stimuli, whereas other neurons in lamina I that express the NK1 receptor respond to highly noxious stimuli. Ablation of the lamina I NK1-expressing neurons sharply decreases the response to highly noxious stimuli and mechanical and thermal hyperalgesia, but leaves responses to mildly painful stimuli unchanged (Mantyh et al., 1997).

15.9.4 Respiratory Control

In their early experiments Euler and Pernow (1956) showed that *SP stimulates breathing* when injected i.c.v. in cats and rabbits. The distribution of SP supports such a role. SP is present in several nerves innervating the lung, and SP is present in the nodosal and petrosal ganglia, and in the tractus solitarius where respiratory movements are integrated. SP is also present in the glomus cells of the carotid body, the afferents from which terminate in the tractus solitarius. Microdialysis of SP levels in the tractus solitarius show that there is a sharp increase in SP levels during hypoxia, an effect that is blocked by denervation of the 9th and 10th cranial nerves that innervate the peripheral chemoreceptors (Lindefors et al., 1986). The role of tachykinins in respiratory control, and especially their pathophysiological roles in asthma, is now under intensive investigation, a topic that is extensively reviewed by Maggi et al. (1995).

Tachykinin receptors are expressed on submucosal gland cells in the respiratory tract and SP is a potent stimulator of *airway mucus secretion* and *microvascular leakage*, resulting in edema of the airway and extravasation of plasma into the lumen. In a comparison of the relative ability of SP, NKA, and NKB to stimulate airway mucus secretion, the rank order is SP >

NKA > NKB. Interestingly, both galanin and somatostatin are effective inhibitors of tachykinin action in the respiratory tract (Wagner et al., 1995).

In the respiratory tract, tissue injury produces *bradykinins* from inactive kinins. Bradykinins are potent arterial vasodilators and venoconstrictors: in the airways, bradykinins selectively cause the release of SP, NKA, and CGRP from pain (nociceptive C) fibers. SP causes mucus hypersecretion, whereas NKA causes bronchoconstriction, microvascular leakage, and bronchial edema, although there are species differences in this classification.

15.9.5 Gastrointestinal Tract

15.9.5.1 Motility

This is a complex subject since the pattern of activity of SP and the other tachykinins on gut motility depends on the species and the level of the gut. NKI receptor immunoreactivity is present in a large number of enteric neurons, with the relative density along the gut being colon > ileum > stomach. SP acts both directly on smooth muscle of the gut and indirectly on the neurons of the myenteric plexus.

Most evidence supports the concept that tachykinins in the gut are excitatory transmitters acting on cholinergic neurons in the myenteric plexus. They act directly on smooth muscle to influence peristaltic movement. The tachykinins SP and NKA interact with the NK1, NK2, and NK3 receptors in a intricate manner: activation of the NK1 receptors results in inhibition of peristalsis, whereas activation of the NK2 and NK3 receptors facilitates peristaltic motor activity (Holzer et al., 1995).

15.9.5.2 Mucus Secretion

In the ileum, but not in the colon, SP acts directly on the mucosal epithelium and also modulates the neurons that innervate the mucosa (Keast, 1987), probably by evoking a slow EPSP in SP-sensitive submucous plexus neurons.

15.9.5.3 Gastrin and Somatostatin Secretion

Tachykinins strongly inhibit gastrin and stimulate somatostatin secretion in the porcine antrum, which contains SP and NKA but not NKB, and tachykinergic nerves mediate inhibitory vagal regulation of gastrin release (Schmidt et al., 1996).

15.9.6 Hypothalamic Integration of Neuroendocrine, Autonomic, and Behavioral Functions

The hypothalamus has an abundant number of tachykinin nerve endings and receptors in pathways that contribute to neuroendocrine, autonomic, and behavioral control. Stimulation of periventricular or hypothalamic NK1 receptors in conscious rats induces an integrated cardiovascular, behavioral, and endocrine response.

The neuroendocrine response to stress is accompanied by an increase in SP levels and in NK1 receptors in specific brain areas. Together with this is the cardiovascular response to increased sympathoadrenal activity, involving an increase in blood pressure and heart rate, mesenteric and renal vasoconstriction, and hindlimb vasodilation (splanchnic shift). The behavioral response consists of increased locomotion and grooming behavior. Taken together, this response is consistent with an integrated stress response to nociceptive stimuli and pain in rodents (Culman and Unger, 1995; Ishikawa and Ozaki, 1997).

From a structure-activity study, it can be seen that the carboxy fragment SP 5–11 is the shortest amino acid sequence that produces the same pattern of cardiovascular and behavioral responses as SP 1–11, and also retains the ability to desensitize the NK1 receptor like SP 1–11 (Tschope et al., 1995). The behavioral responses tested were face washing, hindquarter grooming, and "wet dog shakes." Other tachykinins are also implicated in behavioral responses: the NK3 agonist senktide induces locomotion, rearing, and sniffing when infused into regions of the midbrain that contain DA neurons. Grooming, however, appears to be due to NK1 receptor activation (Stoessl et al., 1991).

15.9.7 Micturition

Tachykinins modulate the micturition reflex at the level of the spinal cord (Lecci and Maggi, 1995). The urinary bladder is innervated by capsaicin-sensitive primary afferent neurons that reach the spinal cord through the pelvic and hypogastric nerves. Peripherally, these neurons also release tachykinins on the urinary bladder. The tachykinin-containing primary afferents are importantly involved in the transmission of sensory stimuli such as pressure, from the bladder and urethra to the spinal cord, and in this manner can affect micturition and mediate bladder pain. Under pathological conditions, these neuropeptides can initiate neurogenic inflammation.

15.9.8 Memory and Recovery from Central Lesions

SP promotes memory and is also reinforcing in normal animals and can counteract age-related performance deficits. These effects seem to be encoded by different SP sequences, since the N-terminal SP 1–7 sequence enhances memory, whereas the C-terminal hepta- and hexapeptide sequences of SP only reinforce. These differential behavioral effects are paralleled by selective and site-specific changes in DA activity in the nucleus accumbens. SP may have neurotrophic as well as memory-promoting effects since SP can also improve functional recovery after unilateral 6-hydroxydopamine lesions of the substantia nigra and after hippocampal lesions (Huston and Hasenohrl, 1995). These effects are reminiscent of the amino acid sequence-specificity of the melanocortins, as discussed in chapter 12.

15.10 Clinical Implications of Tachykinins

The tachykinins, SP, NKA, and NKB, play an important role in pain transmission, smooth muscle contraction, bronchoconstriction, activation of the immune system, and neurogenic inflammation. Neurogenic inflammation may contribute to many disease conditions, such as asthma, inflammatory bowel disease, joint inflammation, and bladder irritation and cystitis.

Tachykinin antagonists have great potential for the clinical management of a number of diseases. Specific nonpeptide antagonists for the three tachykinins and their receptors have been synthesized and have potential benefits in a variety of clinical conditions, including chronic pain, Parkinson's disease, depression, arthritis, irritable bowel syndrome, asthma, and migraine (Khawaja and Rogers, 1996). Since SP metabolism is altered in Alzheimer's disease, this debilitating disease is also a candidate for SP agonists or antagonists. Some individual observations indicate the scope of tachykinin involvement in pathological conditions:

Self-injurious behavior in the *Lesch-Nyhan syndrome* appears to involve an interplay between DA, 5-HT, and the tachykinin neuronal system of the basal ganglia (Sivam, 1996). The lumbar facet joint capsule is innervated by SP-containing nerves and these may be excited or sensitized when the joint is inflamed or exposed to injury-released tissue toxins. The resulting release of SP may account for *idiopathic lower back pain*.

The release of sensory neuropeptides in the nasal mucosa could provide a defensive response to irritants, inducing sneezing, pain, and nasal secretion in animals including humans.

SP and NKA (and CGRP) participate in the *inflammatory reaction in airways of smokers and asthmatics.* NK1 and NK2 receptor mRNA expression is doubled in smokers. NK2 receptor mRNA is quadrupled in asthmatics as compared to nonsmoking controls. These observations have implications for the treatment of both asthma and tobacco smoke–induced airway inflammation (Bai et al., 1995).

15.11 Summary

Tachykinins form a group of endogenous neuropeptides that cause vasodilation, increase vascular permeability, cause hypotension, and induce contraction of smooth muscle. They are found in phyla from the invertebrates to mammals and their functions are similar, although their potencies vary. There are three important mammalian tachykinins, substance P (SP), an undecapeptide, and neurokinin A (NKA) and neurokinin B (NKB), both decapeptides. Tachykinins are found extensively in *peripheral tissues* where due to their vasodilator effects they regulate blood flow, salivation, and micturition. Their ability to cause rapid contraction of smooth muscle involves them in gastric motility and spasms of the smooth muscle of the airways. *Centrally*, tachykinins act as neurotransmitters or neuromodulators in the brain and spinal cord and SP regulates sensory perception in addition to pain. All three tachykinins are found in the CNS, but the pattern of their distribution varies, especially in the spinal cord, and species differences are marked.

SP is widely distributed throughout the CNS, especially in the basal ganglia and nucleus accumbens, in structures involved in the endogenous pain control system, in primary sensory neurons in dorsal root ganglia, and in peripheral neurons concerned with autonomic reflexes. SP is present in substantial amounts in the gut, pancreas, salivary glands, and taste buds, and is colocalized with different neuropeptides or neurotransmitters in various nerve terminals.

There are two *genes* that encode mammalian preprotachykinins PPTs. The PPT-A gene encodes the precursors of several tachykinins, including SP and NKA. Differential splicing results in three different PPT-A mRNAs. The other gene encodes PPT-B and is expressed in different tissues from those in which PPT-A is found; PPT-B is not expressed in most peripheral tissues nor is it found in sensory ganglia. Activity of the preganglionic nerves to the autonomic ganglia inhibits the expression of PPT mRNA and consequently of SP production. Sex steroids mediate the expression of the PPT gene in the anterior pituitary, with males possessing more PPT mRNA than females, but SP and NKA levels in the hypothalamus, anterior pituitary, and plasma are higher in females.

Tachykinin receptors belong to the G protein–coupled superfamily of receptors and contain seven membrane-spanning domains, but they have different affinities which are tissue- and species–specific, as has been demonstrated by selective agonists and antagonists. There are three types of tachykinin receptors: NK1 receptors bind SP, NK2 receptors bind NKA, and NK3 receptors bind NKB, but there is considerable overlap. The receptors activate G(q), which in turn activates the phospholipase C cascade and the release of intracellular Ca^{2+}, as well as opening Ca^{2+} channels in the cell membrane.

SP actions are mediated by NK1 receptors, which are concentrated in laminae I to V of the spinal cord, and in vagal neurons. NK1 receptors are found on submucosal glands and epithelium and in the circular smooth muscle of the intestine, and mediate actions on the cardiovascular system, sympathetic preganglionic neurons, airway secretion, and inflammatory actions in the airways. *NKA actions* are mediated by NK2 receptors, which depolarize tonic neurons in the intestine and mediate bronchial contraction. NKA receptors are involved in the processing of nociceptive information of dorsal horn neurons. *NKB* activates the NK3 receptors, which affect intestinal contractions. NK3 receptors are also found in the endothelium of mesenteric arteries and the NKB-induced vasodilation is mediated by NO.

SP is a *neurotransmitter* in terminals of the primary sensory afferents in the spinal cord, causing a slow long-lasting depolarization which is mediated through a pertussis-resistant G protein. Both SP and NKA are involved in motor pathways, SP acting to prevent the autoinhibition of 5-HT on the stretch reflex, thus maintaining the reflex. SP also facilitates the flexor reflex through increased spinal cord excitability. SP is a *neuromodulator* of ACh action on Renshaw cells in the spinal cord by presynaptically blocking the release of ACh, and modulates the effects of the excitatory amino acids and NMDA in the brain.

SP is the transmitter for the axon reflex and together with NKA increases vascular permeability and vasodilation, and activates immune cells through specific NK1 receptors, resulting in the protective *inflammatory response*. SP release from nerve endings of small diameter pain fibers in the dorsal horn is presynaptically inhibited by met-enkephalin-containing interneurons, which modulate the processing of nociceptive information to higher centers. The administration of capsaicin strongly depletes SP from nerve terminals, decreasing pain sensitivity. SP stimulates respiration, airway mucus secretion, and microvascular leakage in the lungs. The other two tachykinins are less effective. The tachykinins are *excitatory transmitters* in the gut, acting on cholinergic neurons in the myenteric plexus to influence peristaltic movements. Activation of the NK1 receptors inhibits peristalsis, whereas activation of the NK2 and NK3 receptors accelerates peristalsis. Tachykinins modulate the micturition reflex at the level of the spinal cord and the urinary bladder.

The abundant supply of tachykinin nerve endings in the hypothalamus permits the integration of neuroendocrine, autonomic, and behavioral control, especially in response to stress.

SP promotes *memory* in normal animals and can counter age-related performance deficits. Specific sequences of the tachykinin are involved since N-terminal SP 1–7 enhances memory whereas the C-terminal hepta- and hexapeptide sequences improve reinforcement. SP may also have neurotrophic actions in the CNS, improving functional recovery after brain lesions.

Chapter 16 examines the several gut and brain peptides that can be grouped into neuropeptide families: gastrin/CCK, VIP/secretin and glucagon; pancreatic peptide, peptide YY, and neuropeptide Y, bombesin and gastrin-releasing peptide. The individual members of these families, whether produced in the gut or the brain, share many characteristics and if not coded by a single gene, are thought to have arisen from a common ancestral gene. In almost all cases, these neuropeptides have both central and peripheral actions.

Gut and Brain Neuropeptides I. Neuropeptide Families: Gastrin/CCK; VIP/Secretin/Glucagon; PP/PYY/NPY; BN/GRP

16

16.1 The Gut and Brain Neuropeptide Families

Since the fundamental discovery by Bayliss and Starling (1902) that the pancreas secreted a hormone, secretin, in response to intestinal acidification, and their supposition that secretin was a peptide or protein, many other peptides have been identified as regulators of intestinal processes. These peptides, together with the classical neurotransmitters of the autonomic nervous system, ACh and NE, function in an extremely complicated manner to coordinate and control these processes. What is surprising is that the peptides are produced by specialized epithelial endocrine cells in the gastrointestinal tract, by neurons in the gut, and by brain neurons. The APUD hypothesis, based on the presence of histochemical characteristics (*a*mine *p*recursor *u*ptake and *d*ecarboxylation) attempted to explain the production of peptides and amines by a variety of cells located in the nervous system, the gastrointestinal tract, and many other organs from a common origin in the neural crest. However, while certain cells of the thyroid, adrenal medulla, carotid bodies, and autonomic ganglia are derived from the neural crest, the peptide-secreting cells of the gut are not.

Consequently, the actions of the neuropeptides considered in this chapter are not limited to their actions on the gastrointestinal processes but include their many other physiological functions. Conversely, many neuropeptides already discussed in detail in this text have regulatory actions in the gut; while they are included in table 16.1 they are not considered in detail in this chapter apart from their effects on gastrointestinal functions. As these include such important peptides as *somatostatin* (chapter 10), *substance P* (SP, chapter 15), and the *opiate peptides* (chapter 14), it is suggested that the reader refer to these chapters.

16.1.1 Structure and Function of Peptide-Secreting Cells of the Gastrointestinal Tract

The enzyme- and hormone-secreting cells of the gastrointestinal tract have as their overall function the digestion and absorption of food. They are highly specialized morphologically and functionally and although they are found in all regions of the gut epithelium, they are mostly in the base of the mucosa. The cell types can be distinguished by immunocytochemistry, hybridization histochemistry, and receptor visualization. They are described in more detail by Bishop et al. (1988).

The *enterochromaffin (EC) cell* is the most abundant and is found in all regions of the gut. These cells are usually flask-shaped and contain serotonin and various neuropeptides, including SP, motilin, and enkephalin, stored in electron-dense, nonspherical secretory granules. Most of the other neuropeptide-containing cells are more confined to specific gut regions, as outlined below.

16.1.1.1 Stomach

The *enterochromaffin-like (ECL) cells*, unlike EC cells, are restricted to the gastric fundus and contain *hista-*

mine, but so far no peptides have been associated with these cells. Their secretory vesicles are large and surrounded by a thin halo. The stomach fundus also contains the *D cells*, which secrete *somatostatin*. These cells have long cytoplasmic processes in contact with the parietal cells, which lie between the zymogen-containing cells. The *G cells* contain gastrin and are the most abundant endocrine cell type in the antrum; the microvilli on their apical surfaces extend into the gastric lumen enabling them to respond to changes in the gastric contents. The broad base of the G cells contains the secretory granules which are liberated into capillaries. Gastrin in the G cells of the stomach is predominantly in the form of gastrin 17. Gastrin cells are also found in the human duodenum. *A-like cells*, similar to the pancreatic alpha cells, described below, are also found in the stomach mucosa and contain *glucagon*. These cells have not been found in the human stomach.

16.1.1.2 Intestine

D cells are also found in the intestine, especially the colon, and their somatostatin content acts in a paracrine manner on neighboring peptide-containing cells. However, most somatostatin in the intestine is in the extrinsic and intrinsic neurons of the submucosal and muscle layers. More than half of the intestinal somatostatin is somatostatin 28.

Many other neuropeptides can be localized in the duodenum and jejunum. Those cells containing *secretin* are the *S cells*; the related *gastric inhibitory peptide (GIP)* is found in the *K cells*. The *I cells* produce *cholecystokinin (CCK)* and their apical microvilli are immersed in the food-containing contents of the lumen (Buchan et al., 1978b). The upper small intestine also has the *intestinal gastrin (IG) cells* which contain the larger G34 form of gastrin. The *motilin (M) cell* is another distinct cell type found in the upper intestine.

The most numerous cell type in the ileum is the *enteroglucagon (EG) cell*, which contains the precursor molecule *preproglucagon*, which gives rise to glucagon, glycentin, and the glucagon-related peptides GLP-1 and GLP-2. In addition, the EG cell may contain peptide YY (PYY). Most *neurotensin* is found in the *N cells* of the ileum.

a. *Proglucagon-producing cells*

The *L cells* of the mucosa synthesize almost all of the enteric *proglucagon* peptides. The granules of these cells are homogeneous, without halo formation. The L cells also produce the unrelated PYY. Endocrine cells that are indistinguishable from pancreatic alpha cells are found in the intestinal mucosa of some mammals but not in humans. The *A cells* of the mucosa can be distinguished from the L cells by the halos surrounding their granules.

16.1.2 Enteric Nervous System

The enteric nervous system is an autonomous component of the peripheral nervous system. It consists of two ganglionated plexuses, the *myenteric plexus*, which lies between the outer longitudinal and inner circular muscle layers, and the *submucosal plexus* within the submucosa. There are well-known links between the CNS and digestive systems and the brain regulates the emotions that cause digestive responses, such as extreme fright-evoking diarrhea. But most often the gastrointestinal tract functions without the brain and consequently the enteric nervous system is often called the "second brain."

The enteric nervous system is independently situated entirely within the walls of the gut, yet receives input from the central and autonomic nervous systems through the *classical neurotransmitters* ACh and NE, with which neuropeptides are often colocalized.

Table 16.1
Families, origins, and functions of gut peptides[a]

Family	Peptide	Origin	Gastrointestinal tract Regulatory Function[b]
Gastrin-CCK	Gastrin	Antral G cells	Gastric H^+
	CCK	Intestinal I cells	Gallbladder contraction (+)
			Pancreatic secretion (+)
			Pancreatic secretion (+)
			Motility (+ or −)
VIP-secretin-glucagon	VIP	Myenteric neurons	Contractility (−)
			Intestinal secretion (+)
			Pancreatic secretion (+)
	Secretin	Intestinal S cells	Pancreatic secretion (+)
	GIP	Duodenal GIP cells	Gastrin (−) gastric H^+(−)
	Glucagon/GLP-1	Pancreas, intestinal L cells	Gastric H^+(−) insulin (+)
			Insulin (+) glucagon (−)
			Somatostatin (+)
PP-PYY-NPY	PP, PYY	Pancreas, sympathetic neurons	Pancreatic secretion (−)
			Intestinal secretion (−)
			Contractility (−)
	NPY	Gastrointestinal tract, pancreas, liver	Gastric H^+ (−), pancreatic secretion (−)
			Intestinal secretion (−)
Bombesin-GRP	BMB, GRP	Gastric and pancreatic neurons	Gastrin (+) gastric H^+(−)
			Pancreatic secretion (−)
			Contractility (+)
			Somatostatin (+)
Opiates	Enkephalins Dynorphin	Myenteric neurons	Motility (−)
Tachykinins	SP, NKA, NKB	Primary afferents, myenteric neurons, gut endocrine cells	Contraction (+) gastrin (−)
Somatostatin	Somatostatin	Gastric D cells Gastrointestinal tract	General inhibitor of secretion and contractility
Galanin	Galanin	Gastrointestinal tract	Gastric, intestinal, and pancreatic secretion (−), contractility (+ or −)
Motilin	Motilin	Gut endocrine cells	Motility (+)

Table 16.1 (continued)

Family	Peptide	Origin	Gastrointestinal tract Regulatory Function[b]
CGRP	CGRP	Endocrine intestinal cells, extrinsic and intrinsic neurons	Gastric H^+ (−) Pancreatic HCO_3^--secretion (−) Contractility (−)
Insulin	Insulin	Pancreatic beta cells	Liver carbohydrate metabolism
Neurotensin	Neurotensin	Gastric neurons, intestinal N cells	Gastric H^+ (−), pancreatic and intestinal secretion (+), contractility (+ or −)
Endothelin-1	Endothelin-1	Endothelium Neurons, smooth muscle	Vasoconstriction
Motilin	Motilin	Gut endocrine cells	Motility (+)

CCK, cholecystokinin; CGRP, calcitonin gene–related peptide; GIP, gastric inhibitory polypeptide; GLP-1, glucagon-like peptide-1; GRP, gastrin-releasing peptide; NKA, neurokinin A; NKB, neurokinin B; NPY, neuropeptide Y; PP, pancreatic polypeptide; PYY, peptide YY; SP, substance P; VIP, vasoactive intestinal polypeptide.
[a] There may be considerable variation due to species, dosage, experimental conditions, and central vs. peripheral administration.
[b] The predominant effects of the peptides are indicated by + (increase) or − (decrease), but may vary under different conditions and between species.

This input is modified by *enteric neurons* that contain neuropeptides, and by neuropeptides produced by *endocrine cells* in the gastrointestinal tract. 5-HT is also an important neurotransmitter in the gut.

The neurons of the *myenteric plexus* of the enteric nervous system can be divided into two main groups: neurons that contain VIP and nitric oxide synthase, and neurons that contain SP and neurokinin A (NKA), and often also ACh. Groups of VIP neurons also contain bombesin, gastrin-releasing peptide (GRP), neuropeptide Y (NPY), and galanin. The opiates dynorphin and met-enkephalin are found in both groups of neurons. Some neurons also contain somatostatin (Grider, 1994).

The *main function of gastric and intestinal smooth muscle* is to mix and propel the contents of the stomach and intestines in a coordinated manner, to permit proper digestion and absorption, and finally to expel the unabsorbed remains. The peristaltic reflex is responsible for ascending contraction and descending relaxation, movements that are stimulated by distention and mucosal stroking. These important movements are regulated by the autonomic and enteric nervous systems, acting through the many neurotransmitters and neuropeptides that swamp the gastrointestinal tract. In patients with *Hirschsprung's disease*, which is characterized by congenital severe constipation and a distended abdomen, the cause is a lack of enteric neurons in the colon due to failure of embryonic neurons to migrate to this part of the digestive tract.

16.1.3 Gut Sphincters

The gut sphincters, which control the passage of food into the stomach, from the stomach into the duodenum, from the pancreas and gallbladder into the duodenum, and of the feces out of the anus, are densely innervated by peptidergic nerves. Gastrointestinal smooth muscle sphincters, unlike other regions of the gastrointestinal tract, have myogenic tone that is inhibited by neural stimulation. Inhibitory reponses to nerve stimulation remain after blockade of the classical neurotransmitters ACh and NE, due to descending noncholinergic, nonadrenergic input, indicating the role of the colocalized neuropeptides in these nerve terminals. Contraction and relaxation of the sphincters are significantly influenced by several gut and brain neuropeptides.

16.1.4 *Pancreatic Endocrine Cells*

The different endocrine cells of the islets of Langerhans of the pancreas are grouped into individual colonies among the exocrine tissue. The islets represent only 1.0% to 1.5% of the total mass of the pancreas and they contain four main cell types, alpha, beta, delta, and PP cells, which secrete glucagon, insulin, somatostatin, and pancreatic polypeptide, respectively. The islets are innervated by a complex network of autonomic and peptidergic nerves, and receive an abundant arteriolar blood supply. Insulin, glucagon, and somatostatin influence one another's secretions, and the islet cells share junctional specializations. Glucagon stimulates the secretion of insulin and somatostatin; insulin inhibits the secretion of both glucagon and somatostatin and it is very likely that anatomical proximity permits these paracrine regulations (Orci and Perrelet, 1981). The glucagon-producing alpha cells are most abundant at the periphery of the islet, but are less numerous than the insulin-secreting beta cells, which are located more centrally in the islet (the beta cells are described further in chapter 17). Glucagon is unequally distributed in the pancreas, the dorsal pancreas being rich in alpha-cells compared to the ventral pancreas. Like glucagon, somatostatin and pancreatic polypeptide (PP) are distributed around the periphery of the islet but in far smaller amounts than glucagon.

16.1.5 *Pancreatic Exocrine Cells*

The exocrine portion of the pancreas consists of the acinar cells, which produce the enzymes, such as amylase, that are vital for digestion. Both neuropeptides and neurotransmitters influence pancreatic secretion, whether from the acinar cells or from the endocrine cells. Receptors on the pancreatic cell membrane are activated by these ligands and set in play the cascade of second-messenger pathways that ultimately result in secretion. This is depicted schematically in figure 16.1.

16.2 The Gastrin and Cholecystokinin Family

The discovery of gastrin and CCK soon followed that of secretin, and these three peptide hormones formed the acknowledged classical triad of gastric hormones. The resemblance in structure between gastrin and CCK, and the similarity in the arrangement of their genes, suggest that the two peptides arose from a common precursor gene (figure 16.2). Even though they are located on different chromosomes, with human CCK being on chromosome 3 and gastrin on chromosome 17, it is possible that separation of the two genes could have occurred by chromosomal duplication followed by translocation of either or both genes (Haun et al., 1989). Similar neuropeptides belonging to this family, the *ceruleins*, have been isolated from the skin of frogs, and because they are sulfated

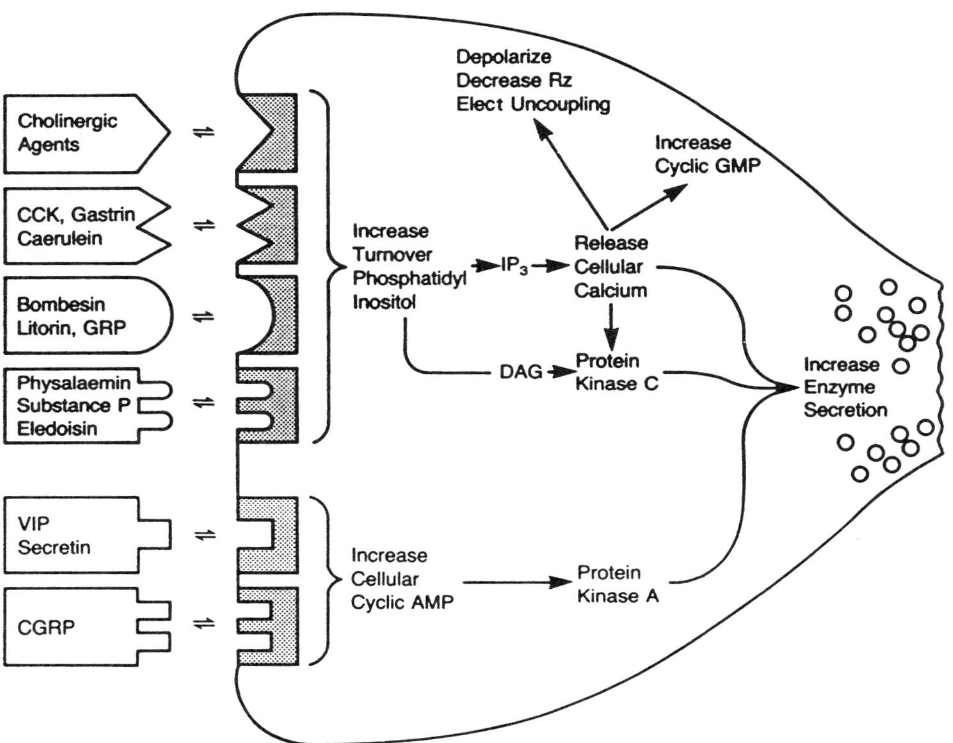

Figure 16.1
Diagram of the pancreatic acinar cell, including the different classes of receptors for secretogogues and the postreceptor mechanisms that couple receptor occupation to stimulation of pancreatic enzyme secretion. CCK, cholecystokinin; GRP, gastrin-releasing peptide; VIP, vasoactive intestinal polypeptide; CGRP, calcitonin gene-related peptide; GMP, guanosine monophosphate; IP_3, inositol 1,4,5-triphosphate; DA6, diacylglycerol. (From Gardner and Jensen, 1990.)

at the same tyrosine residue as CCK, they are of the CCK type.

The amidated C-terminal pentapeptide, Gly-Trp-Asp-Met-Phe-NH_2, which confers biological activity, is identical in gastrin and CCK. As gastrin can bind to the CCK receptor, it has weak CCK activity, and as CCK can bind to the gastrin receptor, it has weak gastrin activity. A recently developed gastrin-specific antibody will help to distinguish these two peptides.

16.2.1 Gastrin

Gastrin is produced by the G cells of the gastric antrum in response to food, especially peptides and amino acids, and from distention of the stomach. Increased acid in the stomach lumen inhibits gastrin production, as does the local production of somatostatin. Under normal physiological conditions, gastrin is an important regulator of gastric acid secretion and

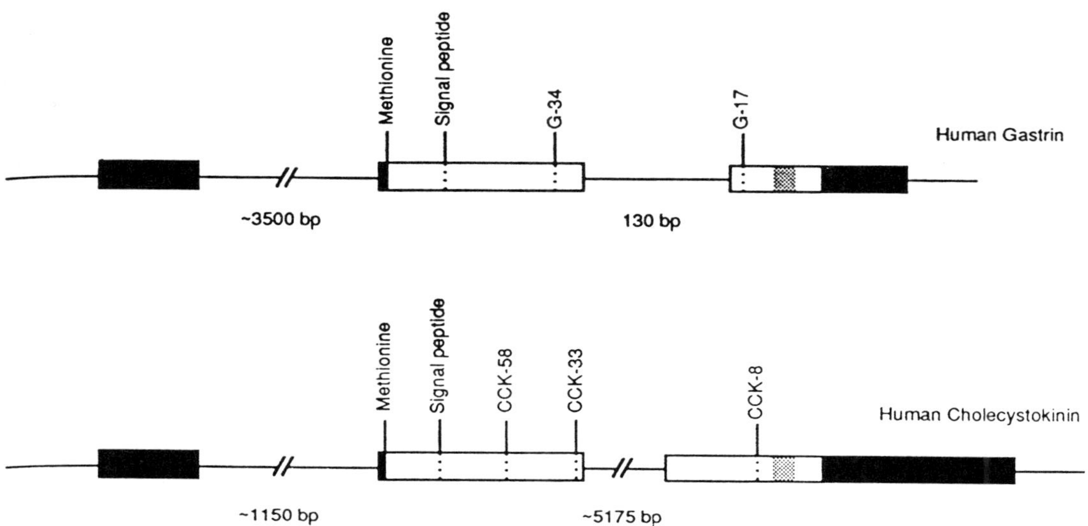

Figure 16.2
Comparison of the human gastrin and cholecystokinin genes. The putative initiator methionines in the second exons and the conserved pentapeptides of the prehormones are schematically aligned. Open boxes indicate translated exons, shaded boxes indicate untranslated exons, and gray boxes indicate conserved amino acids in the preprohormones. (Data compiled from Deschenes et al., 1985, and Takahashi et al., 1986, and modified from Haun et al., 1989. From Liddle, 1994b.)

of proliferation of the acid-secreting segment of the gastric mucosa.

16.2.1.1 Structure of Gastrin

Two forms of gastrin with identical 17–amino acid sequences have been isolated and synthesized: gastrin II, which has a sulfated tyrosine side chain, and gastrin I, which is nonsulfated. The sulfation apparently has no effect on the acid-stimulating effect of gastrin. The C-terminal tetrapeptide sequence contains all the chemical determinants necessary for full gastrin activity (Morley et al., 1965). Most mammalian gastrins are very similar, as shown by the structures of human, porcine, bovine, and canine gastrin 17. The common active C-terminal tetrapeptide is in *italics*; the variations in amino acid sequences from human gastrin are in **boldface**.

Human Gln-Gly-Pro-Trp-Leu-Glu-Glu-Glu-Glu-Glu-Ala-Tyr-*Gly-Trp-Met-Asp-Phe-NH*$_2$

Porcine Gln-Gly-Pro-Trp-**Met**-Glu-Glu-Glu-Glu-Glu-Ala-Tyr-*Gly-Trp-Met-Asp-Phe-NH*$_2$

Bovine Gln-Gly-Pro-Trp-**Val**-Glu-Glu-Glu-Glu-**Ala**-Ala-Tyr-*Gly-Trp-Met-Asp-Phe-NH*$_2$

Canine Gln-Gly-Pro-Trp-**Met**-Glu-Glu-Glu-Glu-**Ala**-Ala-Tyr-*Gly-Trp-Met-Asp-Phe-NH*$_2$

16.2.1.2 Gastrin Gene Expression and Precursor Processing

The human gastrin gene, found on chromosome 17, consists of two introns, one 5′ to the region that codes for preprogastrin, and one that codes for the N-terminal part of gastrin-34 (Ito, et al. 1984), as shown in figure 16.2.

Human *preprogastrin* is arranged as shown below, with the number of amino acids in each segment in parentheses:

Signal peptide	spacer	gastrin-34	C-terminal extension
(21)	(37)	(34)	(9)

The signal sequence is cleaved from preprogastrin to yield *progastrin,* which then is processed by endoproteolysis at dibasic amino acid sequences. Together with the action of basic amino acid carboxypeptidase and peptidylglycine α-amidating monooxygenase (PAM), processing produces *gastrin-34* and *gastrin-17* (Dougherty and Yamada, 1989). Sulfation and phosphorylation occur in the trans-Golgi apparatus region and are followed by amidation, which occurs in immature secretory granules (Varndell et al., 1983). Most active gastrin in gastrointestinal tissues is in the form of the sulfated and nonsulfated forms of gastrin-34 and gastrin-17. Almost half of intestinal gastrin in the adult human is in the sulfated form.

The gastrin gene in mammals is *expressed* mainly in the mucosa of the stomach antrum and the upper small intestine. Pituitary neurons and corticotrophs also express gastrin (Rehfeld et al., 1984). Gastrin precursor peptides are found in the pancreas and spermatozoa, and large amounts of gastrin mRNA are found in several types of human tumors, but these cells do not produce a biologically active gastrin (Bardram et al., 1989).

Both the luminal contents of the stomach and somatostatin regulate gastrin gene expression. Ingestion of proteins or amino acids increases antral gastrin mRNA and decreases antral somatostatin mRNA, suggesting an inverse relationship between gastrin and somatostatin (Karnik et al., 1989). Somatostatin may also inhibit gastrin transcription in pituitary cells.

The *release* of gastrin into the circulation is promoted by foods, especially proteins, peptides, and amino acids, and by GRP from nerve fibers that innervate the antral mucosa. Acid in the lumen of the stomach inhibits gastrin release, probably through local secretion of CGRP 27 and somatostatin. This appears to be a feedforward release of somatostatin by CGRP, which in turn causes acid-mediated feedback inhibition of gastrin release and acid secretion (Manela et al., 1995). Gastrin synthesis and release are prevented by prolonged fasting, and by the release of CCK (Beglinger et al., 1992). The regulation of gastrin release is further complicated by the involvement of cholinergic and sympathetic pathways (Walsh, 1988). Makhlouf and Schubert (1988) have proposed a model for the release of gastrin in which the noncholinergic route uses GRP as a stimulant to gastrin release, whereas the cholinergic pathway removes the inhibitory influence of somatostatin. Both active and inactive forms of gastrin are found in the circulation and the active forms can stimulate gastrin receptors and acid secretion.

16.2.1.3 Gastrin Receptors and Second messengers

Gastrin and CCK mediate their effects through at least two types of receptors, CCK-A and CCK-B receptors, which have about 50% amino acid homology (Kopin, 1992; Wank et al., 1992, 1994). They possess seven membrane-spanning domains, typical of G protein–binding receptors, and stimulate intracellular calcium and inositol phosphate pathways. The CCK-B gastrin receptor is found in gastric parietal cells and is probably the same as the brain CCK-B receptor. Studies of CCK receptor antagonists or of antisense oligonucleotides to the gastrin receptor suggest that stimulation of gastric acid secretion may involve different receptor subtypes (Rao et al., 1995).

The CCK-A receptor is found on gallbladder smooth muscle cells and pancreatic acinar cells. It has a much higher affinity for CCK than for gastrin. The D cells of the gastric fundus contain both the CCK-A and CCK-B receptors, but stimulation of somatostatin release by CCK appears to involve only the CCK-A receptor. Details about the somatostatin receptors are presented in chapter 10.

16.2.1.4 Actions of Gastrin

The best-known action of gastrin is the *regulation of gastric acid secretion* according to the components of ingested food. Other peptides, apart from somatostatin, are also involved in gastric acid secretion, as shown in table 16.2. Gastrin most probably exerts its effects on the histamine-containing cells (ECL cells) in the nonantral gastric mucosa, acting through a CCK-B type of receptor (Sandvik and Waldum, 1991). The secretion of acid in response to gastrin is markedly diminished by histamine H_2 receptor antagonists, whereas vagal, cholinergic stimulation increases acid secretion. Gastrin also has a *proliferative effect* on the ECL cells, and perhaps on other cells in the gut.

16.2.1.5 Clinical Implications of Gastrin

Chronic increase in gastric acid secretion can lead to esophageal ulcers and esophageal reflux. Histamine H_2 receptor antagonists, such as omeprazole (Prilosec) and ranitidine (Zantac) have found widespread use in alleviating these conditions. Prolonged hypersecretion of gastrin may lead to carcinoid tumors derived from the ECL cells, and gastrin has been implicated in gastric carcinomas which have low- and high-affinity gastrin receptors (P. Singh et al., 1985). Gastrin has also been reported to have a trophic effect on human

Table 16.2
Neuropeptide action on gastric characteristics[a]

Gastrin Release	Gastric Acid Secretion	Lower esophageal sphincter contraction	Gastric emptying
BMB +	BMB +	GAL +	MT + or −
GRP +	GAST +	MT +	SP +
SEC −	GRP +	PP +	PACAP +
CGRP −	CCK −	SP +	CCK −
CCK −	CGRP −	CCK −	CGRP −
GAL −	GAL −	CGRP −	GLP-1 −
SP −	GIP −	SEC −	NT −
SS −	GLP-1 −	SP −	PYY −
	NPY −	NT −	SS −
	NT −	PYY −	VIP −
	PYY −	VIP −	
	SEC −		
	SS −		

BMB, bombesin; CCK, cholecystokinin; CGRP, calcitonin gene–related peptide; GAL, galanin; GAST, gastrin; GIP, gastric inhibitory polypeptide; GLP-1, glucagon-like peptide-1; GRP, gastrin-releasing peptide; MT, motilin; NPY, neuropeptide Y; NT, neurotensin; PACAP, pituitary adenylate cyclase–activating peptide; PP, pancreatic polypeptide; PYY, peptide YY; SEC, secretin; SP, substance P; SS, somatostatin; VIP, vasoactive intestinal peptide; + = increase; − = decrease.

[a] There may be considerable variation due to species, dosage, experimental conditions, and central vs. peripheral administration.

adenocarcinomas of the colon. Serum gastrin levels are elevated in patients with colon cancer (J. P. Smith et al., 1989).

Prolonged gastrin secretion by gastrinomas (Zollinger-Ellison syndrome) is characterized by peptic ulcers, diarrhea, and esophageal disease. The trophic effects of gastrin are also seen as an increase in parietal cells, gastric glands, oxyntic mucosal area, and the

Table 16.3
Neuropeptide action on intestine, pancreas, and gallbladder[a]

Intestinal Secretion	Small Intestinal Contractility	Pancreatic Exocrine Secretion	Pancreatic Endocrine Secretion	Gallbladder Contraction
GIP +	BMB +	BMB +	CCK +	BMB +
SP +	CCK +	CCK +	GIP +	CCK +
VIP +	GRP +	GRP +	MT +	GRP +
CGRP −	MT +	NT +	NT +	MT +
NPY −	NT +[b]	SEC +	SEC +	PP −
PYY −	SP +	SP +	GLP +[d]	PYY −
SS −	CGRP −	VIP +	VIP +	SS −
	GAL −	CGRP −	GAL −	
	NPY −	GAL −	NPY −	
	NT −[c]	INS −	PYY −	
	PYY −	NPY −	SS −	
	SEC −	PYY −		
	SS −	SS −		
	VIP −			

INS, insulin. Other abbreviations and symbols as in table 16.2.
[a] There may be considerable variation due to species, dosage, experimental conditions, and central vs. peripheral administration.
[b] Via acetylcholine and SP.
[c] Direct action.
[d] Stimulates insulin, inhibits glucagon.

ECL cells. Surgical removal of the antrum has been recommended for treatment of this syndrome, but pharmacological treatment with the gastrin–CCK receptor antagonist proglumide, or with the long-acting somatostatin analog octreotide, may block gastrin hypersecretion.

Neuroendocrine tumors of the gastrointestinal tract and pancreas may secrete a wide variety of neuropeptides, but these tumors are difficult to locate and treat. There is a hereditary form of these tumors—multiple endocrine neoplasia type 1, with the genetic defect of this autosomal dominant disease traced to chromosome 11q13 (Scherubl et al., 1996).

16.2.2 Cholecystokinin

CCK is one of many neuropeptides that act on the intestine, pancreas, and gallbladder (table 16.3). The first recognized function of CCK, from which it derived its name, was to cause contraction of the gallbladder. Subsequently, it was discovered that CCK has several other gastrointestinal functions, such as the stimulation of pancreatic enzyme and insulin secretion. Endocrine sources of CCK include endocrine cells of the intestinal mucosa, a subpopulation of pituitary cells, and some cells of the adrenal medulla.

CCK is also found in abundance in the CNS, with unusually high amounts in the cerebral cortex, and with lesser amounts in the hypothalamus and arcuate nucleus. Only very low concentrations of CCK are present in the spinal cord and cerebellum (Crawley, 1985). CCK is colocalized in dopaminergic neurons from the mesencephalon which project to the limbic forebrain and the ventromedial hypothalamus, implicating this neuropeptide in the regulation of food intake (G. P. Smith and Gibbs, 1985). The CCK-DA-containing pathways are also related to human neuropsychopathologies including schizophrenia, Parkinson's disease and drug addiction, topics that are reviewed by Crawley (1991).

CCK is present in many peripheral nerves of the gastrointestinal tract, especially in the circular muscle layer of the colon. CCK-containing nerve terminals are also found in the myenteric and submucosal plexuses, where they stimulate the release of ACh and thus the contraction of smooth muscle (Mangel, 1984). CCK neurons are also found surrounding post-ganglionic nerve terminals surrounding the islets of Langerhans in the pancreas, which may be the way in which CCK stimulates insulin and glucagon release, acting as a neurotransmitter or neuromodulator.

16.2.2.1 Structure of Cholecystokinin

Cholecystokinin was initially purified from porcine intestine as CCK-33 by Mutt and Jorpes (1968). As discussed above, CCK and gastrin possess the identical C-terminal pentapeptide, Gly-Trp-Asp-Met-Phe-NH_2 , which is the essential sequence for biological activity of both molecules. Both gastrin and CCK bind to the CCK–gastrin receptor and thus have weakly overlapping activities.

CCK molecules of different size have been isolated from both intestine and brain of various species. The larger forms of CCK, such as CCK-58, appear to be predominant, but variations in length of the active intestinal CCK molecule range from 58, 39, 33, 25, 18, 8, 7, to 5 amino acids, (Reeve et al., 1986). In the nervous system, CCK is found predominantly as the C-terminal octapeptide (CCK-8) of the gut hormone (CCK-1–33). Despite the considerable variation in size, all these peptides have identical C-termini which, however, does not confer CCK selectivity since it shares this vital sequence with gastrin. Selectivity requires at least 7 amino acids, and full potency requires *sulfation of tyrosine at position* 7 from the C-terminal. All the shorter forms of CCK are proteolytic C-terminal fragments of the largest form of CCK, CCK-58.

In the rat and pig, CCK-8 and CCK-22 predominate, whereas CCK-33 and CCK-58 are the major forms in the human. In the dog, the most active CCK forms are CCK-58, CCK-39, and CCK-8. The relative amounts of the different molecular forms of CCK cannot always be accurately determined, as it may be converted into smaller molecular forms by enzymes or by the steric hindrance of antibody binding to the C-terminus of CCK-58 (figure 16.3). The major endocrine form of CCK, produced by the endocrine cells of the small intestine, is CCK-58 (Reeve et al., 1994).

16.2.2.2 Cholecystokinin Gene Expression, Precursor Processing, and Regulation of Release

The *CCK gene* is about 7 kb in size and is composed of three exons, the third of which encodes the biologically active region of the peptide, including CCK-33. The second exon encodes the signal peptide and the prohormone regions of the peptide. The first exon encodes only the 5′-untranslated portion of the CCK mRNA (Deschenes et al., 1985). The human CCK gene is found on chromosome 3. CCK gene expression is stimulated by feeding and depressed by fasting and by somatostatin.

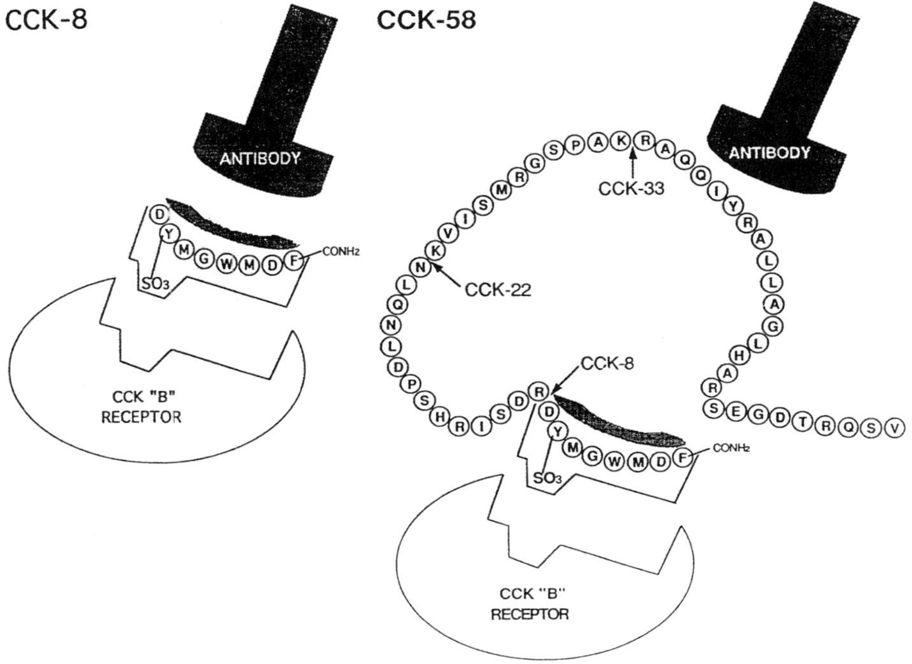

Figure 16.3
The structures of cholecystokin-8 (CCK-8) and CCK-58, as well as how the N-terminal 50–amino acids residue in CCK-58 may influence the activity of its C-terminus, are shown. It can be seen that antibodies and receptors alike have no steric hindrance for binding to CCK-8. However, antibody is sterically hindered from binding to the C-terminus of CCK-58, whereas the CCK-B receptor is not hindered at all. This could possibly be due to a difference in binding orientations. The single-letter code for amino acids is used (see Appendix C). (From Reeve et al., 1994.)

Preprocholecystokinin is a 115–amino acid polypeptide that succumbs to cleavage to first form pro-CCK and subsequently CCK-58, the major processed form of CCK in most tissues (Eng et al., 1990). A vital step in the processing of the CCK molecule is α-amidation of the C-terminal. *O*-Sulfation of Tyr in the seventh position from the amidated C-terminus is essential to the biological activity of CCK, increasing its potency 100-fold. All the shorter forms of CCK are formed by cleavage at monobasic or dibasic residues, and many of these smaller forms are found, together with CCK-58, in various tissues and in blood.

CCK mRNA is found in brain and intestine of many species. CCK is one of the most abundant peptides in the CNS and CCK mRNA levels in cerebral cortex are similar to those identified in the duodenum. As identical cDNAs are made in both tissues, any differences in the final form of CCK must be due to tissue-specific post-translational processing (Gubler et al., 1984).

Depending on the species, CCK mRNA–positive neurons may be present in dorsal root ganglia, and in dorsal horn neurons, especially in the deeper levels of the substantia gelatinosa and lamina III. Of special interest is the predominance of CCK immunoreactivity and mRNA expression in regions related to nociceptive transmission, such as the periaqueductal gray, thalamus, and cortex (Schiffmann and Vanderhaegen, 1991), regions that overlap with the distribution of opiate neuropeptides (Wiesenfeld-Hallin and Xu, 1996). Somatostatin exerts a potent inhibitory effect on CCK gene expression, significantly lowering CCK mRNA levels in the intestine (Liddle, 1994a,b).

CCK, like most gastrointestinal hormones, is released from endocrine cells into the blood after a meal and CCK secretion remains high as long as food is in the stomach. In humans, proteins, amino acids, and fats are the strongest food stimulants to CCK release, but in the rat fat is only a weak stimulant and amino acids do not cause CCK secretion. In the rat, there appears to be a negative feedback mechanism by which trypsin in the intestinal lumen inhibits the release of CCK. A similar mechanism appears to be present in humans (Owyang et al., 1986). Several additional mechanisms are involved in the regulation of CCK secretion: a pancreatic "monitor peptide" (Lu et al., 1989) and an intestinal "CCK releasing factor" (Miyasaka et al., 1989) are stimuli to CCK release. Both these factors require the presence of food in the intestinal lumen to be fully active.

16.2.2.3 Cholecystokin Receptors and Second Messengers

CCK receptors are present throughout the gastrointestinal tract with the exception of the duodenum and jejunum, in the pancreas and gallbladder, and in the brain and some peripheral nerves. CCK receptors in the CNS differ from those found in the periphery. Based on their tissue distribution, the CCK receptors are classified as *CCK-A (alimentary)* or *CCK-B (brain)* receptors (figure 16.4), but there is some overlap as CCK-A receptors are found to a limited extent in the CNS. The characteristics of these receptors have been elucidated through the use of specific CCK receptor antagonists (Gardner and Jensen, 1984; Liddle et al., 1989).

CCK-A receptors are somewhat heterogeneous, with the binding subunit of CCK estimated to be 85 to 95 kD in the human gallbladder but 70 to 85 kD in the bovine gallbladder (Schjoldager et al., 1989). The receptor belongs to the family of G protein–linked, seven transmembrane-spanning domain family of peptides. Receptors in the pancreas and gallbladder are highly specific for CCK, demanding *O*-sulfation of the Tyr residue, so that gastrin has only weak effects upon these organs.

CCK-B receptors are the most prevalent CCK receptors in the nervous system and there is 90% homology between the human and rat CCK-B receptor sequences. However, the CCK-A and CCK-B receptors are clearly distinct gene products since the rat CCK-B receptor is only 48% identical to the rat CCK-A receptor. Functionally, the CCK-B receptors differ considerably from the CCK-A receptors in that they do not have the selectivity of the CCK-A receptor for the sulfated forms of CCK. Consequently, the CCK-B receptor binds CCK-8, desulfated CCK-8, CCK-4, and gastrin with almost equal affinities (Saito et al., 1980).

The *second-messenger system* chiefly used by the CCK receptors is the phosphatidylinositol pathway, with the formation of diacylglycerol and the resulting increase in intracellular Ca^{2+}. There is some evidence that CCK increases cGMP.

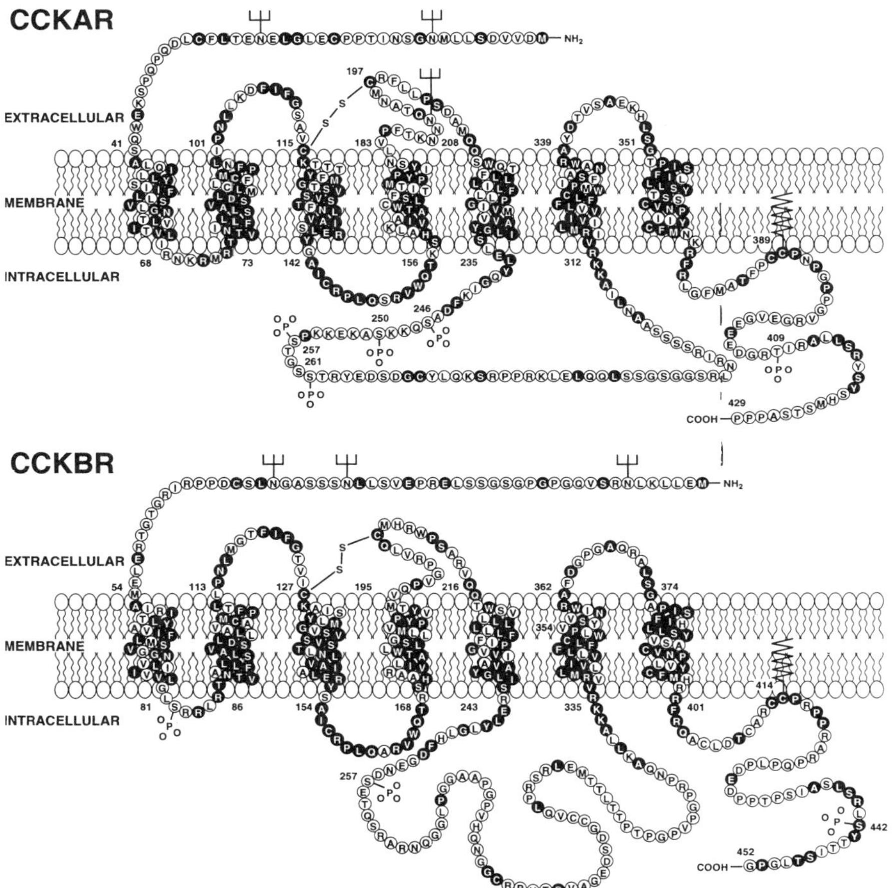

Figure 16.4
Schematic models of rat cholecystokinin A and B receptors (CCKAR, CCKBR). Deduced amino acid sequences (using amino acid letter codes) of rat CCKAR and CCKBR showing putative transmembrane helices, consensus sites for putative *N*-linked glycosylation (tridents), serine and threonine phosphorylation by protein kinase C and A (-PO_3), and conserved cysteines in the first and second extracellular loops possibly forming a disulfide bridge (-S-S-) and a conserved cysteine in the cytoplasmic tail possibly palmitoylated (jagged line extending into the membrane) -NH_2, N-terminus; -COOH, C-terminus. Residues in filled circles are conserved (identical) between CCKAR and CCKBR. (From Wank, 1995.)

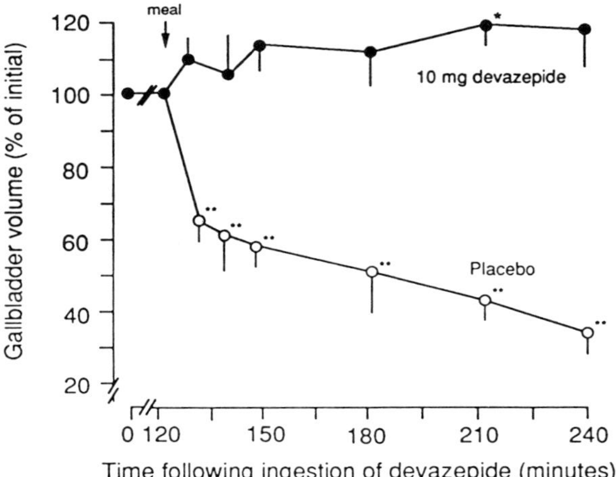

Figure 16.5
Effect of the cholecystokinin (CCK) receptor antagonist devazepide on gallbladder volume. CCK receptor blockade completely inhibits meal-stimulated gallbladder contraction. (From Liddle et al., 1989.)

16.2.2.4 Actions of Cholecystokinin on the Gastrointestinal Tract

Gallbladder contraction is regulated by CCK, and the amount of CCK secreted after a meal is sufficient to cause postprandial gallbladder contraction. Contraction can be completely inhibited by the administration of the CCK receptor antagonist devazepide acting on CCK-A receptors on gallbladder smooth muscle (figure 16.5).

CCK is the major hormone responsible for *stimulating pancreatic enzyme secretion*: extremely small amounts of CCK are effective stimulants to the release of amylase and serine proteases. CCK acts on both the *pancreatic acini* and on *CCK-sensitive afferent nerve fibers* in the pancreas, which bring sensory information to the CNS, which then stimulates pancreatic secretion via a vagal efferent pathway (Owyang, 1996). Thus CCK may act on the pancreas either as a neurotransmitter acting on cholinergic neurons, or as a hormone binding to the CCK-A receptor of the acinar pancreatic cell. Several other secretogogues also act to induce pancreatic secretion (see figure 16.1). CCK also *modifies gene expression* of other pancreatic enzymes, such as trypsinogen and chymotrypsinogen. In contrast to its stimulatory effect on pancreatic secretions, CCK inhibits the release of gastrin through the release of somatostatin, thus *decreasing gastric acid secretion* (Beglinger et al., 1992).

CCK *potentiates* the action or release of several pancreatic secretions, such as the action of secretin on pancreatic bicarbonate release, the amino acid–stimulated release of insulin from islet beta cells that have CCK receptors, and the release of glucagon and PP. CCK also *modulates* the antinociceptive and gastrointestinal actions of morphine (L. Singh et al., 1996).

Gut motility is affected by endocrine secretion of CCK and CCK released by nerve endings in the gut, but the effects vary considerably in different species. In the *upper gastrointestinal tract*, CCK regulates lower esophageal sphincter pressure and slows the rate at which food is emptied from the stomach. However, in humans, CCK is reported to stimulate antropyloroduodenal motility, mainly through reactions with cholinergic neurons in the antropyloric region, and through reactions with smooth muscle receptors in the duodenum (Katchinski et al., 1996). This increases intestinal motility and the transit of food through the intestine is accelerated. CCK acts directly as a neurotransmitter on the smooth muscle of the intestine to cause contractility and indirectly as a neuromodulator of ACh release from parasympathetic postganglionic nerves. CCK also induces relaxation of the sphincter of Oddi, which regulates the passage of pancreatic and biliary secretions into the duodenum.

CCK-8 evokes a marked *gastric mucosal hyperemia*, a response that is brought about by a vagovagal reflex that involves ACh, CGRP, and NO as vasodilator messengers (Heinemamn et al., 1996).

CCK has a *trophic effect* on the pancreas, increasing the secretory capability of the gland through an increase in cell number and size, an effect that is prevented by CCK receptor antagonists (Niederau et al., 1987).

16.2.2.5 Actions of Cholecystokinin on the CNS

Endogenous CCK plays an important role in the regulation of short-term food intake and the sensation of satiety. The first demonstration of decreased food intake resulting from CCK administration was provided by Gibbs et al., (1978). Both i.c.v. and peripheral administration are effective, but the integrity of the vagal nerve is essential to the satiety signal after peripheral injection. The pathway appears to be from the abdominal afferent vagus to the hypothalamus through the nucleus tractus solitarius and the area postrema (Edwards and Ritter, 1981). CCK-A receptor antagonists increase food intake in animals (Brenner and Ritter, 1996) and decrease feelings of satiety in humans (Wolkewitz et al., 1990).

CCK has a *modulatory effect on nociception*, antagonizing the analgesia evoked by the opiates, as has been shown after the exogenous administration of opiates, and after the release of endogenous endorphins by acupuncture or electric shock (Han et al., 1986). This antianalgesic action is confirmed by CCK antagonists, which intensify opiate-induced analgesia.

CCK tetrapeptide (Trp-Met-Asp-Phe) has been linked to anxiety, inducing panic-like attacks in humans when administered as an i.v. bolus injection. Behavioral studies show a facilitative effect of CCK on the hyperlocomotion induced by DA and it is possible that the anxiogenic effect of CCK may be through mesocorticolimbic DA neurons (Crawley, 1991).

CCK, CCK mRNA, and CCK-B receptor mRNA are all upregulated in dorsal root ganglia cells after axotomy, as are two other neuropeptides, galanin and NPY (Hökfelt et al., 1994). Taken together with the neuroprotective and neuroregenerative influences of the melanotropic neuropeptides on spinal motorneurons, discussed in chapter 12, there is a growing body of evidence to show that a plethora of neuropeptides is called upon in response to nerve injury.

16.2.2.6 Clinical Implications of Cholecystokinin

Most of the putative therapeutic applications for CCK come from animal studies. The use of CCK-A receptor antagonists may be useful in reducing esophageal reflux, as CCK causes relaxation of the lower esophageal sphincter. CCK receptor blockade reduces intestinal motility and may be of help in cases of irritable bowel syndrome.

The involvement of CCK in food ingestion raises important possibilities for treatment of eating disorders, for example, CCK receptor blockade to increase appetite or CCK agonists for control of obesity. However, no abnormalities accompany excessive CCK secretion in humans. A decrease in CCK blood levels occurs in celiac disease, in which there is atrophy of the intestinal mucosa and defective gallbladder contraction. Similarly, a low level of CCK is found in bulimic patients who experience no feeling of satiety after eating. CCK levels return to normal after treatment and disappearance of the binge eating but whether the abnormality in CCK levels is the causative factor is unknown (Mitchell et al., 1986).

As CCK antagonists do not potentiate morphine-related respiratory depression, they might be used together with opiates to enhance analgesia and reduce tolerance, especially in patients with neuropathic pain (Wiesenfeld-Hallin and Xu, 1996), but unfortunately these agents are associated with gallstone production. CCK agonists or antagonists hypothetically could be of use in dopaminergic dysfunctions, as postulated in schizophrenia and drug addiction.

16.3 The Vasoactive Intestinal Polypeptide-Secretin-Glucagon Family

The VIP-secretin-glucagon family is one of the largest families of gastrointestinal regulatory peptides and VIP is its most important member. VIP, a 28–amino acid peptide, and a closely related 27-residue peptide, PHI are derived from the same precursor and have very similar actions (Tatemoto and Mutt, 1981). PHI stands for *p*eptide with *h*istamine at the N-terminus and *i*soleucine amide at the C-terminus (human PHI is sometimes referred to as PHM). VIP and PHI, the pituitary adenylate cyclase–activating peptide (PACAP), a 38-residue peptide with 68% homology with VIP (see chapter 13), gastric inhibitory polypeptide (GIP), and glucagon-like peptide-1 (GLP-1) are also members of this family, all of which possess a C-terminal α-amide group. Unexpectedly, growth hormone–releasing hormone (GHRH) is another peptide belonging to this family on the basis of its similarity of structure.

16.3.1 Vasoactive Intestinal Polypeptide

VIP is involved in many regulatory functions, including vasodilation, gastrointestinal secretion and motility, and glycogenolysis. In the CNS, VIP acts as a neurotransmitter or neuromodulator and plays an important role in CNS development and neuronal survival. VIP was first isolated from porcine intestine by Said and Mutt (1970) as a potent vasodilator affecting systemic arterial blood pressure, as well as a powerful dilator of the bronchi.

16.3.1.1 Structure of VIP

VIP is a highly conserved molecule and VIP sequences in the human, pig, cow, rat, dog, and goat are identical: 28-residue peptides with a C-terminal amide. The amino acid sequence of the common mammalian form of VIP is

His-Ser-Asp-Ala-Val-Phe-Thr-Asp-Asn-Tyr-Thr^{11}-Arg-Leu^{13}-Arg-Lys-Gln-Met-Ala-Val^{19}-Lys-Lys-Tyr-Leu-Asn-Ser-Ile^{26}-Leu-Asn^{28}-NH_2

There are minor variations from this pattern in some other species: guinea pig VIP has four substitutions and opossum VIP has five, as does VIP from dogfish and cod. Most of the substitutions occur in positions 11, 13, 19, 26, and 28, implying that these are not important for biological activity (Dockray, 1994). The amino acid sequence of PHI is similar to that of VIP, but there is more species variation and PHI is not as well conserved as VIP. VIP always coexists and is co-released with PHI, and in many neurons is also colocalized with ACh.

16.3.1.2 VIP Gene Expression, Precursor Processing, and Regulation of Release

The peptides of the VIP family are probably the result of exon duplication coupled to gene duplication. The VIP-PHI gene is 9 kb long and has seven exons, five of which have coding sequences. Three separate exons encode VIP, PHI, and the signal peptide sequence (figure 16.6). The human VIP gene is localized on chromosome 6, specifically 6q24 (Gozes, 1988).

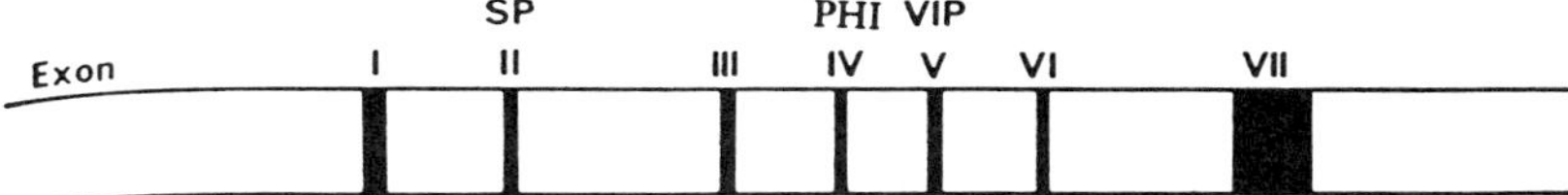

Figure 16.6
Organization of exons and introns of the human vasoactive intestinal polypeptide (VIP)–peptide histodine isoleucine (PHI) gene. There are seven exons (filled boxes), five of which contain coding sequences. There are separate exons for at least three functional domains, the signal peptide (SP), the VIP encoding region, and the PHI encoding region. Introns are shown as open boxes. (From Yamagami et al., 1988.)

The VIP-PHI gene is expressed widely in neurons throughout the *gastrointestinal tract*, in the myenteric and submucous plexuses in the stomach and intestine, and in the sphincters of the gastrointestinal tract of most mammalian species, including the human. Most of the VIP nerve fibers in the gut are of intrinsic origin but there are some extrinsic VIP-containing nerves that innervate the gut, such as the pelvic and vagal nerves. The cerebral cortex and hypothalamus contain significant amounts of VIP. VIP is colocalized with several different peptides and nonpeptide neurotransmitters, in patterns that differ according to tissue and species. In the salivary gland, VIP is colocalized with ACh (see figure 4.4); in the guinea pig ileum, VIP is colocalized with galanin and dynorphin.

VIP mRNA is expressed widely throughout the *central and peripheral nervous systems*. VIP mRNA has been localized to cortical and thalamic neurons and the suprachiasmatic nucleus of the hypothalamus, a brain region involved in the regulation of circadian rhythmicity (Baldino et al., 1989). The expression of the VIP gene is influenced by other hormones, including thyroxine, estrogen, prolactin, and especially by glucocorticoids. The neurotransmitter serotonin is another regulator of VIP gene expression, as is osmotic shock.

Expression of the VIP gene is dramatically regulated during development, with VIP mRNA levels in the developing frontal cortex increasing fivefold in the rat from birth to 3 to 4 days after birth, with an even greater increase at 14 to 16 days. This increase is even more marked in the developing parietal cortex. Developmental regulation of hippocampal VIP mRNA is also considerable, but the hypothalamus starts out at birth with much higher levels of VIP mRNA than would be expected from peptide levels. However, VIP mRNA is detected in the rat intestine as early as 16 days of gestation. VIP receptors are also abundantly distributed throughout the CNS during ontogeny and are increased in many regions undergoing intense cell production (Hill et al., 1994). VIP decreases in the aging brain (Gozes, 1988).

Processing of the VIP-PHI precursor is characterized by cleavage by trypsin-like proteolysis followed by carboxypeptidase B–like removal of basic residues and then by C-terminal amidation. However, there are species- and tissue-specific variations, summarized by Dockray (1994). Different forms of VIP and PHI that are extended at the C-terminus, and that lack the C-terminal amide, still have some biological activity.

Physiological release of VIP ensues from esophageal or intestinal distention. Stimulation of the vagal nerve releases both VIP and PHI, whereas adrenergic sympathetic nerves presynaptically inhibit the release of VIP into the circulation (Sjoqvist and Fahrenkrug, 1986). In vitro, distention of the oral but not the caudal colon causes the release of VIP, in accordance with descending inhibition of the peristaltic reflex (Grider and Makhlouf, 1986).

16.3.1.3 VIP Receptors and Second Messengers

Two VIP receptors have been cloned and characterized. Both VIP receptor 1 (VR1) and VR2 have seven transmembrane domains and have 48% homology with the secretin receptor, all belonging to the G protein–coupled receptor family. The molecular weight of the secretin and VIP receptors is approximately 49 kD, with VIP receptors having a greater weight due to glycosylation. The VR1 gene is located on chromosome 3p22, a position associated with small cell lung cancer. The gene for VR2 is on chromosome 7q36.3. The lung has the highest expression of VR1, whereas VR2 is distributed throughout peripheral tissues. Dense binding sites for VIP are found in discrete locations within the gastrointestinal, respiratory, and genital tracts, correlating in general with the distribution of VIP nerves to epithelia, smooth muscle, and blood vessels (Power et al., 1988).

VIP receptors in the *nervous system* correspond to the profusion of VIP expression sites (Rosselin, 1994). In the CNS, high levels of VIP binding sites are found in the anterior pituitary, pineal body, olfactory bulb, hypothalamus, amygdala, thalamus, hippocampus, suprachiasmatic nucleus, and the brainstem, sites that partially correspond to the physiological actions of VIP in the CNS (Besson, 1988). High-affinity binding sites for VIP, homologous to brain VIP binding sites, are present in lymphocytes and may be involved in the modulation of immune functions, especially in the gastrointestinal immune system (Ottoway, 1988).

The VIP receptors vary in their affinities for different members of the VIP-secretin-glucagon family. In general, VIP receptors bind VIP, PHI, secretin, LHRH, and PACAP, but do not bind glucagon or GIP. The second-messenger pathway is through adenylate cyclase and cAMP.

16.3.1.4 Actions of VIP on Peripheral Tissues

Neurotransmitter and *neuromodulator* actions ascribed to VIP are numerous. VIP appears to act as a noncholinergic, nonadrenergic mediator in the cardiovascular system and respiratory and urinogenital tracts, as well as in the gastrointestinal tract, possibly through the release of NO. PHI is 5 to 10 times less potent than VIP. VIP has strong chronotropic and inotropic effects on cardiac muscle and, through its cAMP-mediated action on vascular smooth muscle, is a potent vasodilator. In the CNS VIP is both a neurotransmitter and neuromodulator, in some instances causing excitation and in others inhibition, the effect probably due to different co-transmitters. VIP, together with NE, controls energy metabolism in astrocytes through stimulation of glycogenolysis (Magistretti et al., 1993).

In the *gastrointestinal tract*, VIP causes relaxation of the stomach and lower esophageal sphincter, acting as a transmitter for inhibitory enteric neurons, and slows peristalsis in the intestine acting through its *depolarizing* effect on ganglion cells in the inferior mesenteric ganglia (figure 16.7).

In the *respiratory tract* VIP acts as an *anti-inflammatory* agent, independent of cholinergic or adrenergic innervation, and as an important neurotransmitter or neuromodulator to relax the smooth muscle of the airways of the lung and pulmonary vessels and to dilate the blood vessels that supply the respiratory system (Said, 1988). This is in contrast to the *proinflammatory tachykinins* which contract the smooth muscle of the lung (Maggi et al., 1995).

In the *reproductive tract* VIP is an active participant in secretion, motility, and blood flow (Fahrenkrug et al.,

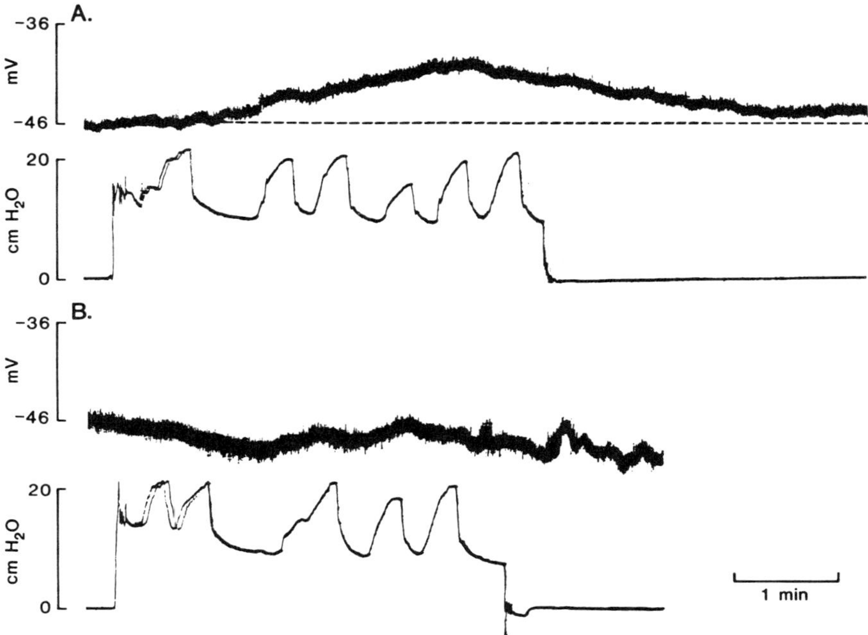

Figure 16.7
Effect of vasoactive intestinal polypeptide (VIP) antiserum on the slow excitatory postsynaptic potential evoked by distention of the distal colon. (In each panel: top trace) Intracellular recording from a neuron in the inferior mesenteric ganglion; (bottom trace) intraluminal pressure in a segment of the distal colon. Throughout this experiment, hexamethonium (2×10^{-4} M) and atropine (2×10^{-6} M) were present in the Krebs solution bathing only the ganglion, eliminating cholinergic and adrenergic responses. A, An increase in colonic intraluminal pressure caused a slow, noncholinergic depolarization 7 mV in amplitude. B, Pressure ejection of VIP antiserum blocked the distention-induced slow depolarization. Recordings A and B were made from the same neuron. (From Love et al., 1988.)

1988). The male and female reproductive tracts are abundantly supplied with VIP-containing nerve fibers and VIP is stored and released from large spherical, dense-core vesicles in the nerve terminals. In the female, VIP influences the passage of the ovum through the ovarian duct, relaxes uterine smooth muscle during pregnancy, and through increased blood flow and lubrication, increases sexual arousal. In the male, VIP acts as a neurotransmitter in penile erection (figure 16.8), an effect that is blocked by a VIP antagonist (Gozes et al., 1995).

VIP has potent *secretory* and *transport effects* and VIP-containing nerves supply all *exocrine glands*, including the salivary, lacrimal, and tracheobronchial glands, increasing their blood supply and enzyme and water secretion. VIP stimulates transport of chloride in the intestine and airways, and of water and bicarbonate in the pancreas. In some species, including humans, VIP

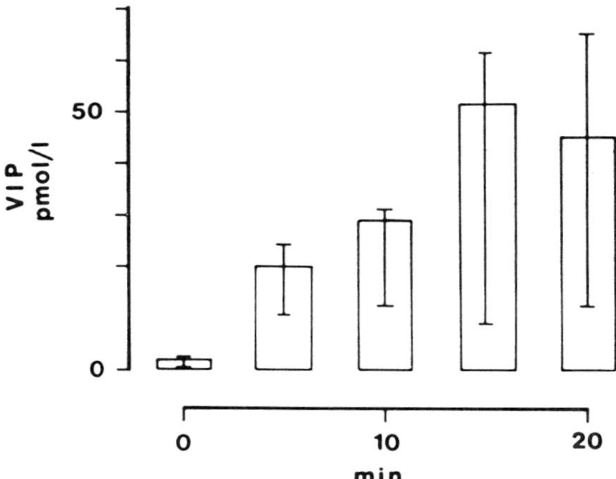

Figure 16.8
Concentration of vasoactive intestinal peptide (VIP) in corpus cavernosum at rest and during full erection or tumescence (figures are median and interquartile ranges of results obtained in 11 experiments in eight men). Stimulation was started immediately after 0 minutes. Tumescence or erection was obtained after 2 to 4 minutes and was unchanged during the period of observation. The increase in VIP was significant. (From Fahrenkrug et al., 1988.)

administered i.v. releases insulin and glucagon, but PHI is unable to evoke this response, even in high dosages (Fahrenkrug et al., 1987).

VIP has important secretogogue effects on *neuroendocrine secretions*. VIP from the hypothalamus reaches the anterior pituitary through the portal vessels to regulate the secretion of PRL, GH, LH, ACTH, and consequently corticosterone. These neuroendocrine effects are discussed in detail in the review by Rostene (1984).

In the CNS, VIP is associated with *biological rhythms*, with VIP mRNA in the suprachiasmatic nucleus peaking at night, and being independent of environmental light entraining (Glazer and Gozes, 1994). This raises the intriguing possibility that VIP might be a determinant rather than a result of circadian rhythms.

16.3.1.5 Actions of VIP on Development and Neurogenesis

The remarkable changes in VIP and VIP receptor content in various brain regions during development, as discussed above in section 16.3.1.2, suggest that there may be a transient developmental role for this peptide (Gozes and Brenneman, 1993). In vitro studies show that treatment with VIP stimulates neuronal mitosis, neurite extension, and neuronal survival in sympathetic and neuroblastoma cultures (Pincus et al., 1990). VIP has remarkable effects on glial cells, serving a paracrine function between developing neurons and glia, which results in the release of glial substances required for neuronal survival (Brenneman and Eiden, 1986).

Whole-mouse embryos in culture show a dramatic increase in growth after only 4 hours of exposure to VIP, which regulates mitosis in the neuroepithelium during midgestation (figure 16.9). Treatment of pregnant mice during embryonic days 9 to 11 with a VIP antagonist retards growth strikingly and is accompanied by microencephaly (Gressens et al., 1994). Although VIP receptors are present in the embryonic nervous system during this period, there is no indication of VIP mRNA in the early embryo. Where, then, does the essential VIP come from? It appears that levels of VIP in maternal serum are 6 to 10 times baseline levels during embryonic days 10 to 12, coinciding with the time that embryonic growth is regulated by VIP. VIP is also an important growth regulator in the early postnatal period in the rat; blockade of VIP results in neuronal dystrophy and an increase in both VIP mRNA and VIP binding sites (Hill et al., 1994). VIP-induced growth occurs through high-affinity, GTP–insensitive binding sites

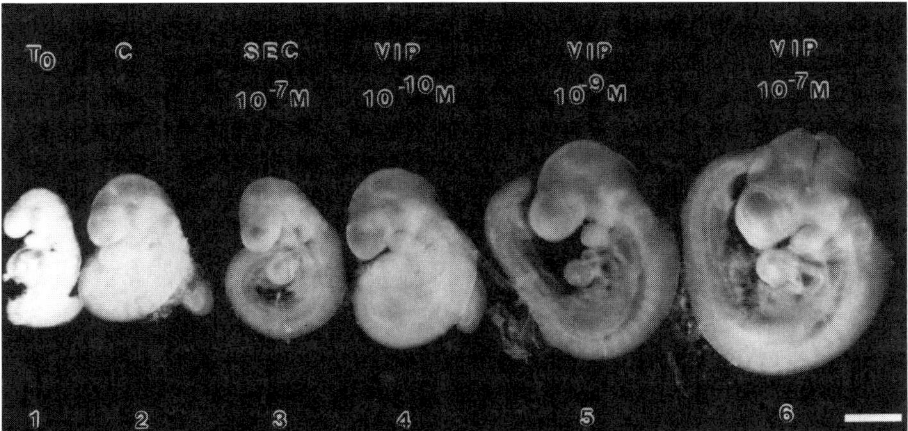

Figure 16.9
Vasoactive intestinal polypeptide (VIP) promotes embryonic growth without inducing macroscopic abnormalities. 1, Typical appearance of explanted whole embryos before the culture (T_o). Note that the yolk sac and ectoplacental core were removed to allow a comparison with the cultured embryos (2–5). These 4-hour cultured embryos were processed in the same experiment and represent the typical macroscopic aspect observed in repeated cultures with 10^{-10}, 10^{-9}, or 10^{-7} M VIP and 10^{-7} secretin (SEC) when compared with control cultured embryos (C). (From Gressens et al., 1993.)

which are localized to the embryonic neuroepithelium (Hill et al., 1997). VIP stimulation of these receptors also causes the release of other growth factors. Thus VIP appears to control neuronal morphology and integrity at critical periods of development, both directly and indirectly. Blocking VIP function in the early postimplantation embryo retards growth and results in microcephaly, and impaired development of complex motor behaviors (Wu et al., 1997).

An interesting approach to the study of VIP functions is the synthesis of a *VIP antagonist (Met-Hybrid)* that is designed to maintain the binding capacity of the parent VIP molecule while losing the agonistic properties to become a classical antagonist. Met-Hybrid consists of a carboxyl fragment of VIP 7–28 and a 6–amino acid fragment of neurotensin (NT 6–11) and is the most potent VIP-preferring receptor antagonist known. The effectiveness of Met-Hybrid in inhibiting VIP functions permits a sharp focus on the widespread actions of VIP. This antagonist powerfully inhibits VIP functions in vivo, blocking VIP potentiation of sexual behavior and impaired learning behavior. Met-Hybrid severely damages neonatal motor development and reflexes, and induces marked microcephaly during gestation if administered to pregnant mice. In addition, the antagonist inhibits VIP-stimulated mitosis in normal and cancer cells (Gozes et al., 1995).

16.3.1.6 Clinical Implications of VIP

Many diseases of the gastrointestinal tract may involve VIP. VIP, acting as a neurotransmitter affecting descending relaxation in the gastrointestinal tract, sphincter relaxation, and intestinal motility, may be involved in some gut motility disorders, such as esophageal spasm, dysphagia, and Hirschprung's disease, conditions associated with a *reduction in inhibitory neural input*. Similarly, many of the major features of cystic fibrosis may be due to a lack of VIP (Heinz-Erian and Said, 1988). Therapeutic use of VIP is hindered by side effects such as secretory diarrhea, cutaneous flushing, hypotension, and tachycardia. The use of specially designed VIP agonists and antagonists with tissue and receptor specificity holds promise for improved and focused drug design (Gozes et al., 1996).

Elevated levels of VIP and PHI are seen in patients with Werner-Morrison syndrome, who suffer from watery diarrhea (Moriarty et al., 1984). Watery diarrhea and intestinal hypersecretion are also seen in the Verner-Morrison (pancreatic cholera) syndrome, in which elevated VIP levels are due to a VIP-secreting pancreatic tumor (Bloom, 1978). Tumor size, VIP levels, and the associated symptoms are all decreased following treatment with a long-lasting somatostatin analog SMS 201–995 (Wood et al., 1985). In patients with Crohn's disease, who suffer from intestinal inflammation and obstruction, abnormalities of VIP-containing intestinal nerves have been identified, together with a variety of immunological disturbances.

The vasodilator effects of VIP may be involved in the pathogenesis of *cluster-type headaches*, as salivary VIP levels are elevated in patients with this type of headache, but not in those with migraine headaches. (Nicolodi and Del Bianco, 1990). Specific VIP antagonists may alleviate some of these symptoms.

A more positive role for VIP is seen in its action as a *neuroprotective agent* of possible use in the treatment of the neurodegeneration characteristic of Alzheimer's disease. In vitro studies of dissociated cereral cortical cultures show that VIP protects against β-amyloid neurotoxicity. In addition, the loss of cholinergic neurons in Alzheimer's disease is correlated with impairment of learning and memory. In animal models of Alzheimer's disease, cholinergic blockade results in the loss of learning and memory abilities, a deficit that is markedly reduced by treatment with VIP. The neuroprotective action of VIP in these models is believed to be due to VIP-elicited release of survival-promoting substances. Of practical importance is that intranasal administration of a lipophilic analog of VIP is an effective and efficient method of treatment since VIP cannot cross the blood-brain barrier and its half-life in the systemic circulation is only minutes (Gozes et al., 1997).

a. *VIP, peptide T, and HIV*

The pattern of distribution of VIP receptors on normal human brain is very similar to that of human immunodeficiency virus (HIV) receptors. The CD4 molecule is the cell surface receptor to which the HIV virus first attaches when gaining cell entry. The virus enters the cell by binding its envelope glycoprotein gp120 to the CD4 antigen present on brain and immune cells. This cell surface recognition molecule is normally modulated by VIP, and HIV has been found to mimic VIP binding via peptide T (4–8). Peptide T, a pentapeptide so named because half of its amino acids are threonine, whose single-letter abbreviation is *T*, inhibits the binding of HIV to human T cells (Pert et al., 1986)

It is believed that the peptide T portion of the HIV envelope and the neuropeptide VIP compete for recognition at the CD4 receptor molecule. The core pentapeptide attachment sequence of HIV is a pharmacological analog of the neuropeptide VIP (Pert et al., 1988).

Peptide T 4–8	Thr-Thr-Asn-Tyr-Thr
VIP (7–11)	Thr-Asp-Asn-Tyr-Thr

Neuronal growth and maintenance are enhanced by VIP and the cortical shrinkage in patients with AIDS may be due to the ability of the viral envelope molecules (gp120) to antagonize VIP's neurotrophic effects. Peptide T, which unlike VIP, can cross the blood-brain barrier, may be useful clinically to halt or attenuate the spread of HIV in infected persons. Limited clinical trials have shown that the peptide is nontoxic and the small number of patients tested appear to show some improvement (Ruff et al., 1988).

16.3.2 Secretin

It had long been known that acid in the proximal small intestine induces pancreatic exocrine secretion, but Bayliss and Starling (1902) were the first to show that the acid caused the release of a substance from the intestinal mucosa that was secreted into the circulation and, on reaching the pancreas, produced a copious pancreatic secretion. They called this substance *secretin*. Secretin was one of the last gastrointestinal hormones to be cloned.

16.3.2.1 Structure of Secretin

Secretin is a basic 27–amino acid peptide with a molecular weight of 3055. The C-terminus is amidated, as are that of so many other gastrointestinal regulatory peptides. Human secretin differs from porcine and bovine secretin in only two residues, Asp^{15} and Ser^{16}, which are replaced by Glu^{15} and Gly^{16}

His-Ser-Asp-Gly-Thr-Phe-Thr-Ser-Glu-Leu-Ser-Arg-Leu-Arg-Asp^{15}-Ser^{16}-Ala-Arg-Leu-Gln-Arg-Leu-Leu-Gln-Gly-Leu-Val-NH_2

16.3.2.2 Secretin Gene Expression, Precursor Processing, and Regulation of Release

The *gene* encoding secretin is divided into four exons with a length of 813 base pairs. The entire secretin sequence is encoded by a single exon, but the secretin gene encodes only a single copy of its biologically active peptide. This differs from the VIP and glucagon genes which are duplicated as glucagon-like peptides and PHI (Kopin et al., 1991). The region near the N-terminus is similar in the members of the VIP-secretin-glucagon family, but the remaining amino acid residues show marked sequence diversity, indicating that there has been extensive divergence of this gene family since the duplication of an ancestral gene (Leiter et al., 1994).

The *preprosecretin* C-terminal peptide is not well conserved and there is only a 39% homology between rat and porcine C-terminal peptide, suggesting that this portion of the precursor is not physiologically important (Kopin et al, 1990).

Expression of the secretin gene is chiefly in the small intestine. It is highest in the ileum which is a considerable distance from gastric acid, supposedly the secretogogue for secretin, indicating that other factors may be involved in evoking secretin secretion (Kopin et al., 1990). Secretin mRNA is not detectable in other regions of the gastrointestinal tract, with the exception of the colon. There may be very low levels of secretin mRNA in the brainstem, hypothalamus, and cortex. Reports of widespread secretin immunoreactivity throughout the CNS are probably due to cross-reactivity of secretin antisera with other members of the secretin-glucagon-VIP family.

During *development*, secretin mRNA and secretin in the intestine reach their highest levels 2 days before birth, and in the pancreas reach maximal levels about day 19 of gestation, falling to undetectable levels in the adult (figure 16.10). Secretin immunoreactivity is localized to insulin-producing beta cells and may influence pancreatic growth and development.

The *release* of secretin is mediated by a secretin-releasing peptide liberated by acid in the duodenum.

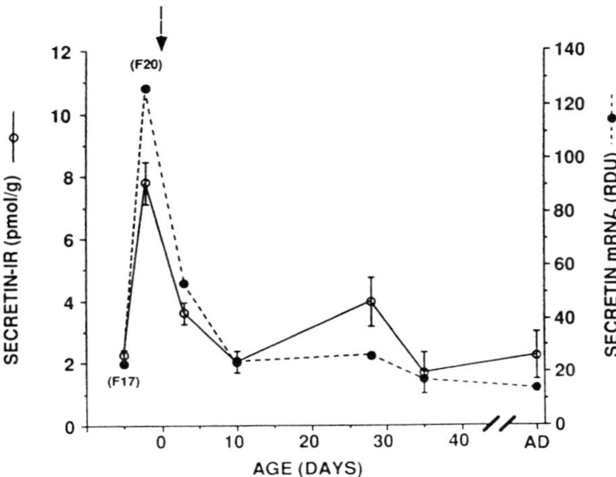

Figure 16.10
Ontogeny of secretin immunoreactivity (IR) and mRNA in developing rat duodenum. Secretin immunoreactivity is shown as mean ±SEM. Secretin mRNA levels were quantitated from the autoradiographs of Northern blots by scanning densitometry and are shown as relative densitometry units (RDU). An arrow indicates the day of birth. F17 and F20, days 17 and 20 of fetal gestation, respectively; AD, adult animals. (From Kopin et al., 1991.)

Secretin stimulates the releases of pancreatic juice, including a protease which then abolishes the activity of the secretin-releasing peptide, forming an efficient feedback loop to inhibit further secretin release (Li et al., 1990). The release of secretin from duodenal cells is mediated through mechanisms involving cAMP, Ca^{2+}, and protein kinase C.

16.3.2.3 Secretin Receptors and Second Messengers

The secretin receptor belongs to the G protein–coupled receptor family, and has seven hydrophobic transmembrane domains and five potential N-linked glycosylation sites. The receptor consists of 427 amino acids with a molecular weight of 48 kD or as much as 51 or 62 kD depending on the extent of glycosylation (Ishihara et al., 1991). Other members of this peptide family may act as secretin receptor agonists, and secretin may, in turn, act as an agonist to the other peptide family members. There seem to be two types of secretin receptors, a high-affinity secretin receptor, which binds secretin preferably, and a low-affinity secretin receptor, which has a higher affinity for VIP. The situation may be more complex, with as many as four secretin-VIP receptor subtypes possible (Bissonnette et al., 1984). The *second-messenger* system utilized by the secretin receptor is G protein activation of adenylate cyclase and cAMP.

16.3.2.4 Actions of Secretin

Physiological doses of secretin, administered peripherally, *increase the secretion of pancreatic water and bicarbonate*, an action that is potentiated by CCK. Secretin also stimulates the secretion of *alkaline bile* and the secretion from *submucosal duodenal glands* (Brunner's glands) in rats but not in humans. There is also considerable interaction between secretin and ACh produced by vagal innervation of the pancreas. Secretin is found in low amounts in the brain and centrally administered secretin increases the volume of pancreatic secretion and bicarbonate output considerably more that i.v. infusion of a comparable dosage. Thus central secretin may be involved in the regulation of the endocrine pancreas (Conter et al., 1996)

In the stomach, the action of secretin is *inhibitory*, inhibiting gastric secretion of acid, the release of gastrin, and gastric emptying. Secretin may also influence the release of other gut hormones such as insulin, glucagon, somatostatin, PP, parathyroid hormone, and calcitonin. Whether the action of secretin is inhibitory or stimulatory depends on the dosage, the species, and the health of the recipient (Leiter et al., 1994).

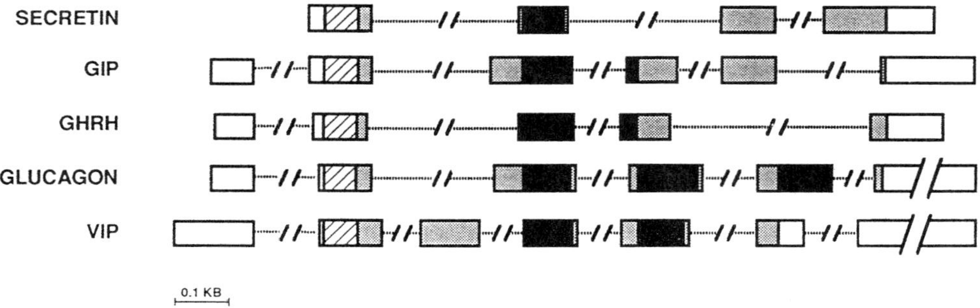

Figure 16.11
Structural organization of the genes encoding members of the secretin-glucagon family. Exons encoding similar functional domains are aligned and shown as boxes drawn to scale for the glucagon (rat), growth hormone–releasing hormone (GHRH) (rat), vasoactive intestinal polypeptide (VIP) (human), and gastric inhibitory peptide (human) genes. Introns are depicted as broken lines. Untranslated regions are indicated by open boxes. Crosshatched boxes denote signal peptides. Biologically active peptides are shown as solid boxes. N- and C-terminal peptides are indicated by shaded boxes. (From Kopin et al., 1991.)

16.3.3 Gastric Inhibitory Polypeptide

GIP is a duodenal peptide named for its ability to inhibit gastric acid secretion, but its most potent effects are its ability to release insulin and its strong insulin-like effects on adipose tissue and liver.

16.3.3.1 Structure of GIP

GIP has been highly conserved, indicating its important role as an anabolic hormone, and may have a role in the regulation of insulin secretion. Human and porcine GIP immunoreactivities contain components of molecular weights 5 kD and 8 kD, respectively, with only minor differences between human, porcine, and bovine sequences (T. W. Moody et al., 1984). GIP contains about 42–amino acid residues and thus is longer than the related neuropeptides VIP, PHI, and secretin, which consist of about 30–amino acid residues. Porcine GIP differs from human GIP shown below in only two positions: Arg^{18} and Ser^{34} replace His^{18} and Asn^{34}. There is only a single amino acid substitution in bovine GIP, with Ile^{37} replacing Lys^{37} (Jörnvall et al., 1981).

Tyr-Ala-Glu-Gly-Thr-Phe-Ile-Ser-Asp-Tyr-Ser-
Ile-Ala-Met-Asp-Lys-Ile-His^{18}-Gln-Gln-Asp-Phe-
Val-Asn-Trp-Leu-Leu-Ala-Gln-Lys-Gly-Lys-Lys-
Asn^{34}-Asp-Trp-Lys^{37}-His-Asn-Ile-Thr-Gln

16.3.3.2 GIP Gene Expression, Precursor Processing, and Regulation of Release

The exon-intron organization of this gene is very similar to the genes of the other members of this superfamily (figure 16.11) and it has been suggested that the GIP precursor contains the sequences of both insulin-stimulatory and insulin-inhibitory peptides (Takeda et al., 1987). While the genes of this VIP-secretin-glucagon superfamily are remarkably similar in organization, they are localized on different chromosomes: glucagon on chromsome 2, VIP on chromosome 6, and GIP on chromosome 17. The human GIP gene consists of six exons separated by five introns. Exons 3 and 4 encode the mature human GIP

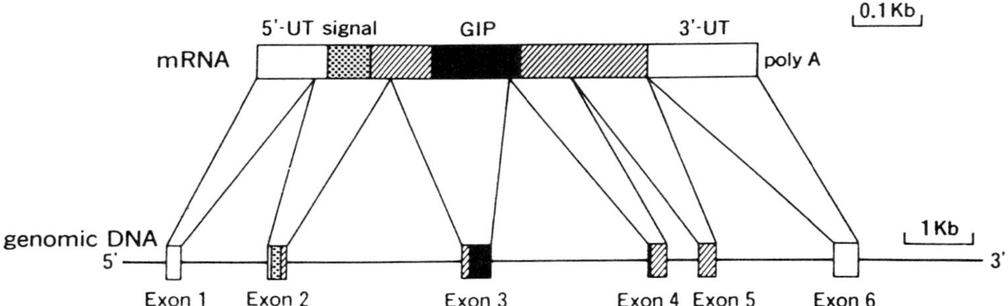

Figure 16.12
Organization of the human gastric inhibitory peptide (GIP) gene (bottom line) and mRNA (top line). The six exons and five introns are represented by boxes and lines, respectively. The 5′ untranslated region (5′UT) and 3′ untranslated region (3′-UT) are indicated by open boxes. The putative signal peptide is indicated by a dotted box. Shaded areas represent the N- and C-terminal peptides. The black box represents GIP. (From Inagaki et al. 1989.)

(figure 16.12) and the 5′-flanking region contains a number of possible regulatory elements (Inagaki et al., 1989).

Human prepro-GIP is a 153–animo acid protein with a molecular weight of 17 kD *Processing* at single Arg residues at either end of the GIP sequence yields GIP 1–42. GIP *release* is stimulated by glucose ingestion and is followed by the release of insulin within 5 minutes. Long-chain fatty acids stimulate a longer and greater release of GIP (figure 16.13).

GIP mRNA has been detected only in the K cells of the duodenum, where the GIP-containing cells are interspersed with other peptide-containing cells such as secretin, glucagon, somatostatin, and neurotensin (Buchan et al., 1978a). There does not appear to be any colocalization of peptides within a single intestinal endocrine cell, in contrast to the colocalization of several peptides within neurons of the enteric nervous system (Costa et al., 1986a,b).

16.3.3.3 GIP Receptors and Second Messengers

The GIP receptor is a monomer of 59 kD. Two types of GIP binding sites have been identified on pancreatic beta cells, a high-affinity and a low-affinity binding site, neither of which binds glucagon, secretin, or VIP (Amiranoff et al., 1985). The second messengers involved appear to be the cAMP and phosphatidylinositol intracellular pathways.

16.3.3.4 Actions of GIP

The physiological importance of GIP as an *inhibitor of gastric secretion* is debatable. GIP may inhibit acid secretion in part by inhibiting gastrin secretion, and a vagal cholinergic mechanism may be involved since GIP does not inhibit acid secretion if the vagus is cut. GIP may act through the local release of somatostatin, and the opiate peptides and the sympathetic nervous system may also be involved. It is difficult, therefore, to dissect out the specific contribution of GIP to the inhibition of gastric acid secretion.

The potent *insulinotropic action* of GIP, while predominantly on the pancreatic islet beta cells, may involve an intraislet regulation of alpha cells since adding alpha cells to cultures of purified beta cells considerably increases the effect of GIP. GIP-induced insulin release is highly dependent on glucose metab-

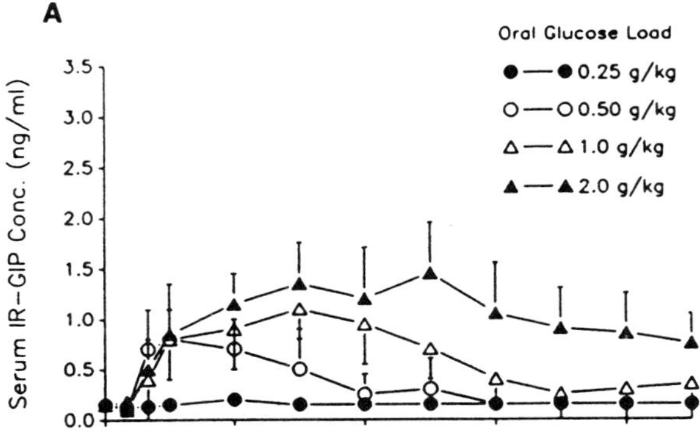

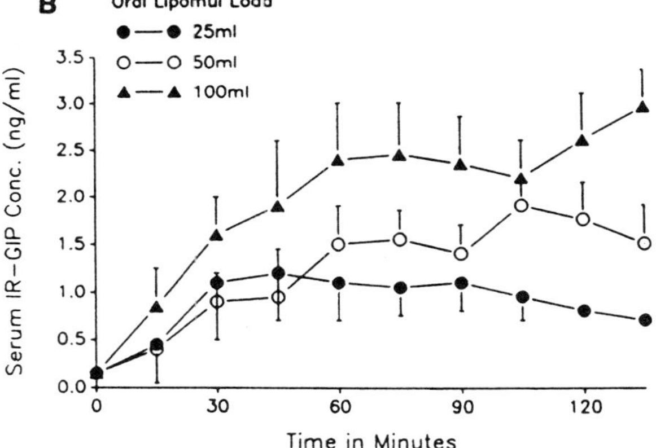

Figure 16.13
Immunoreactive gastric inhibitory peptide (IR-GIP) responses to ingestion of graded oral doses of A, glucose, B, triglycerides (lipomul) in the dog. (From Pederson et al., 1975.)

olism and beta cell Ca^{2+} transport, although the exact mechanism is unclear. Through its robust stimulation of insulin release, GIP affects *carbohydrate metabolism*, inhibiting glucagon-stimulated hepatic glycogenolysis and reducing hepatic glucose production. It has also been suggested that GIP may facilitate the rapid secretion of glucagon-like peptides from the intestine.

Again, through its action on insulin release, GIP promotes *triglyceride synthesis* in adipose tissue, although GIP may also influence fatty acid synthesis directly by acting on adipocytes and fat metabolism (Ebert and Creutzfeldt, 1987).

16.3.3.5 Clinical Implications of GIP

GIP may be involved in the development of obesity since it increases fat storage in adipocytes, both directly through its action on the pancreatic beta cell and indirectly through its release of insulin.

16.3.4 Glucagon and Glucagon-like Peptide-1

Glucagon is primarily a pancreatic peptide, produced by the alpha cells and acting directly on the beta cells of the pancreas to regulate insulin secretion. It has an important role in carbohydrate, fat, and protein metabolism. However, proglucagon is differentially processed in the pancreas, where it yields glucagon, and in the intestine where it remains uncleaved to form *glucagon-like peptides GLP-1 and GPL-2*. Of these, GLP-1 is the more important peptide, acting indirectly on glucose metabolism through its effects on pancreatic and glucagon secretion; GLP-1 also has inhibitory effects on gastric acid secretion and motility. The function of GPL-2 is not known.

16.3.4.1 Structure of Glucagon

Glucagon, a 29–amino acid neuropeptide mainly produced by the alpha cells of the pancreas but also by the A-like cells of the gastric mucosa, has maintained a high degree of conservation during evolution, with the primary structure the same in all mammals tested, except for the guinea pig.

His-Ser-Gln-Gly-Thr-Phe-Thr-Ser-Asp-Tyr^{10}-Ser-Lys-Tyr-Leu-Asp-Ser-Arg-Arg-Ala-Gln^{20}-Asp-Phe-Val-Gln-Trp-Leu-Met-Asn-Thr^{29}

Avian glucagons differ from the mammalian by only a few amino acids. The biological activity of glucagon requires the integrity of the whole molecule; the C-terminal moiety is required for binding and the N-terminal region for selective binding and effector coupling (Christophe, 1996). The N-terminal histidine, essential to biological activity, is the same as in secretin and VIP.

16.3.4.2 Structure of GLP-1 and GPL-2

GLP-1 is a 29–amino acid peptide, the full sequence of which represents proglucagon 72–108 (Ørskov et al., 1989). However, the naturally occurring *truncated GPL-1 (tGPL-1)*, which is the proglucagon sequence 78–107, is the more potent stimulator of insulin secretion. GLP-2 corresponds to amino acids 126–158 of proglucagon and this sequence probably came later in evolution since fish proglucagon contains only GLP-1 (Lund et al., 1982).

The enteric proglucagon peptides are produced by the L cells, most of which are in the ileum. Very little true glucagon is produced in the gastrointestinal tract, mostly by gastric endocrine A-like cells of some species, but A cells are lacking in the human.

16.3.4.3 Glucagon Gene Expression, Precursor Processing, and Regulation of Release

In all species, except for the anglerfish, which has two glucagon genes encoding two different glucagon mRNAs, there is only a single gene for preproglucagon. The mRNAs for transcription are identical in the pancreas and intestine, indicating that the differences between the glucagon-related peptides in these tissues must be due to differential tissue processing (Mojsov et al., 1986). The proglucagon gene is also expressed in the CNS, mostly in the nucleus of the tractus solitarius and in the hypothalamus (Drucker and Asa, 1988).

The *preproglucagon gene* is a 9.4-kilobase polynucleotide, composed of six exons and five introns, and is located on chromosome 2. The preprohormone contains a 20–amino acid signal peptide sequence followed by the 160–amino acid proglucagon sequence.

Proglucagon formed in the alpha cells of the pancreas, contains, in addition to glucagon (proglucagon 33–62), a *glucagon-related pancreatic peptide (GRPP)*, and a single large molecule, the major *proglucagon fragment (MPGF)* that contains the two glucagon-like peptides GLP-1 and GLP-2.

Pancreatic Proglucagon GRPP–glucagon–MPGF

cleaved to

GRPP + glucagon + GLP-1 + GLP-2

In the L cells of the intestine, GLP-1 and GLP-2 are formed and secreted separately, and the N-terminal portion, known as *glycentin*, remains intact. GLP-1 and GLP-2 are separated by a third peptide, *intervening peptide-2 (IP-2)*. Glycentin, consisting of 69 amino acids, is the major intestinal peptide with glucagon-like immunoreactivity and contains the glucagon sequence at position 33–61 (Ørskov et al., 1986). Glycentin also contains *oxyntomodulin* (glycentin 32–69), which contains the characteristics of the whole hormone.

Processing of the intestinal peptides also yields *miniglucagon*, or glucagon 19–29, which has opposing effects to glucagon on glucagon targets: miniglucagon evokes a negative inotropic effect on cardiac myocytes, decreasing their contractility, and inhibits insulin release from pancreatic beta cells. Miniglucagon is effective at extremely low concentrations, in the picomolar range, whereas glucagon acts in the nanomolar range (Bataille et al., 1996).

Intestinal Proglucagon Glycentin–GLP-1–IP-2–GLP-2

cleaved to

Glycentin + GLP-1 + IP-2 + GLP-2

cleaved to

Oxyntomodulin + Miniglucagon

The primary *regulator* of pancreatic alpha cell secretion of glucagon is a reduction in blood glucose, whereas insulin is a potent inhibitor of glucagon secretion. *Pancreatic glucagon* acts as a hyperglycemic factor to maintain glucose homeostasis, but is tightly coupled with insulin secretion in the normal person, making it difficult to evaluate their actions separately. However, it appears that insulin suppression of glucagon is dominant, since glucagon secretion rises dramatically as soon as a neutralizing antiinsulin serum enters the microcirculation of the pancreatic islets (figure 16.14).

Secretion and release of the intestinal and pancreatic glucagons occurs synchronously, and the chief glucagons are secreted in equimolar amounts (Ørskov et al., 1986). The release of *intestinal glucagons* is stimulated by an ordinary mixed meal, and the microvilli of the L cells are stimulated by the unabsorbed nutrients in the intestinal lumen; secretion of GLP-1, tGPL-1, and GLP-2 increases rapidly. This is reflected in the sharp rise in the plasma levels of these enteroglucagons after a meal. The rapidity of the response may be facilitated by the duodenal hormone, GIP.

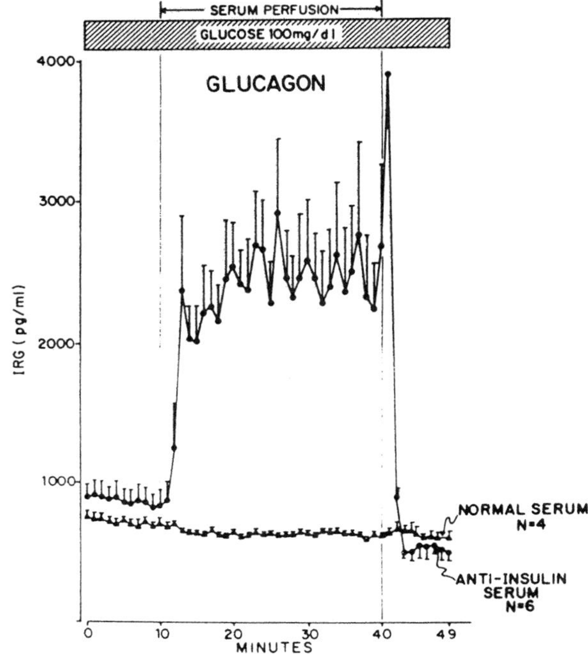

Figure 16.14
The effect of antiinsulin serum (closed circles) on glucagon secretion (mean ± SEM) in the isolated perfused rat pancreas. Normal guinea pig serum (closed triangles) was used as a control. IRG, immunoreactive glucagon. (From Maruyama et al., 1994.)

There is an important "anticipatory response" with an initial secretion of glucagon and insulin occurring at the beginning of exercise, initiated by signals from the activated adrenergic signals from the lateral hypothalamus. This rapid response depends on the innervation of the pancreatic islets by adrenergic, cholinergic, peptidergic, and purinergic nerves and results in the prevention of hypoglycemia rather than its correction, providing glucose levels adequate for the exercise.

16.3.4.4 Glucagon and GLP-1 Receptors and Second Messengers

The rat glucagon receptor gene contains 12 exons, seven of which code for the seven transmembrane segments. The hepatic *glucagon receptor* is a glycoprotein of 63 kD, containing four N-linked glycans and it belongs to the large family of G protein binding receptors, and also fits into a smaller subset of homologous receptors for the related neuropeptides such as VIP, GIP, GRP, PACAP, and GHRH. In addition, there is considerable homology with nonrelated peptides such as CRH, parathyroid hormone, and calcitonin (Segre and Goldring, 1993). While the primary target tissue of glucagon is the liver, glucagon receptor mRNA is present not only in hepatic tissue but also in the kidney, heart, stomach, pancreatic islets, spleen, thymus, adrenal, and skeletal muscle. The physiological function of these receptors is, as yet, unknown (Hansen et al., 1995).

Glucagon, acting through G protein binding receptors, stimulates adenylate cyclase, which increases intracellular cAMP. This is followed by activation of cAMP-dependent protein kinase and phosphorylation, which ultimately results in *glycogenolysis* in liver cells. This sequence in adipose tissue results in *lipolysis* through the activation of lipases which release glycerol and free fatty acids. Glucagon also acts through inositol phosphate–mediated pathways, perhaps using a *second glucagon receptor GR-1*, and its effects on glycogenolysis, gluconeogenesis, and ureagenesis may be the result of phosphorylation of key enzymes using both pathways (Unger and Orci, 1990).

GLP-1 does not react with glucagon receptors but has its own specific receptors. The GPL-1 receptor is a protein with a molecular weight of 63 kD. GPL-1 binds to rat insulinoma cells through G protein binding receptors associated with adenylate cyclase. The GPL-1 receptor is also synthesized in rat pituitary, hypothalamus (especially the ventromedial nucleus, hippocampus, olfactory cortex, and choroid plexus, indicating that these neurons play an important role in glucose sensing (Alvarez et al., 1996). GLP-1 receptors are *not* found on hepatocytes. GLP-1 does not bind or stimulate glucagon-secreting cells so it is postulated that the inhibitory effect of GLP-1 on glucagon secretion may be through stimulated secretion of somatostatin on islet cells (Fehmann and Habener, 1991). No receptors for glycentin have been described as yet, and both insulin-stimulating and insulin-inhibiting effects have been reported.

16.3.4.5 Actions of Glucagon and GLP-1

Pancreatic glucagon has important regulatory functions for *glucose and amino acid metabolism* and consequently for blood glucose. Glucagon acts as a *hyperglycemic factor* by stimulating hepatic glucose release either through glycogenolysis or gluconeogenesis. Gluconeogenesis is achieved through the conversion of amino acids, or of glycerol, to glucose under the influence of glucagon acting on the hepatic enzymes involved in these reactions. These effects are the opposite of those of insulin, a potent hypoglycemic peptide.

Adipose tissue is the other main target of glucagon, which acts as a *lipolytic agent* to liberate free fatty acids and glycerol, which circulate to the liver where they can serve as substrates for gluconeogenesis. Thus, through lipolysis, glucagon acts as a hyperglycemic factor. This action is usually only demonstrable in the absence of insulin, which is a potent inhibitor of lipolysis, but can be demonstrated in diabetic patients. Glucagon exerts positive inotropic and chronotropic effects on cardiac muscle, acting through cAMP.

Intestinal GPL-1 and *tGPL-1* simultaneously *stimulate insulin secretion* and *inhibit glucagon secretion*. Truncated GPL-1 also stimulates *somatostatin secretion* from isolated pancreatic islet cells and slows gastric emptying. No specific physiological functions have been assigned to the remaining products of intestinal proglucagon processing.

Glucagon infusions have a central effect, *suppressing food intake*, specifically of carbohydrates. Centrally administered GLP-1 *inhibits food and water intake* in rats (Tangchristensen et al., 1996) and reduces body temperature (Oshea et al., 1996).

16.3.4.6 Clinical Implications of Glucagon and GLP-1

During fasting, glucagon plays an important role in raising blood sugar, coordinated with the hyperglycemic action of adrenal catecholamines. Glucagon contributes to the pathogenesis of *diabetes* so a potent and long-acting glucagon antagonist could be beneficial clinically. The difficulty is that the entire glucagon molecule is required for effectiveness.

There are many clinical conditions in which large amounts of unabsorbed nutrients reach the intestine and cause *elevated levels of intestinal proglucagon peptides*. These increased levels are found in acute infectious diarrhea, and in patients in whom the gastric contents are rapidly emptied into the duodenum (dumping syndrome). A fashionable operation, in which a jejunoileal bypass is performed to treat morbid obesity, results in large amounts of unabsorbed nutrients reaching the ileum, with consequent increases in the enteroglucagon levels (Sarson et al., 1981). These levels are similarly elevated in patients with malabsorption resulting from tropical diseases or from celiac disease.

GLP-1 has a marked *antidiabetogenic effect* and has a possible role in the treatment of non–insulin-dependent diabetes mellitus (Gutniak et al., 1992). High levels of tGPL-1 in patients with accelerated gastric emptying are accompanied by increased insulin secretion and resulting hypoglycemia (Jarhult et al. 1981; Miholic et al., 1991).

16.4 The Pancreatic Polypeptide Family

The evolutionary connections among members of the PP family were considered in chapter 1. The PP family of structurally related peptides has been isolated from both the gut and the brain, but the three members of this family show remarkable tissue specificity. *Pancreatic polypeptide* is expressed only in the pancreatic islets, *peptide YY (PYY)* is found in the endocrine cells of the duodenum and exocrine pancreas, and *neuropeptide Y (NPY)* is widely distributed in neural tissue. The basic endocrine effect of PP is to inhibit pancreatic exocrine secretion and to relax the gallbladder, that of PYY is to inhibit gastric emptying and secretin-stimulated pancreatic secretion. NPY has many diverse effects that will be considered later in this chapter but its actions on the gastrointestinal tract are primarily inhibitory.

16.4.1 Pancreatic Polypeptide and Peptide YY

16.4.1.1 Structure of PP and PYY

In almost all species, PP is a 36–amino acid residue peptide with an amidated tyrosine residue at the C-terminus, removal of which destroys all biological activity. The entire C-terminal amidated hexapeptide is required for biological activity. PYY is also an amidated 36–amino acid residue peptide, 16 of which differ from PP. PYY was named based on the presence of tyrosine residues at both its C- and N-termini, using the single-letter code for tyrosine (*Y*) (Tatemoto et al., 1981). The amino acid sequence of porcine PP is shown; that of the PYY sequence has the identical residues in italic.

PP Ala-Pro-Leu-Glu-Pro^5-Val-Tyr-Pro-Gly-Asp^{10}-Asp-Ala-Thr-Pro-Glu^{15}-Gln-Met-Ala-Gln-Tyr^{20}-Ala-Ala-Glu-Leu-Arg^{25}-Arg-Tyr-Ile-Asn-Met^{30}-Leu-Thr-Arg-Pro-Arg^{35}-Tyr-NH_2

PYY Tyr-*Pro*-Ala-Lys-*Pro*^{5}-Glu-Ala-*Pro-Gly*-Glu^{10}-*Asp-Ala*-Ser-*Pro-Glu*^{15}-Glu-Leu-Ser-Arg-*Tyr*^{20}-Tyr-*Ala*-Ser-*Leu-Arg*^{25}-His-*Tyr*-Leu-*Asn*-Leu^{30} -Val-*Thr-Arg*-Gln-*Arg*^{35}-*Tyr*-NH_2

16.4.1.2 PP and PYY Gene Expression, Precursor Processing, and Regulation of Release

The common structure of the genes for PP, PYY, and NPY are illustrated in figure 16.15. The *PP gene* consists of four exons and three introns. The first exon encodes the 5′ untranslated region; the signal sequence and the PP sequence are encoded by the second exon (Leiter et al., 1985). The *prepro-PP* is a 95–amino acid molecule from which is cleaved the prohormone sequence 1–36 with a C-terminal extension. The sequential action of processing enzymes removes the extension, leaving behind the amidated tyrosine residue at the C-terminus. The PP gene is expressed within most cells of the pancreas with most PP-containing cells in the head of the pancreas.

The *PYY gene*, like the PP gene, consists of four exons and three introns. Exon 1 contains the 5′-untranslated region; exon 2, the translational initiation site, the signal peptide, and the PYY sequence, minus the C-terminal tyrosine residue. Exon 3 encodes the Tyr residue. Exon 4 encodes part of the

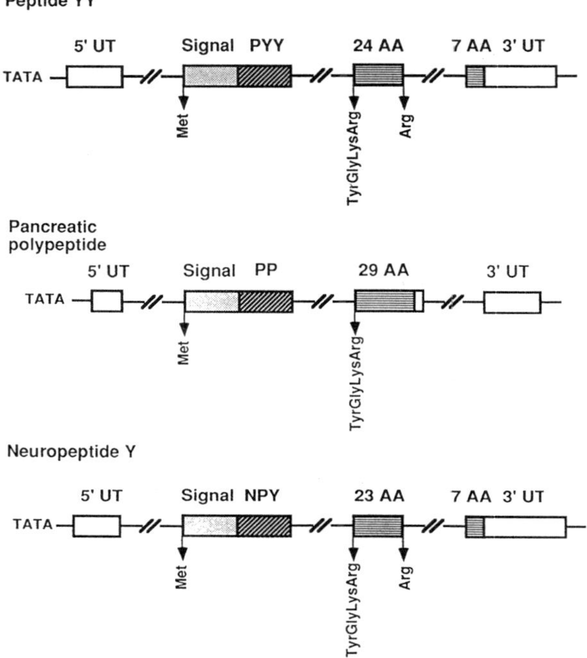

Figure 16.15
Structural organization of the rat genes in the pancreatic polypeptide (PP) family. Exons are indicated as boxes. Protein coding regions are shaded. Flanking and intron sequences are shown as solid lines. TATA, Goldberg-Hogness promotor; 5′ UT and 3′ UT, 5′- and 3′-untranslated regions of the mRNA; Signal, signal peptide; PYY, peptide YY. AA, amino acid. (From Krasinski et al., 1990.)

C-terminal extension and the 3′-untranslated region. The precursor structure is highly conserved and shared by all three members of this family. It consists of a signal peptide, a 36–amino acid mature hormone, a Gly-Lys-Arg sequence followed by a C-terminal peptide of about 30 residues (Krasinski et al., 1990). The major forms of PYY processed from the precursor are PYY 1–36 and PYY 3–36. PYY is expressed in the distal small intestine, colon, and rectum, and only rarely in the stomach and duodenum. PYY colocalizes with proglucagon in some L cells in the intestine.

The initial release of PP is a complex of cephalic-vagal stimulation (presence of food in the mouth) and gastric distention caused by food in the stomach. This is followed by a more prolonged response which involves other peptides such as CCK. Insulin hypoglycemia is the most potent stimulus to PP release and vagotomy completely abolishes this response (Jahrhult et al., 1981). PYY is released by fat in the duodenum and is also considerably increased after rapid gastric emptying following vagotomy. The PYY released acts as a feedback mechanism to slow the rate of gastric emptying. There is a considerable time difference in the response of PP and PYY to a meal, as PYY levels rise much more slowly and are not dependent on vagal stimulation (figure 16.16).

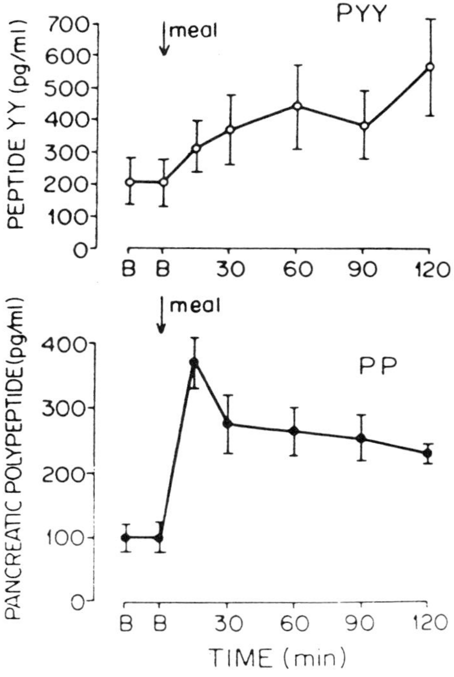

Figure 16.16
Comparison of the pancreatic polypeptide (PP) and peptide YY (PPY) responses to a 15% liver extract meal in dogs. (From Taylor, 1985.)

16.4.1.3 PP and PYY Receptors and Second Messengers

No PP receptors have been identified on pancreatic acini in mammals, but high-affinity PP receptors are present in the area postrema and nucleus tractus solitarius of the brain. These are regions with fenestrated capillaries, which permit the passage of circulating PP into the brain (Whitcomb et al., 1990). These investigators also identified specific binding of PP to the dorsal nucleus of the vagus. This raises the intriguing concept that PP acts indirectly to inhibit pancreatic secretion by preventing ACh release centrally at the level of the vagal nuclei and peripherally on cholinergic nerve fibers or peripheral ganglia. This completes a feedback loop whereby PP released peripherally by vagal stimulation inhibits the central vagal nuclei. Other PP receptors have been found in the adrenal medulla, small intestine, and liver. PYY receptors are present in the intestine.

16.4.1.4 Actions of PP and PYY

PP inhibits pancreatic secretion of enzymes, bicarbonate, and water, and may play a role in negative feedback control of the pancreas through its inhibitory action on vagal ACh release. PP *increases the tonic contraction* of lower esophageal sphincter pressure, both indirectly through intrinsic cholinergic neurons and directly on the smooth mucle of the sphincter. PP may improve gallbladder filling during the interdigestive period by relaxing the gall bladder.

PYY is a potent inhibitor of many gastrointestinal functions. PYY inhibits secretin-stimulated pancreatic secretion in many species, but apparently not in humans. PYY inhibits gastric secretion of acid and pepsin, acting on the cephalic phase of gastric secretion through a neural mediator. PYY inhibits gastric emptying and, in the intestine, PYY inhibits prostaglandin E_2–induced secretion of fluid and electrolytes from the jejunum, an action probably mediated through NPY receptors (Saria and Beubler, 1985). Fat in the intestine slows intestinal transport and delays gastric emptying, a phenomenon called the *ileal brake*. PYY is probably one of the factors involved in this mechanism as it inhibits gut motility, especially in the colon. In addition, PYY is a powerful *vasoconstrictor* of cerebral and splanchnic blood vessels.

16.4.1.5 Clinical Implications of PP and PYY

PP is produced by some pancreatic and intestinal tumors, but no clinical syndrome has been associated with elevated PP levels. The elevated levels of PYY seen in patients suffering from malabsorption may delay gastric emptying and movement of food through the intestines.

16.4.2 Neuropeptide Y

NPY is widely distributed in the central, peripheral, and enteric nervous systems of species extending from insects to humans (McDonald, 1988). NPY has many distinct physiological actions ranging from direct inhibitory actions on the gastrointestinal tract to complex regulation of endocrine, metabolic, and behavioral functions specifically related to nutrient and energy homeostasis, and consequently of body weight (Leibowitz, 1994). NPY also is involved in the regulation of cardiovascular responses, circadian rhythms, and pituitary release of hormones. Many of these diverse actions may be accounted for by the coexistence and interaction of NPY with other transmitters and neuropeptides in the brain (Aoki and Pickel, 1990).

16.4.2.1 Structure of NPY

NPY is a 36–amino acid peptide, the most biologically active form of which is amidated. Like PYY it was named according to its terminal tyrosine (*Y*) at the C- and N-terminals of the peptide (Tatemoto et al., 1981).

Tyr^{1}-Pro-Ser-Lys-Pro-Asp-Asn-Pro-Gly-Glu^{10}-Asp-Ala-Pro-Ala-Glu-Asp-Leu-Ala-Arg-Tyr^{20}-Tyr-Ser-Ala-Leu-Arg-His-Tyr-Ile-Asn-Leu^{30}-Ile-Thr-Arg-Gln-Arg-Tyr^{36}-NH_2

16.4.2.2 NPY Gene Expression, Precursor Processing, and Regulation of Release

The *NPY gene* spans 7.2 kb pairs and contains four exons and three introns in an arrangement similar to that of the PP gene. Exon 1 encodes the 5′-untranslated region; the signal peptide and most of NPY are encoded by exon 2. The human NPY gene is located on chromosome 7. The rat NPY preprohormone consists of 98 amino acids from which is cleaved a 69–amino acid residue pro-NPY which is then amidated (Larhammar, 1987). There is complete homology of NPY in guinea pig, rabbit, rat, and human (O'Hare et al., 1988).

The NPY gene is *expressed* throughout the gastrointestinal tract of most mammals, especially in the lower esophageal sphincter and upper gut. The NPY-containing fibers are of both extrinsic and intrinsic origin and NPY is co-localized with NE in sympathetic neurons (Lee et al., 1985). In nonadrenergic nerves of the small intestine NPY is colocalized with VIP and PHI (Ekblad et al., 1984). In descending interneurons NPY is usually colocalized with bombesin and NO synthase, but never with 5-HT or somatostatin (Uemura et al., 1995). NPY is also expressed in the pancreas, liver, heart, and spleen, and in endothelial cells of blood vessels.

In the CNS, NPY and NPY mRNA are found in all brain subregions tested, and NPY is densely concentrated in the hypothalamus, which also contains high levels of mRNA and receptor sites for NPY (Merchanthaler et al., 1993). NPY is synthesized by neurons of the arcuate nucleus and secreted from their terminals in the PVN and ventral hypothalamus, regions that govern energy balance and neuroendocrine regulation.

The *release* of NPY is strikingly increased by food deprivation, which initiates a marked increase in NPY mRNA and NPY, specifically in the arcuate and paraventricular nuclei. NPY is also involved in the natural rhythm of feeding behavior, which is strongest during the active feeding cycle (dark cycle) in rats. NPY levels in the PVN peak at the onset of the active feeding cycle, preceded by an increase in NPY mRNA or NPY in the arcuate nucleus. This peak is probably dependent on the diurnal rise of corticosterone (Ponsalle et al., 1992).

16.4.2.3 NPY Receptors and Second Messengers

NPY receptors belong to the superfamily of G protein binding receptors and interact with G_i to inhibit the production of cAMP. There are five NPY receptor subtypes (Y1–Y5) but most information is available about Y1 and Y2. These receptors can be distinguished by their ability to bind specific peptide or nonpeptide analogs (Kirby et al., 1997) or by their different pre- and postjunctional effects. The subtype Y3 binds NPY but not PYY with high affinity. Receptors that bind both NPY and PYY are found in discrete areas of the brain, especially in the cortex and hippocampus. Peripheral tissues with NPY receptors include the gut, heart, spleen, and kidney.

In the CNS, high concentrations of NPY receptors are found in the PVN and arcuate nucleus. NPY synthesis in vitro is increased by the administration of substances that stimulate the production of cAMP and in vivo central administration of dibutyryl cAMP increases NPY levels, exclusively in the arcuate nucleus and medial PVN (Akabayashi et al., 1994).

16.4.2.4 Actions of NPY

The *inhibitory actions of NPY on the functions of the gastrointestinal tract* are manifold. NPY inhibits both acid and pepsin secretion by the stomach, pancreatic secretion, and intestinal fluid and electrolyte secretion. NPY inhibits motility in the gut (figure 16.17), probably by inhibiting excitatory NE pathways in the gut wall (Holzer et al., 1987). In some species, however, NPY may cause contraction of the intestine.

NPY has a strong *stimulatory effect on food intake*, increasing the size and duration of the meals, particularly of carbohydrate-rich meals. In very low dosages (picograms) NPY can stimulate the animal to eat half of its daily food intake in 1 hour (Stanley et al., 1985). These actions are associated with high levels of corticosterone and insulin, the release of which is stimulated by NPY (Fuxe et al., 1989).

The involvement of NPY in obesity is clearly demonstrated in experiments with genetically obese mice (*ob/ob*). The mutation has been mapped to the gene encoding carboxypeptidase E, a processing enzyme that removes C-terminal–paired basic residues from peptides derived from prohormones. As a result of this mutation NPY is overproduced in the hypothalamus. The obesity syndrome in these mice results

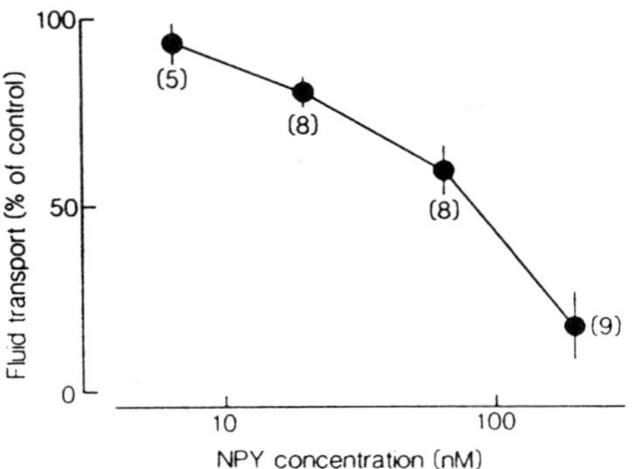

Figure 16.17
Effect of neuropeptide Y (NPY) on the peristaltic reflex in segments of the guinea pig small intestine. The segments were perfused with Tyrode's solution via their vascular supply, and NPY was administered by intra-arterial infusion. Abscissa, Final concentration of NPY in the vascular perfusion medium. Ordinate, Propulsion of fluid. Mean ± SEM, number of experiments as indicated in parentheses. (From Holzer et al., 1987.)

from a deficiency of *leptin*, a hormone produced by fat cells that acts centrally to suppress feeding and stimulate metabolism, and which normally inhibits the expression and release of NPY (Stephens et al., 1995; Schwartz et al.,1996). Erickson et al.(1996) generated *ob/ob* mice that were deficient in NPY. These double mutants weighed less than obese mice but more than normal mice, and the loss of NPY did not completely reverse other indicators of metabolism, indicating that other neuromodulators are involved in the regulation of energy balance. One of these is MSH and the *melanocortin-4 receptor (MC4-R)* (see chapter 12).

This revelation is due to a fascinating series of experiments with mutant mice, the *ob* and *agouti* mice. The *ob* mice lose their appetites when injected with synthetic melanocortins that bind to the MC4-Rs, even when they are given additional NPY to spur their food intake. In a different mouse mutant, the *agouti* mouse, which is bright yellow due to an agouti protein that blocks the MC4-R needed to produce the melanin for normal dark fur, also gets very fat. Fan et al., (1997) in Roger Cone's laboratory, showed that the agouti protein also blocked the MC3-R and MC4-R in the hypothalamus, the site of action for leptin and NPY production. If the MC4-Rs are blocked by the agouti protein, the animals rapidly regain their appetites. Knockout mutant mice in which the MC4-R has been knocked out show the same weight gain as the agouti mutants (Huszar et al., 1997).

The link between NPY, MSH, the MC4-Rs, and leptin is becoming clearer. Increased fat deposition increases leptin levels, decreasing food intake and increasing energy expenditure provided that MSH and the MC4-Rs are available. This allows the body to maintain constant stores of fat. In agouti mice, which lack leptin and have blocked MC4-Rs, food intake soars and the animals become obese. In normal animals, NPY is an important mediator in the response to starvation, increasing food intake, whereas MSH and the MC4-R, working through the hypothalamic response to leptin, decrease food intake to maintain normal weight in response to increased fat stores.

Recently another factor in the complex control of food intake has been identified. Two appetite-stimulating peptides, named *orexins* from the Greek word for appetite, are synthesized in the lateral hypothalamus (LH). Injection of the orexins into the LH causes rats to devour from three to six times as much food as control rats. Further confirmation of the importance of these neuropeptides in the control of appetite is shown by the upregulation of orexins in starved animals (Sakuri et al., 1998). The orexins may be important regulators of the LH as a feeding center, and may work synergistically with another LH appetite-stimulating hormone, melanin concentrating hormone (MCH) (see section 12.2.5.2). The role of MCH in appetite control, however, is conflicting. Qu et al. (1996) report that MCH injected into the lateral ventricles of rats increases food consumption. In contrast, several other investigators have found MCH to be an anorectic peptide, inhibiting food intake (Rovere et al., 1996; Presse et al., 1996).

NPY also enhances memory processes in mice, a phenomenon that can be separated from the increased feeding elicited by this neuropeptide. A critical portion of the NPY molecule for improving memory involves amino acids 20–26. Feeding requires either all 36 amino acids or at least a fragment longer than NPY (20–36). It may be that the intact NPY molecule, but not short fragments, acts at postsynaptic Y1 receptors, whereas NPY and long fragments act at the Y2 presynaptic receptors (Flood and Morley, 1989).

NPY has an important role in *central cardiovascular regulation*. NPY 1–36, given centrally, causes hypotension due to a decrease in mean arterial blood pressure and a drop in heart rate, mediated by the Y1 receptors. In contrast, the shorter fragment NPY 13–36 produces a vasopressor response through activation of the Y2 receptors (Fuxe et al., 1990).

The neuroendocrine effects of NPY are generally stimulatory. Injection of NPY into the PVN or i.c.v. injection increases the secretion of insulin, corticosterone, and VP. NPY is an important regulator of *secretion of anterior pituitary hormones*, especially in the regulation of reproductive functions, by controlling the episodic basal release of LH and, in some species, the preovulatory LH surge. NPY acts on both the hypothalamus and the anterior pituitary, involving an amplification of NE stimuli, and is dependent on the specific gonadal steroid environment (see section 10.4.2). In amphibians, NPY inhibits α-MSH secretion (Danger et al., 1990).

NPY can act as a *neurotransmitter, neuromodulator*, or a *neurohormone*. NPY has both pre- and postsynaptic actions in peripheral tissues, such as vascular smooth muscle and the vas deferens, and is a potent inhibitor of excitatory transmission in the hippocampus in vitro (Colmers, 1990).

16.4.2.5 Clinical Implications of NPY

NPY is implicated as a mediator of the hyperphagia, low metabolism, and endocrine changes that accompany leptin deficiency. However, obese humans, as well as rodents, have high levels of leptin and therefore it is possible that leptin "resistance" may be the cause of the obesity (Considine et al., 1996). Therapy aimed at leptin receptors may hold promise for some forms of human obesity, but the MC4-Rs are smaller and probably easier to bind and stimulate, to decrease appetite.

16.5 The Bombesin and Gastrin-Releasing Peptide Family

Bombesin is a neuropeptide first discovered in the skin of amphibians of the genus *Bombina* (Erspamer et al., 1972). Subsequently, the mammalian counterpart, gastrin-releasing peptide, was identified in extracts of mammalian gut and brain (Walsh et al., 1979) and in carcinoid tumors of the lung. This extract shares with bombesin the ability to stimulate gastrin release and gastric acid secretion and is very similar in amino acid sequence to bombesin. The neuropeptides *ranatensin* and *neuromedin B* belong to a subfamily of the bombesin-GRP superfamily. Neuromedin B was named for the initial letter of *b*ombesin by Minamino et al. (1988). It was thought at one time that there would be a neat delineation between the neuropeptides found in frogs (bombesin and ranatensin) and those found in mammals (GRP and neuromedin B). However, frogs have both bombesin and GRP and mammals appear to possess four or more bombesin-like peptides.

16.5.1 Structure of Bombesin, Gastrin-Releasing Peptide, and Related Neuropeptides

Whereas bombesin is a peptide consisting of 14 amino acid residues and GRP contains 27 residues, the 10 C-terminal residues differ only in 1 amino acid, resulting in similar biological properties of the two peptides. In the following structural formulas, the amino acids identical to those in the bombesin sequence are shown in *italics*.

Bombesin	pGln-Gln-Arg-Leu-*Gly-Asn-Gln-Trp-Ala-Val-Gly-His-Leu-Met*-NH_2
GRP 27	Ala-Pro-Val-Ser-Val-Gly-Gly-Gly-Thr-Val-Leu-Ala-Lys-Met-Tyr-Pro-Arg-*Gly-Asn-His-Trp-Ala-Val-Gly-His-Leu-Met*-NH_2

Two shorter forms of GRP, GRP 23 and GRP 10, in addition to GRP 27, have been isolated from canine intestine. GRP 10 is also found in spinal cord.

Ranatensin, an 11–amino acid peptide isolated from the frog *Rana pipiens*, and *neuromedin B*, its 32–amino acid mammalian counterpart found in spinal cord, are structurally related to bombesin and GRP.

Bombesin	pGln-Gln-Arg-Leu-*Gly-Asn-Gln-Trp-Ala-Val-Gly-His-Leu-Met*-NH_2
Ranatensin	pGln-Val-Pro-*Gln-Trp-Ala-Val-Gly-His*-Phe-*Met*-NH_2
Neuromedin B	Ala-Pro-Leu-Ser-Trp-Asp-Leu-Pro-Gln-Pro-Arg-Ser-Arg-Ala-Gly-Lys-Ileu-Arg-Val-His-Pro-Arg-Gly-Asn-Leu-*Trp-Ala*-Thr-*Gly-His*-Phe-*Met*-NH_2

16.5.2 Bombesin, Gastrin-Releasing Peptide, and Neuromedin B Gene Expression, Precursor Processing, and Regulation of Release

There is a single human *GRP gene*, located on chromosome 18, comprised of three exons and two introns. Alternative splicing gives rise to three distinct RNAs. All three RNAs encode for GRP 27 but differ in their encoding of variable C-terminal extension peptides (Sausville at al. 1986). The human *neuromedin B gene* is on chromosome 15.

Prepro-GRP consists of 147 amino acid residues that constitute a signal peptide, then a single copy of GRP 27, followed by a C-terminal extension peptide (CTEP)

Signal peptide, *GRP*-27, CTEP . . . 850 bases

Preproneuromedin B 32 has a single copy of neuromedin B following the signal peptide and is flanked by the C-terminal extension peptide

Signal peptide, *neuromedin B* 32, CTEP . . . 648 bases

Preprobombesin consists of a signal peptide, with a single copy of bombesin sandwiched between an N-terminal extension peptide (NTEP) and a C-terminal extension peptide.

Signal peptide, NTEP, *bombesin*, CTEP . . . 648 bases

Preproranatensin is organized like preprobombesin, with a single copy of ranatensin between the N-terminal and C-terminal extension peptides.

Signal peptide, NTEP, *ranatensin*, CTEP . . . 405 bases

Expression of GRP has usually been determined using antibodies to bombesin and GRP. GRP is found throughout the gastrointestinal tract. GRP-immunoreactive nerve fibers richly innervate the stomach, the myenteric plexus, submucosal plexus, and longitudinal muscle of the small and large intestine. Intestinal cell bodies may be identified as containing GRP reactivity after colchicine treatment. Pancreatic nerve fibers and cell bodies also express GRP and bombesin and are closely associated with exocrine acini but not with the endocrine islets (Moghimazadeh et al., 1983).

In the CNS, a small proportion of neurons of spinal dorsal ganglia express bombesin, which is *not* colocalized with SP. After colchicine treatment, nerve cell bodies that express bombesin are found in many brain areas, especially in the hypothalamus. Moderate amounts of bombesin and GRP are present in the thalamus, midbrain, medulla and pons, striatum, cortex, and hippocampus. Very little is found in the olfactory bulb and spinal cord. Discrete localization of bombesin and GRP is present in the PVN, suprachiasmatic nucleus, central gray region of the midbrain, the trigemimal complex, the dorsal vagal nucleus, and the nucleus of the tractus solitarius, all regions that cooperate in regulating autonomic functions (A. U. Moody et al., 1988).

Bombesin or GRP is expressed generously in the epithelium of the lungs of the fetus and neonate, but few bombesin-expressing cells are found in the adult except in lung tumors (Yamaguchi et al., 1983).

In the CNS, expression of *neuromedin B* is highest in the pituitary gland, with lesser concentrations in the hypothalamus, hippocampus, dorsal root ganglia, dentate gyrus, and olfactory bulb, in contrast to GRP, which is expressed mainly in the forebrain (Namba et al., 1985; Wada et al., 1990). In the gut, the highest concentration of neuromedin B is in the esophagus and rectum.

The *release* of bombesin, GRP, and neuromedin B has not been extensively investigated. Electrical stimulation of the vagus causes the release of GRP from perfused pig stomach and pancreas. Electrical stimulation of the splanchnic nerve releases immunoreactive bombesin into the plasma of the calf, but not the pig (Bloom and Edwards, 1984).

16.5.3 Bombesin, Gastrin-Releasing Peptide, and Neuromedin B Receptors and Second Messengers

There are two distinct receptors for the bombesin-GRP family and the ranatensin-neuromedin B subfamily. Pancreatic acinar cells express the GRP-preferring receptor, whereas esophageal and gastric smooth muscle cells express a receptor that binds preferentially to neuromedin B, but these cells also express the separate GRP-preferring receptor (Battey and Wada, 1991). The two types of receptors have been cloned and the GRP-preferring receptor has a molecular weight of 43 to 45 kD, a size that is considerably increased by glycosylation to 75 kD. The GRP receptor contains seven putative membrane-spanning domains and thus is a member of the G protein–coupled receptor family. This receptor is highly expressed in the hypothalamus. Activation of protein kinase C is involved in the proliferative reponse of fibroblasts to bombesin, together with phosphorylation and the rapid mobilization of intracellular calcium (Erusalimsky et al., 1988).

The neuromedin B–preferring receptor is also a member of the G protein–coupled receptor family, has a molecular weight of 43 kD, and is glycosylated. The greatest density of neuromedin B receptors is in the central thalamic and olfactory regions.

16.5.4 Actions of Bombesin, Gastrin-Releasing Peptide, and Neuromedin B

Both bombesin and GRP are powerful stimulants for the *release of gastrin and gastric acid*, which is clearly shown by the inhibition of gastric secretion resulting

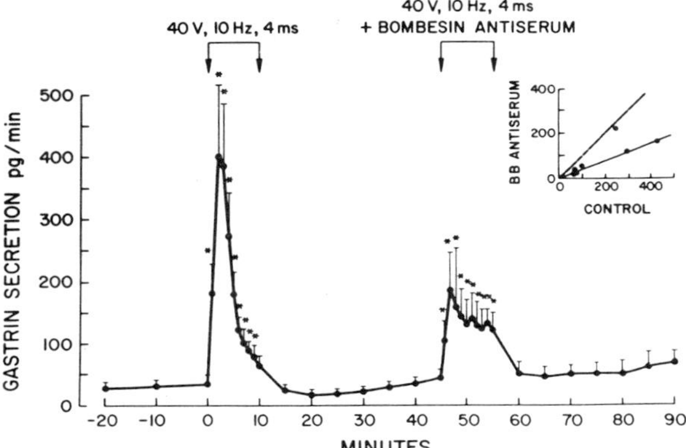

Figure 16.18
Inhibitory effect of antiserum against bombesin on gastric secretion induced by electrical field stimulation (arrows) of the antral region of the vascularly perfused rat stomach. Inset, Control response plotted against response in the presence of antiserum against bombesin (BB antiserum) in six experiments. Brackets, 1 SE; $*P < .05–.01$. (From Schubert et al., 1985.)

from the administration of an antiserum against bombesin (figure 16.18). The GRP-associated peptides that are produced by alternative splicing of mRNA are not able to excite gastric secretion. The pathway for secretion appears to be vagal stimulation of the antral mucosa, which partly through a noncholinergic mechanism, that is, the release of GRP, induces gastrin release. This response is inhibited by somatostatin.

Bombesin and GRP also release an *inhibitor of gastric acid secretion*, which is probably somatostatin, so that the final amount of acid secreted is a balance between the stimulatory and inhibitory effects of these neuropeptides (Schubert and Hightower, 1989).

Pancreatic exocrine secretion is stimulated by bombesin and GRP and again this response is complex, partly mediated by another neuropeptide, intestinal CCK, and partly due to a direct binding to receptors on the pancreatic acinar cells. Immunoreactive GRP is released from the stimulated vagus onto acinar cells, which respond with a profuse, protein-rich exocrine secretion (Knuhtsen et al., 1985). Bombesin and GRP also *increase gastrointestinal contractility*, and contractility of the *gallbladder*, both directly and by mediation of vagally induced gastric contraction.

Central administration of bombesin and GRP into the ventricles has the opposite effect of peripheral administration, strongly *inhibiting gastric acid secretion* (Taché et al., 1988). The hypothalamic nuclei are particularly sensitive to bombesin, a not surprising observation given the dense concentration of bombesin receptors in these structures. Bombesin-containing neurons are found in nerve terminals of the nucleus of the tractus solitarius and the dorsal motor nucleus of the vagus, but the inhibitory pathway seems to involve the sympathetic nervous system.

Bombesin acts as a neurotransmitter or neuromodulator with significant autonomic and behavioral effects; for example, bombesin, GRP, and neuromedin B are implicated in the control of food intake. Bombesin and GRP, but not neuromedin B, suppress NaCl intake (Flynn, 1996). Bombesin given i.c.v. has profound effects on thermoregulation in the rat and induces hyperglycemia.

Bombesin and GRP excite the release of several other neuropeptides, such as CCK, gastrin, somatostatin, pancreatic glucagon, and GIP. GRP inhibits the release of GH and PRL by dopaminergic mechanisms that involve increased somatostatin secretion in the hypothalamus and depression of PRL release from the pituitary (see chapters 9 and 10) (Kentroti and McCann, 1996).

Bombesin and GRP have trophic effects on the pancreas and gut, increasing mucosal DNA content and causing hyperplasia of cells in the pancreas, stomach, and colon. Bombesin and neuromedin B are produced by small cell lung cancers and act in an autocrine fashion to stimulate growth of the cancer cells.

Neuromedin B was originally isolated on the basis of its ability to cause contraction of guinea pig ileum and rat uterus (Minamino et al., 1988), and it has very weak bombesin-like effects on pancreatic secretion. Neuromedin B may participate in some central regulatory processes but definitive evidence is lacking.

16.5.5 Clinical Implications of Bombesin and Gastrin-Releasing Peptide

Hypersecretion of bombesin-like peptides by small cell lung carcinomas suggests that the trophic effect of these neuropeptides may initiate or maintain the growth of these cells. Antibodies to the C-terminal region of bombesin or GRP specifically inhibit this type of carcinoma only. Use of such antibodies or bombesin antagonists may be appropriate clinical therapy (Coy et al., 1988).

16.6 Summary

Peptide-containing cells are found throughout the gastrointestinal tract and can be identified by their morphological and immunohistochemical characteristics. The enteric nervous system is an autonomous component of the peripheral nervous system and consists of the myenteric and submucosal plexuses. These receive input from the central and autonomic nervous systems through nerve terminals that contain either ACh and NE, often colocalized with neuropeptides. Gut sphincters, which control the passage of food into and out of the stomach, and of feces out of the anus, are regulated by peptidergic nerves in combination with the classical neurotransmitters. Pancreatic endocrine cells in the islets of Langerhans secrete peptides which are released into the circulation and also have important paracrine effects. Pancreatic exocrine cells, which produce the digestive enzymes, are regulated by both neuropeptides and neurotransmitters.

The *gastrin and cholecystokinin family* consists of the well-known gastric hormones, although their effects are now known to extend far beyond actions on the gastrointestinal tract. While the genes for these two neuropeptides are on different chromosomes, their structural similarities indicate that they may have arisen from a common precursor gene. Both neuropeptides possess an identical amidated C-terminal pentapeptide, which results in some overlapping of functions. The *gastrin gene* is expressed in the gastric antrum and upper small intestine, pituitary corticotrophs, and pancreas. Processing of progastrin yields gastrin-34 and gastrin-17. Sulfated gastrin 17 (gastrin I) is the most prevalent form. Gastrin II is nonsulfated, but is as potent as gastrin I in stimulating gastric acid secretion.

The *CCK gene* is composed of three exons, the third of which encodes the biologically active region of the peptide. CCK gene expression is stimulated by feeding, depressed by fasting, and by somatostatin. Prepro-CCK is cleaved to pro-CCK, then to CCK-58. α-Amidation of the C-terminal is essential to activity. Shorter CCK forms are produced by cleavage at monobasic or dibasic residues and are proteolytic C-terminal fragments of CCK-58. The differently sized CCK molecules vary considerably in tissue distribution according to species. CCK mRNA is found in the intestine and brain of many species. CCK-8 is the predominant form in the CNS; CCK-33 is the gut hormone. In the CNS, CCK mRNA is expressed in regions related to nociceptive transmission, overlapping with the distribution of opiate neuropeptides. CCK-containing nerve terminals are found throughout the gastrointestinal tract, including the myenteric and submucosal plexuses. CCK is released from endocrine cells into the blood after a meal, and there are several factors that inhibit CCK release from these cells.

Gastrin and CCK receptors are of two main types, CCK-A and CCK-B, products of two different genes. The CCK-A receptor is found on gallbladder smooth muscle cells and pancreatic acinar cells, has a much higher affinity for CCK than for gastrin, and is highly specific for the sulfated form of CCK. Inhibition of somatostatin release is only through the CCK-A receptor. The CCK-B receptor is present in gastric cells and in the brain and is much less selective than the CCK-A receptor, binding gastrin and several forms of CCK equally well. These receptors are typical G protein binding receptors and stimulate intracellular calcium and inositol phosphate pathways.

Gastrin is produced in the gastric antrum in response to food and is an important regulator of gastric acid secretion, which in turn, inhibits gastrin production. Local somatostatin also inhibits gastrin secretion. GRP and foods, especially proteins, peptides, and amino acids, promote the release of gastrin into the circulation, a release that is prevented by fasting, CCK, and somatostatin. Cholinergic and adrenergic pathways are also concerned in gastrin release.

CCK regulates gallbladder contraction after a meal and stimulates pancreatic enzyme secretion and the secretion of insulin and glucagon. In contrast, CCK inhibits the release of gastrin and consequently decreases gastric acid secretion. Gut motility is increased by CCK acting on cholinergic nerve terminals to release ACh for muscle contraction, as well as by a direct action on intestinal smooth muscle. CCK has a trophic effect on the pancreas and causes a reflex gastric mucosal hyperemia. In the CNS, CCK decreases food intake by inducing satiety, antagonizes the analgesia evoked by opiates, and is one of several neuropeptides upregulated in dorsal root ganglia after axotomy.

The *vasoactive intestinal polypeptide, secretin, and glucagon family* is one of the largest families of gastrointestinal regulatory peptides, of which VIP is the most important member, with wide-ranging effects on the CNS and on development. Other neuropeptides that are structurally related to this family include PACAP and GHRH, which were discussed in chapter 10.

VIP is the most important neuropeptide of this large family. It is a highly conserved molecule consisting of 28 residues with a C-terminal amide. PHI is a closely related 27–amino acid peptide, derived from the same gene and precursor as VIP and with similar actions. VIP and PHI always coexist and are coreleased. The VIP-PHI gene is expressed throughout the gastrointestinal tract and VIP nerve fibers are both intrinsic and extrinsic. In the CNS, VIP mRNA is found in cortical and thalamic neurons and the suprachiasmatic nucleus. VIP coexists with several different neuropeptides and neurotransmitters in different tissues, such as with ACh in the salivary glands.

The *expression* of the VIP gene is strikingly regulated during development, increasing sharply through the first two postnatal weeks in the rat. Expression is regulated by many hormones, especially glucocorticoids. Processing is tissue- and species-specific, producing different forms of bioactive VIP and PHI. Physiological release of VIP is from esophageal or intestinal distention, which stimulates the vagal nerves to release both VIP and PHI. Adrenergic stimulation presynaptically inhibits VIP release.

There are several distinct *VIP receptors*, all belonging to the G protein–coupled receptor family, with different affinities for different members of the VIP-secretin-glucagon family. The second-messenger pathway utilizes adenylate cyclase and cAMP. Binding is high in the gastrointestinal, respiratory, and genital tracts, and in lymphocytes. In the CNS, high levels of VIP binding sites are found in the anterior pituitary, pineal body, olfactory bulb, hippocampus, suprachiasmatic nucleus, and brainstem. VIP acts as a noncholinergic, nonadrenergic mediator in the systems listed above, increasing the rate and strength of cardiac contractions and causing a potent vasodilation. VIP acts as an anti-inflammatory agent in the respiratory tract, and is an important stimulus to secretion, motility, and blood flow in the male and female reproductive tracts. VIP increases secretion of almost all exocrine glands through its vasodilator actions and stimulates ion and water transport. VIP regulates mitosis in early embryos, accelerating growth and regulating normal neuronal organization.

Secretin was first discovered in 1902, but it was one of the last gastrointestinal peptides to be cloned. Secretin is a 27–amino acid peptide with an amidated C-terminus. The secretin gene encodes only one copy of the neuropeptide, and only the region near the N-terminus is similar to the other members of the VIP-secretin-glucagon family. Expression of the gene is mainly in the ileum and low levels are found in some regions of the CNS. Secretin receptors belong to the G protein–coupled family and there may be several secretin receptor subtypes, which use adenylate cyclase and cAMP as the second-messenger system. Secretin release into the circulation is mediated by a secretin-releasing peptide liberated by acid in the duodenum. Secretin, in turn, stimulates the secretion of pancreatic juice, including a protease which closes the feedback loop by abolishing the activity of the secretin-releasing peptide.

The main function of secretin is to stimulate the secretion of pancreatic water and bicarbonate, an action potentiated by CCK. There may be central actions of brain secretin, acting through vagal innervation of the pancreas, on the regulation of pancreatic secretin. In the stomach, secretin inhibits gastric secretion of acid, the release of gastrin and gastric emptying, and may also inhibit the release of many other gut hormones.

Gastric inhibitory polypeptide inhibits gastric secretion and potently releases insulin from the pancreas. GIP is a 42–amino acid peptide which has been highly conserved. The organization of the GIP gene is very similar to that of the other members of this neuropeptide family, but these genes are located on different chromosomes. GIP mRNA is found only in the duodenum and GIP does not seem to be colocalized with other neuropeptides. There are two types of GIP receptors found on pancreatic cells and they use cAMP and phosphatidylinositol intracellular pathways. The physiological significance of inhibition of gastric secretion by GIP is unsure but the most important function of GIP is its ability to release insulin and thus affect carbohydrate and lipid metabolism.

Glucagon is a pancreatic peptide that stimulates insulin secretion but *glucagon-like peptide* is produced in the intestine. Glucagon is another highly conserved 29–amino acid peptide. There is only a single gene for preproglucagon and the mRNAs are identical for glucagon produced in the pancreas and intestine. However, differential processing produces mainly glucagon in the pancreas and GLP-1 in the intestine. The gene is also expressed in the CNS. In the pancreatic alpha cells, proglucagon is processed not only to glucagon but to a glucagon-related pancreatic peptide and GLP-1 and GLP-2. A truncated form of GLP-1 (tGPL-1) is also produced. In the intestine, proglucagon is processed to glycentin, GLP-1, and GLP-2; glycentin is then cleaved to form oxyntomodulin and miniglucagon (glucagon 19–29), which has effects on glucagon targets opposite to those of glucagon. A fall in blood glucose stimulates the release of glucagon from the pancreas, whereas insulin secretion inhibits glucagon release. All the enteroglucagons are secreted and released by intestinal cells in response to a meal.

The glucagon receptor has considerable homology with the receptors for VIP, GIP, GRP, PACAP, and GHRH. It is found mainly in the liver but also in adipose tissue and many peripheral organs. The second-messenger pathway is through adenylate cyclase and cAMP, and through the inositol phosphate–mediated systems. GLP-1 has its own receptors and they are found on insulin-producing cells, the pituitary, hypothalamus, olfactory cortex, and choroid plexus, but not on hepatocytes.

Pancreatic glucagon is a hyperglycemic and lipolytic factor which stimulates the release of glucose from the liver, and fatty acids and glycerol from adipose tissue, which also contributes to gluconeogenesis. Glucagon infusions suppress carbohydrate intake. Intestinal GPL-1 and tGPL-1 stimulate insulin secretion and inhibit glucagon secretion, and tGPL-1 also stimulates ST secretion. Centrally, GPL-1 inhibits food and water intake and may be involved in the regulation not only of feeding but also of water and salt homeostasis.

Pancreatic polypeptide, neuropeptide Y, and *peptide YY* have important evolutionary connections and have been isolated from both the gut and the brain. However, they show remarkable tissue specificity. The structures of the genes for these three related neuropeptides are very similar, as are the precursor structures, which are highly conserved, as discussed in section 1.5.2.4. However, PP is *expressed* only in the pancreatic islets, PYY in the endocrine cells of the duodenum and exocrine cells of the pancreas, whereas NPY is extensively distributed in the CNS, especially in the arcuate nucleus and PVN, and in the periphery. PP *receptors* are present in the area postrema and nucleus tractus solitarius of the brain, and the dorsal nucleus of the vagus. PYY receptors are present in the intestine. There are several types of NPY receptors, and high concentrations are found in the PVN and arcuate nucleus. NPY receptors that bind both NPY and PYY are found in specific brain areas, especially the cortex and hippocampus. The receptors for this family of neuropeptides use adenylate cyclase and cAMP as second messengers.

Hypoglycemia is the most potent stimulus for PP *release*, and food in the mouth and stomach releases PP through cephalic-vagal stimulation, which is followed more slowly by the release of other neuropeptides such as CCK. PYY release is initiated by fat in the duodenum, an action independent of vagal stimulation. NPY is released by food deprivation and peaks at the onset of the active feeding cycle, preceded by an increase in NPY mRNA or NPY in the arcuate nucleus.

PP inhibits pancreatic secretion of enzymes, bicarbonate, and water, inhibits vagal ACh release, and increases the tone of the lower esophageal sphincter. PYY inhibits many gastrointestinal functions, including inhibition of gastric secretion of acid and pepsin, gastric emptying, and secretion of fluid and electrolytes from the jejunum. PYY is involved in mechanisms that inhibit gut motility and is also a powerful vasoconstrictor of cerebral and splanchnic blood vessels. NPY inhibits gastric, intestinal, and pancreatic secretions, and gut motility.

NPY stimulates food intake, especially of carbohydrates, and is involved in obesity, as shown by mouse mutants that overproduce NPY. Leptin, a hormone produced by fat cells, is believed to be the normal inhibitor of NPY production. The MC4 receptors in the hypothalamus appear to be the site of action for leptin and NPY. NPY 1–36 decreases blood pressure and heart rate acting through Y1 receptors, whereas NPY 13–36 has a vasopressor effect through activation of Y2 receptors. NPY stimulates the neuroendocrine system, increasing the secretion of insulin, corticosterone, and VP. NPY is an important regulator of LH, acting on both the hypothalamus and pituitary, actions dependent on gonadal steroids. NPY acts as a neurotransmitter or neuromodulator, or both, in the the CNS and peripheral tissues.

Bombesin and gastrin-releasing peptide both stimulate gastrin release and gastric secretion, and are very similar in amino acid sequence. *Ranatensin* and *neuromedin B* belong to a subfamily of the bombesin-GRP superfamily. GRP is the mammalian counterpart to bombesin, a neuropeptide first discovered in amphibian skin, but there is some overlap in this distribution. Bombesin is a 14–amino acid peptide; GRP contains 27 amino acids of which the 10 C-terminal residues differ from those of bombesin by only 1 amino acid. Ranatensin and neuromedin B belong to a subfamily of the bombesin-GRP family, structurally related to bombesin and GRP. There is a single bombesin-GRP-neuromedin B gene, and alternate splicing gives rise to three distinct mRNAs, all of which encode for GRP 27 but differ in their encoding of variable C-terminal extension peptides.

GRP mRNA is *expressed* throughout the gastrointestinal tract, and in pancreatic nerves associated with exocrine acini. In the CNS, spinal dorsal ganglion cells express GRP which is not colocalized with substance P. GRP is present in many brain regions, especially the forebrain, hypothalamus, and regions that control autonomic functions. In the fetus GRP is expressed in the lung, and again in lung tumors in the adult. Neuromedin B is expressed chiefly in the pituitary, with lesser amounts in the hypothalamus, hippocampus, dentate gyrus, olfactory bulb, and dorsal root ganglia. In the gut, most neuromedin B is in the esophagus and rectum.

The GRP-preferring *receptor* is expressed by pancreatic acinar cells and centrally is most highly expressed in the hypothalamus. The neuromedin B–preferring receptor is found in esophageal and gastric smooth muscle cells, which also express the GRP-preferring receptor. Both receptor types belong to the G protein binding receptor family and activate protein kinase C, phosphorylation, and the mobilization of intracellular Ca^{2+}.

Bombesin and GRP *release* gastrin and gastric acid secretion via vagal stimulation of the antral mucosa, which, through the release of GRP, induces gastrin secretion. Somatostatin, which is released by bombesin and GRP, inhibits this response. Gastric acid secretion, therefore, is a balance between the stimulatory and inhibitory effects of these neuropeptides. Bombesin and GRP stimulate pancreatic exocrine secretion, aided by intestinal CCK. Bombesin and GRP increase gastrointestinal and gallbladder contractility, both directly and through the vagus. Central administration of bombesin or GRP has opposite effects to that of peripheral administration, inhibiting gastric acid secretion. These neuropeptides act as neurotransmitters or neuromodulators in the regulation of food intake, suppression of NaCl intake, thermoregulation, and response to hyperglycemia. Bombesin and GRP excite the release of CCK, gastrin, somatostatin, pancreatic glucagon, and GIP, but inhibit GH and PRL release. Bombesin and GRP cause hyperplasia in the pancreas, stomach, and colon and are produced by small cell lung cancers. Neuromedin B has weak bombesin properties.

Chapter 17 continues with the discussion of those brain and gut neuropeptides which, with the exception of insulin, do not fall into neat neuropeptide families. They include galanin, motilin, calcitonin gene–related peptide, and neurotensin.

Gut and Brain Neuropeptides II. Insulin, Galanin, Motilin, CGRP, Neurotensin

17

17.1 Insulin

Insulin was first isolated from pancreatic tissue by Banting and Best (1922) and very soon after its initial isolation, extracts containing increasingly pure insulin were administered to diabetic patients with dramatic results, lowering blood glucose and ameliorating many of the symptoms of the disease. Yet, despite many years of intense investigation, there are still aspects of insulin biosynthesis and structure that are not well understood. The major action of insulin is on glucose homeostasis, but it has other complex physiological effects, stimulating carbohydrate, protein, and lipid metabolism, DNA and RNA synthesis, and promoting growth. The chief targets for insulin regulation of glucose homeostasis are the liver, skeletal muscle, and adipose tissue. However, insulin also stimulates glucose metabolism in other tissues that do not seem to be involved in glucose homeostasis.

The role of insulin in the brain has been a subject of controversy but more recent evidence indicates that insulin from the circulation reaches the brain via a specialized blood-brain transport system and is an important afferent CNS signal that regulates normal energy balance (Schwartz et al., 1992).

A chain
Gly-Ile-Val-Glu-Gln-*Cys*^{6}-Cys^{7}-Thr-Ser-Ile-*Cys*^{11}-Ser-Leu-Tyr-Gln-Leu-Glu-Asn-Tyr-Cys^{20}-Asn

B chain
Phe-Val-Asn-Gln-His^{5}-Leu-Cys^{7}-Gly-Ser-His^{10}-Leu-Val-Glu-Ala-Leu^{15}-Tyr-Leu-Val-Cys^{19}-Gly-
Glu-Arg-Gly-Phe-Phe^{25}-Tyr-Thr-Pro-Lys-Thr^{30}

Figure 17.1
The primary structure of human insulin, showing the A chain (21 amino acids) and B chain (30 amino acids). The two polypeptide chains are connected by two disulfide bridges, A7 to B7, and A20 to B19. In addition, a third disulfide bridge links positions 6 and 11 in the A chain.

17.1.1 Evolution of Insulin and Insulin-like Growth Factors

Insulin is found in nonmammalian vertebrates, invertebrates, and in unicellular organisms, and its primary structure has been relatively well conserved throughout evolution, although not as well as that of glucagon (see chapter 16). Nevertheless, the biological activity of insulin has remained consistent in all mammals, including the human, but excepting the guinea pig, in which the insulin gene has acquired mutations which decrease the metabolic efficiency of the hormone. The three-dimensional structure of insulin has remained fairly constant throughout evolution and is believed to be responsible for this stability.

Insulin belongs to the superfamily of peptide hormones which contains *insulin-like growth factors* (*IGFs*) I and II, relaxin, and certain invertebrate peptides. The genes of these neuropeptides may have evolved from a common ancestral insulin gene more than 550 million years ago as the peptides have similar primary and tertiary structures and all are involved in growth regulation and metabolism. IGFs were discussed in chapter 13, section 13.5.2.3, together with growth hormone.

17.1.2 Structure of Insulin

The insulin molecule consists of two polypeptide chains, A and B. The A chain of 21 amino acids is linked to the B chain containing 30 amino acids by two disulfide bridges. These connect A7 to B7, and A20 to B19; a third disulfide bridge connects positions 6 and 11 in the A chain (figure 17.1). In 1972 the three-dimensional structure of insulin was clarified through the use of x-ray crystallography, showing insulin to be a compact, globular polypeptide (Blundell et al., 1972). Insulin circulates mainly as a monomer, with a molecular weight of 6000, but two monomers may aggregate to form a dimer, or three dimers may aggregate in the presence of two zinc atoms to form a hexamer. In the monomer, the residues at the C-terminal portion (see below) of the B chain (Gly^{23}-Phe^{24},Phe^{25}) are exposed at the surface to form a configuration that is essential to biological activity.

17.1.3 Insulin Gene Expression, Precursor Processing, and Regulation of Release

In most species, the insulin gene exists as a single copy, except in the rat and mouse which have two nonallelic and functional insulin genes. In the human,

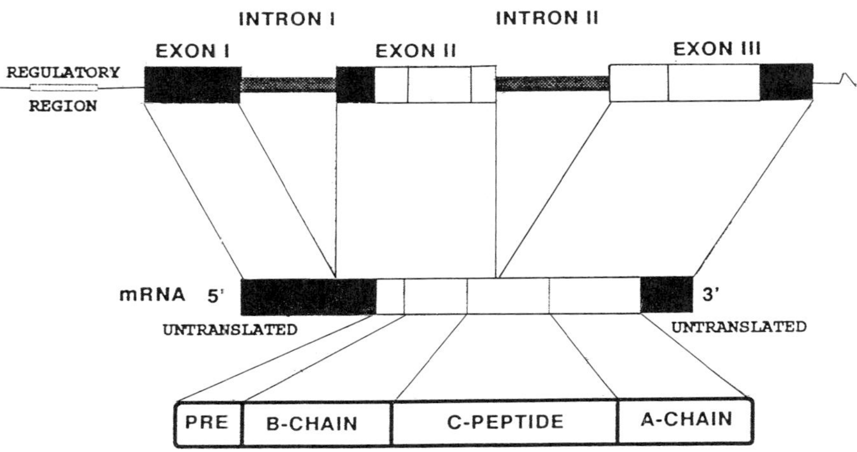

Figure 17.2
The preproinsulin gene and mRNA. The gene is shown above the fully spliced mRNA below. Regions of the mRNA encoding the different parts of the preproinsulin molecule are as indicated beneath the mRNA. (From Schoelson and Halban, 1994.)

the insulin gene is located on the short arm of chromosome 11 and it consists of three exons and two introns (figure 17.2). The first exon is highly conserved and is present in all mammalian insulin genes sequenced. The second exon is found in all sequenced genes, except the mouse and rat, and is much more variable in length than exon 1.

Expression of the insulin gene and the biosynthesis of insulin are remarkably tissue-specific, being restricted to the beta cells of the pancreatic islets, perhaps to the fetal liver, and some insulin-related material in the brain (LeRoith et al., 1983). The beta cells form a central core within the islets of Langerhans, mainly in the dorsal lobe of the pancreas. They are larger and more polyhedral in shape than the alpha cells, and contain a rich population of neuropeptide-containing secretory granules, in addition to insulin. Other islet cells also get insulin-rich blood from an internal portal system so that autocrine, paracrine, and local circulation interactions between insulin, somatostatin, and glucagon balance plasma glucose levels within a finely delimited range.

Preproinsulin is processed, by removal of the signal peptide, to *proinsulin*, which forms a continuous chain from the N-terminal region of the B chain to the C-terminal portion of the A chain. A connecting peptide, the C peptide, links the C-terminus of the B chain to the N-terminus of the A chain (figure 17.3). The secretory pathway for insulin biosynthesis, as revealed by Orci (1988), has formed the basis for our present understanding of universal peptide synthesis and intracellular trafficking (see chapter 3). Proinsulin, which is never glycosylated, is transported from the *cis*-cisternae of the Golgi apparatus to the *trans*-cisternae where the immature secretory granules are covered with a clathrin coat. It is within these immature granules of the beta cell that the final conversion of proinsulin to insulin occurs. In addition to insulin, proinsulin conversion yields the C peptide and two pairs of basic amino acids. Consequently,

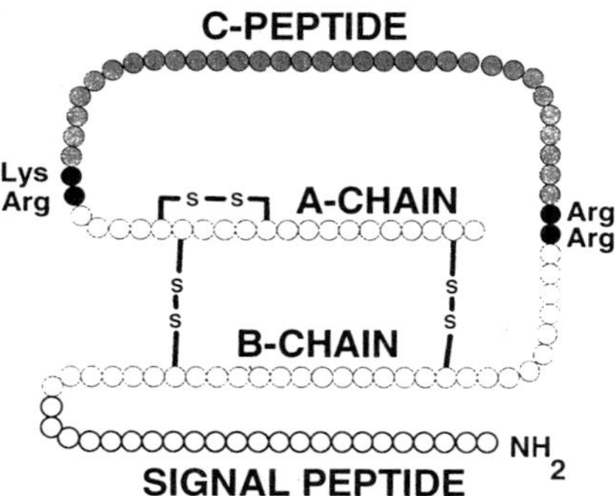

Figure 17.3
Preproinsulin. The initial high-molecular-weight precursor of insulin consists of four distinct domains. The signal peptide occupies the first 23 residues and is cleaved off within the lumen of the rough endoplasmic reticulum to produce proinsulin. Conversion of proinsulin to insulin arises at the pair of basic residues linking the two insulin (A and B) chains to the C (connecting) peptide. (From Schoelson and Halban, 1994.)

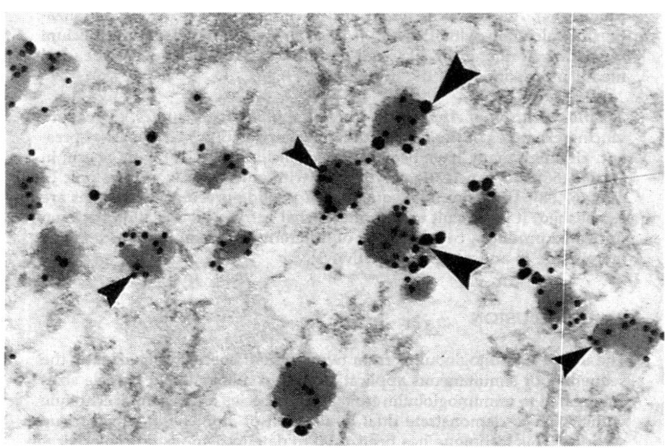

Figure 17.4
Coexistence of C peptide and insulin in pancreatic beta cell granules immunostained to show antigenic sites. C-peptide (40-nm gold, large arrowheads) and insulin (20-nm gold, small arrowheads) are co-localized in some secretory granules. (From Varndell and Polak, 1984.)

both the C peptide and insulin coexist in many of these granules (figure 17.4). The C peptide is released into the circulation in amounts equimolar to those of insulin, and it has recently been shown to have important biological effects, restoring impaired nerve conduction, vascular permeability, and Na^+, K^+-ATPase values in the diabetic rat and human to normal (Ido et al., 1997).

Glucose is certainly the most important *regulator* of insulin secretion, acting at both the transcriptional and post-transcriptional levels, but there are many factors that increase insulin secretion and release. These can be divided into the *initiators* and the *potentiators* (Henquin, 1994). The initiators increase insulin secretion in the absence of any other stimulus and include D-glucose, D-glyceraldehyde, D-mannose, L-leucine, D-fructose, certain amino acids, fatty acids, and certain pharmacologic agents. Figure 17.5 illustrates the changes in electrical activity of a beta cell that result from administration of increasing concentrations of glucose. The depolarizing action of glucose on beta cells activates channels that generate Ca^{2+}-dependent action potentials. This results in Ca^{2+} influx and the release of insulin by Ca^{2+}-regulated exocytosis. The proper functioning of these voltage-dependent Ca^{2+} channels is dependent on ATP-sensitive K^+ channels, which act as "metabolic sensors" and close as a consequence of glucose metabolism, depolarizing the cell membrane and permitting the activation of the Ca^{2+} channels. A rare neonatal disorder that is characterized by uncontrolled hypersecretion of insulin is associated with the absence of functional ATP-sensitive K^+ channels (Dunne et al., 1997).

The potentiators can increase insulin secretion only in the presence of an initiator, especially glucose. Potentiators include glucagon, CCK, gastric inhibitory peptide (GIP), and glucagon-like peptide-1 (GLP-1),

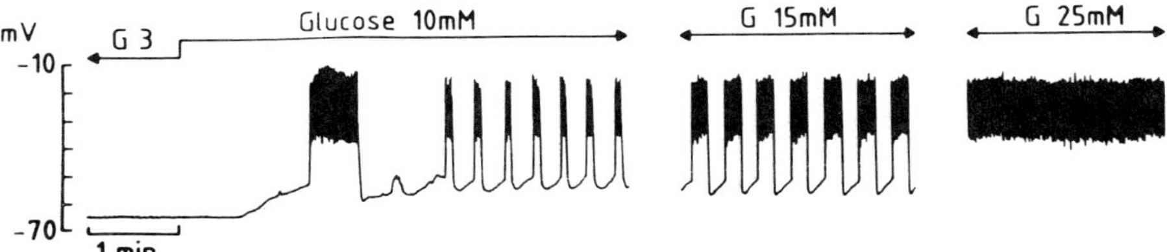

Figure 17.5
Changes in the membrane potential of a mouse beta cell induced by successive increases in glucose concentration in the perfusion medium. The three recordings were obtained in the same cell with an intracellular electrode. (From Henquin, 1994.)

all gastrointestinal, neuropeptides that are released from intestinal endocrine cells after a meal. Other neuropeptides that have weakly stimulatory effects on insulin secretion include gastrin, secretin, VIP, gastrin-releasing peptide (GRP), VP, and OT. Galanin and somatostatin are inhibitors of insulin secretion. CGRP and opiate peptides also decrease insulin secretion, but their physiological role is unclear.

The pancreatic islets are innervated by both cholinergic and sympathetic neurons and insulin secretion is stimulated by ACh but inhibited by α-adrenergic input. It is not certain whether these neurotransmitters act directly on beta cells or whether they affect intrinsic pancreatic peptidergic nerves that subsequently modulate insulin release. Interestingly, both parasympathetic and sympathetic stimulation increase glucagon secretion and suppress somatostatin secretion (Kurose et al., 1990). There is a negative feedback between somatostatin and insulin. Insulin deficiency induces hypersecretion of somatostatin, and long-term treatment with somatostatin results in a mild hyperglycemia.

The secretion of insulin is pulsatile, occurring every 1.5 to 2.0 hours in the basal state but amplified by a meal, especially after breakfast. Insulin secretion is reduced in persons who exercise regularly, but their glucose tolerance is normal, indicating that insulin sensitivity is improved by exercise (O'Meara and Polonsky, 1994).

Glucose fails to stimulate the beta cells of persons with insulin-dependent diabetes mellitus (IDDM or type I diabetes), who are insulin-deficient. In patients with non–insulin-dependent diabetes (NIDDM or type II), there is often an increased secretion of insulin, which is nevertheless inadequate for the circulating glucose levels, in some cases due to insulin resistance based on receptor or glucose transport protein defects.

Whether insulin is expressed in the brain or whether the immunoreactive insulin present in the brain is really only insulin bound to receptors is uncertain. Insulin mRNA has been reported in neonatal brain and in brain neurons in culture. Insulin in the CSF and brain may be the result both of local synthesis in the CNS, and uptake from the peripheral blood through the BBB. Most evidence points to the conclusion that insulin in the adult brain is predominantly of pancreatic origin, entering the brain across the BBB (Schwartz et al., 1992), possibly mediated by a specific transport system coupled to insulin receptors in cerebral microvessels and circumventricular organs (Plata-Salaman, 1991).

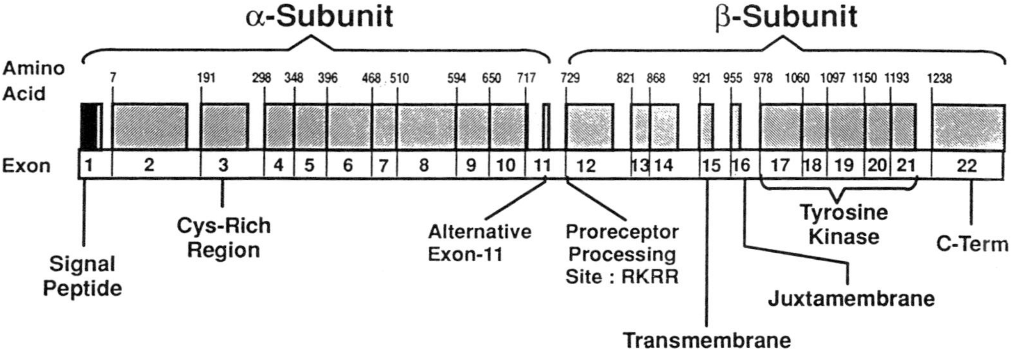

Figure 17.6
The exon structure of the insulin receptor gene. The first amino acid encoded by each exon is indicated (R, arginine; K, lysine). The approximate location of important structural features is also displayed. (From White and Kahn, 1994.)

17.1.4 Insulin Receptors and Second Messengers

The *insulin receptor gene* is located on the short arm of chromosome 19 and is more than 150 kb in length, containing 22 exons (figure 17.6). Exon I encodes the signal peptide. Exons 2 to 10 encode the α subunit. Exons 12 to 22 encode the β subunit. Exon 11 undergoes alternative slicing to yield two distinct mRNA species that encode α subunits with different C-terminal tails (Seino and Bell, 1989), which may explain some of the heterogeneity of insulin binding. A portion of the β subunit region of the gene incorporates the tyrosine kinase section, resulting in the classification of the insulin receptor as one of the tyrosine kinase receptors for many growth factors. The *insulin-like growth factor-I (IGF-I) receptor,* which is encoded by exon III of the insulin receptor gene, is closely related to the insulin receptor, as shown in figure 6.12. However, the insulin receptor is mainly involved in regulating metabolism, whereas the IGF-I receptor is implicated in regulating growth and development.

The *insulin receptor* is a protein kinase located on the cell surface and the kinase activity is essential to tyrosine residues in its acceptor substrate. Kinase activity is dependent upon divalent cations (Mg^{2+} and Mn^{2+}). The human insulin receptor is a heterodimer consisting of two α subunits (135 kD) and two β subunits (95 kD), joined by disulfide bonds to form a β-α-α-β heterotetramer (see chapter 6, section 6.5, and figure 6.12). The two α subunits, positioned entirely outside the cell, are linked by disulfide bonds and contain the insulin binding site(s). The β subunit is the transmembrane portion that contains the insulin-regulated tyrosine protein kinase activity. Both subunits are glycosylated.

Insulin receptors are widely *expressed* in almost all tissues in all species studied (LeRoith et al., 1983), being especially concentrated in liver, skeletal muscle, and adipose tissue, an expected finding in view of the pleiotropic effects of the peptide. CNS insulin receptors are present in highest concentration in the olfactory bulb, followed in decreasing order of concentration by cerebral cortex, hippocampus, hypothalamus, amygdala, and septum. Many other brain regions contain lesser amounts of the receptor. Insulin levels and insulin receptor numbers in the brain are independent of peripheral insulin levels (Havrankova et al., 1979), unlike the peripheral insulin receptors which are downregulated by elevated insulin levels and upregulated by a decrease in insulin.

The insulin receptor has remarkable homologies with the structure and function of oncoproteins of the *Src* family and insulin can induce changes in the expression of proto-oncogenes in certain cell lines, but the functional significance of this altered expression is unclear.

Activation of the insulin receptor occurs when insulin binds to the α subunit, and is greatly enhanced by insulin-stimulated autophosphorylation of the β subunit (Wilden et al., 1992). The phosphorylated β unit becomes an activated tyrosine kinase. Phosphorylation, in turn, allows binding of other proteins that have SH2 domains to regulate the associated catalytic activities that mediate the insulin response (White and Kahn, 1994). Many insulin actions are propagated through a series of protein phosphorylations and dephosphorylations of serine residues of proteins. The receptor also has an important ATP binding site.

Surprisingly, the second-messenger system by which insulin elicits its many responses is not known for certain. Logically, the intrinsic tyrosine kinase activity of the insulin receptor should be the preferred pathway, but several other pathways have been proposed, including Ca^{2+}, since insulin stimulates phosphorylation of calmodulin, which in turn appears to be linked to insulin binding and insulin receptor phosphorylation, and may be part of the receptor itself (Graves et al., 1986).

Internalization of the insulin receptor occurs by receptor-mediated endocytosis (see chapter 3), stimulated by the binding of insulin. Subsequently the insulin molecule dissociates from the receptor and is degraded while the receptor itself is dephosphorylated, which inactivates its catalytic activity (Backer et al. 1989). Internalized insulin receptors may be recycled back to the cell surface or they may be degraded by lysosomes.

17.1.5 Actions of Insulin

The primary action of insulin is to regulate glucose homeostasis. Active transport of glucose in the intestine and in the proximal convoluted tubules of the kidney requires Na^+-coupled glucose co-transporters, which use the energy supplied by the Na^+ gradient to move glucose against its concentration gradient, either into the cells of the intestinal mucosa, or out of the lumen of the renal tubule back into the peritubular efferent arterioles. These transporters do not appear to be affected by insulin or altered in diabetes. However, insulin stimulates the synthesis of the facultative, passive glucose transporters, especially GLUT4, large glycoproteins with 12 membrane-spanning regions, and translocation into the cell membrane. Consequently, a chronic effect of insulin lack is a decreased response of the transport system, resulting in high levels of blood glucose that cannot be utilized by the cells. The mechanism by which the activation of the insulin-receptor kinase is coupled to the translocation of the transporter is unknown (White and Kahn, 1994).

Muscle, liver, and fat are the principal targets for insulin disposal of glucose, first increasing transport into cells, then activating the enzymes involved in intracellular utilization of glucose, amino acids, and fatty acids. Simultaneously, insulin inhibits gluconeogenesis and the catabolic processes leading to the breakdown of glycogen, fat, and protein. These are immediate effects of insulin, occurring within seconds or minutes after insulin stimulation.

White and Kahn (1994) cite several enzyme systems that are more slowly activated or inhibited by insulin, since they involve action on gene transcription. These long-term effects may take hours or days and include insulin stimulation of DNA synthesis, cell proliferation, and cell differentiation, processes that may require the combined action of insulin and IGF-1.

Central effects of insulin can be seen in the hyperphagia resulting from the administration of insulin to obese type II diabetic patients. In baboons, however, central administration of insulin reduces food intake (Woods and Porte, 1983). The hypothalamic-hypophyseal axis is implicated in the reduced ACTH-cortisol responses during hypoglycemia in IDDM patients (Kinsley and Simonson, 1996) and the HPA axis is chronically stimulated in the NIDDM rat (Tojo et al., 1996).

17.1.6 Clinical Implications of Insulin

The tremendous importance of insulin in the treatment of type I diabetes is well-known. Many drugs affect insulin secretion and insulin action. These include α- and β-adrenergic antagonists, clonidine, benzodiazepines, and opiates, and this interaction should be taken into consideration when these drugs are administered to persons with diabetes. A judicious combination of insulin and C peptide may improve the therapy of diabetes in unexpected ways.

Mutations that occur in the insulin gene can be associated with several pathological conditions. Point mutations that prevent the proper processing of proinsulin to insulin result in familial hyperproinsulinemia, inherited as an autosomal dominant phenotype; the affected individuals are not diabetic. Mutations in the insulin receptor gene account for only a small proportion of cases of NIDDM. Three different mutations within the A or B chains decrease insulin binding to its receptors and may be the cause of some cases of type II diabetes. Hyperinsulinism is often associated with obesity, and may be due to a reduction in the number of insulin receptors.

Insulin is essential to the growth of most types of tumor cells and malignant cells require less insulin than normal cells for their growth in culture. Many human tumors produce insulin which may then act as an autocrine factor favoring their proliferation.

Autonomic and peripheral *neuropathies* are commonly associated with diabetes mellitus and in rodent models there are deficits in nerve growth factor (NGF) and its high-affinity receptor, trkA. This leads to a decreased retrograde axonal transport of NGF and decreased support of NGF-dependent sensory neurons, with reduced expression of their neuropeptides, SP and CGRP. Treatment of diabetic rats with NGF normalizes these defects. The ameliorative action of Org 2766, the ACTH 4–9 analog, on sensorimotor and autonomic neuropathy in streptozocin-induced diabetes mellitus in rats (Kappelle et al., 1994), and its improvement of the vibration threshold in diabetic humans (Bravenboer et al., 1994), suggests a possible therapeutic use for Org 2766 in peripheral neuropathies (see chapter 12). NGF and insulin have also been considered as therapy for diabetic patients with peripheral neuropathy (Tomlinson et al., 1996) and a similar function for IGF is indicated (Zhuang et al., 1996).

Impairment of cognitive functions is associated with IDDM in children, with those children developing IDDM before 5 years of age being the most affected. This may be due to the disruptive effect of chronic hyperglycemia on myelinization (Northam et al., 1995). In adults with NIDDM, decreased visual cognitive function is associated with the autonomic neuropathy.

The method of insulin administration is not perfect: oral administration is not feasible as the peptide is destroyed in the gastrointestinal tract and several daily injections require frequent self-monitoring of glucose levels. Implantable minipumps are under investigation, as are implantable grafts of pancreatic islets and pancreas transplants. Diet and exercise are important elements in the treatment of diabetes.

17.1.7 *Relaxin*

The primary structures of insulin and relaxin are similar, both containing A and B chains with similarly placed disulfide bonds. The peptides probably arose from gene duplication, although there is only about 40% homology between them. A relaxin-like peptide is found in shark ovaries that resembles mammalian insulin more than mammalian relaxin, and which, like relaxin, relaxes the pubic symphysis in mammals. What it does in the shark is unknown.

The effects of relaxin on the mammalian reproductive system are the best understood. In mammals relaxin is produced by the corpus luteum, and in primates relaxin is also found in the endometrium and placenta. Plasma levels of relaxin increase greatly during pregnancy and drop just before parturition. The increase in relaxin is correlated with increased cervical dilation and the transformation of the cartilaginous tissue of the pubic symphysis to a more flexible structure. Relaxin acts on the estrogen-primed uterus to inhibit myometrial contractions, and as relaxin levels decline at the end of gestation, the relaxing effect on uterine contractions is removed. Relaxin may have further helpful effects in pregnancy and parturition: collagen degradation in fetal membranes to assist in their rupture, synergistic action with GH in stimulating mammary gland growth, and increased blood flow to the fetus. Relaxin probably uses the adenylate cyclase, cAMP intracellular messenger pathway.

However, the central effects of relaxin have now been clearly demonstrated. Relaxin receptors are found not only in the uterus and cervix but also in discrete regions of the olfactory system, neocortex, hippocampus, thalamus, amygdala, midbrain, and medulla of the male and female rat brain. In addition, relaxin binds to the subfornical organ, the paraventricular (PVN) and supraoptic nuclei (SON) (Osheroff and Phillips, 1991). These anatomical findings support the observations that exogenous relaxin causes the release of OT and VP, which can be correlated with increased firing of SON neurons, increased water consumption (Way and Leng, 1992), and involvement of the central angiotensin II system (Geddes et al., 1994). The subfornical organ may also be involved in the pressor effects of relaxin and in central mediation of the events that lead to delivery in the rat (Summerlee and Wilson, 1994). What is not clear is whether endogenous relaxin has any significant physiological role in males and nonpregnant females.

17.2 Galanin

Galanin appears to be a phylogenetically old peptide as it is also present in submammalian species and in invertebrates. Galanin was first isolated from porcine intestine and subsequently found to be widely distributed throughout the gastrointestinal tract, where it may be colocalized with VIP in the ileum. Galanin is present in many other organ systems, including the respiratory tract, pancreas, liver, urogenital tract, adrenal gland, thyroid, heart, visual tract, and oral region. Like NPY, galanin is densely concentrated in the brain, especially in the hypothalamus where it is colocalized with GnRH. (Merchenthaler et al., 1993) Galanin is also found in peripheral nerves innervating skin and muscles. Galanin was named on the basis of its N-terminal glycine and C-terminal alanine residues (Tatemoto et al.,1983).

This widespread distribution is reflected in the many functions now attributed to galanin, affecting almost all central and peripheral systems, including motility and secretion in the gastrointestinal tract, inhibition of insulin secretion, release of GH and PRL, modulation of the HPA axis, regulation of body weight, and modulation of nociceptive stimuli.

17.2.1 Structure of Galanin

Galanin is a 29–amino acid residue peptide (30 in humans). The N-terminal region, consisting of residues 1–15, is fully conserved in all species studied, whereas the C-terminal half is more variable and is probably responsible for species-specific variations. It does not belong to any known neuropeptide family.

Pig galanin has the following structure:

Gly^{1}-Trp-Thr-Leu-Asn-Ser-Ala-Gly-Tyr-Leu-Leu-

Gly-Pro-His-Ala^{15}- Ile^{16}-Asp^{17} -Asn-His-Arg-Ser-
Val^{16}-Gly^{17}

Phe-His^{23}-Asp-Lys-Tyr^{26}-Gly-Leu-Ala^{29}-NH_2
Ser^{23} *Asn*^{26} *Thr*^{29} *Ser*^{30}-NH_2

Human galanin differs from pig galanin in positions 16, 17, 23, 26, and 29, as indicated by the residues shown in italic beneath those of the porcine galanin. Only human galanin has an additional amino acid, Ser, in position 30.

17.2.2 Galanin Gene Expression, Precursor Processing, and Regulation of Release

Galanin is encoded by a single gene, but its structure has not yet been described in detail. The galanin gene consists of six exons. The first exon encodes the untranslated part of galanin mRNA, exon 2 encodes a leader sequence rich in hydrophobic residues, exon 3 encodes most of the N-terminal conserved part, and exons 4 to 6 encode the variable C-terminal part of galanin, another peptide of unknown function and the 3′-untranslated region of the mature mRNA (Kaplan et al., 1991; Strauss and Kaplan, 1991).

The mature galanin mRNA has been cloned and is approximately 0.85 to 0.95 kb in size. It encodes a 123– or 124–amino acid precursor, *preprogalanin*. Different species-specific forms of galanin are produced during processing, some of which are shortened by removal of the C-terminal (galanin 1–19) or N-terminal (galanin 5–29). There are also tissue-specific sex differences (Gabriel at al., 1989) that appear during puberty in the anterior pituitary, intermediate lobe, and median eminence that result in higher levels of galanin in females (figure 17.7). Galanin mRNA levels are increased in GnRH neurons during the gonadotropin surge of the estrous cycle, suggesting a tight coupling of galanin biosynthesis and release to the state of activity of GnRH neurons (Rossmanith et al., 1996). Galanin mRNA in the CNS is upregulated by interference with neuronal activity such as nerve crush, nerve section, or drugs (Hökfelt et al., 1987).

Expression of the galanin gene corresponds well with the distribution of galanin throughout the peripheral and central nervous systems and the organ systems listed above. However, there are some inconsistencies which may be due to differences in the methods used to localize the message (Rökaeus, 1994). The galanin pathway is through neurons in the medial preoptic area and PVN which project locally and to the median eminence. Galanin expression and synthesis in these areas is influenced by fat intake, estrogens, thyroxine, and glucocorticoids.

Galanin release in the gastrointestinal tract is precipitated by distention of the gut or the presence of

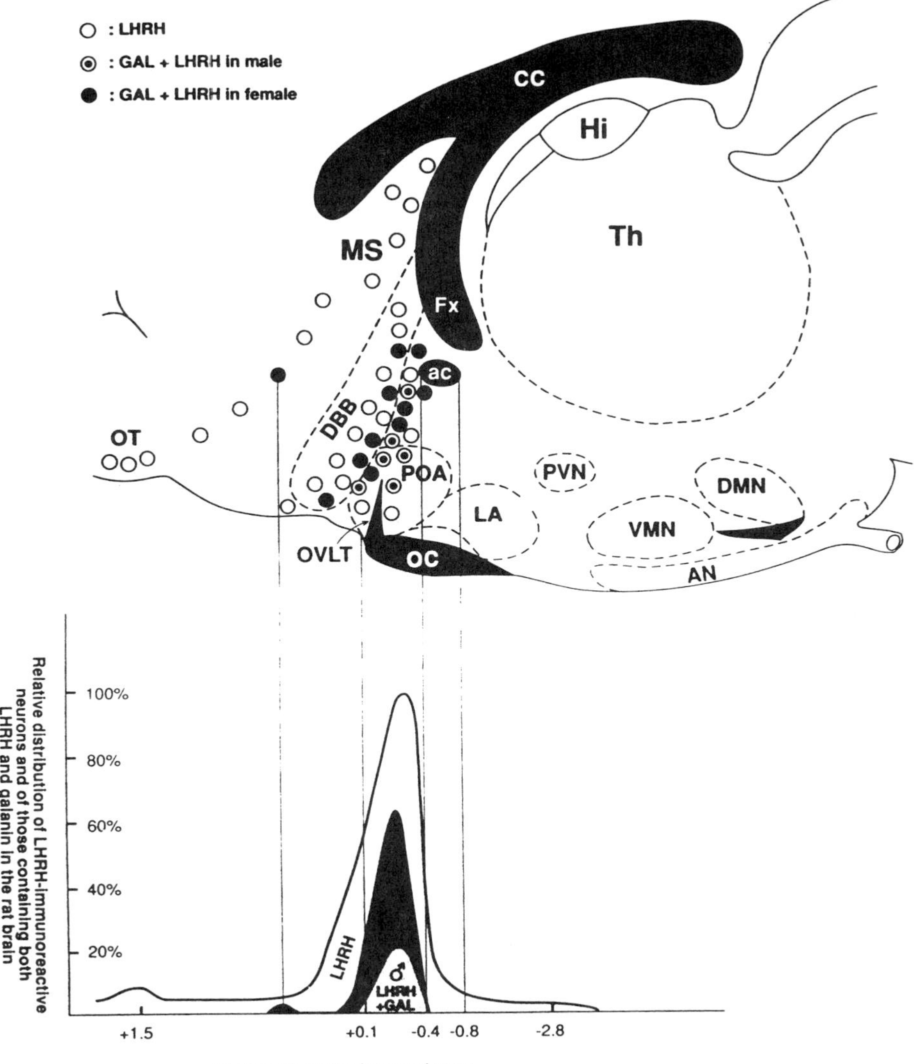

Figure 17.7
Schematic representation of the incidence of neurons co-localizing galanin (GAL) and luteinizing hormone–releasing hormone (LHRH) in the female and male rat brain. The upper panel is a diagrammatic sagittal section of the rat brain, indicating regions containing LHRH perikarya expressing GAL. The majority of these neurons are located in the transition between the (DBB) and preoptic area (POA) at the level of the organum vasculosum of the lamina terminalis (OVLT). Note that in the female rat, scattered cells co-expressing GAL and LHRH are seen in the anterior paraolfactory area, just anterior to the DBB. The lower panel indicates the relative distribution of LHRH-immunoreactive neurons and those containing both LHRH and GAL in female and male rat brains. Note the higher degree of colocalization of these neuropeptides in female rats. ac, anterior commissure; AN, arcuate nucleus; CC, corpus callosum; DMN, dorsomedial nucleus; Fx, fornix; Hi, hippocampus; LA, lateral hypothalamus; MS, medial septum; OC, optic chiasm; PVN, paraventricular nucleus; Th, thalamus; VMN, ventromedial nucleus. (From Merchenthaler et al., 1991.)

bile, amino acids, acid, and hypertonic saline or glucose. Sympathetic nerve stimulation may cause some release of galanin from the intestine, liver, and adrenal gland. Galanin released from pituitary cells is secreted in a pulsatile manner into the median eminence and thence into the portal blood, which contains about 30% of the total level of galanin in peripheral serum (López et al., 1991).

17.2.3 Galanin Receptors and Second Messengers

The galanin receptor from brain and pancreatic beta or alpha cells is approximately 53 and 54 kD. There are differences in receptor structure depending on the species and tissue, and several putative tissue-specific receptor subtypes have been proposed. The receptor isolated from insulin-secreting cells and from the brain is specific for the N-terminal, species-conserved part of the galanin molecule, but the rest of the molecule is needed for full binding properties (Lagny-Pourmire et al., 1989). In the rat gastrointestinal tract and the sphincter of the iris of the eye, the binding sites on smooth muscle are C-terminal–dependent, but the N-terminal region is needed for full binding efficiency. The second-messenger system appears to be a pertussis toxin–sensitive GTP binding protein acting through adenylate cyclase and cAMP to reduce the intracellular Ca^{2+} concentration. Newly developed synthetic peptide-type galanin receptor antagonists are helping to elucidate the function of galanin in many systems, as well as distinguishing putative subtypes of galanin receptors.

17.2.4 Actions of Galanin

17.2.4.1 Peripheral Effects

In the gastrointestinal tract galanin increases salivation, inhibits gastric acid secretion and pancreatic and intestinal secretion, and in humans suppresses the postprandial rise in glucose and many gastrointestinal peptides. The motility of the gastrointestinal tract is affected by galanin but there are considerable differences among species as to the response, which also varies according to the region of the intestine. Galanin may produce excitatory effects on certain gut smooth muscle and inhibitory effects on others. Some of the actions are dependent upon the C-terminal part of galanin, others on the N-terminal portion, but the whole molecule is needed for full biological activity. These different responses are summarized by Rökaeus (1994). In the human, the overall action of administered galanin is delayed contractility and increased transit time through the gastrointestinal tract (Bauer et al., 1989).

Galanin causes hyperglycemia in most mammalian species due to its inhibitory action on insulin secretion. Galanin also is a potent inhibitor of somatostatin. However, although in vitro studies show galanin to inhibit insulin secretion in human pancreatic tissues, it has no effect in humans in vivo. Conflicting results also are reported for the pig, in which galanin has been shown to either stimulate or inhibit insulin secretion (Messell et al., 1990; Hermansen et al, 1989).

17.2.4.2 Central Effects

The central endocrine effects of galanin are mainly inhibitory: following administration into the PVN galanin decreases pituitary secretion of ACTH and thus blood levels of corticosterone. I.c.v. injections of galanin inhibit VP release and impair cognitive performance. Galanin may act as an essential autocrine regulator of GnRH neurons since it may be coreleased with GnRH and act presynaptically on GnRH neurons, potentiating GnRH-induced secretion of LH (figure 17.8). In this manner galanin may coordinate GnRH release in its distinctive pulsatile

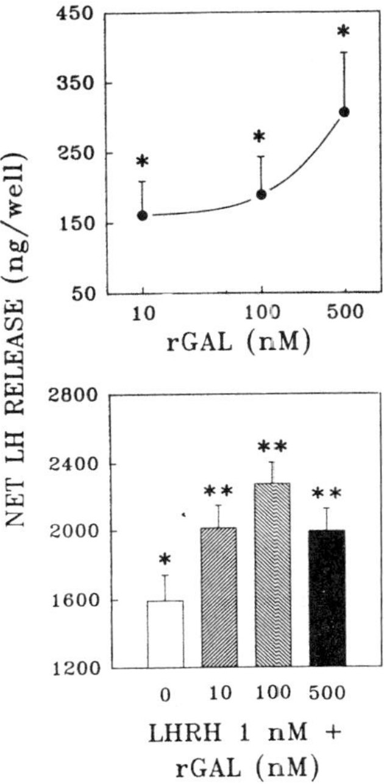

Figure 17.8
Above, Galanin (GAL) stimulates luteinizing hormone (LH) secretion and potentiates LH-releasing hormone (LHRH)–induced LH secretion from anterior pituitary cells in vitro. Below, Galanin potentiates the LHRH-induced LH release from dispersed pituitary cells. (From López et al. 1991.)

fashion (Rossmanith et al., 1996). In the absence of galanin, GnRH is released in a continuous manner, which is ineffective in evoking the LH surge (see chapter 10, figure 10.14). In the spinal cord galanin inhibits excitability and potentiates the analgesic effects of morphine (Bedecs et al., 1995).

Hypothalamic peptides control an animal's choice of nutrients (Leibowitz and Myers, 1987). Galanin influences food intake in a manner distinctly different from that of NPY, since galanin acts preferentially on the ingestion of fat and reduces energy expenditure, thus increasing fat deposition. Galanin levels rise during the mid to late hours of the active feeding cycle. This is in contrast to the pattern of NPY release which increases carbohydrate appetite at the start of the active feeding period (see chapter 16). Galanin also is increased during development and puberty, at which time fat appetite is sharply increased and carbohydrate intake declines. At puberty, there is a positive feedback loop between galanin in the medial preoptic area and the PVN, and estradiol, linking nutrient balance and reproduction (Leibowitz, 1994).

Feeding behavior requires complex integration between neuroendocrine pathways, sensory inputs, and motor outputs. The suggested mechanism by which galanin induces preferential fat intake is through galanin release of DA. Injection of galanin into the PVN increases the release of DA into the nucleus accumbens, which reinforces feeding behavior, in this case preferential fat intake (Hoebel et al., 1994).

17.2.5 Clinical Implications of Galanin

The role of galanin and NPY and their receptors in normal and abnormal feeding patterns is being elucidated through the use of peptide receptor antagonists, antisera, and antisense oligodeoxynucleotides. These techniques permit the correlation of altered peptide levels in specific brain areas with resulting behavioral and hormonal changes (Sabol and Higuchi, 1990). It is feasible that these techniques will lead to a better understanding of the complex interaction of neural and hormonal control of aberrant eating patterns such as anorexia, bulimia, and pathological obesity.

17.3 Motilin

Motilin was discovered by John Brown in 1967, and its sequence published a few years later (Brown et al., 1973). Brown named it *motilin* because it increased motility in stomach pouches. Interestingly, in 1903, Enriques and Hallion suggested motilin as a hypothetical humoral agent that stimulated intestinal peristalsis. It was, then forgotten, rediscovered, and sequenced by Brown more than 60 years later. Motilin is another of the gut-brain peptides found in the endocrine cells of the gut and in central neurons.

17.3.1 Structure of Motilin

Motilin is a 22–amino acid peptide, folded into an α helix from Glu^9 to Lys^{20}, with a wide turn in the N-terminal part over the first six residues (Edmondson et al., 1990). Porcine and human motilin are identical.

Phe-Val-Pro-Ile-Phe-Thr-Tyr^7-Gly^8-Glu-Leu-
His^7-Ser^8

Gln-Arg^{12}-Met^{13}-Gln^{14}-Glu-Lys-Glu-Arg-Asn-
Lys^{12}-Ile^{13}-Arg^{14}

Lys^{20}-Gly-Gln^{22}OH

There is considerable heterogeneity in motilin structure in mammalian species. Canine intestinal motilin differs in positions 7, 8, 12, 13, and 14, as shown in italic by the residues beneath those of human and porcine motilin. Rat motilin structure seems to differ from other mammalian motilin and has a different contractile effect on duodenal muscle fibers. The N-terminal amino acid sequence 1–10 is essential to the contractile characteristics of motilin (Poitras et al. 1992; Peeters et al, 1992).

17.3.2 Motilin Gene Expression, Precursor Processing, and Regulation of Release

The structure of the motilin gene is unusual in that the bioactive peptide is encoded by two distinct exons, exons 2 and 3. The human motilin gene is mapped to chromosome 6 and consists of five exons separated by four introns spanning about 9 kb of genomic DNA (Daikh et al., 1989; Yano et al., 1989).

Human *prepromotilin* is composed of a 25–amino acid signal peptide, followed by *promotilin* 1–89. The 22–amino acid bioactive molecule, *motilin*, is followed by a 65–amino acid sequence of no known function (Poitras, 1994). As only one mRNA species has been identified, the multiple forms of motilin found must result from post-translational processing of the single motilin precursor.

Motilin mRNA is present in the gut of many animal species, with maximal concentrations in the duodenum, predominantly in the lower portion of the intestinal crypts (Daikh et al., 1989; Yano et al., 1989). The presence of motilin in the mammalian brain remains highly controversial, although there is clear evidence that peripherally administered motilin can evoke CNS responses.

The basal *release* of motilin in the fasting dog is cyclic, with peaks in plasma motilin concentrations occurring every 80 to 120 minutes, synchronous with the initiation of phase III of the *migrating motor complex (MMC)*. The MMC refers to the contractile activity of four cycles in the stomach, duodenum, and jejumum in the interdigestive (fasting) state. Phase III is a group of strong contractions with maximal contractile force.

The MMC may act as the hypothetical "clock" regulating the activity of the motilin-secreting duodenal cell. However, this cyclic release is highly variable in individual animals and humans. In the dog, these cycles are barely influenced by food, but in the human the ingestion of fat is a potent stimulus to motilin release, and carbohydrates decrease motilin levels. Many factors, including several neuropeptides and muscarinic receptors, have been suggested as regulators of the clock regulating the cycle of motilin release, but species and individual variations have made definitive studies difficult.

17.3.3 Motilin Receptors

Motilin receptors are found in the antrum, duodenum, and colon of the rabbit, with the greatest density being in the distal colon (Depoorte et al., 1991). In the human, the greatest density of motilin receptors is in the antrum of the stomach and it decreases aborally through the gastrointestinal tract. There seem to be two types of motilin receptors, those that are located in the smooth muscle of stomach and intestine, as shown by in vitro muscle strips, and others that are neural, as shown by in vivo investigations. When motilin is administered intra-arterially to dogs, the stimulatory action is blocked by atropine or tetrodotoxin, indicating a neurogenic action of motilin activating a motilin receptor on intrinsic nerves. The mechanism involved appears to be muscarinic transmission and perhaps a nicotinic preganglionic synapse with a noncholinergic nerve (Poitras et al., 1990).

17.3.4 Actions of Motilin

The most important action of motilin is as a circulating hormone inducing *gastroduodenal contractions* that mimic phase III of the MMC (figure 17.9). The contractions last for 10 to 30 minutes and stop spontaneously even if motilin administration is continued. Exogenous motilin stimulates contraction of the lower esophageal sphincter, and in some species accelerates gastric emptying.

Synthetic motilin agonists, such as 13-Nle-motilin, weakly stimulate *pancreatic secretion*, induce strong tonic contractions of the gallbladder, and increase the contractility of the colon. Again, these observations are species-specific and neither pancreatic secretion nor gallbladder contractions are observed in humans following motilin administration.

Motilin acts as a *neuroregulator* despite its absence from neuronal cells. *Feeding behavior* is affected by motilin: it stimulates eating in fasted rats and inhibits eating in satiated rats (Olsen et al., 1980). Motilin has direct effects on *neuronal excitability*, depressing the firing of neurons in the lateral vestibular nucleus of rabbits (Chan-Palay et al., 1982), yet stimulating corticospinal neurons in the rat (Phillis and Kirkpatrick, 1980).

17.3.5 Clinical Implications of Motilin

Hypermotilinemia has been found in many clinical conditions, such as carcinoid tumors, irritable bowel syndrome, and Zollinger-Ellison syndrome, the last a complex of peptic ulcers, extreme gastric hyperacidity, and gastrin-secreting pancreatic tumors. However, none of the patients with these conditions had symptoms that could be associated with the increased motilin levels. Similarly, patients with low levels of motilin do not display any expected clinical symptoms such as delayed transit through the gastrointestinal tract and constipation. There is some association of elevated motilin levels in diabetic patients with autonomic abnormalities. The pathophysiological significance, therefore, of altered motilin levels remains obscure at this time.

17.4 Calcitonin-Gene–Related Peptide, Amylin, and Adrenomedullin

CGRP is a neuropeptide formed by the alternative splicing of the mRNA transcribed from the calcitonin gene and consequently named *calcitonin gene–related*

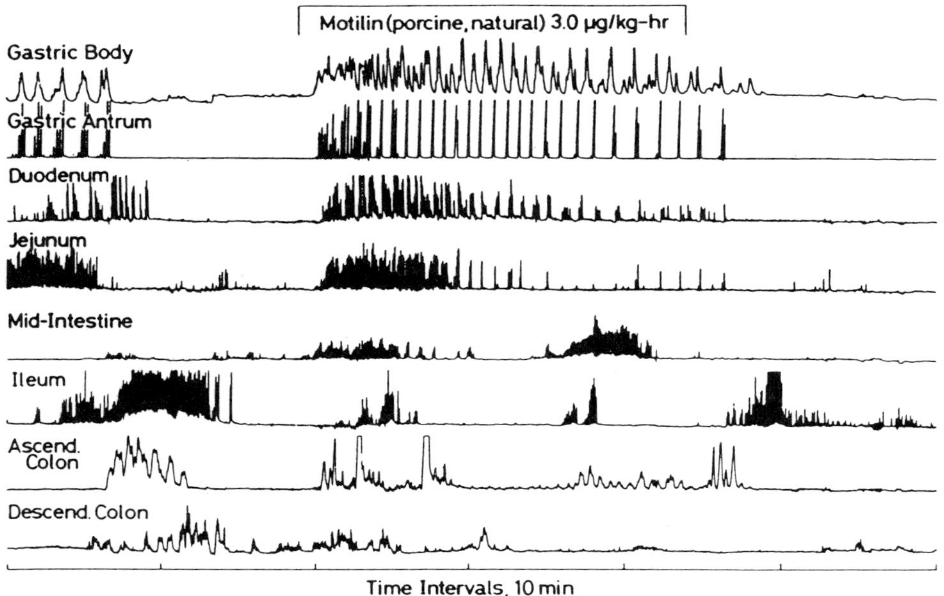

Figure 17.9
Effect of a large dose of motilin (3.0 μg/kg/hour) on gastric contractile activity in a dog. Soon after the initiation of IV infusion, strong contractions are evoked simultaneously in the stomach, duodenum, and upper small intestine. Colonic motor activity seems to be stimulated. Note that the frequency of contractions in the stomach is higher than the natural contractions. (From Itoh, 1990.)

peptide. In the thyroid C cells the primary RNA transcripts are processed to mRNA for calcitonin, whereas mRNA for CGRP is found mainly in the CNS and in autonomic nerves throughout the gastrointestinal tract. CGRP is a potent relaxant of smooth muscle, and affects blood flow, gastrointestinal secretion, and motility. CGRP also has central actions that affect food intake, gastric acid secretion, and the motor activity of the gastrointestinal tract. Calcitonin is discussed in detail in chapter 18. Other CGRP-related peptides are amylin and adrenomedullin. These two peptides, together with CGRP and calcitonin, contain two N-terminal cysteines that form a disulfide bridge resulting in an N-terminal loop, plus a C-terminal amide (Wimalawansa, 1996). All four peptides have been highly conserved and may have arisen from gene duplication.

17.4.1 *Structure of CGRP*

CGRP is a 37–amino acid polypeptide, with slight differences in sequence homology between different mammalian species and birds. All forms of CGRP, however, have a disulfide bridge between Cys^2 and Cys^7 and an amidated C-terminal Phe^{37}. There are two forms of CGRP, CGRP-I and CGRP-II (sometimes termed CGRP-α and -β) which differ slightly in amino acid composition.

Human CGRP I (CGRP-α) Ala-Cys^{2}-Asp^{3}-
Asn^{3}

Thr-Ala-Thr-Cys^{7}-Val-Thr-His^{10}-Arg-Leu-Ala-

Gly-Leu-Leu-Ser-Arg-Ser-Gly^{20}-Gly- Val^{22} -Val-
Met^{22}

Lys- Asn^{25} -Asn-Phe-Val-Pro-Thr^{30}-Asn-Val-Gly-
Ser^{25}

Ser-Lys-Ala-Phe^{37}-NH_2

Human CRGP II differs from CRGP I in positions 3, 22, and 25, as indicated by the amino acids in italic beneath those for CRGP I. Rat CGRP I differs from human CGRP I in positions 3, 25, and 35, and bovine CRGP I has five substitutions in the amino acid sequence.

17.4.2 CGRP Gene Expression, Precursor Processing, and Regulation of Release

The calcitonin gene encodes both calcitonin and CGRP. It contains genomic regions that represent the discrete hormone-encoding domains which will be expressed differently in thyroid and nervous tissue (figure 17.10). This is a tissue-specific process since in the thyroid C cells, the primary RNA transcripts are processed to yield calcitonin mRNA, and in neural tissue the primary product is mRNA for CGRP (Amara et al., 1982). In rat and in the human, there are two calcitonin genes, both of which encode CGRP I and CGRP II. Other mammalian species appear to have only one form of CGRP. In the human, the calcitonin gene is on the short arm of chromosome 11, near the insulin gene.

The calcitonin-CGRP gene comprises six exons. In the thyroid, the first four exons are spliced to form calcitonin mRNA, whereas in nervous tissue the first three exons are spliced to the fifth and sixth exons to generate CGRP-I (CGRP-α) mRNA. The second calcitonin-CGRP gene produces CGRP-II (CGRP-β) which is expressed in small amounts in both thyroid C cells and in brain. CGRP is expressed in sensory systems, including the olfactory and gustatory systems, in the hypothalamic and limbic areas, as well as in intrinsic and extrinsic neurons throughout the digestive system, indicating an integrative action of CGRP on food intake.

In the stomach, the CGRP I–containing nerve fibers are mostly axons from primary afferents that originate from dorsal root ganglia (figure 17.11), whereas in the intestine both spinal afferents and intrinsic enteric neurons supply CGRP II (Sternini and Anderson, 1992). CGRP usually coexists with SP in afferent nerve fibers, and CGRP is co-localized in enteric neurons with choline acetyltransferase, CCK, somatostatin, and NPY (Costa et al., 1986). The pancreas and mesenteric arteries are richly innervated by primary afferents containing CGRP.

CGRP is distributed in endocrine cells in the anterior pituitary (especially the gonadotrophs), adrenal medulla, and in thyroid C cells. The extensive CGRP innervation of most organs, especially around arteries and veins, explains its involvement with cardiovascular homeostasis.

CGRP was the first neuropeptide to be identified in both the cell bodies of *motor neurons* and their neuromuscular junctions in mammals, and the level of CGRP is upregulated during nerve injury and regeneration.

Release of CGRP is effected by stimulation of primary afferent nerve endings by capsaicin (see chapter 15) and by lowering stomach pH to 6 (Geppetti et al.,

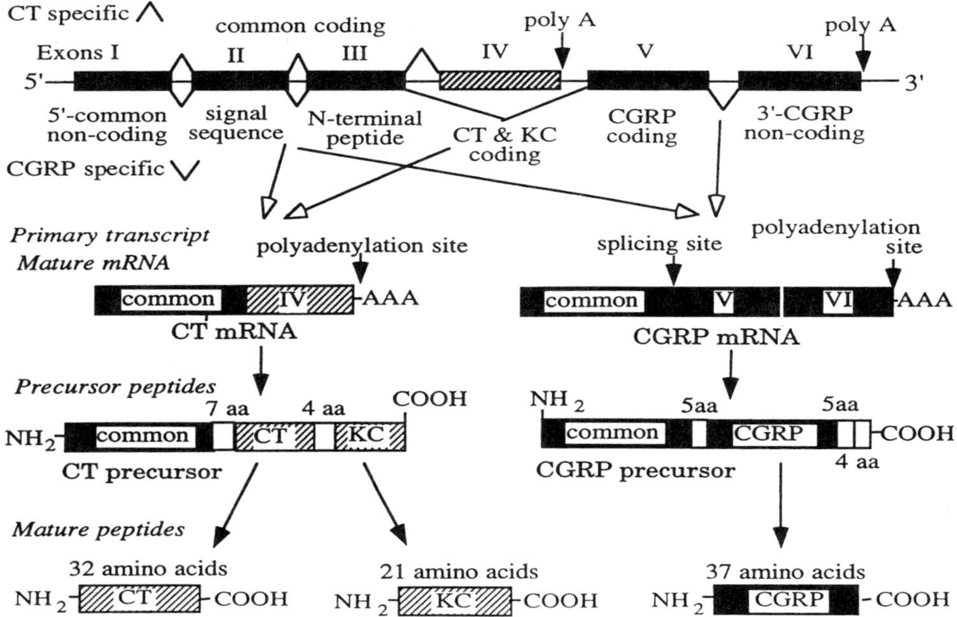

Figure 17.10
A schematic representation of the structural organization of the human calcitonin (CT) and calcitonin gene–related peptide (CGRP) gene. Two different mRNAs may be produced from the alternative processing of the single primary transcript and use of two polyadenylation sites: one coding for the CT precursor (crosshatched boxes) and the other coding for the CGRP precursor (black boxes). Post-translational modifications include intramolecular disulfide bridge formation at the N-terminal and amidation of the C-terminal residue. KC, katacalcin; (From Wimalawansa, 1996.)

1991). Colonic distention also releases CGRP from afferent nerve terminals in the inferior mesenteric ganglion. CGRP released from fibers around the mesenteric arteries and arterioles in the gastrointestinal tract is probably an important source of circulating CGRP. The CGRP antagonist CGRP 8–37 blocks the effects of CGRP released from these sources.

17.4.3 CGRP Receptors and Second Messengers

The common CGRP receptor has been cloned (Aiyar et al., 1996), has a molecular weight of about 66 kD, and consists of only one subunit (Wimalawansa, 1992, 1996). Several CGRP receptors have been identified and classified as $CGRP_1$ and $CGRP_2$ receptors, on the basis of their recognition of different CGRP antagonists (Dennis et al. 1990). One of the most important pharmacological tools for the study of CGRP receptors is the antagonist, CGRP 8–37, which is specific for $CGRP_2$. $CGRP_2$ receptors mediate the relaxant effects on intestinal smooth muscle and the inhibition of gastric acid secretion in the rat. $CGRP_2$ receptors mediate vasodilation but their effects vary according to the specific vascular bed (Bauerfeind et

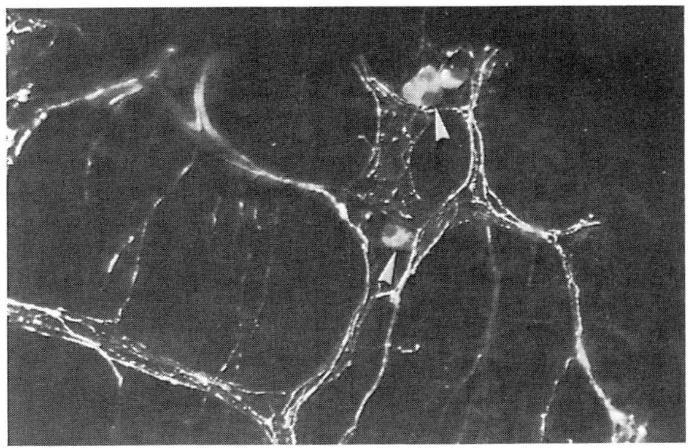

Figure 17.11
Fluorescence photomicrograph of muscle strip showing calcitonin gene-related peptide-immunoreactive cells in the myenteric ganglia (arrowheads) of the duodenum of a colchicine-treated rat. X200. (From Lee et al., 1987.)

al., 1989) and $CGRP_1$ receptors are the primary activators of vasodilation. In some tissues both CGRP I and CGRP II interact with the same receptor.

Calcitonin uses a different receptor from CGRP since the latter causes relaxation of smooth muscle, whereas calcitonin increases tension (Chakder and Rattan, 1990). Amylin probably acts through the CRGP receptors in potential target tissues. The adrenomedullin receptor has been cloned and has been shown to be a member of the G protein–linked receptor superfamily (Kapas et al., 1995).

CGRP receptors are widely distributed in the nervous system: receptors are present in discrete brain areas, especially the cerebellum, the nucleus accumbens, and the tail of the caudate nucleus. Very high levels of CGRP receptors are seen in solitary, vagus, hypoglossus, and dorsal medullary reticular nuclei, and the area postrema. Moderate levels are found in the dorsal and ventral spinal cord, the cardiovascular system, the adrenal, anterior pituitary, exocrine pancreas, kidney, liver, bone, and skeletal muscle. Sites for CGRP binding are present throughout the gastrointestinal tract, especially in the smooth muscle and endothelium of arteries and arterioles of the small intestine and the internal anal sphincter (Gates et al., 1989).

The transduction mechanisms used by CGRP are complex. CGRP receptors in the liver, pancreas, gastric D cells, gastric smooth muscle, vascular smooth muscle, and vascular endothelium use the adenylate cyclase pathway to activate cAMP. The long-lasting depolarization of myenteric neurons is dependent on a decrease in the resting membrane conductance for K^+. The relaxation of vascular smooth muscle may involve both cAMP and changes in K^+ conductance, plus the release of mediators such as NO (Marshall, 1992).

17.4.4 *Actions of CGRP*

CGRP is a potent and long-lasting vasodilator, causing *increased blood flow* in vascular beds, due to its relaxant effects on vascular smooth muscle. Consequently CGRP causes a prolonged hypotension (figure 17.12). In addition to its effects on vasomotion, CGRP acts on the cardiovascular system to regulate microvascular permeability, protects the heart against ischemia, and has hypertrophic effects on the heart.

In the gastrointestinal tract, the increased blood flow through the stomach, which is seen after back-diffusion of acid through a damaged gastric mucosal barrier, is mediated by CGRP released from afferent nerve fibers and NO (Holzer et al., 1994). This additional blood flow protects the gastrointestinal mucosa from further injury. This concept is supported by the development of gastric mucosal damage in rats exposed to ethanol but immunized against CGRP (Forster and Dockray, 1991).

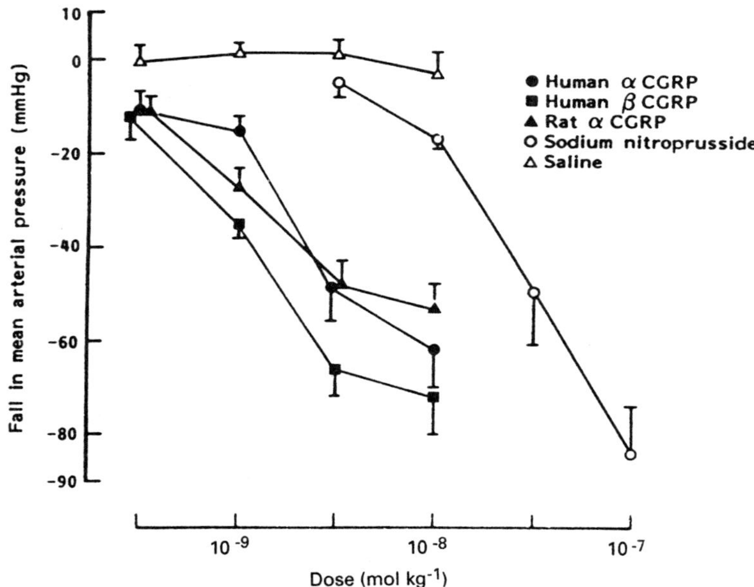

Figure 17.12
Effect of human α- and β-calcitonin gene–related peptide (α CGRP, β CGRP) and sodium nitroprusside, given by IV bolus, on blood pressure in conscious normotensive rats. Points represent mean ± SEM in groups of six rats. (From Marshall, 1992.)

CGRP relaxes precontracted esophageal, gastric, and intestinal smooth muscle, and inhibits spontaneous phasic contractions of the colon (Maggi et al., 1996). CGRP also relaxes the lower esophageal sphincter and the internal anal sphincter. The effect of CGRP on the esophageal sphincter is partially neuronal and partially a direct effect of CGRP on smooth muscle, whereas the relaxant effect on the anal sphincter is directly on smooth muscle (Rattan et al., 1988).

CGRP strongly *inhibits gastric acid secretion* by a central action that modulates parasympathetic outflow to the stomach, presumably increasing gastric blood flow and thus protecting the gastric mucosa against lesions. CGRP also inhibits gastric secretion following peripheral administration through specific release of gastric somatostatin and by a decrease in ACh transmission in the enteric nervous system (Taché, 1992).

Ion and fluid transport in the intestine is affected in some species by CGRP. In the guinea pig colon, CGRP increases chloride secretion by depolarizing myenteric neurons. In the rat colon, CGRP has an antisecretory effect, which may be mediated by somatostatin.

CGRP may play a role in *peripheral nerve regeneration*, as indicated by the increase in CGRP-immunoreactive neurites that extend into the distal part of the injured nerve a few days after nerve crush, presumably to be released from the growth cone into the surrounding endoneural tissue (Dumoulin et al., 1992). CGRP is one of many neuropeptides that are affected by nerve section (figure 17.13) and CGRP

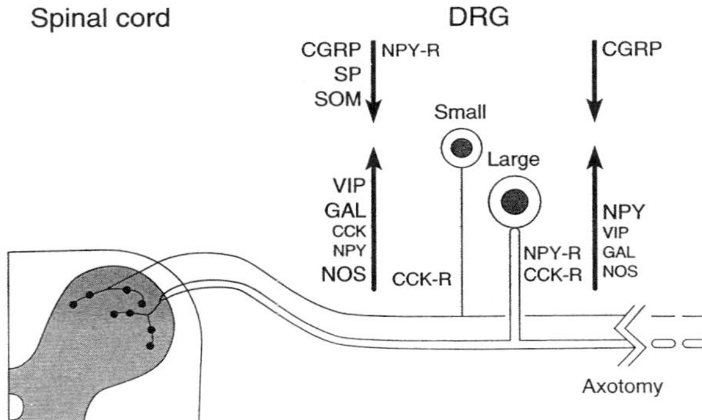

Figure 17.13
Schematic drawing of a small and large primary sensory neuron in a dorsal root ganglion (DRG) sending a central branch to the dorsal horn of the spinal cord, and with a peripheral branch that has been sectioned (axotomy). The changes occurring in levels of peptides and of both peptide and peptide receptors mRNAs are indicated by arrows. Thus, in small, unmyelinated DRG neurons, calcitonin gene–related peptide (CGPR), substance P (SP), and somatostatin (SOM), as well as neuropeptide Y receptor (NPY-R) mRNA are downregulated, whereas vasoactive intestinal peptide (VIP), galanin (GAL), cholecystokinin (CCK), NPY, and nitric oxide synthase (NOS), as well as CCK_B receptor (CCK-R) mRNA are upregulated. In the large, myelinated neurons, CRGP is downregulated whereas NPY, VIP, GAL, and NOS, as well as both the NPY and CCK receptor mRNAs are upregulated. Larger letters indicate pronounced changes; smaller letters denote modest changes. (From Hökfelt et al., 1994.)

may have a special role in that it modulates the effects of SP, with which it is coreleased, as well as directly affecting dorsal horn neurons (Hökfelt et al., 1994). These neuromodulatory effects may be integrated with CGRP effects on the neuromuscular unit since CGRP receptors are present on muscle cells and the neuropeptide has several consequential effects on skeletal muscle, improving contractile efficiency and regulating ACh receptor α subunit biosynthesis (Changeux et al., 1992).

Central, but not peripheral administration of CGRP *increases body temperature and decreases food intake*. The effects on food intake are not abolished by a potent CCK A receptor antagonist, indicating a possible independent role for CGRP in satiation (Morley et al., 1996).

17.4.5 Clinical Implications of CGRP

There is little specific information on gastrointestinal functions being affected by deficiencies or hyperproduction of CGRP. There are some associated pathological conditions: some mucosal ulcers are associated with a depletion of CGRP; streptozotocin-induced diabetes selectively damages myenteric CGRP neurons in the rat intestine; and CGRP levels are decreased in colitis and in patients with inflammatory bowel disease (Eysselein et al., 1992). CGRP is secreted by several neuroendocrine tumors, including medullary thyroid carcinoma. Aging is associated with the disappearance of CGRP-containing nerve fibers in the stomach, which is accompanied by a loss of the hyperemic response to gastric acid challenge. As a consequence, the gastric mucosa of aged rats becomes more vulnerable to acid injury (Grønbech and Lacy, 1995). The advent of specific CGRP antagonists should produce more definite evidence for a physiopathological role for CGRP.

17.4.6 Amylin and Adrenomellulin

Amylin (islet amyloid polypeptide) and *adrenomedullin* are coded for by separate genes, different from the calcitonin-CGRP gene. The gene encoding amylin is in the short arm of chromosome 12 in the human. Amylin shares a 46% amino acid homology with CGRP. Amylin is found in the beta cells of the pancreatic islets and is a predominant component of amyloid deposits in the pancreas of patients with NIDDM.

Amylin is synthesized and released in parallel with insulin and may act as a paracrine agent influencing the pancreatic islets (Bretherton-Watt et al., 1992). Amylin probably activates CGRP receptors. Adrenomedullin was initially isolated from the human pheochromocytoma but is found in the adrenal, brain and many peripheral tissues. It has been purified and its cDNA cloned.

Adrenomedullin is a 52-amino acid vasoactive peptide, encoded by a gene on chromosome 11 in the rat and pig. Rat adrenomedullin is a 50-amino acid peptide with 2 amino acid deletions and 6 substitutions compared to the human peptide, whereas porcine adrenomedullin is identical to the human peptide, except for one amino acid substitution in position 40. Adrenomedullin shares about 27% homology with CGRP and has similar, potent hypotensive effects on the cardiovascular system, which are mediated by NO (Kitamura et al., 1995). Adrenomedullin has profound natriuretic effects, acting directly on the renal tubules and increasing renal blood flow. Adrenomedullin and related peptides regulate adrenal mineralocorticoid secretion, acting through CGRP receptors. Centrally, adrenomedullin may modify the HPA axis to inhibit water drinking and salt appetite, as well as inhibiting the release of VP, suggesting that the peptide may interact with brain mechanisms regulating fluid and electrolyte homeostasis (Nussdorfer et al., 1997; Samson and Murphy, 1997). Adrenomedullin has specific G protein-coupled receptors in the brain different from those of CGRP, indicating that adrenomedullin may serve centrally as a neurotransmitter or neuromodulator (Sone et al., 1997).

17.5 Neurotensin

Neurotensin (NT) was found serendipitously by Susan Leeman during the isolation of substance P from bovine hypothalami (Carraway and Leeman, 1973). This fraction possessed vasodilator and cyanotic effects and an identical fraction was subsequently isolated from bovine and human intestines. NT is present thoughout the animal kingdom and exerts a variety of physiological effects, including vasodilation, cyanosis, increased histamine release, effects on gastrointestinal smooth muscle activity, increased intestinal secretion, and mediation of many of the effects that follow fat ingestion.

17.5.1 Structure of Neurotensin and Related Neuropeptides

NT is a 13–amino acid peptide, and has a strongly conserved C-terminal sequence, the bioactive sequence, which it has in common with NT from several other species. Human, bovine, canine, porcine, and rat NT are identical.

Neurotensin

Glu-Leu-Tyr-Glu-Asn-Lys-Pro-Arg-Arg-*Pro-Tyr-Ile-Leu*

Neuromedin

Lys-Ile-*Pro-Tyr-Ile-Leu*

The biological activity of NT resides in the last 5 or 6 C-terminal residues. Substitution of Trp for Tyr in position 11 increases biological activity. Several NT-related peptides have been sequenced, including *xenopsin* from frog skin, and peptides from turkey, dog, and rat, all of which share the C-terminal sequence Pro-Trp-Ile-Leu. *Neuromedin N* (NmN) is a 6–amino acid peptide which shares C-terminal sequence and biological activity with NT. Chick LANT-6 is also a hexapeptide that is similar to NmN except that Ile^2 is replaced by Asn^2.

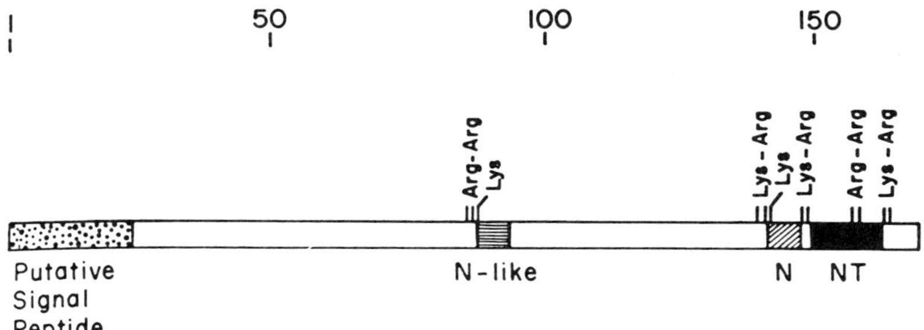

Figure 17.14
Schematic diagram of preproneurotensin and neuromedin N. The position of neurotensin (NT) (solid), neuromedin N (cross-hatched), neuromedin N-like (horizontally lined), and putative signal peptide (stippled) coding domains are indicated. The positions of all paired, basic amino acid residues are shown. The amino acid numbers are indicated. (From Dobner et al. 1987.)

17.5.2 Neurotensin Gene Expression, Precursor Processing, and Regulation of Release

Both NT and NmN are synthesized from a common 170–amino acid precursor in mammalian brain and intestine. The gene encoding NT and NmN has 10.2 kb pairs, with four exons and three introns. Exon 4 encodes NT and NmN (Kislauskis et al., 1988). Two mRNAs of different length (1.0 and 1.4 kb) have been found, with the ratios varying in different tissues and species, but the functional significance of the variation is not known.

The *precursor NT-NmN* consists of a signal peptide, both NmN and NT sequences, and a 5–amino acid "tail peptide" (Carraway et al., 1992) (figure 17.14). In the intestine most of the NmN is stored as the high-molecular-weight, extended peptide of 125 residues. In the brain, however, it is mostly the hexapeptide form of NmN that is found. The tail peptide is present in both the ileum and brain, but its function is unknown. In some tissues NT 6–13 is found. Most of the NT (>90%) is expressed in the gut, mainly in the ileum, to a lesser extent in the jejunum, and very little in the duodenum. NT is found in the endocrine N cells of the intestine, which are open cells with their apical microvilli exposed to the luminal contents. Some gut NT is localized in the myenteric plexus (Sundler et al., 1982).

NT is found in nerve cells, fibers, and terminals in the brain, mainly in the arcuate nucleus and the preoptic area of the hypothalamus, and also in extrapyramidal and limbic regions, such as the striatum and nucleus accumbens. NT release from the last two structures, as measured by in vivo microdialysis, is mediated by dopaminergic D_2 receptors (Wagstaff et al., 1996) and NT, in turn, appears to regulate dopminergic transmission along the nigrostriatal and mesolimbic pathways (Li et al., 1995).

Most of the NT peptides in the circulation are metabolites. This, together with the number of different NT peptides found in brain and gut, supports the concept that NT is degraded during secretion.

Release of NT is evoked chiefly by fat in the jejunum, supplemented by a local humoral or neural stimulus that releases NT from the ileum. The neural mechanism is cholinergic, but independent of the vagus, since section of the vagus does not abolish the release of NT. Several other factors induce NT secretion, such as bombesin, carbachol, catecholamines, and SP.

17.5.3 Neurotensin Receptors and Second Messengers

The NT receptor belongs to the G protein–coupled receptor family and consists of 424 amino acids with a molecular weight of 47 kD. When glycosylated, its molecular weight rises to 100 kD (Vincent, 1995). NT receptors have been localized throughout the brain and brainstem, by both autoradiographic and immunohistochemical techniques. The receptor is expressed in highest concentrations in the cerebellum, hippocampus, piriform cortex, and neocortex of the mouse brain (Mazella et al., 1996). As some regions of the brain have NT binding sites that can be identified only by autoradiography, it appears that in some species, but not in humans, there may be two molecularly distinct forms of the receptor. Some brain regions show receptors on perikarya, dendrites, and axons, indicating that NT may act both presynatically and postsynaptically (Boudin et al., 1996).

NT receptor mRNA is expressed in the intestine at only about 10% of the level found in brain (Tanaka et al., 1990). It is interesting to note that most of the NT is found in the gastrointestinal tract, but the densest concentration of NT receptors is in the brain and brainstem. Receptors that mediate contraction in the duodenum and colon are related but not identical to NT receptors that subserve relaxation in these organs, as determined by specific NT antagonists (Mule et al., 1996). The second messenger activated by the NT receptors is the inositol phosphate pathway.

17.5.4 Actions of Neurotensin

NT acts as a local hormone or paracrine agent in the periphery, and as a neurotransmitter or neuromodulator, or both, in the spinal cord, where it depresses the activity of most neurons (figure 17.15). However, central or peripheral injections of NT produce completely different pharmacological effects. The electrophysiological effects of NT in the brain are inconsistent: NT increases the in vitro firing rate of DA neurons in the mesencephalon and cortex but appears to inhibit the firing rate of neurons in the thalamus, and has variable effects on hippocampal neurons. Some of these responses are discussed by Lambert et al. (1995).

In the gastrointestinal tract, NT causes *relaxation* of the ileum by direct action, and contraction of its smooth muscle by an indirect mechanism. Relaxation is tetrodotoxin-resistant and is blocked by NT antagonists. Contraction is through cholinergic and SP mediators.

NT affects *secretion* in different ways, inhibiting gastric acid secretion but stimulating secretion by the intestine and pancreas. Similarly, NT decreases blood flow through adipose tissue but increases blood flow through the intestine. The effects of NT are probably *potentiating* rather than independent; NT potentiates the stimulatory effects of secretin and CCK on pancreatic secretion. NT stimulates gastric mucosal prostaglandin secretion, an action that may be mediated by NT release of histamine (Zhang et al., 1989).

NT affects *gastrointestinal motility*. After a fat-rich meal, NT lowers esophageal sphincter pressure, slows gastric emptying, and inhibits the MMC, actions that are partly dependent on vagal cholinergic mechanisms (Hellstrom, 1986).

There is a direct neural pathway from NT-containing neurons in the arcuate nucleus to the subfornical organ, as determined by anterograde tracer studies, so this pathway may be involved in the *modulation of cardiovascular and body fluid homeostasis* (Rosasarellano et al., 1996). High doses of NT cause hypertension, whereas low doses elicit hypotension.

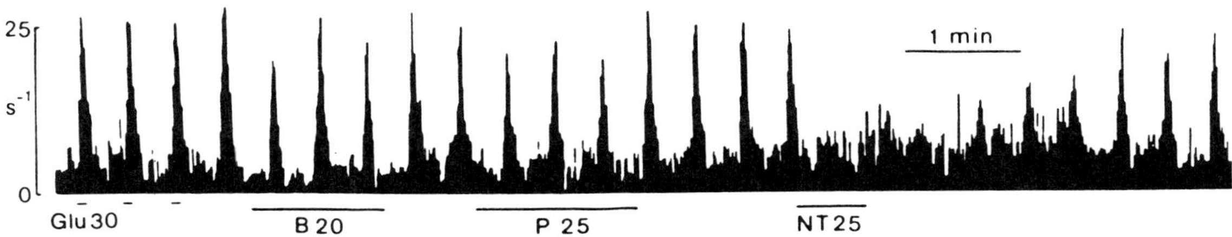

Figure 17.15
Depressant effect of neurotensin on a wide-dynamic-range neuron in lamina IV of the dorsal horn of the spinal cord. Pen recorder tracing shows the output from a gating ratemeter counting the activity and displaying it as spikes on the ordinate. This unit was responding reproducibly to automatically controlled periodic applications of glutamate (Glu) by iontophoresis (the first three applications indicated by short horizontal bars below the records). Iontophoretic application of a potent benzodiazepine (B) and of an endogenous peptide (P) failed to alter the excitatory response to glutamate or basal discharge rate, seen as the activity between responses to glutamate. Neurotensin, on the other hand, abolished the response to glutamate, and the glutamate response only gradually returned over a period of 2 to 3 minutes. Long horizontal bars below the records indicate periods of drug application. Numbers represent current in nanoamperes. (From Henry, 1982.)

NT excites neurons in the amygdaloid nucleus through specific NT receptors so that NT may be involved in amygdaloid function. Microinjections of high dosages of NT into the preoptic area, which is involved in the regulation of body temperature, and which is rich in NT, cause hypothermia; low dosages, on the other hand, result in hyperthermia. If NT is injected into the posterior hypothalamus, which controls sympathetic output, NT produces *hypothermia* at all dosages tested (Benmoussa et al., 1996) (figure 17.16). NT is also considered to be a *hyperanalgesic* agent.

NT produces many behavioral effects after central administration. These include reduced food intake, catalepsy, and alterations in locomotor activity, phenomena that mimic the effects of neuroleptics and suggesting that NT may an endogenous neuroleptic-like peptide. Many of these effects may be due to a modulating action of NT on selective brain DA systems (Lambert et al., 1995). Normally, NT is released after fat ingestion; defects in the processing of NT may lead to the development of obesity, as food intake remains high.

17.5.5 Clinical Implications of Neurotensin

NT may inhibit the formation of gastric ulcers induced by stress (Nemeroff et al., 1983). The NT gene is expressed only briefly during the development of the fetal colon but it is reexpressed in almost one quarter of human colon cancers, indicating that dedifferentiation may occur in certain types of colon cancer (Evers et al., 1996). Hypersecretion of NT is usually found in neuroendocrine tumors that are producing large amounts of other peptides, especially VIP, which makes it difficult to assign a specific role to NT. No clinical dysfunctions can be attributed to NT in patients whose tumors produce only NT. Consequently, the physiological role of NT is probably that of a supportive actor in the theatre of gut regulatory peptides.

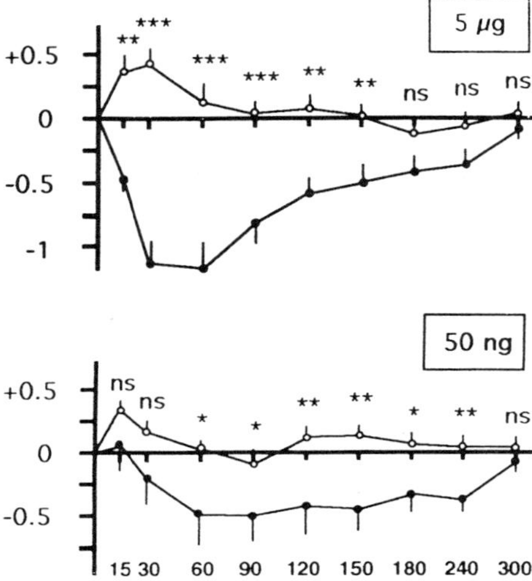

Figure 17.16
Thermal effects of neurotensin in the posterior nucleus of the hypothalamus. In abscissa, time in minutes; in ordinates, temperature variations in degrees Celsius Neurotensin, black circles, controls, open circles. *$P < .05$, **$P < .01$, ***$P < .001$. (From Benmoussa et al., 1996.)

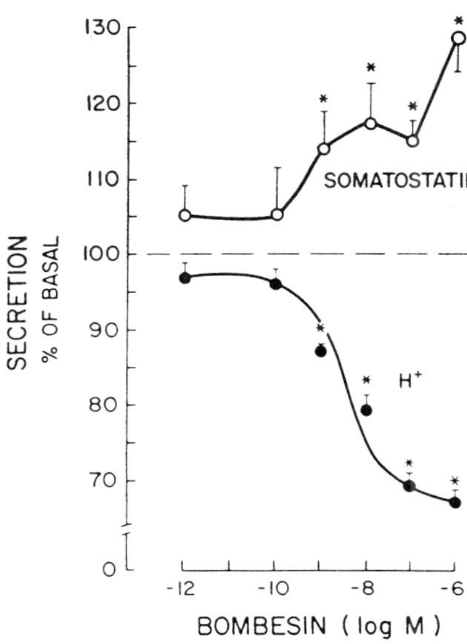

Figure 17.17
Concentration-response curve for the effect of bombesin on the secretion of basal acid (black circles) and somatostatin (open circles). Values are expressed as a percentage of the control basal secretion. Asterisks denote significant difference from control basal secretion. Mean ± SE of 4 to 14 experiments with each concentration. (From Schubert and Hightower, 1989.)

17.6 Somatostatin as the Final Common Path for Neuropeptide Inhibition

Tables 16.2 and 16.3 clearly show the surprisingly large numbers of neuropeptides that have similar inhibitory actions on gastric, intestinal, and pancreatic functions. Many of these neuropeptides may have direct effects on their target organs, but many of them may indirectly inhibit through their well-documented stimulation of *somatostatin*, a general inhibitor (figure 17.17). The VIP-secretin-glucagon family, for example, all inhibit gastric acid secretion in vivo, have no effect on gastric parietal cells in vitro, but all stimulate somatostatin release (Schubert, 1991; Schubert and Hightower, 1989). Gastrin, CCK, CGRP, GIP, calcitonin, and bombesin-GRP are other neuropeptides that influence somatostatin release.

The administration of somatostatin, in many cases, directly mimics that of the individual neuropeptide. This may be an example of physiological redundancy, or a fail-safe mechanism, by which the overlapping gastrointestinal functions of these neuropeptides are conserved because they are linked to portions of the molecule that are needed for other, more individual functions, some of which are, perhaps, yet to be discovered. The considerable degree of species-specificity indicates that variation in neuropeptide function in the gastrointestinal tract is well tolerated.

17.7 Vagal Integration of Gastrointestinal Functions

The functions of the gastrointestinal tract are integrated in a most complex manner by peripheral neuropeptides acting as hormones or local paracrine factors, by the intrinsic neuronal networks in the myenteric and submucosal plexuses, and by positive and negative feedback on central nuclei controlling the vagus. In the stomach, the vagus innervates three separate subpopulations of myenteric neurons that contain different neuropeptides. The first group comprises the gastrin-rich cells in the antrum and oxyntic mucosa of the corpus of the stomach; the second group is in the myenteric plexus and longitudinal muscle layer and contains GRP; and the third group of neurons contains VIP. This provides the basis for the physiological vagal control of gastrin release, gastric acid secretion, and gastric motility (Berthoud, 1996).

These feedback loops involve neuropeptides, including somatostatin, acting directly on central neurons, or activating or inhibiting peripheral nerve terminals of the afferent vagus. The vagus, in turn, stimulates somatostatin release, although this again is species-specific, and simultaneously stimulates the release of bombesin so that the two neuropeptides may have coordinated effects on the target gastrin cell (figure 17.18). Figure 17.19 illustrates the interaction of some gut peptides on the two main regulators of gut motility, somatostatin and ACh, and a model proposed by DuVal et al. (1981) for the release of gastrin. In this model the noncholinergic route uses CGRP as a stimulant for gastrin release, whereas the cholinergic pathway removes the inhibitory influence of somatostatin.

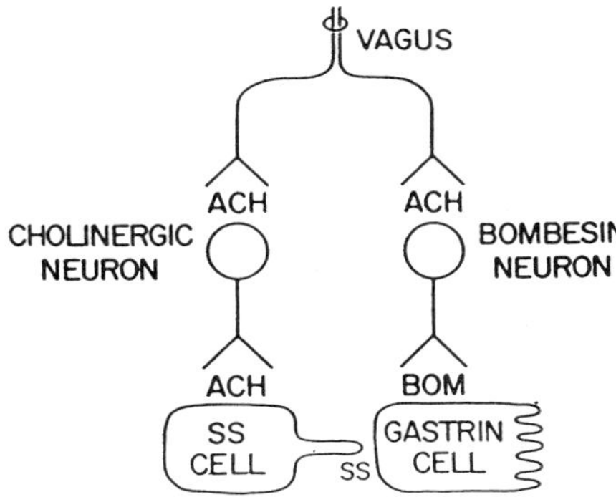

Figure 17.18
Model for the regulation of gastrin secretion by intramural cholinergic and noncholinergic (bombesin-containing) neurons. The somatostatin (SS) cell in the rat antrum is anatomically coupled to the gastrin cell by cytoplasmic processes. The influence of the cholinergic neuron is mediated by inhibition of somatostatin secretion, which eliminates the basal constraint exerted by somatostatin on gastrin secretion. The noncholinergic pathway is mediated by release of bombesin (BOM) on or near the gastrin cell. The two pathways act synergistically: elimination of the restraint mediated by somatostatin makes it possible for the full effect of bombesin to be exerted on the gastrin cell. ACH, acetylcholine. (From DuVal et al., 1981.)

17.8 Summary

Insulin is best known for its effects on glucose homeostasis but also affects protein and lipid metabolism. Insulin belongs to the superfamily of neuropeptides that consists of IGFs, relaxin, and certain invertebrate peptides. These peptides have similar primary and tertiary structures and all are involved in growth and metabolism. There is only one insulin gene, except for the rat and mouse, which have two, and its expression is limited to the beta cells of the pancreas, and perhaps to the fetal liver and some areas of the brain. The insulin molecule consists of two polypeptide chains, A

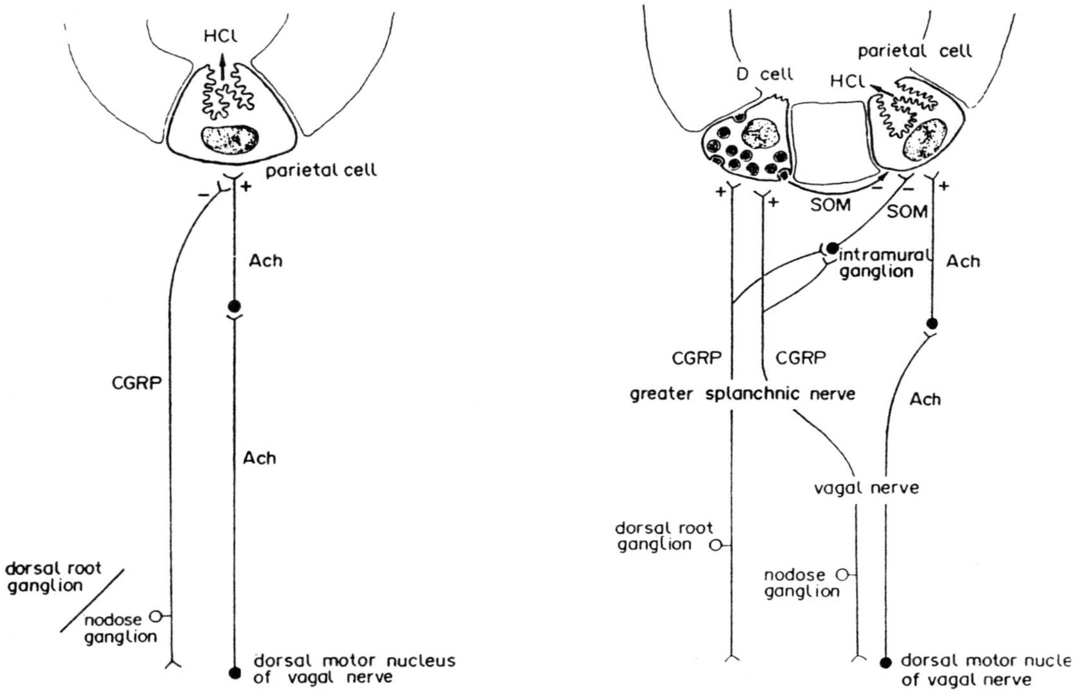

Figure 17.19
Schematic drawings showing the mechanisms of the inhibition of the basal and stimulated acid secretion by calcitonin gene–related protein (CGRP). (Left) CGRP fibers originating from the nodose ganglion presynaptically affect the cholinergic post-ganglionic parasympathetic terminals. (Right) Somatostatin (SOM) inhibits here; two possibilities are indicated: CGRP stimulates SOM secretion from D cells or intramural SOM neurons. SOM released from these cells inhibits gastric secretion. Ach, acetylcholine. (From Ishida-Yamamoto and Tohyama, 1989.)

and B, which are linked by two disulfide bridges, while a third bridge connects amino acids 6 and 11 in the A chain. The prohormone contains a C peptide that connects the A and B chains and that is removed during final processing to insulin.

Insulin receptors are heterogeneous and widely distributed, accounting for the extensive effects of insulin, but they are especially concentrated in liver, skeletal muscle, and adipose tissue. The insulin receptors are one of the family of tyrosine kinase receptors for many growth factors, including IGF-1. The insulin receptor is a heterodimer, consisting of two α and two β subunits joined by disulfide bonds, and containing an insulin binding site and an insulin-regulated tyrosine protein kinase region. Activation of the latter site initiates phosphorylation, essential to the catalytic activities that mediate the insulin response. The receptor is internalized after binding with insulin. Specific intracellular second-messenger systems for insulin have not been positively identified.

Insulin secretion is mainly *regulated* by glucose, acting at both transcriptional and post-transcriptional levels, but initiators and potentiators affect insulin secretion and release. The initiators include D-glucose, D-glyceraldehyde, D-fructose, D-mannose, and L-leucine, and their presence is required for a potentiator to increase insulin secretion. The potentiators are other neuropeptides, chiefly CCK, GIP, and GLP-1. Glucose fails to stimulate insulin secretion in patients with IDDM. ACh stimulates insulin secretion, which is inhibited by α-adrenergic input. There is a negative feedback between insulin and somatostatin, with insulin deficiency increasing somatostatin secretion, and somatostatin inhibiting insulin secretion. Insulin secretion is pulsatile and is amplified by a meal.

The primary action of insulin is the regulation of glucose homeostasis, which is promoted by the ability of insulin to increase the synthesis of the passive glucose transporters required to move glucose into the cell. In skeletal muscle, liver, and fat, insulin increases glucose utilization and decreases gluconeogenesis. Long-term effects on gene transcription may require the cooperation of IGF-1. Centrally, insulin affects food intake and the HPA axis.

Relaxin, a peptide produced by the corpus luteum of mammals, and the endometrium and placenta of primates, has structural similarities to insulin and the two peptides may have evolved from a common ancestral gene. In the mammalian reproductive system, rising levels of relaxin during pregnancy facilitate parturition by softening the cartilage of the pubic symphysis, degrading fetal membranes to assist in their rupture, and increasing blood flow to the fetus. Receptors for relaxin are in the uterus and cervix, and in several brain regions, including the subfornical organ, the PVN, and SON. Exogenous relaxin causes the release of OT and VP, and consequent pressor changes and increased water consumption.

Galanin is another phylogenetically old peptide, found in invertebrates and submammalian species as well as in mammals. Galanin affects almost all physiological systems including the gastrointestinal tract and the HPA axis. Galanin is a 29–amino acid peptide (30 in humans), the N-terminal region galanin 1–15 being fully conserved, whereas the C-terminal half is more variable. Galanin is encoded by a single gene and preprogalanin is processed in a tissue- and species-specific manner to produce different forms of galanin. Galanin mRNA is is widely distributed throughout the gastrointestinal tract, in most organ systems, and in peripheral nerves innervating skin and muscle. Galanin is densely concentrated in the hypothalamus, where it is colocalized with GnRH, and in other brain areas, including the pituitary. Regulation of galanin mRNA appears to be linked to the activity of GnRH neurons during the estrous cycle, by fat intake, estrogens, thyroxine, and glucocorticoids. Galanin release from the gastrointestinal tract is evoked by distention of the gut, or the presence of bile, amino acids, acid, hypertonic saline, or glucose. Galanin released from pituitary cells is secreted in a pulsatile way into the median eminence and the portal vessels.

Galanin receptors differ in structure according to species and tissue. Receptors isolated from brain an pancreatic alpha or beta cells are specific for the N-terminal portion of galanin, whereas the receptors of the gastrointestinal tract and iris of the eye are specific for the C-terminal portion. The second-messenger system is through adenylate cyclase and cAMP. *Peripherally*, galanin increases salivation but inhibits most gastrointestinal secretions, and has variable effects on gut motility, depending on species and gut region. As a result of galanin inhibition of insulin secretion, it has a hyperglycemic effect. *Centrally*, the effects of galanin are mostly inhibitory, decreasing pituitary secretion of VP and ACTH and consequently of blood levels of corticosterone. Galanin may act presynaptically on GnRH neurons to coordinate the pulsatile release of GnRH. Galanin increases fat intake and reduces energy expenditure and thereby increases fat deposition.

Motilin is another of the gut-brain peptides found in the endocrine cells of the gut and in central neurons. Its clearest action is to increase intestinal motility. Motilin is a 22–amino acid peptide folded into an α helix, with considerable structural heterogeneity in mammalian species. The N-terminal sequence 1–10 is essential to biological potency. The *motilin gene* is unusual in that the bioactive peptide is encoded by two of its five exons. There is only one promotilin, which contains the 22–amino acid sequence of motilin, followed by a long sequence of no known function. Consequently, the different forms of motilin must result from post-translational processing of this single motilin precursor.

Motilin mRNA is present in the gut, with maximal concentrations in the duodenum. It is uncertain whether there is any motilin in the brain, although exogenous motilin can evoke CNS responses. *Motilin receptors* are in the gastrointestinal tract, varying in distribution in different species. One type of receptor is located in smooth muscle of stomach and intestine, and another type is neural. The most important function of motilin is the induction of gastroduodenal contractions which last from 10 to 30 minutes. Motilin also stimulates contraction of the lower esophageal sphincter and may accelerate gastric emptying. Central effects of exogenous motilin include effects on feeding, and direct depression of neurons in the lateral vestibular nucleus, but stimulation of cortical neurons.

Calcitonin-gene-related peptide, amylin, and *adrenomedullin.* CGRP is formed by alternative splicing of the mRNA transcribed from the calcitonin gene. CGRP is a 37–amino acid peptide with a disulfide bond and an amidated C-terminal Phe^{37}. The *calcitonin gene* encodes both calcitonin and CGRP and contains regions that are differently expressed in the thyroid to yield calcitonin mRNA, and in neural tissue to express mRNA for CGRP. There are two forms of CGRP, CGRP I and II, both of which, in the rat and human, are encoded by two different genes. CGRP is expressed in sensory systems, including the hypothalamic and limbic areas, in neurons throughout the digestive system, and in the primary afferent nerves of pancreatic and mesenteric arteries. CGRP is usually colocalized with SP in afferent nerve fibers, and in enteric neurons CGRP coexists with choline acetyltransferase, CCK, somatostatin, and NPY. CGRP is also expressed in endocrine cells in the small intestine, pancreas, the gonadotrophs of the pituitary, the adrenal medulla, and to a small extent in thyroid C cells. CGRP is expressed in cell bodies of motorneurons and the peptide is found in their neuromuscular junctions. CGRP is upregulated by nerve injury and during nerve regeneration. CGRP *release* occurs through stimulation of primary afferent nerve endings, by increased acid in the stomach, and by colonic distention.

CGRP receptors are distributed throughout many areas of the brain, especially the cerebellum, nucleus accumbens, and caudate nucleus. Binding sites for CGRP are present throughout the gastrointestinal tract, especially in the smooth muscle and endothelium of arteries and arterioles, as well as in skeletal muscle. Several CGRP receptors can be recognized on the basis of their functional response to different CGRP antagonists. $CGRP_1$ receptors mediate the relaxant effects on intestinal smooth muscle and the inhibition of gastric acid secretion. $CGRP_2$ receptors mediate vasodilation. Several transduction mechanisms are used by CGRP depending on the site of action. They include adenylate cyclase, a decrease in the resting membrane K^+ conductance, or both these mechanisms plus the release of NO.

Owing to its potent relaxant effects on vascular smooth muscle, CGRP is a long-lasting vasodilator, causing prolonged hypotension. CGRP regulates microvascular permeability and protects the heart against ischemia. In the gastrointestinal tract CGRP protects the mucosa from acid hyperemia by increasing blood flow and inhibiting gastric acid secretion. CGRP relaxes gastrointestinal smooth muscle and the various gastrointestinal sphincters. The peptide causes the release of somatostatin, and many of the inhibitory effects, including inhibition of pancreatic and colonic secretion, attributed to CGRH may be indirect, through somatostatin release. CGRP may be involved in peripheral nerve regeneration, modulating the effect of SP with which it is co-released, as well as acting directly on dorsal horn neurons, and at the neuromuscular junction. Centrally, CGRP increases body temperature and decreases food intake.

Amylin and *adrenomedullin*, like calcitonin and CGRP, contain two N-terminal cysteines that form an N-terminal loop and a C-terminal amide. All four peptides are highly conserved and may have arisen from gene duplication. Amylin and adrenomedullin are coded for by separate genes, different from the calcitonin-CGRP gene. Amylin is found in the beta cells of the pancreas and is a component of amyloid deposits in the pancreas of patients with NIDDM. Adrenomedullin is a 52 amino acid vasoactive peptide found mainly in the adrenal medulla, endothelium, and smooth muscle of blood vessels, and in the anterior pituitary and CNS. Adrenomedullin has hypotensive effects similar to those of CGRP, has profound natriuretic effects, and acts centrally to inhibit water drinking and salt appetite. Both amylin and adrenomedullin probably activate CGRP receptors, but adrenomedullin has its own G protein-coupled receptor in the brain.

Neurotensin is found throughout the animal kingdom, first identified by its vasodilator and cyanotic effects. Neurotensin is a 13–amino acid peptide with a strongly conserved, bioactive C-terminal sequence which it has in common with NT from other species. Several NT-related peptides also have this sequence: neuromedin N (NmN), frog xenopsin, and chick LANT-6. Both NT and NmN are synthesized from a common precursor in mammalian brain and intestine, which contains both NT and NmN sequences and a "tail" peptide of unknown function. Almost all mRNA for NT is in the endocrine cells of the gut, with lesser amounts of NT in nerve cells, fibers, and terminals in the brain, especially the arcuate nucleus, POA, striatum, and nucleus accumbens. NT *release* from brain is mediated by dopaminergic D_2 receptors, whereas NT release from the gastrointestinal tract is evoked by fat in the jejunum, together with a local humoral or neural stimulant from the ileum.

NT receptors belong to the G protein–coupled receptor family and are located throughout the forebrain. There may be two forms of the NT receptor, but not in humans. Receptors are found on cell bodies, dendrites, and axons, indicating a presynaptic and postsynaptic action of NT. NT receptor mRNA is expressed in the gastrointestinal tract at only 10% of its level in brain, in contrast to the relevant levels of NT mRNA in these tissues. The second messenger activated by NT receptors is the inositol phosphate pathway.

NT lowers esophageal sphincter pressure, slows gastric emptying, and inhibits the MMC. NT may cause relaxation of ileal smooth muscle directly, or contraction via an indirect mechanism. It also has different effects on secretion, inhibiting gastric secretion, but stimulating intestinal and pancreatic secretion, probably by potentiating the effects of secretin and CCK. *Centrally*, NT modulates cardiovascular and fluid homeostasis, possibly through NT-containing neurons that synapse in the arcuate nucleus. NT inhibits food intake, produces hypothermia, and is a hyperanalgesic agent.

Many of the neuropeptides have similar inhibitory actions on gastrointestinal tract functions, some of which may be direct, but many could be through the stimulation of somatostatin secretion, which may be the final common path for neuropeptide inhibition. The administration of somatostatin, in many cases, directly mimics that of the individual neuropeptide. In addition, the integrative role of the vagus in gastrointestinal functions cannot be overlooked. A series of feedback controls involving neuropeptides, including somatostatin, may act directly on central neurons, or peripherally on nerve terminals of the afferent vagus. The vagus, in turn, may cause the release of neuropeptides, including somatostatin.

Chapter 18 is the last chapter on vertebrate neuropeptides and includes the cardiac, renal, thyroid, and parathyroid hormones. These are the natriuretic hormone family, angiotensin, calcitonin and thyroxine, parathyroid hormone, and parathyroid-related hormone. As the reader will expect by now, these primary sites of neuropeptide production are supplemented, or exceeded in importance in some cases, by their production in neural tissues.

Cardiac, Renal, Parathyroid, and Thyroid Neuropeptides: ANH, AT, CT, PTH, PRH-rP, T_3, T_4

18

All of the neuropeptides discussed in this chapter are intimately involved in physiological regulation of water and electrolyte homeostasis, with the exception of thyroxine (T_4), which is an important regulator of overall tissue metabolism. While the primary site of production of these peptides is peripheral, they are all produced in neural tissue as well and have profound effects on the CNS.

18.1 Natriuretic Hormone Family

For many years it was believed that the sodium and water diuresis caused by distention of the atria of the heart was caused by a neural reflex that suppressed VP release. It took many years, from the first observation by Kisch (1956) that the atria contained granules visible under the electron microscope and that these granules appeared to be secretory (de Bold, 1979), to the definitive experiment by de Bold et al. (1981) in which these authors injected crude atrial extracts into rats and observed both diuresis and natriuresis. This conclusively showed the heart to be an endocrine organ.

The active substance is known by several names: atrial natriuretic factor (ANF), atrionatriuretic peptide (ANP), atriopeptin, and *atrial natriuretic hormone (ANH)*, which is the term used in this text. It has now been extensively investigated, its molecular biology elucidated, as well as its physiological and pathological significance. On a molar basis, ANH is 10,000 times more potent than any currently available diuretic agent. ANH has several other physiological functions in addition to its effects on water and salt diuresis. Its control over water and salt homeostasis, together with its vasodilator effects and ability to increase vascular permeability, give ANH an important role in the regulation of blood pressure. This is compounded by the ability of ANH to inhibit aldosterone and renin secretion. In addition, ANH has central effects which include drinking behavior, inhibition of the release of certain neuropeptides at the central level, and is itself released from the hypothalamus into the hypophyseal portal system.

18.1.1 The Natriuretic Peptide System

ANH is only one member of the family of neuropeptides involved in the central regulation of endocrine and autonomic functions. ANH was purified and its amino acid sequence identified in 1984 by Kangawa and Matsuo. This led to a search for related compounds and Sudoh et al. (1990) found a peptide in brain with similar structural and physiological properties to ANH. This was named *brain natriuretic peptide (BNP)*, but subsequent studies have shown BNP to be produced mainly in the ventricles of the heart. Like ANH, BNP has potent effects on diuresis and natriuresis, and is an effective vasodilator.

C-type natriuretic peptide (CNP) is the third important member of this system. CNP was first isolated in the CNS, where it is found in much higher concentrations than either ANH or BNP (Sudoh et al., 1990). Like BNP, CNP has a much wider distribution than first thought and is also found in macrophages, kidney, and endothelial cells. CNP has a comparatively weaker effect on diuresis and natriuresis than ANH or BNP, but it acts as a venodilator and inhibits smooth muscle proliferation in vitro. The structures of the three natriuretic peptides are depicted in figure 18.1. Structure activity studies of ANH, BNP, and CNP show that the natriuretic and arterial dilator properties of ANH reside in its C-terminal tail. CNP lacks this structure and is devoid of both arterial and natriuretic effects. The biological activity of CNP is dependent on its ring formation. ANH and BNP are of cardiac origin and are released into the circulation

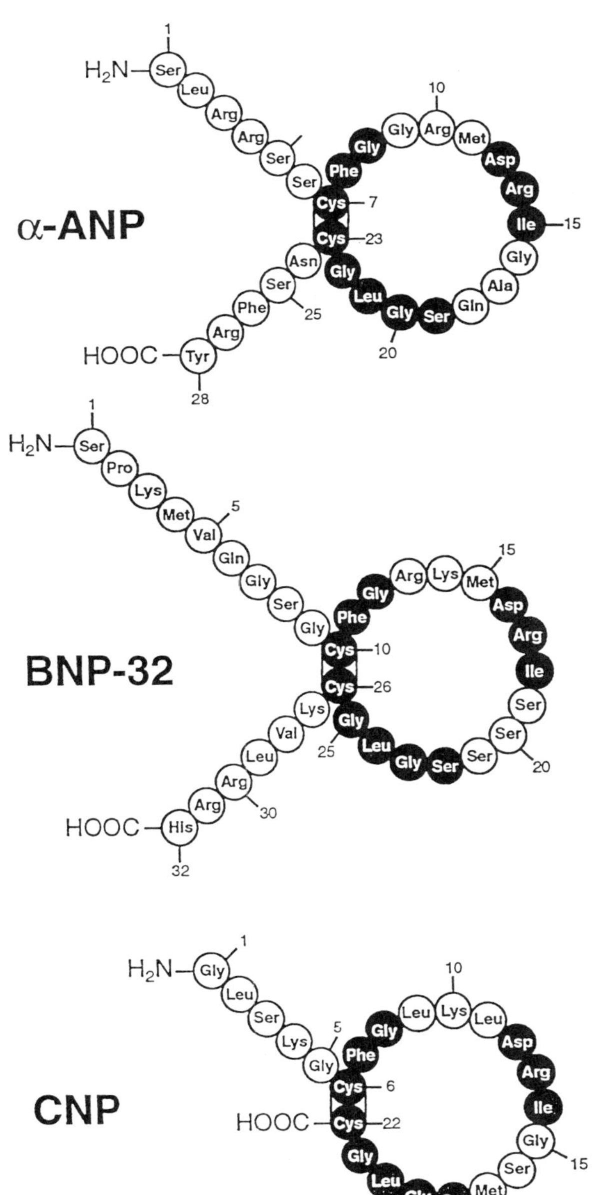

to act on target tissues distant from the site of production and release. On the other hand, CNP and its receptors are found in brain and peripheral blood vessels and may act together with nitric oxide and the prostaglandins to form a system of vasodilators with paracrine activity (Barr at al., 1996).

The evolutionary aspects of these natriuretic peptides are interesting. Each is derived from a separate gene. Unlike ANH and CNP, the structure of BNP shows considerable species diversity, indicating that it is an evolutionary older peptide than the other two. In the euryhaline teleost, CNP is the major form and is important for the adaptation of fish from seawater to water with half the salinity of the sea. Hypothalamic CNP increases at this time, while hypothalamic angiotensin II (AT II) levels decrease. The opposing effects of these two neuropeptides on osmoregulation permits the adaptation of these fish to different salinities. Galli and Phillips (1996) suggest that as animals moved from an aquatic to a terrestrial environment, ANH evolved as a volume-regulating hormone, while retaining its sodium-regulating properties.

18.1.2 Atrionatriuretic Hormone

18.1.2.1 ANH Gene, Precursor Processing, Expression, and Regulation of Release

The structure of the rat *ANH gene* is depicted in figure 18.2. In the human, rat, mouse, and cow, the genomic

Figure 18.1
Structures of human natriuretic peptides: atrionatriuretic hormone (ANP), brain natriuretic peptide (BNP), and C-type natriuretic peptide (CNP). Shaded circles indicate identical amino acids that recur as a regular pattern of 11 ring members. Each ring structure is stabilized by a disulfide bond. The C-terminal tail is essential to the arterial dilator and natriuretic properties of atrionatriuretic hormone. The tail is absent in CNP, which lacks these biological properties. (From Barr et al., 1996.)

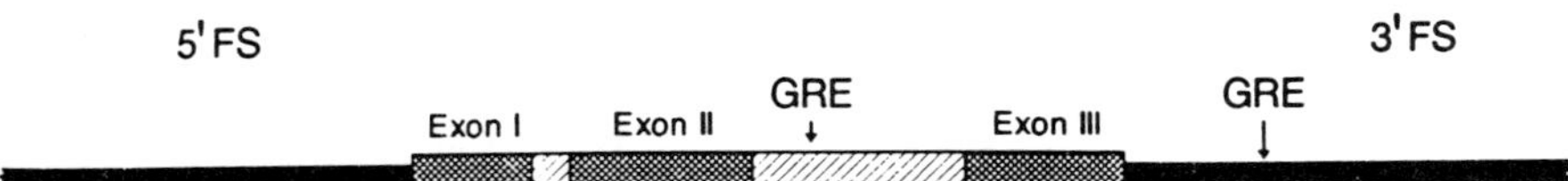

Figure 18.2
Structure of the rat atrionatriuretic hormone gene. Transcribed portions of the gene, represented as a thick line, include the exon (checked pattern) and intron (diagonal lines) sequences. 5′-FS and 3′-FS (flanking regions) are also shown. Relative positions of DNA sequences with putative homology to glucocorticoid regulatory elements (GRE) are identified. (From Gardner et al., 1988.)

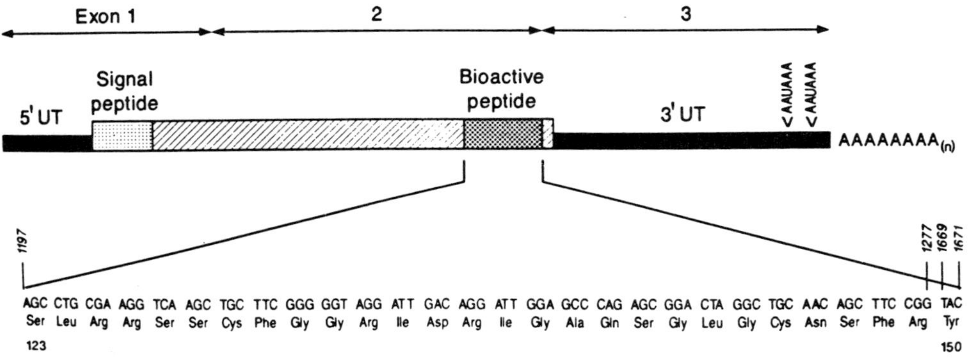

Figure 18.3
Structure of the rat atrial natriuretic hormone (ANH) mRNA. Prepro-ANH coding sequences, depicted by the broad line, include the signal peptide at the N-terminus, the N-terminal portion of the pro-ANH molecule (diagonal lines), and the bioactive ANH peptides at the C-terminus. The 5′-untranslated (UT) and 3′-UT regions are represented by thin dark lines. Two cleavage-polyadenylated signals (AAUAAA) present in the 3′-UT region also are depicted. Sequence contribution of each of the three exons to the ANH mRNA structure are shown above. Detailed DNA sequence of the coding (messenger) strand from that portion of the ANH gene representing the bioactive peptide is presented below. The sequence is arranged in triplets together with the appropriate encoded amino acid. Amino acid positions correspond to amino acids 123–150 in prepro-ANH. (From Gardner et al., 1988.)

DNA sequences are present as single-copy genes, simply organized with three exons and two introns. Exon 1 encodes the 5′-untranslated region, the signal peptide, and the first 16 amino acids of the pro-ANH molecule. Exon 2 encodes most of the prohormone, including the bioactive sequence (figure 18.3). Exon 3 encodes the terminal Tyr (amino acid 151 in human and dog), or Tyr-Arg-Arg in the rat and other mammals. The human ANH gene is assigned to chromosome 1.

Prepro-ANH represents a 149 to 153 amino acid protein, depending on the species (rat and mouse, 152; human, 151; dog, 149). Cleavage of the signal peptide from the human prepro-ANH results in the 126–amino acid *pro-ANH molecule.* In the C-terminal region containing the bioactive ANH sequence, there

1 10 20
Asn Pro Val Tyr Ser Ala Val Ser Asn Thr Asp Leu Met Asp Phe Lys Asn Leu Leu Asp-
(Met) (Asn) (Ala)
30 40
His Leu Glu Glu Lys Met Pro Val Glu Asp Glu Val Met Pro Pro Gln Val Leu Ser Glu Gln-
(Leu) (Val) (Pro)
50 60
Thr Asp Glu Ala Gly Ala Ala Leu Ser Ser Leu Ser Glu Val Pro Pro Trp Thr Gly Glu Val-
(Asn Glu) (Pro) (Pro)
70 80
Asn Pro Ser Gln Arg Asp Gly Gly Ala Leu Gly Leu Gly Arg Gly Pro Trp Asp Pro Ser Asp-
(Ser) (Ala) (Ser)
90 100
Arg Ser Ala Leu Leu Lys Leu Arg Ala Leu Leu Ala Gly Pro Arg Ser Leu Arg Arg Ser Ser-
(Thr Ala)
110 120 126
Cys Phe Gly Gly Arg Ile Asp Arg Ile Gly Ala Gln Ser Gly Leu Gly Cys Asn Ser Phe Arg Tyr
(Met)

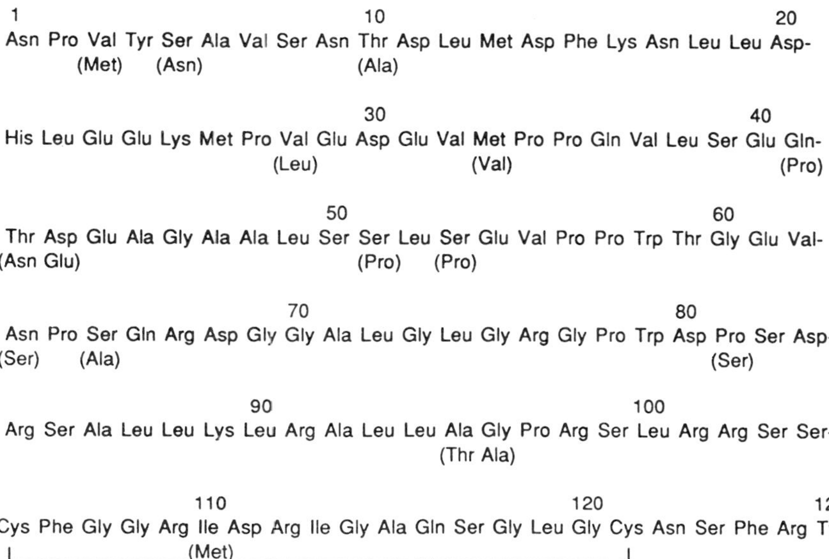

Figure 18.4
Sequences of pro–atrial natriuretic hormone. The prohormone sequence is for the rat; differences for humans at each position are noted in parentheses. (From Adams, 1987.)

is 93% homology between the human, rat, mouse, dog, and rabbit (Oikawa et al., 1985). There is considerably less homology in the introns of the gene.

a. Peptides derived from pro-ANH

The ANH system is a series of peptides of variable size and function that are derived from a 126–amino acid prohormone (figure 18.4). The prohormone, which has a disulfide bridge between Cys^{105} and Cys^{121}, is synthesized in the myocytes of the cardiac atrium and stored in granules for release into the circulation. Cleavage of pro-ANH by proteases results in the formation of the ANH 1–28 sequence at the C-terminal, corresponding to positions 99–126 of the prohormone. The sequence 1–30 is the *long-acting natriuretic peptide (LANP)*; sequence 31–67 acts as a vasodilator; sequence 79–98 has potassium-excreting (kaliuretic) properties. These peptides all have hypotensive, diuretic, natriuretic, or kaliuretic properties, individually or combined, to varying degrees (Overton and Vesely, 1996), and whereas all of them are found in the circulation, ANH 1–28 is the most prevalent circulating form (Gower et al., 1994).

Deletion of the extreme C-terminal Arg-Tyr dipeptide decreases vasodilator properties tenfold; removal of the C-terminal Phe-Arg-Tyr tripeptide decreases vasodilator activity 100-fold and natriuretic-diuretic activity up to 1000-fold (Geller et al, 1984). N-terminal deletions appear to be less important.

There is a considerable difference in the half-lives of these peptides in plasma: ANH and kaliuretic peptide are completely degraded in plasma within 2 hours, whereas LANP and vessel dilator are not significantly degraded after 24 hours' incubation in plasma (Overton and Vesely, 1996).

Expression of ANH is mainly in the atria. In the atrial secretory vesicle, most ANH is present as the 126–amino acid precursor. ANH mRNA transcripts also appear to a much lesser degree in the ventricles, aortic arch, autonomic ganglia, lung, hypothalamus, and in many other brain areas (Gardner et al., 1988), including olfactory regions (Ryan and Gundlach, 1995). A detailed description of mRNA in the brain is provided by Standaert et al. (1988). ANH is also found in lymphoid tissues, in which the immunoreactive form is ANH 5–28, a truncated form of the circulating ANH 1–28. Interestingly, thymic ANH is colocalized in macrophages with β-endorphin (Throsby et al., 1994).

b. ANH peptides in the CNS

The major forms of ANH in the CNS differ from those in the atria and plasma. In atrial extracts, the major form of the prohormone is the 9 kD form, whereas in the brain the lower-weight forms, 1.5 to 1.8 kD, predominate. These are chiefly the 1–24 and 1–25 sequences, in contrast to the ANH 1–28 found in heart and plasma. This difference suggests that tissue-specific processing achieves different ANH peptides and that neural ANH may have quite different functions from peripheral ANH (Samson, 1987).

Release of both the C-terminal and N-terminal ANH prohormone peptides results from atrial stretch. Each of the atrial natriuretic peptides acts as a negative feedback on the other peptides. For example, ANH inhibits the release of LANP, vessel dilator, and kaliuretic peptide (Vesely et al.,1994).

18.1.2.2 Natriuretic Receptors and Second Messengers

Three different natriuretic peptide receptors have been identified (figure 18.5). They are all trans-

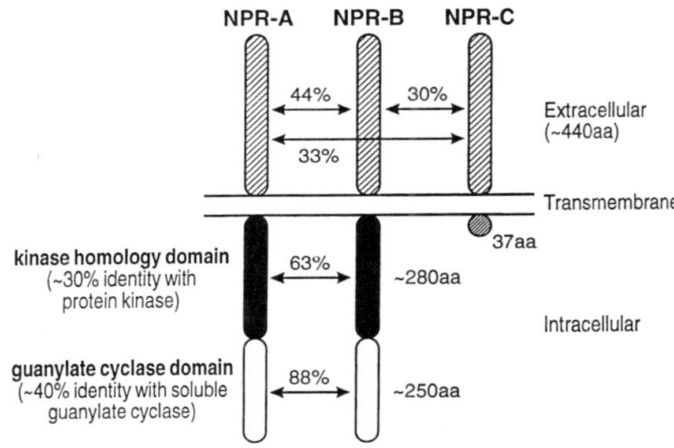

Figure 18.5
Diagram of the natriuretic peptide receptor (NPR) family. Percentages indicate the degree of sequence identity within protein domains for the human receptors. In addition to interaction between the natriuretic peptides and the extracellular domain (hatched), the kinase homology domain (black) plays an important role in regulating enzyme activity. It is this region that includes the binding site for ATP which allows interaction between cyclic guanosine monophosphate production and cellular ATP levels. The natriuretic peptide clearance receptor NPR-C, with its short cytoplasmic tail, binds and internalizes natriuretic peptides prior to their hydrolyzation within lysosomes. (From K. J. Koller and Goeddel, 1992.)

membrane proteins, two of which, *natriuretic peptide receptors (NPR)-A* and *NPR-B*, activate guanylate cyclase and thereby increase cyclic guanosine monophosphate (cGMP) (Nakao et al., 1992). *NPR-C* is the third type of receptor, a "clearance receptor": it does not generate cGMP and instead removes natriuretic peptides from the blood, a rather novel function for a receptor. The clearance receptor has a large N-terminal extracellular domain, a single transmembrane domain, and a short cytoplasmic tail, and binds both native and various truncated forms of ANH with high affinity. (Porter et al., 1989) and removes them by the internalization of the receptor-ligand complex, followed by lysosome hydrolysis. The NPR-C receptor is then rapidly recycled to the cell surface (Nuzzenzeig et al., 1990). NPR-C is widely expressed in kidney, heart, adrenal, and brain (Wilcox et al., 1991). Unlike NPR-A and NPR-B, NPR-C does not stimulate guanylate cyclase but instead inhibits adenylate cyclase and stimulates phosphoinositol hydrolysis, and activates the metabolic clearance and degradation of natriuretic peptides.

The extracellular domains of NPR-A and NPR-B are 44% homologous, and only 30% identical to the C receptor (see figure 18.5). NPR-A and NPR-B contain an important kinase homology domain that includes a binding site for ATP that permits the interaction of cellular ATP with cGMP, for in addition to the relative affinities, the response of a cell to the natriuretic peptides is modulated by cellular ATP levels.

The affinities of the three receptors for their ligands, as determined through the amount of cGMP produced, varies. The order of potency for the formation of cGMP via NPR-A is ANH $\geq$ BNP $\gg$ NPR-C. For NPR-B the order is CNP $>$ ANH $\geq$ BNP. For NPR-C the binding affinity is ANH $>$ CNP $>$ BNP. None of these receptors is preferentially activated by BNP (Suga et al., 1992). There is considerable species variation in the structure and action of BNP and consequently there is some confusion about the relative affinity of the NPR-B for BNP.

a. ANH receptors and second messengers

The rat ANH receptor is a transmembrane glycoprotein, with the ANH binding site on the cell surface. Its molecular weight varies from 140 kD to 65 kD depending on the tissue and species examined. This receptor heterogeneity suggests that more than one form of the receptor may exist in different tissues. For example, there are four distinct molecular forms of the ANH receptor in endothelial cells (Jacobs and Vlasuk, 1987). For most ANH receptors the *second-messenger* pathway for ANH activity is guanylate cyclase and cGMP, with the guanylate cyclase activity located on the cytoplasmic side of the plasma membrane (Kuno et al., 1986), but in some tissues ANH decreases cAMP. The variety of receptor forms may explain the differential degree of response to ANH by various tissues.

Smooth muscle cells of the vasculature are heavily supplied with ANH receptors, about 500,000 per aortic muscle cell (Schenk et al., 1985). ANH receptors are found in the zona glomerulosa of the adrenal gland, the region in which synthesis and secretion of aldosterone occurs. ANH receptors are present in the renal cortex, including the glomeruli and renal artery; in the renal pelvis; and in intermedullary tissue, including the collecting tubule. The number of glomerular receptor sites for ANH varies with the salt intake: a low salt intake upregulates these receptors; dehydration depresses ANH synthesis and augments receptor number, indicating that ANH is a circulating hormone that participates in the regulation of extracellular fluid volume (Jacobs and Vlasuk, 1987).

ANH receptors are present in the CNS, especially in the hypothalamus and the circumventricular organs, as well as in many other CNS sites, including the pituitary and cerebellum (Quiron et al., 1986).

18.1.2.3 Actions of ANH

ANH has important regulatory actions on the cardiovascular system, integrated with water and electrolyte homeostasis. Increased atrial pressure or atrial volume stimulates the release of ANH from atrial myocytes. This results in vasodilation and a shift of fluid into the interstitial spaces. ANH also increases

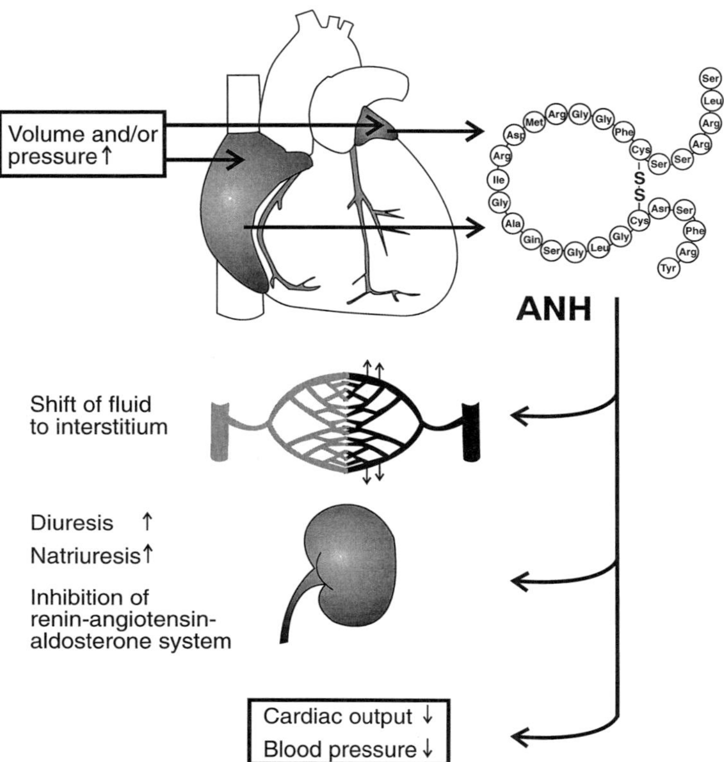

Figure 18.6
Atrial natriuretic hormone (ANH) is secreted from the cardiac atria in response to increased atrial pressure or volume. Circulating ANH acts on the microvasculature to induce a shift of fluid into the interstitial space. ANH also increases fluid loss from the kidneys and inhibits the renin-angiotensin-aldosterone system. The combined effects of ANH on various organs causes a reduction in cardiac output and systemic blood pressure. (From Christensen, 1995.)

diuresis and natriuresis, through direct action on renal glomerular filtration rate and through decreased medullary hypertonicity. In addition, ANH is a potent antagonist of the renin-angiotensin-aldosterone system, inhibiting angiotensin-mediated vasoconstriction. The consequent loss of water and salt, together with the shift of fluid out of the systemic circulation, rapidly decreases atrial pressure, resulting in a fall in cardiac output and blood pressure (figures 18.6 and 18.7.).

ANH acts as a *neuromodulator* in the brain where it participates in cardiovascular control. Most ANH-containing cell bodies are found in the anteroventral third ventricle (AV3V) region which is involved in the maintenance of cardiovascular function and in fluid and electrolyte balance. ANH has a general de-

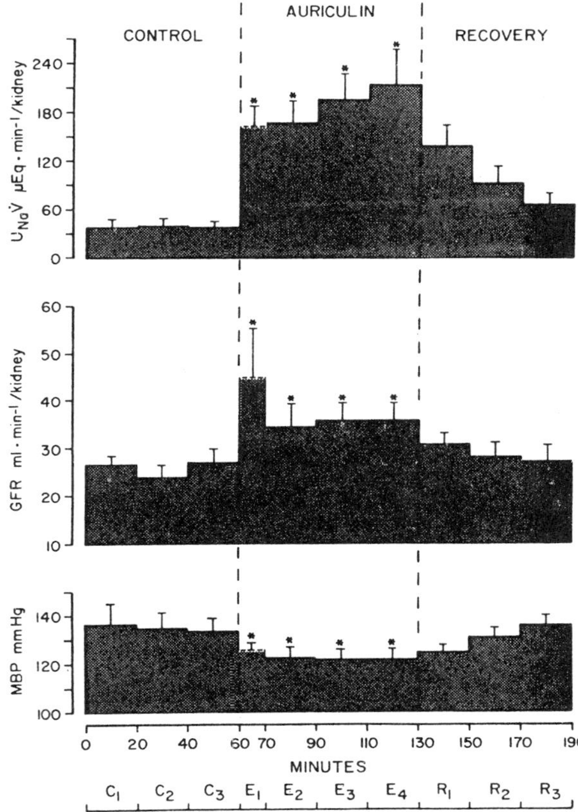

Figure 18.7
Time course of effects of synthetic atrial natriuretic hormone (auriculin) on mean blood pressure (MBP), glomerular filtration rate (GFR), and sodium excretion ($U_{Na}\dot{V}$) in anesthetized dogs. ANH was given as a 1.0 μg/kg prime followed by a constant infusion of 0.1 $\mu g.kg^{-1}.minute^{-1}$. C, control; E, experimental; R, recovery periods. (From Maack et al., 1984.)

pressant effect on central neurons. ANH inhibits the firing of PVN neurons causing a depressor effect on the AV3V region, and lowering blood pressure through this central mechanism (Ku and Zhang, 1994). The AV3V region also receives important afferent input from ascending serotoninergic axons which activate ANH release (Reis et al., 1994). ANH also affects cardiac electrophysiological indices, including heart rate, intra-atrial conduction time, and the refractory period. These effects are both direct on cardiac tissue and indirect through ANH's vagoexcitatory and sympathoinhibitory actions (Clemo et al., 1996).

In most instances, ANH acts as an inhibitory hormone. It inhibits POMC synthesis and the release of ACTH. This occurs as ANH passes from the hypothalamus into hypophysial portal blood where most ANH is in the form of ANH 5–28, in contrast to circulating ANH 1–28 (Lim et al., 1994). In the pancreas, ANH inhibits glucagon release by a mechanism that involves cGMP and an inhibition of Ca^{2+} uptake (Verspohl and Bernemann, 1996).

Behavioral effects of ANH, apart from regulation of water intake, include anxiolytic effects, which are antagonized by an endogenous indole, *isatin*.

18.1.2.4 Integration of ANH Actions with VP and Angiotensin II

The central effects of ANH appear to be well integrated with the actions of two other neuropeptides, VP (ADH) and AT II. The distribution of ANH and ANH receptors in the CNS suggests that ANH may influence fluid and electrolyte balance at several levels, two of the most important being inhibition of water intake and suppression of VP release.

a. *Inhibition of water intake*

AT II is a potent stimulus to drinking, an action mediated partly through receptors in the subfornical

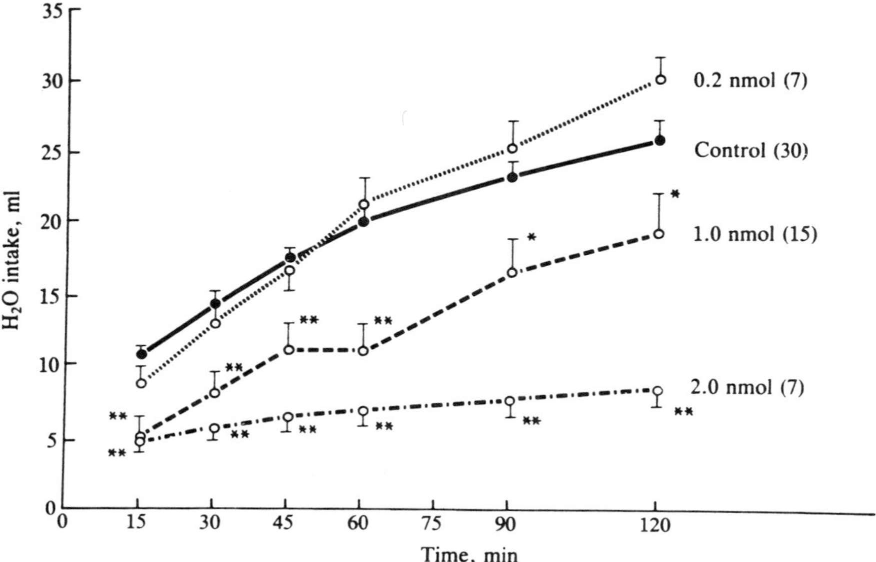

Figure 18.8
Cumulative water intake following third cerebroventricular infusion of 2 μL saline (control) or saline-containing atrial natriuretic hormone in overnight, water-deprived rats. $^{*}P < .01$; $^{**}P < .001$. (From Antunes-Rodrigues et al., 1985.)

organ. Central administration of ANH inhibits spontaneous drinking (figure 18.8) and antagonizes the dipsogenic and dehydrating effects of AT II (Lappe et al., 1986).

b. Suppression of VP release from the posterior pituitary

The antidiuretic effects of VP are in contrast to the diuretic actions of ANH, and central or peripheral administration of ANH inhibits the basal secretion of VP. This is probably a direct action of ANH on VP neurons since pressure microinjection of ANH on VP neurons in the PVN causes a long-lasting inhibition of neuronal firing (figure 18.9). These three neuropeptides, VP, ANH, and AT II, form a close neuronal network along a subfornical organ-preoptic-hypothalamic axis to regulate body fluid volume (Palkowits et al., 1995).

18.1.2.5 Integration of ANH with Endothelin

Endothelin (ET) is a 21–amino acid peptide that belongs to a family of isopeptides (ET-1, ET-2, and ET-3) with strong vasoconstrictor activity and which modulates the circulating levels of other neuropeptides, including the natriuretic peptides and VP (Fukada et al., 1988; Shichiri et al., 1989). The endothelins are synthesized by endothelial cells and differ only slightly from each other. Endothelin receptors are found in several tissues, including the heart, lungs, kidney, adrenal, pituitary, and CNS. In the CNS, endothelin receptors are localized in areas concerned with water and electrolyte balance, including the

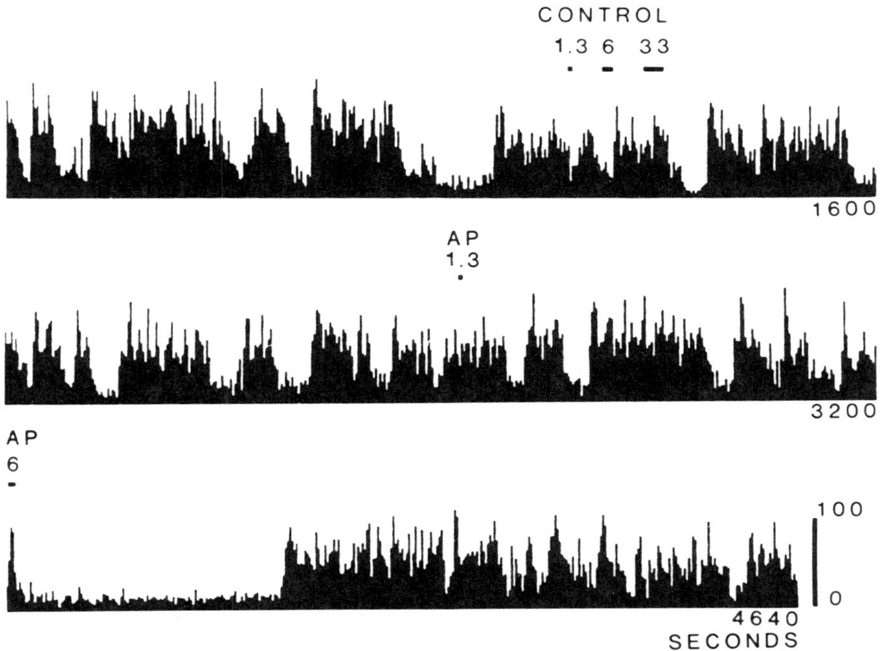

Figure 18.9
A continuous-time histogram to show the effect of atrial natriuretic hormone (ANH) on the activity of presumptive vasopressin (VP) units in the posterior magnocellular part of the paraventricular nucleus. The phasic firing pattern is typical of VP neurons. An inactive analog of ANH (control) applied by pressure microinjection in quantities of 1.3 and 6 fmol had no effect on neuronal firing. Application of 1.3 fmol of ANH was also ineffective, but the 6-fmol dose of ANH promptly caused a profound and long-lasting inhibition of firing, followed immediately by a spontaneous return of the neurons to their previous firing rate. AP, action potential. (From Standaert et al., 1988.)

PVN and supraoptic nucleus (SON), and the posterior pituitary. ET is released from the posterior pituitary in response to water deprivation, and ICV injections of ET increase the secretion of OT and VP and activate the sympathetic nervous system. These antidiuretic effects oppose the actions of ANH and imply that ET may balance the actions of ANH on water and salt homeostasis (Antunes-Rodriques, 1993).

18.1.3 Brain Natriuretic Peptide

18.1.3.1 The BNP Gene and Its Expression

BNP is derived mainly from cardiac ventricular cells and has structural and physiological similarities to ANH (see figure 18.1). The human *BNP gene* is located on chromosome 1, as is the ANH gene. The mouse BNP gene is organized into three exons and two introns. BNP transcripts are found predominantly in the ventricles, but are also present in the CNS and in many peripheral tissues, including the lung, thyroid, adrenal, kidney, spleen, small intestine, ovary, uterus, and striated muscle, suggesting that BNP has paracrine or autocrine functions in these organs. There are some differences in the expression of ANH and BNP transcripts in rat and human tissues.

18.1.3.2 Release of BNP and Its Actions

BNP is released simultaneously with ANH in response to atrial stretch, but its physiological role is still to be ascertained. BNP secretion is greatly increased in patients with congestive heart failure or hypertensive heart disease with cardiac hypertrophy. This increased secretion may be considered a compensatory mechanism against ventricular overload, since the natriuretic, diuretic, and vasodilator actions of ANH and BNP reduce both cardiac preload and afterload.

In patients with essential hypertension, both BNP and ANH are released in response to sodium restriction (which decreases their release) and sodium loading (which augments their release), inplying that the two neuropeptides form a dual peptide system contributing to the maintenance of sodium balance and blood pressure. BNP also has natriuretic properties, which are not as effective as those of ANH. The vasodilator effects of BNP are seen in arteries constricted by AT II or endothelin: BNP has potent relaxing effects on rat and human arterial tissue, with a considerably weaker relaxing effect on veins.

18.1.4 C-Type Natriuretic Peptide

CNP, the third member of the natriuretic family, was originally identified in the CNS, where it is present in much higher concentrations than either ANH or BNP (Sudoh et al., 1990). CNP is structurally homologous with atrial and brain natriuretic peptides (see figure 18.1) but its gene and precursor molecules are different from the ANH gene and precursor. CNP is the dominant active natriuretic peptide in the hypothalamus and the anterior pituitary has the highest concentration of CNP anywhere in the body. CNP has also been detected in the systemic circulation. In addition, CNP is produced by vascular endothelial cells, the kidney, seminal fluid, the uterus, intestine, and immune system. Its widespread distribution in the endothelium of peripheral blood vessels extends its action beyond that of involvement in the control of blood pressure and salt and water homeostasis, to include that of a vasodilator acting on vasculature at or near its site of production.

18.1.4.1 The CNP Gene, Precursor Processing, and Regulation of Release

The *CNP gene* has at least two exons in the coding region for prepro-CNP. The gene is flanked in the 5′-region by regulatory elements that are not part of the ANH or BNP genes, indicating different transcription mechanisms for the CNP gene. CNP-22 is derived from a preprohormone of 126 amino acids, and a pro-CNP, which is processed to form CNP-53 and CNP-22 (figure 18.10). CRP-22 has a molecular weight of about 2200 and incorporates a ring structure that is common to all the natriuretic peptides and which conveys biological activity, but it lacks the C-terminal tail necessary for arterial vasodilator and diuretic properties (see figure 18.1). The predominant form of CNP in the circulation is CNP-22; that found in endothelium is CNP-53, which is sometimes referred to as the storage form of CNP-22, but has also been reported to have venodilator properties. CNP-53 is present in human urine in greater concentrations than CNP-22 (Mattingly et al., 1994).

Many factors regulate the transcription of the CNP gene and *release* of the active CNP. The cytokines, tumor necrosis factor, interleukin-1, and transforming

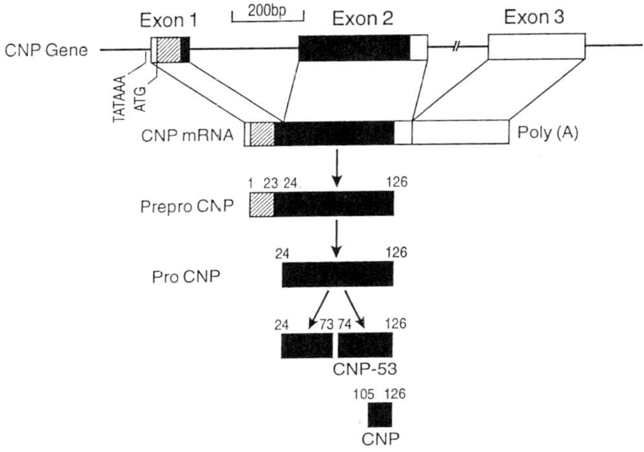

Figure 18.10
Gene structure and biosynthetic pathway of human C-type natriuretic peptide (CNP). The putative transcriptional start site and exon 3 are indicated by the open boxes. The first two stages take place within the cell nucleus. Prepro-CNP, pro-CNP, and CNP-53 have all been identified within the cell, but CNP-22 does not appear to be found within the cell. Hatched bar is the signal peptide sequence; black bar is the prohormone sequence. (From Barr et al., 1996.)

growth factor, influence CNP release in culture (Suga et al., 1993), and CNP, in turn, modulates the effects of the cytokines on vascular cell proliferation and migration. Both ANH and BNP stimulate CNP secretion but BNP has 20 times the stimulatory effect of ANH.

18.1.4.2 CNP Receptors and Second Messengers

Both ANH and CNP produce vasodilation through increasing cGMP in arterial smooth muscle cells, activating two distinct receptors, *natriuretic peptide receptor-A (NPR-A)* and natriuretic *peptide receptor-B (NPR-B)*. The NPR-B receptor, present in the adrenal medulla, pituitary, and cerebellum (Wilcox et al., 1991), is highly specific for CNP, binding CNP with an affinity three times greater than either ANH or BNP.

In the hypothalamus CNP binds to NPR-B, which is found throughout the hypothalamus, including the neurons of the PVN, the subfornical organ, and the SON. mRNA for natriuretic peptide B receptor is also present in the posterior pituitary. As these areas are all intimately concerned with neuroendocrine regulation, CNP may well be integrated into these complex regulatory mechanisms (Langub et al., 1995).

18.1.4.3 Actions of CNP

CNP is a potent vasorelaxant, causing marked vasodilation. CNP relaxes venous tissue but is not always effective on arterial tissue. CNP does, however, relax bronchial smooth muscle. The effects of CNP on natriuresis are uncertain. The hemodynamic effects of CNP are species-dependent: in rats and dogs, but not in humans, administration of low dosages of CNP causes systemic hypotension due to a fall in blood pressure and cardiac output.

Unlike ANH, CNP does not affect the renin-angiotensin system but does induce catecholamine production in the adrenal medulla (Tsutsui et al., 1994). CNP has been reported to inhibit the release of LH in the pituitary (Samson et al., 1993), and the extremely high levels of CNP in the pituitary portend other important endocrine actions for this peptide.

18.1.5 Clinical Implications of Natriuretic Peptides

Increased levels of circulating ANH and BNP, but not CNP, are associated with congestive heart failure. It is not understood why the elevated ANH levels are related to the retention of salt and water in these patients. However, the kidneys become less responsive to the natriuretic action of the neuropeptide hormone, which may be the critical point for the development of edema and salt retention. Renal hyporesponsiveness is related to the activation of opposing sodium-retaining systems, especially the renin-angiotensin-aldosterone system. Blockers of antinatriuretic factors or agents that decrease the degradation of ANH may be therapeutically useful (Winaver et al., 1995).

Endogenous levels of ANH are increased in patients with essential hypertension, who also have exaggerated renal responses to administered ANH. In patients with dilated cardiomyopathy and severe heart failure, plasma BNH levels are higher than ANH levels, in contrast to BNP levels in healthy persons, which are only about 16% of that of ANH. Consequently, BNP may be involved in physiological processes in a manner different from that of ANH, and the atrium and ventricle may have different functions under various pathophysiological conditions (Makino et al., 1996).

Transgenic mice that overexpress the BNP gene have a 10- to 100-fold increase in plasma BNP and an elevated plasma cGMP concentration. These transgenic mice have significantly lower blood pressure than their nontransgenic littermates, indicating that a role for BNP, perhaps, as a long-term therapeutic agent (Ogawa et al., 1994), may be useful.

18.2 Angiotensin

18.2.1 The Renin-Angiotensin Systems

18.2.1.1 Peripheral Angiotensin Systems

The first component of the renin-angiotensin system was discovered in 1898 by Tigerstedt and Bergman who found that a kidney extract increased blood pressure. The active component was named *renin*, which is synthesized and released into the circulation by the juxtaglomerular cells of the kidney. Renin acts as an protease to cleave the relatively inert liver protein, *angiotensinogen*, present in the circulation, to a decapeptide, *angiotensin I* (figure 18.11). Angiotensin I is converted by *angiotensin-converting enzyme (ACE)* to the highly active octapeptide *AT II*. ACE is present in many tissues such as the lung and kidney. Circulating AT II acts on peripheral high-affinity AT II receptors in vascular smooth muscle, the zona glomerulosa of the adrenal gland, and the kidney to cause vasoconstriction, aldosterone secretion, and sodium retention, affecting blood volume and blood pressure, and water and salt homeostasis.

Angiotensinogen is the limiting factor in the production of AT II, so that control of renin secretion is pivotal to the renin-angiotensin system. Renin is secreted by the juxtamedullary cells in the afferent arteriole of the renal glomerulus, in response to hypovolemia or hypertonicity of the blood. The renin response is modified by the chemoreceptors of the macula densa in the distal convoluted tubule. Together, the juxtamedullary cells and the macula densa

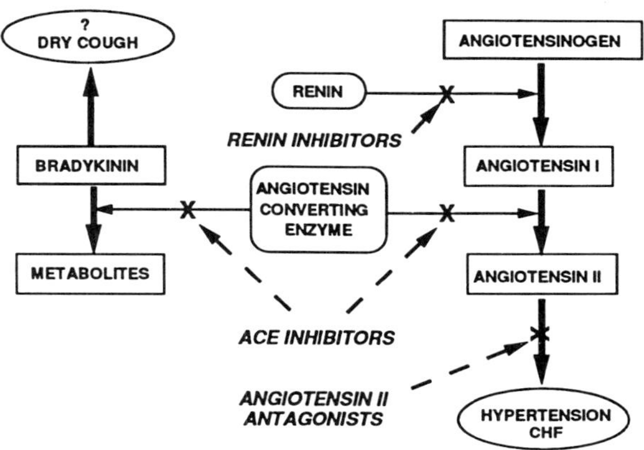

Figure 18.11
Schematic diagram of the components of the renin-angiotensin system, showing the points of inhibition of several classes of drugs. ACE, angiotensin-converting enzyme; CHF, congestive heart failure. A side effect of ACE inhibitors may be a dry cough, due to ACE-inhibitor stimulation of bradykinin. (From Brooks and Ruffolo, 1994.)

cells form the juxtaglomerular apparatus which controls renin secretion.

The production of renin has classically been considered as limited to the kidney but it is now realized that local AT II generating systems exist in many organs such as the brain, kidneys, adrenals, testes, and arterial wall. AT II and its receptors have now been found in many different tissues, including the arterial wall, kidney, adrenal heart, gonads, and pituitary gland (Inagami et al., 1988), raising the likelihood that AT II may have autocrine, paracrine, and even intracellular actions.

18.2.1.2 Brain and Pituitary Angiotensin System

Circulating AT II has central effects, increasing blood pressure by a direct action on CNS receptors, but AT II is also produced locally in the brain and pituitary to form a central angiotensin system that is vital to the control of cardiovascular functions; fluid homeostasis, including water intake; and the release of pituitary hormones (Saavedra, 1992). Angiotensinergic neurons with cell bodies in the rostral hypothalamus project into the ME, releasing AT II into the hypophyseal portal vessels to inhibit the release of PRL, GH and TSH from the anterior pituitary (Franci et al., 1997). AT II is also implicated in the pathophysiology of several diseases, including hypertension and congestive heart failure. The ability of central administration of AT II to elicit drinking behavior (Fitzsimons, 1969) initiated considerable interest in the central neural systems and mechanisms that mediated these effects, studies that are continuing today.

18.2.2 Phylogenetic Distribution of Angiotensin Peptides

An angiotensin I–like molecule with a 78.5% homology with the N-terminal part of human angiotensinogen has been purified from the leech (Laurent et al., 1995). AT II–like immunoreactivity and ACE-like enzyme activity are also present in tissues of the crab. The presence of these molecules in invertebrates, and in vertebrates from fish to primates, reflects the high degree of conservation of angiotensins in evolution and their importance in water and electrolyte homeostasis and volume control.

18.2.3 Structure of Angiotensins

There are several native AT peptides and AT receptor subtypes.

AT I	Asp-Arg-Val-Tyr-Ile-His-Pro-Phe-His-Leu
AT II	Asp-Arg-Val-Tyr-Ile-His-Pro-Phe
AT III	Arg-Val-Tyr-Ile-His-Pro-Phe
AT IV	Val-Tyr-Ile-His-Pro-Phe

AT I is inactive and the other three angiotensins interact with different receptor subtypes: AT II binds primarily at the AT_1 site, but also interacts at the AT_2 receptor site; AT III acts at the AT_1 and AT_2 receptor sites, and AT IV acts primarily at the AT_4 site but may also bind at the AT_1 and AT_2 sites.

The angiotensins have different potencies for various physiological parameters. AT II and AT III are equipotent in evoking maximum pressor responses and drinking behavior, but AT IV is far less effective. The puny effects of AT IV are attributed to its preferential binding to the AT_4 receptor, which does not appear to be involved in these physiological and behavioral responses (Wright et al., 1996).

18.2.4 Angiotensinogen Gene Expression; Angiotensin Precursor Processing and Regulation of Release

The *angiotensinogen gene* has been cloned and angiotensinogen mRNA is expressed in the brain and the liver. In studies of normotensive and hypertensive rats, there is a 28% greater expression of the angiotensinogen gene in the anteroventral hypothalamus, preoptic area, and medial septum of the hypertensive strain. Interestingly, there were no differences between strains in gene expression in the liver. The enhanced activity of the brain angiotensin system in the hypertensive rats may be due to differences in the brain angiotensinogen gene (Yongue et al., 1991).

Processing of angiotensin I by peptidases results in the formation of the different angiotensins. ACE converts the decapeptide AT I to the octapeptide AT II. In the brain, AT II is converted by amino peptidase A by N-terminal cleavage to AT III, which is the active form of angiotensin in the central control of cardiovascular functions (Wright et al, 1996). This conversion of AT II to AT III is also required for the release of VP by AT II and makes AT III one of the main effector peptides of the renin-angiotensin system in the control of VP release (Zini et al. 1996). Angiotensin I can also produce AT III by a metabolic pathway independent of ACE activity. Aminopeptidase N is responsible for the N-terminal cleavage of AT III to produce AT IV.

Release of AT II is regulated by volume and osmotic changes; hypovolemia or hypo-osmolarity result in an increase in both peripheral and central AT II, with increased blood pressure resulting from arterial vasoconstriction. AT II-induced secretion of aldosterone and VP (and perhaps OT) diminish the loss of sodium and water through increased reabsorption in the kidney, thereby restoring extracellular water and electrolyte stores. These peripheral effects are integrated with central effects that increase drinking and salt appetite. The consequent restoration of fluid volume terminates the release of AT II. AT II release is also modulated by glucocorticoids, which increase the number of AT II receptors following adrenalectomy and potentiate the dipsogenic action of AT II, and by minerocorticoids, which increase AT II receptor expression and enhance sodium appetite (Fluharty and Epstein, 1983). Catecholamines, dopamine, and estrogen are all considered to play a role in AT II release.

18.2.5 Angiotensin Receptors and Second Messengers

The *AT_1 receptor gene* is represented as a single-copy gene in most species, except for rodents, which have two gene copies that encode highly homologous AT_1 receptors in rat and mouse. This is probably due to gene duplication occurring following the branching of the rodent order from the mammalian phylogenetic tree, but prior to the divergence of the rat and mouse (figure 18.12). The probable gene duplication

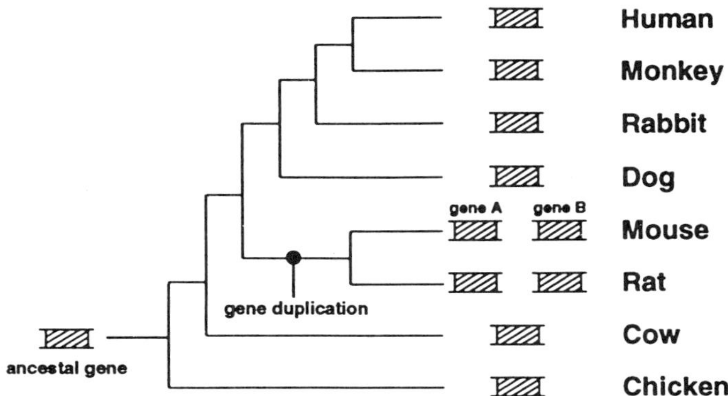

Figure 18.12
The evolution of the angiotensin II type T (AT_1) receptor gene. Phylogenetic relationships are constructed based on hemoglobin amino acid sequence data. The period wherein the proposed duplication occurred is indicated by the circle. (From Czelusniak et al., 1990.)

occurred approximately 24 million years ago. Human chromosome 3 bears the single AT_1 receptor gene in the human genome. There is 34% homology between the AT_1 and AT_2 receptor subtypes. The amino acid sequences encoded by the genomic DNA of all species consists of 359 amino acid residues with a molecular weight of approximately 41 kD.

The AT_1 and AT_2 receptors have seven transmembrane domains, characteristic of the superfamily of G protein–coupled receptors (Mukoyama et al., 1993). All AT_1 receptors possess four cysteine residues, suggestive of two disulfide bridges (figure 18.13). The AT receptors are a heterogeneous group, consisting of at least four different subtypes, AT_1, AT_2, AT_3, and AT_4, which mediate the different functions of the three angiotensins. Most is known about the AT_1 binding site, which mediates the classical angiotensin responses concerned with water balance and the maintenance of blood pressure. There is considerable evidence that there may be more than one AT_1 receptor subtype.

Less is known about the AT_2 site, which binds both AT II and AT III and may be involved in vascular growth. The AT_3 site was discovered in cultured neuroblastoma cells and the AT_4 site preferentially binds AT IV and is involved in memory acquisition and retrieval, as well as the regulation of blood flow (Wright and Harding, 1994). From this incomplete description it is obvious that there are still many questions to be answered concerning the functions of the different AT receptor subtypes. All the known functions mediated by AT II receptors seem to be mediated by AT_1 receptors and the functions of the AT_2 receptors is unclear. *Second-messenger pathways* for the AT_1 and AT_2 receptors differ. AT_1 receptors use the phospholipase C–induced calcium mobilization as well as the inhibition of adenylate cyclase. The AT_2 receptor signal transduction system involves inhibition of cGMP.

These receptor subtypes are differentially *expressed*. The proportional distribution of AT_1 and AT_2 receptors is tissue- and species-dependent, but in all

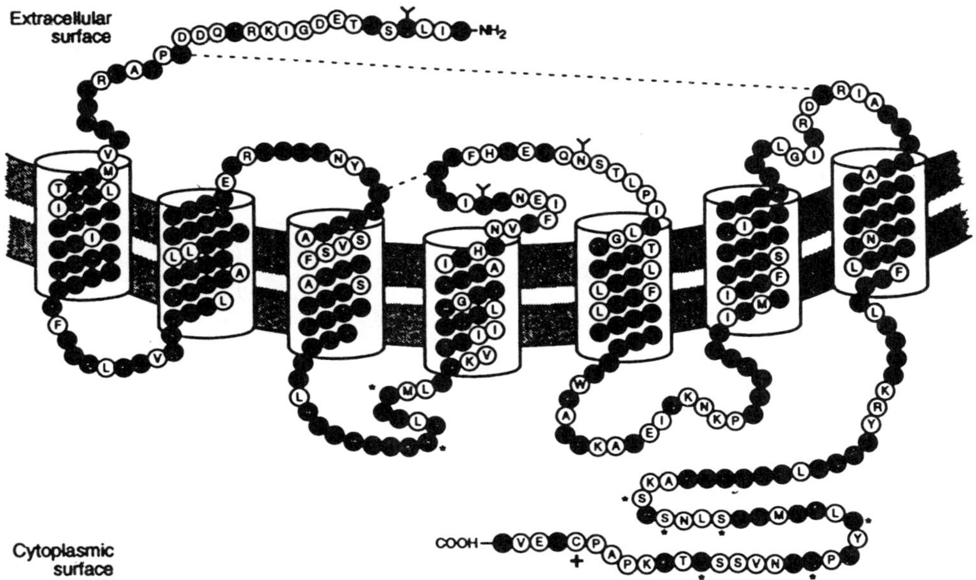

Figure 18.13
Secondary structure model for the distribution of the human angiotensin II (AT_1) receptor in the plasma membrane. The amino acids in the seven transmembrane-spanning domain helices are depicted within cylindrical columns embedded within the membrane. Also shown are amino acid sequences connecting the successive helices and forming loops in the cytoplasmic and extracellular space. The darkened residues denote amino acids conserved between the human AT II receptor and a cloned amphibian AT II receptor. Potential sites for post-translational glycosylation are marked above the sequence by a Y; potential disulfide bridges between extracellular cysteine residues are indicated by dashed lines; asterisks denote potential phosphorylation sites; the cross indicates a possible palmitoylation site. Letters indicate codes for amino acids (see appendix C). (From Bergsma, 1994.)

species the major physiological functions, such as cardiovascular, fluid, and electrolyte regulation, are mediated by the AT_1 receptor. It is interesting that in fetal and neonatal tissue, AT_2 receptors are more highly concentrated than in adult tissue, suggesting that AT II may be involved in fetal growth and differentiation

Most AT II receptors are found in the heart and blood vessels and these are primarily AT_1-type receptors. In most species, the predominant form in the adrenal cortex is the AT_1 receptor; in the adrenal medulla of some species there may be more AT_2 binding sites (Edwards and Ruffolo, 1994). The kidney contains AT II receptors in the glomerulus, proximal tubule, vasa recta, and juxtaglomerular cells, most of which are of the AT_2 type. The lung and reproductive organs also express mRNA for AT II receptors. In the CNS, AT_2 receptor mRNA is high in the lateral septum, thalamic nuclei, locus ceruleus, and the inferior olive, as well as in several brain nuclei and numerous brainstem nuclei (Lenkei et al., 1996).

Regulation of the AT_1 receptor is by several mechanisms: downregulation by AT II, which follows the rapid internalization of AT II; regulation of gene expression by AT II, aldosterone, and glucocorticoids; and regulation of the signal transduction mechanisms involving G protein coupling.

18.2.6 Angiotensin-Converting Enzyme and Angiotensin II Receptor Antagonists

There are many ACE inhibitors, the best known of which is captopril, the first ACE inhibitor to be investigated. The disruption of the renin-angiotensin system by ACE inhibitors has provided an effective therapy for several diseases, such as hypertension and congestive heart failure. The development of antagonists to specific AT receptor subtypes has had great importance in delineating the functions of these receptors. Effective nonpeptide antagonists to AT_1 receptors include losartin and SK&F 108566, which are able to block all functions mediated by AT II. Another group of AT II receptor antagonists is specific for the AT_2 receptor and includes the nonpeptide PD123319. These antagonists are very useful in characterizing the AT II receptor subtypes, but as the functions of AT II all seem to be mediated by the AT_1 receptors, little therapeutic benefit is foreseen for the AT_2 antagonists.

18.2.7 Actions of Angiotensins

18.2.7.1 Peripheral Angiotensin II Functions

AT II has a potent direct vasoconstrictor effect on vascular smooth muscle, as well as an indirect action evoked through the sympathetic nervous system. The vascular responsiveness to AT II is increased by increased sodium intake and decreased by sodium restriction. The renin-angiotensin system has the dual capability of simultaneously regulating arterial vasomotion and extracellular blood volume, thus exerting a fine control over blood pressure and water and salt balance.

AT II stimulates vascular smooth muscle cell hypertrophy and proliferation in normal and in injured arterial walls in animals, but this action has not been clearly demonstrated in humans. AT II also has direct and indirect effects on the kidney. There are three main direct effects on the kidney (Ichikawa and Harris, 1991). AT II decreases renal blood flow by acting on the afferent and efferent arterioles and has variable effects on glomerular filtration rate (figure 18.14). AT II has an important third function as a modulator of proximal tubule reabsorption, in general increasing reabsorption through its dual actions on receptors in the efferent arteriole smooth muscle and on proximal tubule epithelial cells (figure 18.15). Consequently, AT II is a highly efficient regulator of net proximal fluid transport. AT II also suppresses renin formation through a short negative feedback loop. All these actions of AT II are inhibited by ANH, AT II antagonists, or by ACE inhibitors. The indirect effects of AT II are through stimulation of the zona glomerulosa of the adrenal gland to secrete aldosterone, which also increases tubular reabsorption of Na^+.

AT II has effects on carbohydrate metabolism through stimulation of the biosynthesis of glucocorticoids by the zona fasciculata or reticularis of the adrenal. AT II may be involved in the regulation of blood glucose by stimulating hepatic gluconeogenesis and glycogenolysis.

18.2.7.2 Central Actions of Angiotensins

AT II has an important role in physiological drinking behavior and salt appetite. AT II, together with afferent neural input from cardiovascular baroreceptors, stimulates thirst and salt intake in rats. This is inhibited

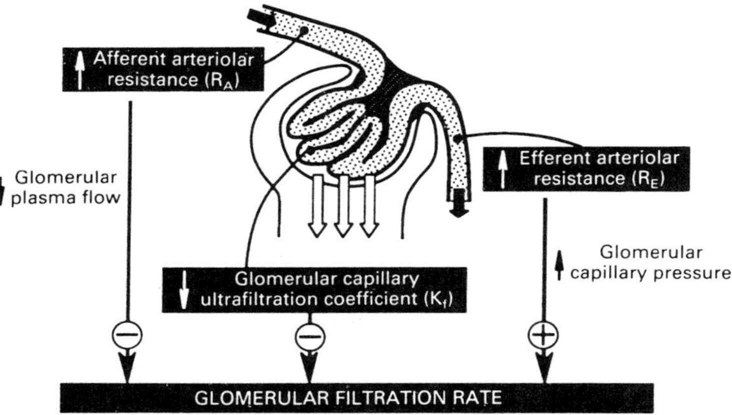

Figure 18.14
Effector sites of angiotensin II (AT II) within the glomerular microcirculation. The constrictor action of AT II raises afferent (R_A) and efferent (R_E) resistances and reduces the glomerular capillary ultrafiltration coefficient (K_f). While an increase in R_A and reduction in K_f tend to reduce glomerular filtration rate (GFR), an increase in R_E, in some circumstances, serves to raise (or prevent reduction in) GFR. The magnitude of the constrictor effect of AT II on these targets is not uniform among different pathophysiological states for reasons largely unknown, the net effect of AT II being to raise, lower, or have no impact on GFR. (From Ichikawa and Harris, 1991.)

by central OT administration. The circumventricular organs appear to be the site of action for circulating AT II on the dipsogenic response (Simpson, 1981).

AT II, AT III, and AT IV all evoke pressor responses, drinking behavior, and salt appetite when centrally administered, but the effects of AT II and AT III are more potent than those of AT IV. These effects are all mediated through the AT_1 receptor subtype (Wright et al., 1996). AT II applied iontophoretically excites vasomotor neurons in the rostral ventrolateral medulla that regulate blood pressure (L. C. S. Silva et al., 1993). The increased firing of these neurons is greater in spontaneously hypertensive rats than in normotensive rats, indicating that a heightened sensitivity to AT II may underlie the hypertension in these rats (Chan and Wong, 1995).

AT II acts as a *neuromodulator.* Within the CNS, AT II increases sympathetic activity, facilitates the release of epinephrine from sympathetic nerve terminals, and stimulates transmission in the adrenal medulla and sympathetic ganglia. The release of epinephrine is facilitated by presynaptic actions on prejunctional AT_1 receptors. The resulting hypertension is due to neurally mediated vasoconstriction (Reid, 1992).

AT II has central neuroendocrine effects, altering the release of pituitary and hypothalamic neuropeptides. AT II releases ACTH from the pituitary by a direct action on the corticotrophs and indirectly by stimulating CRH or by its potent ability to release VP. AT II also stimulates PRL and LH release, the latter effect being modulated by estrogen levels. This seems to be the first evidence of a role for the AT_2

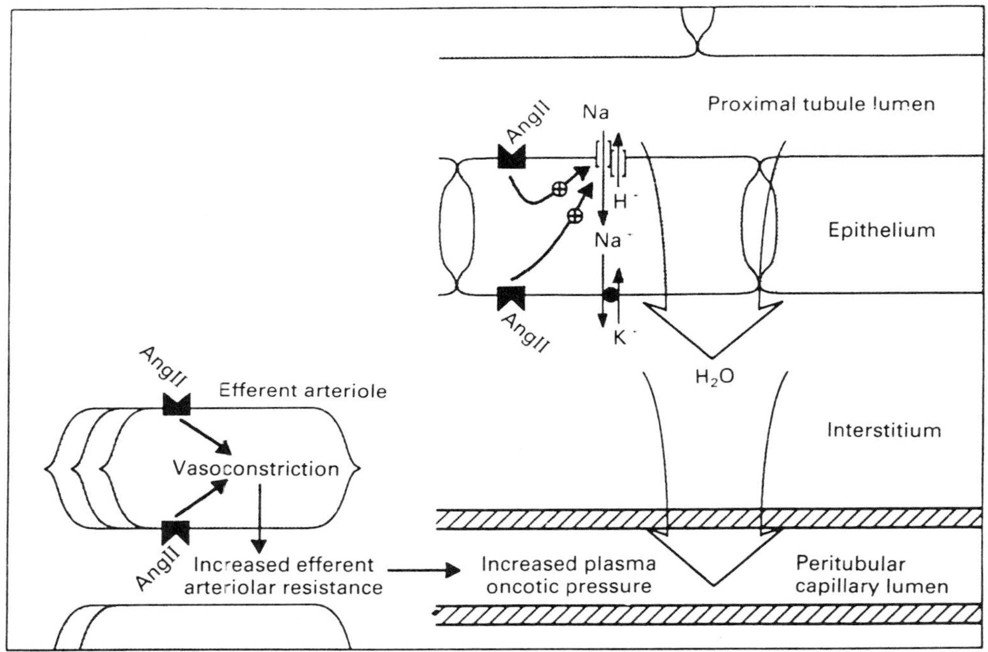

Figure 18.15
Effect of angiotensin II (AngII) on proximal tubule transport. Angiotensin II, through specific receptors present in both postglomerular vascular smooth muscle cells (i.e., efferent arteriole) and proximal tubule epithelial cells, regulates not only the transepithelial fluid transport but also the transcapillary fluid transport. These two transport processes are series-linked, that is, transport from tubule lumen to interstitium, and from interstitium to peritubular capillary compartment. Angiotensin II activates Na^+, H^+ transport in the proximal tubule, and assists transport into the peritubular capillary lumen through constriction of the efferent arteriole and increased oncotic pressure. (From Ichikawa and Harris, 1991.)

receptor subtype, as both AT_1 and AT_2 receptor antagonists block AT II–induced PRL and LH secretion (Stephenson and Steele, 1992).

The *behavioral effects* of AT II extend to actions beyond those involved in drinking and salt appetite, including changes in cognitive function, anxiogenesis, and reduced male sexual behavior. The cognitive actions are demonstrated by central administration of AT II, or of renin, which can generate brain AT II, with resulting defects in passive avoidance behavior (M. Koller et al., 1975). Both cognitive effects and anxiogenesis are prevented by ACE inhibitors.

18.2.8 Clinical Implications of Angiotensin

The therapeutic effects of blocking the production of AT II through the inhibition of ACE have been evaluated in many diseases. ACE inhibitors, such as captopril, are extremely effective as hypotensive drugs. They prevent the formation of AT II and lower blood pressure by systemic arteriolar dilation in patients with essential hypertension. The advantage of the ACE inhibitors is that they decrease total peripheral resistance but do not affect heart rate or cardiac output. The ACE inhibitors are also extremely useful in the management of congestive heart failure. There is some evidence that ACE inhibitors provide protection against myocardial infarction in hypertensive patients with elevated plasma renin levels (Alderman et al., 1991). Captopril was shown to have an remarkably beneficial effect on patients with chronic renal failure associated with diabetes (Lewis et al., 1993).

The AT_1 receptor antagonists losartan and SK&F 109566 are also highly effective antihypertensive drugs. Losartan is active following oral administration and has fewer side effects than ACE inhibitors because it antagonizes the renin-angiotensin system at the level of the AT receptor (Freed et al., 1994), thus providing a sharper focus for its action. The human angiotensinogen gene has recently been identified; mutations cause an increase in angiotensinogen, a condition that results in hypertension.

18.3 Calcitonin

Calcium metabolism is regulated by three hormones, *calcitonin* (CT), *parathyroid hormone (PTH)*, and *calcitriol*, a metabolite of vitamin D_3. Calcitonin was discovered and named by Copp (Copp and Cameron, 1961) as a hormone released by high calcium perfusion of the thyroid and parathyroid, and which lowered plasma calcium. Copp believed that CT was secreted by the parathyroid, but later experiments, in which the parathyroid glands were excised, clearly demonstrated that the source of CT was the thyroid (Foster et al., 1964). CT acts principally on bone, but has a direct action on the kidney and gastrointestinal secretory activity, and has both direct and indirect actions on the CNS.

18.3.1 Phylogenetic Distribution of Calcitonin

CT is an ancient peptide, found in unicellular organisms such as *Escherichia coli* through amphibians, fish, reptiles, and mammals, including humans. The structures that produce CT also vary considerably in different species. In mammals, they are primarily found in the thyroid gland; in fish, amphibians, reptiles, and birds, the ultimobranchial body is the source of CT. CT-producing cells may also migrate during development to other sites. In the lizard, C cells in the lung form an important source of CT, and in humans active C cells are present in the lungs, adrenals, thymus, and brain (O. L. Silva and Becker, 1981).

18.3.2 Structure of Calcitonin

The number of amino acid residues and the structure of the chain ends are identical in all CTs and are essential to biological activity. It is the central portion of the chain that has considerable variation. The CTs consist of a chain of 32 amino acid residues with a disulfide bridge between Cys^1 and Cys^7 which forms a ring of 7 amino acid residues at the N-terminal. Another CT characteristic is the presence of a proline amide group at the C-terminus. The molecular weight of CT is about 3500. The main CTs are divided into three groups according to their primary structure, which surprisingly does not reflect similarities of function.

The first group encompasses the *artiodactyls* (pig, ox, and sheep); the second group is that of *mammals* (human, rat), and the third group includes *fish* (salmon, eel). Most of the amino acid residues 1–9 are common to groups 1 and 2, although residues 2 and 9 show some variation. Residues 28 and 30 are common to all three groups. The structure of human CT is shown below:

Cys-Gly-Asn-Leu-Ser-Thyr-Cys-Met-Leu-Gly^{10}-
Thr-Tyr-Thr-Gln-Asp-Phe-Asn-Lys-Phe-His^{20}-
Thr-Phe-Pro-Gln-Thr-Ala-Ile-Gly-Val-Gly^{30}-
Ala-Pro-NH_2

18.3.3 Calcitonin Gene Expression, Precursor Processing, and Regulation of Release

Both CT and CGRP are expressed by the *CT–α-CRGP gene* which includes coding regions for both CT and CGRP (see chapter 17). The human CT–α-CRGP gene is located on the short arm of chromosome 11, that of the mouse on chromosome 6. CT is the main product of the thyroid C cells and is a hypocalcemic hormone. CGRP is expressed mainly in neural tissue and acts as a neurotransmitter exerting potent vasodilator effects, as discussed in chapter 17.

Transcription of the CT gene leads to a large RNA, which is alternatively spliced and polyadenylated into either a CT-encoding mRNA or a CGRP- encoding mRNA, a tissue-specific process that results in the formation of CT in thyroid cells and CGRP in the brain. CT is derived from the post-translational *processing* of the precursor *preprocalcitonin*. Removal of the signal peptide produces *procalcitonin*; removal of its N-terminal region forms a 57–amino acid peptide that contains the CT sequence linked to the 21–amino acid residues of *katacalcin*. The CT molecule is then liberated by amidating cleavage at the Gly-Lys-Lys-Arg site (figure 18.16). Katacalcin is also called *calcitonin carboxyl-adjacent peptide (CCAP)*, and is secreted synchronously with CT but has no known physiological function. However, CCAP is useful, as is CT, as a diagnostic marker of medullary thyroid carcinoma, a tumor of the C cells.

The main *expression of CT* is in the parafollicular (C cells) of the thyroid. These cells differ histologically and cytochemically from the T_4-secreting cells. CT is also found in many other tissues, such as the liver,

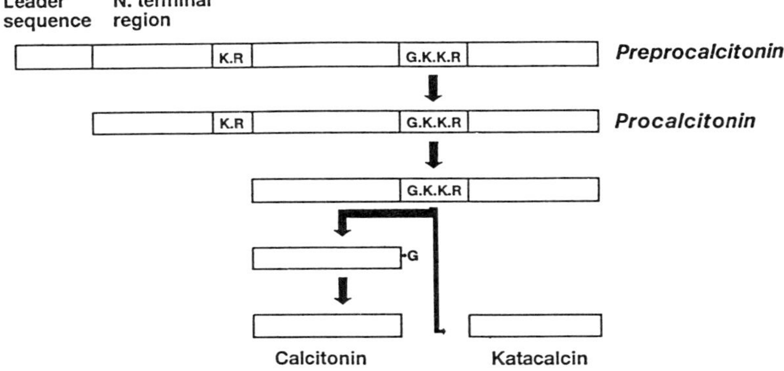

Figure 18.16
Schematic representation of the biosynthetic pathway of calcitonin in thyroid C cells. Amino acids are represented by the one-letter code (see appendix C). (From P. Motté et al., 1990.)

where it may be bound to receptors and acts as a reservoir for CT release. CT is also found in the CNS, including the medulla oblongata, which suggests involvement of CT in the regulation of autonomic functions. The *release* of CT is regulated chiefly by elevated serum calcium levels.

18.3.4 Calcitonin Receptors and Second Messengers

The CT receptor is a member of the G protein–coupled receptors, which coupling activates several signaling pathways. There are multiple receptor subtypes or isoforms found in bone, brain, and kidney, and they vary in their ability to bind CT.

In bone, CT receptors are found in osteoclasts (Chambers and Moore, 1983), the main function of which is the resorption of bone; in osteocytes, which assist in bone synthesis; and in certain bone marrow cells. Kidney CT receptors are found in the cortex and outer and inner medulla, especially in the ascending loop of Henle. CT receptors in the CNS are found in various brain regions, including the nucleus accumbens, preoptic areas and the PVN of the hypothalamus, the arcuate nucleus, lymph cells, and some types of tumor cells, and in the pituitary. This distribution in pituitary and hypothalamic areas suggests that CT may have *neuroendocrine analgesic* or general *neuromodulator* effects in the CNS. The CT receptor has two isoforms, $C1_a$ and $C1_b$, which overlap considerably in their distribution in the brain.

All these receptors mediate their effects through *adenylate cyclase*, but the various isoforms of CT receptors may activate several signaling proteins, including protein kinase C, cAMP-dependent protein kinase, and calcium-calmodulin–dependent kinase (Horne et al., 1994). Salmon and eel CT bind to both receptors with equal affinity, but human CT binds only to the $C1_a$ receptor (Hilton et al., 1995). Synthetic salmon and eel CTs have the greatest affinity for all types of CT receptors and also have the greatest hypocalcemic effects.

18.3.5 Actions of Calcitonin

CT is involved in the regulation of mineral metabolism, especially calcium homeostasis, with its main target being the osteoclasts of bone. CT rapidly inhibits osteoclast activity and decreases plasma concentrations of calcium if bone turnover is high. CT affects the number of osteoclasts by inhibiting production of the osteoclast precursor. This antiosteolytic effect retards bone demineralizarion and breakdown of the bone matrix. CT is also involved in physiological states that require high calcium levels, such as periods of rapid bone growth, pregnancy, and lactation.

Not only is CT involved in bone formation and resorption, but its actions are influenced by the hypercalcemic actions of PTH (see section 18.4) and vitamin D metabolites such as calcitriol (vitamin D_3) which play an important role in calcium homeostasis. Other hormones that interact with CT include estrogens, which prevent the onset of postmenopausal osteoporosis; corticosteroids, which reduce osteoblast activity and thereby inhibit bone formation; and T_4, which stimulates both osteoblasts and osteoclasts.

In the kidney, which has specific CT receptors distinct from VP and PTH receptors, CT elicits a direct and rapid increase in urinary excretion of water and various ions, including calcium, phosphate, sodium, potassium magnesium, and chloride.

The principal action of CT on the gastrointestinal tract is a general inhibition of gastric and secretory activity, and an inhibition of gallbladder contraction. Very high dosages of CT increase the secretion of water and ions into the intestinal lumen and stimulate intestinal absorption of CT. Lower physiological doses have no effect. CT stimulates the release of somatostatin, which may be the final common path for these inhibitory mechanisms. This may be integrated centrally with decreased vagal activity (see chapter 17, section 17.7). By inhibiting many of these gastrointestinal functions, CT protects the gastrointestinal tract, preventing the development of gastric ulcers in animals exposed to stress.

Centrally, CT reduces food intake, resulting in anorexia. CT has antinociceptive effects which have been variously attributed to involve central cholinergic systems, β-adrenergic receptors, serotonin (5-HT) and GABA receptors, but not opiate receptors.

On a more general level, CT has complex physiological roles which are still not well understood. Apart from its direct effects, outlined above, CT is involved in the regulation of functions controlled by Ca^{2+}. These include cellular permeability, enzyme activation, muscle contractility, transmitter and endocrine secretion, cardiac function, and blood coagulation.

18.3.6 Clinical Implications of Calcitonin

Low CT levels may result in osteoporosis, which is characterized by a generalized diminution of bone tissue mass, weakening the skeleton and resulting in bone fragility and crush fractures. Osteoporosis is common in the elderly, and following menopause or ovariectomy. Natural porcine CT and synthetic salmon, eel analog, and human CTs are the forms of the hormone used therapeutically to counteract the disorders of bone loss, such as Paget's disease, some types of hypocalcemia, and high bone turnover osteoporosis. Acute pancreatitis is also treated with CT.

The analgesic effects of CT are used to counteract the pain associated with osteoporosis, certain malignancies, and other nonosteogenic pain, usually in combination with morphine. A major problem has been the route of CT administration: the usual method has been by injection, but new pharmaceutical formulations, such as nasal preparations, are now available and may supplant the older methodology.

Raised CT levels may result in several disorders, especially malignancies, most of which involve tumors of the thyroid or other tissues containing C cells, such as the human lung.

18.4 Parathyroid Hormone and Parathyroid Hormone–Related Protein

Functioning together with calcitonin and vitamin D to maintain calcium homeostasis are PTH and *parathyroid hormone-related protein (PTH-rP)*. PTH is produced chiefly by the parathyroid glands and responds to a minute drop in blood calcium levels by increasing plasma calcium levels, acting in a classical endocrine manner. PTH acts on bone, kidneys, and intestine as a hypercalcemic factor. PTH-like peptides are found in a variety of extraparathyroidal sites, including the brain and hypothalamus, and may have a neuroendocrine role in the regulation of pituitary function. Because of the crucial role of Ca^{2+} in cellular functions, PTH is essential to life. Deaths that occurred after thyroidectomy in the early days of endocrinology were really a result of removal of the parathyroids, which are embedded on the surface of the thyroid gland.

PTH-rP is a protein with strong PTH-like activity, which acts on PTH receptors in bone and kidney. PTH-rP is synthesized in the brain and several other normal tissues such as vascular smooth muscle, but was first isolated from lung tumors and renal carcinomas associated with hypercalcemia. High concentrations of PTH-rP are also found in milk and the placenta, suggesting that it may be involved in the transport of calcium into milk during lactation, and that PTH-rP may participate in calcium homeostasis in the fetus. PTH-rP does not circulate, implying that it probably acts as a paracrine or autocrine factor.

18.4.1 Phylogenetic Distribution of PTH and PTH-rP

PTH and PTH-like peptides are present in primitive vertebrates (hagfish), fish, amphibians, reptiles, birds, and mammals, as well as in the sensory ganglia of an invertebrate, the pond snail. PTH and PTH-rP are closely related evolutionarily, but have distinct physiological roles. As neither the hagfish nor the snail have parathyroid glands, the actions of PTH on calcium flux in invertebrates may precede its role in calcium homeostasis in higher vertebrates.

18.4.2 Structure of PTH and PTH-rP

PTH is an 84–amino acid peptide, the sequence of which is shown in figure 18.17. The primary structures of PTH are highly homologous in mammals and the 84–amino acid sequence is the chief form in which PTH is secreted by the parathyroids. It is cleaved in the peripheral circulation into two fragments, the physiologically active one being PTH 1–34.

PTH-rP is a protein containing 141 amino acids with a molecular weight of 16 kD. The N-terminal region has a high homology with PTH, 8 of the first 13 amino acids being identical. There is no similarity, however, in the remainder of the sequence. Nevertheless, a synthetic fragment of PTH-rP (PTH-rP 1–34), has effects similar to several actions of PTH 1–34 and these two peptides react with the same receptor with similar affinities. There is now evidence that there are three separate regions of these peptides that have their own distinct biological actions (Mallette, 1991), as indicated in figure 18.18 and table 18.1.

There is an interesting homology between PTH 15–25 and α-MSH. These sequences contain small homologous domains that contain much of the information that directs PTH receptor binding and most of the α-MSH (ACTH 1–11 rather than ACTH 1–13) sequence, respectively. There is sufficient homology to permit each peptide to weakly interact with the receptor of the other peptide (Rafferty et al., 1983).

18.4.3 PTH and PTH-rP Gene Expression, Precursor Processing, and Regulation of Release

The PTH gene has two introns which interrupt the coding sequence at the region of the mRNA. Exon 2 codes for the signal sequence and exon 3 encodes PTH and the 3′-untranslated region of its mRNA. There is considerable homology in the human, rat, and bovine PTH genes. The gene for human PTH is on the short arm of chromosome 11.

Prepro-PTH contains a fourfold internal homology that probably represents four copies of a primitive gene (Mallette, 1994). It consists of 115 amino acids containing a signal peptide of 31 amino acids, of which 25 are proteolytically removed to yield *pro-PTH* (90 amino acids), which in turn is processed to *PTH 1–84.* The biological activity of PTH is contained within the first 34 amino acids. Almost all *PTH expression* is in the parathyroid glands, with considerably less in hypothalamic structures, in which PTH mRNA is restricted to the PVN and SON (Fraser et al., 1990). There is complete homology between parathyroid and brain cDNA fragments and the mRNA for the brain PTH gene is identical in size to that of parathyroid PTH.

	1 2 3 4 5 6 7 8 9 10 11 12 13 14 15 16
Human-PTH:	NH_2-SerValSerGluIleGlnLeuMetHisAsnLeuGlyLysHisLeuAsn
Bovine-PTH:	Ala. . . . . Phe. . . . . Ser
Pig-PTH:	. . . . Phe. . . . . Ser
Rat-PTH:	Ala. . . . . Ala
	17 18 19 20 21 22 23 24 25 26 27 28 29 30 31 32 33
	SerMetGluArgValGluTrpLeuArgLysLysLeuGlnAspValHisAsn
	. . . .
	. . .Leu. . . . .
	. . .Val. . . . . MetGln. . . . .
	34 35 36 37 38 39 40 41 42 43 44 45 46 47 48 49 50
	PheValAlaLeuGlyAlaProLeuAlaProArgAspAlaGlySerGlnArg
	. . . . .SerIle. . . Tyr. . . . . GlySer. . . . .
	. . . . .SerIleVal. His. . . . . Gly. . . . .
	. . . . . Ser. . . . . ValGlnMet. . .Ala. . .GluGlySerTyr. . . . .
	51 52 53 54 55 56 57 58 59 60 61 62 63 64 65 66 67
	ProArgLysLysGluAspAsnValLeuValGluSerHisGluLysSerLeu
	. . . . .Gln. . . . . . .
	. . . . .Gln. . . . . . .
	. . .Thr. . . . . .AspGlyAsnSer. . . . . . .
	68 69 70 71 72 73 74 75 76 77 78 79 80 81 82 83 84
	GlyGluAlaAspLysAlaAspValAsnValLeuThrLysAlaLysSerGln -COOH
	. . . . Asp. . . . .Ile. . . . . Pro. . . .
	. . . . .Ala. . .Asp. . . . .Ile. . . . . Pro. . . .
	. . . . . Gly. . . . . Asp. . . . .Val. . . . .

Figure 18.17
Amino acid sequence of human, bovine, porcine, and rat parathyroid hormone (PTH). (From Blind et al., 1990.)

Release of PTH from the parathyroid glands and from neural tissue is similarly dependent on depletion of extracellular calcium, and suppressed by vitamin D_3. Degradation of intact PTH is by cleavage in the liver and kidneys, and in its peripheral target tissues, between amino acids 34 and 37. This yields fragments which contain either the C-terminal or N- terminal sequence, but only the N-terminal sequences contain the biologically active form of PTH (Slatopolsky et al., 1982). The active fragments have a short half-life as they are rapidly cleared from the circulation. Brain PTH-degrading enzymes also are present in brain tissues.

The gene that encodes PTH-rP is on the short arm of chromosome 12, in a position that is homologous to the position of PRH on chromosome 11, two chromosomes that are believed to have evolved from one another (Craig et al., 1986). The PTH gene may have

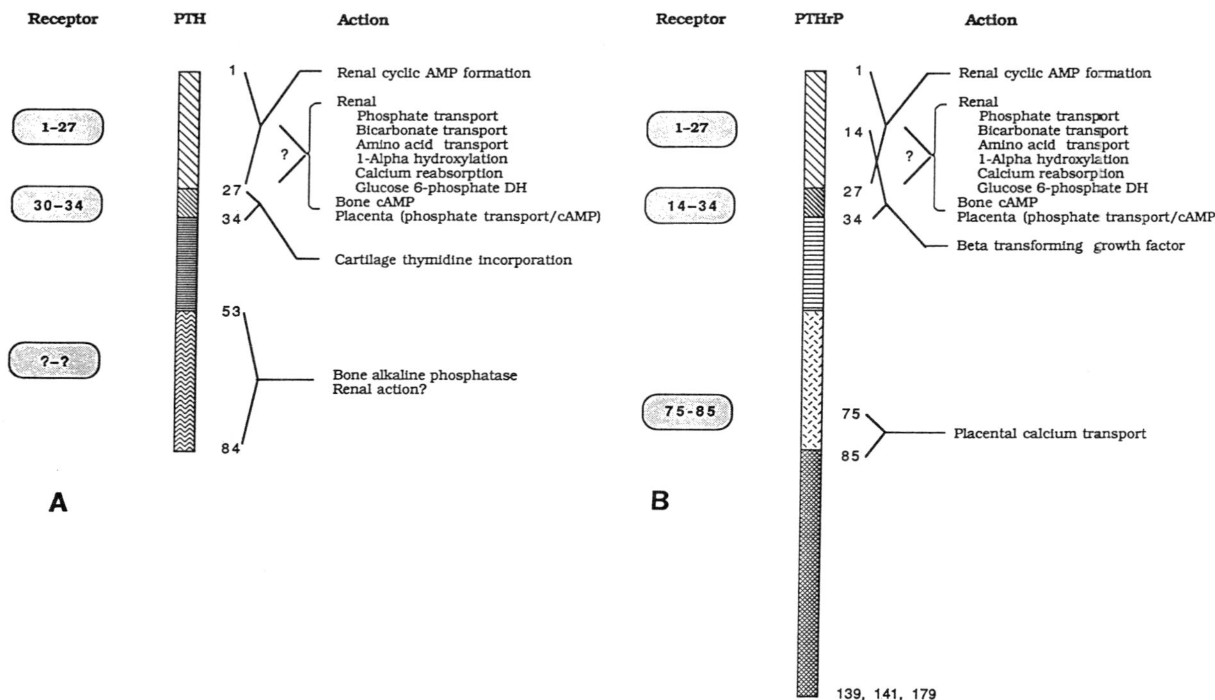

Figure 18.18
Stylized diagram to indicate distinct functional regions of parathyroid hormone (PTH) (A) and PTH-releasing protein (PTHrP) (B), and their documented or postulated receptors. The hormone molecules are diagrammed in linear fashion, with different shadings to indicate roughly the extent of the different functional domains that can be differentiated. Putative or demonstrated receptors for the various regions are indicated at the left of each diagram. The structural features of the 1–34 region necessary for several actions of PTH and PTH-rP have not yet been clarified. (From Mallette, 1991.)

evolved by a twofold genetic reduplication, producing four copies which then diverged in structure, so that the 53–84 region of PTH is homologous with the 1–34 region (Mallette et al., 1986).

The human PTH-rP gene is on chromosome 12 (figure 18.19), whereas the PTH gene is on chromosome 11. These two chromosomes are believed to be related in evolutionary terms and there are several examples of similarly related proteins the genes of which are located on chromosomes 11 and 12 (Martin et al., 1991). The human PTH-rP gene is a single-copy gene with nine exons, much more complex than the PTH gene with only three exons, and also much more complex than the PTH-rp of rodents and chicks (figure 18.20). There is remarkable conservation of the primary sequence up to residue 111, after which there is considerable divergence between the species.

The PTH-like biological activity of PTH-rP, like that of PTH, is contained within the first 34 amino acids. Shortening PTH-rP to 1–29 reduces its activity

Table 18.1
Multiple actions of the parathyroid polyhormones

Line	PTH	PTH-rP[a]	Region	Biological activity	Site of Action
1	+++	+++	1–27	Stimulate cAMP formation	Proximal renal tubule
2	+++	+++	1–34	Phosphaturia, bicarbonaturia	Proximal renal tubule
3	+++	+++	1–34	25-Hydroxyvitamin $D_{1\alpha}$ hydroxylation	Proximal renal tubule
4	+++	+++	1–34	Glucose-6-phosphate dehydrogenase	Proximal renal tubule
5	+++	+++	1–34	Increase calcium reabsorption	Distal renal tubule
6	+++	?	1–34	Increase cAMP, alter phosphate transport	Placental membranes
7	+	+++	1–34	Bone resorption, bone cAMP	Osteoblast
8	+	+++	1–34	Stimulate cAMP formation	Dermal fibroblast
9	–	+++	75–85	Increase transfer of Ca^{2+} and Mg^{2+}	Placenta
10	–	+++	14–36	β-Transforming growth factor	Dermal fibroblast, NRK 49F
11	+++	?	53–84	Increase alkaline phosphatase	Osteoblast-like cell
12	+++	?	53–84	Possible, not yet defined	Renal tubule
13	+++	?	30–34	Increase thymidine incorporation	Chondrocyte

From Mallette (1991).
PTH, parathyroid hormone; PTH-rP, parathyroid hormone–releasing protein; cAMP, cyclic adenosine monophasphate.
+ = increase; – = decrease.
[a] The ? indicates that the biological effect has not been tested with PTH-rP.

to 10% of that of PTH-rP 1–34, and shorter fragments are inactive; thus the PTH-like actions of PTH-rP are mediated through the N-terminal sequences, which show some limited sequence homology with PTH (Kemp et al., 1987). The PTH-rP gene is subjected to a wide variety of physiological and pharmacological controls, including estrogen.

PTH-rP gene expression is mainly in the brain, being highest in the supramamillary nucleus of the hypothalamus and medial superior olivary nucleus, with lesser amounts in many other brain regions (Weaver et al., 1995). There is a startling difference in the amounts of PTH and PTH-rP mRNA expressed in brain and hypothalamus as compared to that in the parathyroids: neural PTH and PTH-rP mRNA is less than 0.2% of that expressed in the parathyroid glands (Nutley et al., 1995). PTH-rP is expressed in meningeal cells but not in astrocytes; however, astrocytes and not meningeal cells synthesize the mRNA for the PRH-rP receptor, indicating a paracrine meningo-astrocytic loop by which PRH-rP may influence astrocyte differentiation (Struckhoff and Turznski, 1995).

There is at present no indication that PTH-rP has a function as a circulating hormone in the adult, but high levels of PTH-rP are found in the fetal parathyroid and in the placenta, and this neuropeptide may be the circulating PTH during ontogeny (Rodda et al., 1988).

Additional forms of PTH-rP have been isolated from different tumors and probably arise from alternative splicing that gives rise to three mRNA species that encode three proteins that differ at the C-terminus and have different molecular weights

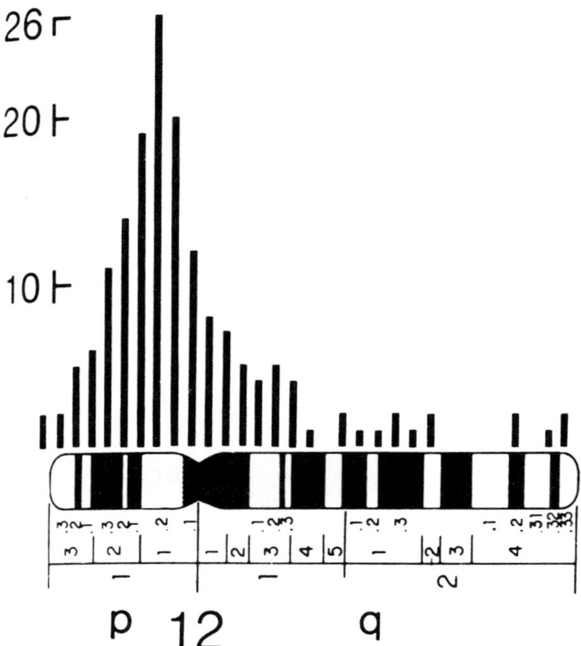

Figure 18.19
Chromosomal localization of the parathyroid hormone–releasing protein gene using in situ hybridization. Grains scored over prophasic chromosome 12. Of the grains 61% is over a large region consisting of the short arm and the proximal quarter of the long arm over sub-bands 12p11.2 and 12p.11.1, and the peak of grains is over sub-band 12p11.2. (From Suva et al., 1989.)

(Mangin et al., 1988). These three forms consist of 139, 141, or 173 amino acids, but their N-terminal regions 1–139 are identical (Suva et al., 1989).

18.4.4 PTH and PTH-rP Receptor and Second Messengers

There is a single type of cloned receptor for the N-terminal portion of PRH and PRH-rP in the CNS. This receptor is a protein of 593 amino acids, with the same primary structure whether cloned from osteoclasts, kidney, or cerebellum. Although PTH and PTH-rP receptor mRNA is widely distributed in rat tissues (Urena et al., 1993), its highest concentration is in the parathyroids, implying a paracrine or autocrine regulation of PTH and PTH-rP in these glands. In the brain, most PTH and PTH-rP receptor mRNA is present in the trigeminal nucleus and ganglion, the reticular and pontine regions, the hypoglossal nuclei, and the area postrema (Weaver et al., 1995). The neural receptors have the same functional properties as the receptors from non-neural tissues and their widespread distribution in the brain implies that PRH-rP may have biological functions yet to be identified (Eggenberger et al., 1996). These, too, probably include paracrine or autocrine actions.

PTH stimulates the generation of *phosphoinositol triphosphate* and induces an increase in intracellular Ca^{2+}. The second-messenger system for PRH-rP is less clear. There may be a dual signaling system in the brain with some neurons using cAMP and others using only cytosolic Ca^{2+} (Fukayama et al., 1995).

18.4.5 Actions of PTH and PTH-rP

Peripherally, PTH interacts with receptors in bone to stimulate osteoclast activity by increasing their number, activity, and life span to increase serum calcium. In this manner PTH acts as a hypercalcemic agent encouraging bone resorption. Calcium absorption in the gut is altered by the increased 1α-hydroxylation of 25-hydroxyvitamin D by PTH. In the kidney PTH inhibits tubular reabsorption of phosphate and bicarbonate, thus affecting minerals other than calcium.

Centrally, PTH inhibits the firing of neurons of the ventromedial nucleus of the hypothalamus through a postsynaptic mechanism mediated by PTH receptors, and counteracts hypocalcemia, indicating a possible

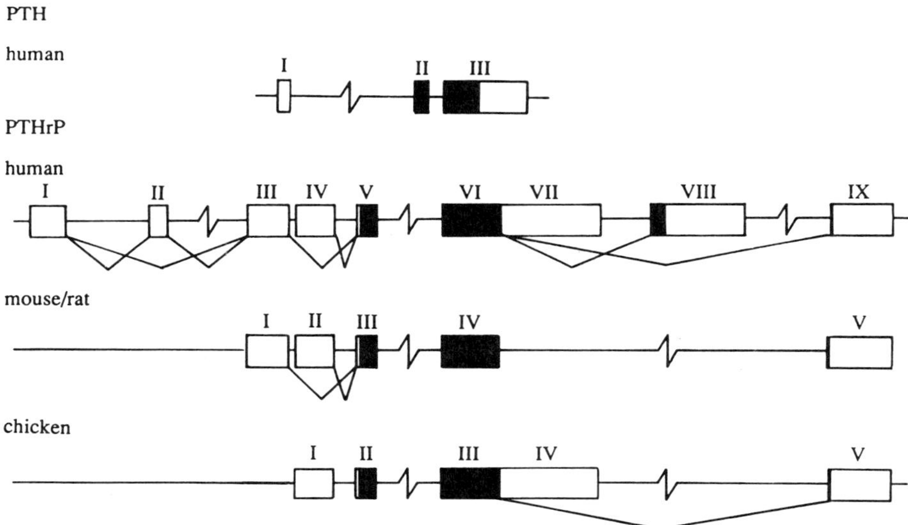

Figure 18.20
Comparison of the genomic organization of the human parathyroid hormone (PTH) and parathyroid hormone–releasing protein (PTHrp) genes with those from mouse and rat, and chicken. The coding regions and untranslated sequences are indicated by the closed and open boxes, respectively. The human PTH-rp gene has been aligned below the human PTH gene at the common intron-exon boundary 5′ to their respective coding regions, whereas the mouse-rat and chicken structures are aligned over areas of sequence homology within the exon regions of the human gene sequence. Potential alternative splicing events of the human, mouse-rat, and chicken genes are indicated below. (From Martin et al., 1991.)

central regulatory role for PTH in calcium homeostasis.

PTH-rP 1–34 has the same effect as PTH 1–34 on bone modeling but PTH-rP 1–34 has β-transforming growth factor activity not possessed by PTH 1–34. In addition, PTH-rP may be considered a hormonal growth factor. PTH-rP from the fetal parathyroid gland is associated with normal fetal growth and differentiation, as well as the regulation of fetal calcium, and may be the physiologically active form in the fetus (Rodda et al., 1988)

An additional function for both PTH and PTH-rP is that of vasorelaxation and as PTH-rP is present in abundance in aortic vascular smooth muscle, locally synthesized PTH-rP may antagonize vasoconstrictors in smooth muscle (Hongo et al., 1991). The multiple actions of PTH and PTH-rP are listed in table 18.1.

18.4.6 Clinical Implications of PRH and PTH-rP

The most frequent cause of primary hyperparathyroidism is a parathyroid adenoma. It is accompanied by hypercalcemia and hypophosphatemia. Subtotal removal of the parathyroids may be indicated since hypercalcemic crisis is an acute disease with high lethality. Hypoparathyroidism results in hypocalemia, hypocalciuria, and hyperphosphatemia. This severe mineral imbalance leads to convulsions, tetany, intracranial hypertension, changes in nails and teeth, and depressive or psychotic behavior. There are several causes of this disorder, among them trauma of the neck, more rarely metastic tumor of the parathyroids, and even more rarely, hereditary absence of the parathyroids. Treatment with calcium combined with calcitriol is extremely effective.

PTH-rP is implicated in the hypercalcemia of certain tumors, especially prostatic adenocarcinomas which secrete PTH-rP. PTH-rP was first isolated from lung and rectal tumors that were secreting large amounts of calcium.

18.5 Thyroid Hormones

The importance of the thyroid gland in the occurrence of goiter and cretinism was appreciated in the late nineteenth century, to be followed by the discovery that triiodothyronine (T_3) and thyroxine (T_4) are the most potent thyroid hormones, and that iodine deficiency led to deficiencies in the synthesis of these hormones. Subsequently, it was realized that the growth and development of the nervous system are dependent upon a normal metabolic state, regulated by an appropriate supply of thyroid hormones. As the common denominator for thyroid hormone action is stimulation of cellular protein synthesis, thyroid hormones are involved in almost all physiological processes. In addition, thyroid hormones are permissive for the proper functioning of other hormones, and thereby exert an essential regulatory role in an extremely diverse series of functions throughout life, including metabolism, growth, development, reproduction, and behavior.

18.5.1 Phylogenetic Distribution of Thyroid Hormones

The thyroid hormones are among the oldest hormones, being found in sponges, the most primitive or simply organized of multicellular animals, and the hormones have assumed different functions throughout phylogeny. The major role of the thyroid hormones in fish is ion regulation, involving activation of the sodium pump and production of ATP within the mitochondria. The profound effects on metamorphosis of amphibian larvae, such as the frog tadpole, by thyroid hormones are well-known. Removal of the thyroid glands prevents metamorphosis, whereas implantation of the thyroids or administration of thyroid hormones accelerates development. As in mammals, the secretion of thyroid hormones is dependent upon adequate stimulation of the thyroid gland by TSH from the anterior pituitary. In fish, amphibians, reptiles, and birds, thyroid hormones increase metabolic activity to varying degrees, but their action on metabolism is most marked in birds and in mammals, where they play an essential part in thermogenesis by increasing the activity of the sodium pump to produce more energy and thus heat, vital in the evolution from poikilothermy to homeothermy.

18.5.2 Structure of Thyroid Hormones

Thyroid hormones are formed from iodinated amino acids, (mono-, di-, tri- or tetraiodotyrosine) characterized by a diphenylether function. Phenolic hydroxyl is present on one of the benzene rings and an alanyl chain on the other (see figure 13.6). The thyroid hormones are incorporated into a glycoprotein, *thyroglobulin (Tg)*, which is synthesized by the follicular cells of the thyroid and stored in the colloid spaces. The hormones are released as free molecules of T_4 and

T_3 into the circulation, where they are bound to thyroid hormone transport proteins.

18.5.3 Thyroid Hormone Synthesis, Regulation of Release, and Metabolism

The thyroid hormones are complexed through covalent bonds to iodine, which is trapped as iodide by thyroid follicular cells and transported against an electrical gradient across the cell. At the luminal surface of the cell iodide is converted by a peroxidase to an oxidized species of iodine. The iodide is incorporated into tyrosyl groups of thyroglobulin as monoiodotyrosine or diiodotyrosine. Oxidative coupling then produces T_4 and T_3 (see figure 13.6). The T_3 form is considered to be the most potent physiological thyroid hormone, although T_4 is produced in much greater amounts than T_3. Much of T_4 is converted within target cells to T_3 by type I 5′-deiodinase (outer ring deiodinase).

Thyroid hormone synthesis and release from the thyroid follicles are regulated by the TRH-TSH axis, which is inhibited by thyroid hormones at both the hypothalamic and anterior pituitary levels, as discussed in chapter 13, sections 13.3.4 and 13.3.5. Tg synthesis is also regulated by TSH and a large supply of iodine and of thyroid hormones is stored in the Tg molecule. Mutations in the Tg gene cause a structurally defective protein which has severe functional consequences (Medeiros-Neto et al., 1993). T_3, T_4, and other iodinated amino acids are freed from the Tg molecule by the action of lysosomal proteolytic enzymes and thus made available for secretion into the circulation. The thyroid hormones are inactivated in the thyroid itself, or in extrathyroidal tissues, chiefly the liver, kidney, muscle, and brain, by deiodination, the iodide being excreted in the urine or feces, or reabsorbed and reused.

Thyroid hormones are also found in the CNS, distributed throughout the brain, with the highest levels of T_4 found in the cerebellum and thalamus, the highest T_3 levels in the thalamus.

18.5.4 Thyroid Hormone Binding Proteins and Transport of Thyroid Hormones

18.5.4.1 Binding Proteins in the Blood

Thyroid hormones circulate in the blood bound to several plasma proteins that differ considerably in their concentration and ability to bind thyroid hormones. Steady-state thyroid hormone levels in plasma are composed predominantly of hormones synthesized in the thyroid, mainly T_4, and tissue iodothyronine metabolites, mainly T_3 and reverse T_3, a metabolite actively formed from T_4 within the brain. These hormones circulate in noncovalently bound complexes with the carrier proteins and consequently T_3 and T_4 remain in the plasma much longer than most hormones.

The three major *thyroid hormone transport proteins are T_4-binding globulin, transthyretin* (TTR), (so named for its role in the transport of the retinol-binding protein), and *albumin.* TTR is synthesized in the liver and also in the choroid plexus. Mutations in the genes for these binding proteins may result in pathological thyroid homone conditions (Bartalena, 1990). TTR evolved much earlier in the brain than in the liver, and the domains of TTR involved in T_4 binding have been completely conserved for 350 million years.

18.5.4.2 Role of the Choroid Plexus

The *choroid plexus* accumulates thyroid hormones, especially T_4 (figure 18.21). Unbound T_3 and T_4 are transported into the brain mainly across the blood-brain barrier, but also across the choroid plexus–CSF

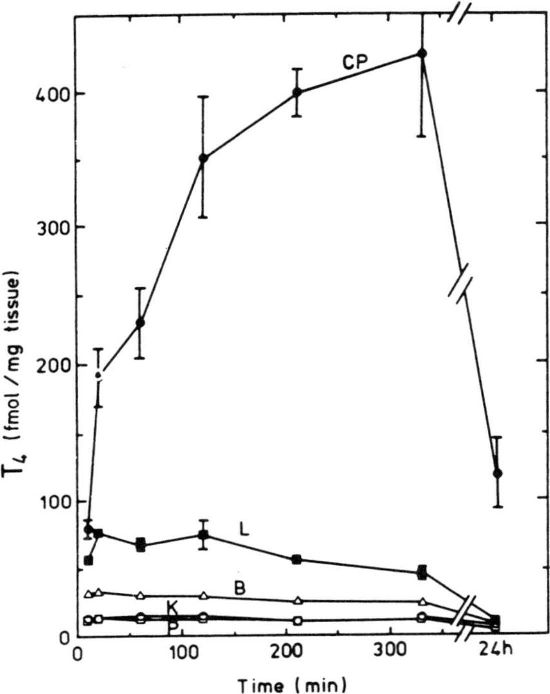

Figure 18.21
Kinetics of uptake of i.v. injected ^{125}I-thyroxine into choroid plexus (CP), liver (L), kidney (K), brain (B) and pituitary (P). (From Dickson et al., 1987.)

barrier. The choroid plexus is also the site of synthesis of TTR. This may allow the formation of a T_4-TTR complex which is secreted into the CSF and distributed to the brain. In this manner, the concentration of T_4 in the CNS may be controlled and T_4 converted to T_3 by specific deiodinases (Dickson et al., 1987). T_3, which is believed to be the physiologically active form of thyroid hormone, especially in the brain, can then react with receptors in the cell nuclei, regulating gene transcription.

18.5.4.3 Transport Through the Placenta

Placental transfer of maternal T_4 to the fetus occurs in a variety of mammals, including humans. Disturbances in the intrauterine thyroid environment result in several biochemical dysfunctions, for example, of phosphate metabolism and of two enzyme systems associated with growth control, protein kinase C and ornithine decarboxylase. Lower levels of important enzymes involved in transmitter metabolism, such as acetyltransferase and dihydroxyphenylalanine (DOPA) decarboxylase also occur (Ekins et al., 1994). These critical biochemical dysfunctions result in irreversible brain damage to the fetus.

18.5.4.4 Cellular Entry and Binding

T_3 and T_4 enter the cell mainly by passive diffusion. Whereas most neuropeptides activate membrane-bound receptors, the thyroid hormones are small enough to penetrate the cell membrane. Some thyroid hormones may penetrate the cell by a transport process involving membrane binding sites and receptor-mediated internalization of T_3 and T_4 (Krenning et al., 1983). Serum free T_3 and free T_4 are immediately available and almost all transport protein-bound T_3 and T_4 ultimately is freed to enter the cell if intracellular free hormone levels decline. Additional T_3 becomes available to the cell since it is produced from intracellular T_4, which seems to act as a prohormone for T_3. Once inside the cell, T_3 and T_4 are bound to intracellular components in the cytosol, including cytoplasmic proteins, microsomes, and mitochondria, but this mechanism probably serves as a buffer and storage for the thyroid hormones and is not characterized by any of the specific criteria for receptors (Oppenheimer, 1985). The bulk of intracellular T_3 and T_4 is stored in the cytoplasm and only about 10% of the cell content is present in the nucleus. There is a remarkable exception, however, in

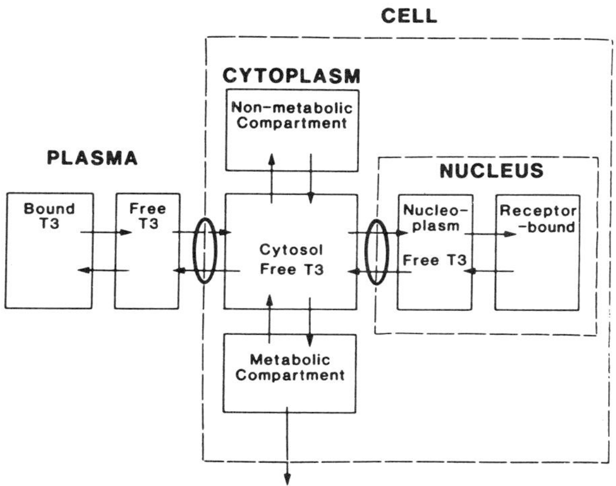

Figure 18.22
Schematic representation of equilibrium relationships of triiodothyronine (T3) between plasma and cytosol T_3, and between the cytosol and other cellular components, including the nucleus. Ringlike structures enclosing transport (arrows) show the presumed site of operation of two stereospecific transport systems. (From Oppenheimer and Schwartz, 1985.)

pituitary cells in which about 50% of intracellular T_3 is in the nucleus. From the cytoplasm, T_3 enters the nucleus by diffusion or by a transport mechanism in the nuclear membrane (figure 18.22).

18.5.5 Thyroid Hormone Receptors

The receptors for thyroid hormones are high-affinity *nuclear receptors* within the chromatin, with intrinsic DNA-binding properties. They have a molecular weight of approximately 50 kD with an affinity for T_3 10 times that for T_4, about 10^{-10}M. The thyroid hormone receptors share several characteristics of steroid hormone receptors: they recognize specific DNA sequences in the promoter region of the genome, they

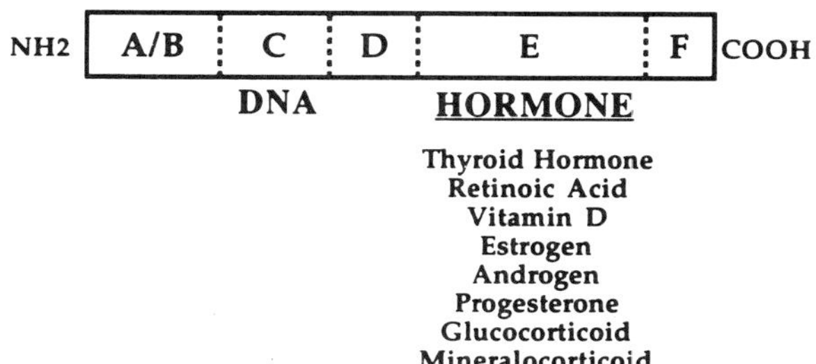

Figure 18.23
Steroid and thyroid hormone receptor superfamily. The prototypal nuclear hormone receptor is shown. The domains are labeled A to F; the C domain is the DNA binding domain. The indicated receptors have similar structures. (From Lazar, 1993.)

have a nuclear site of action, and they regulate gene transcription. The T_3 nuclear receptor also has been identified by molecular cloning as the normal product of an oncogene, the *c-erbA gene*. Consequently, the thyroid hormone receptors have been placed in the same receptor superfamily as the steroid hormones and certain oncogene receptors (figure 18.23).

There are multiple thyroid hormone receptor isoforms across a variety of species, formed from the thyroid hormone receptor α and β genes. The expression of the isoforms is regulated transcriptionally and post-transcriptionally, with the mRNA for each isoform subject to individual tissue-specific and hormonal regulation. The receptors are synthesized in the cytoplasm and guided to the cell nucleus under the control of a signal sequence in the D domain (see figure 18.23). In the nucleus the receptors interact with T_3, target genes and other proteins. Thyroid hormone receptors regulate the transcription of target genes in the presence of physiological concentrations of T_3.

The most highly regulated thyroid hormone receptor isoform is $\beta 2$, the mRNA for which is abundant in the anterior pituitary and detectable in the arcuate, paraventricular, and ventromedial nuclei of the hypothalamus. In pituitary cells, T_3 down-regulates $\beta 2$ mRNA, as does TRH to a lesser degree (Hodin et al., 1990). The mRNAs encoding the other isoforms are found in almost all tissues, but are differentially distributed: Thyroid hormone receptor $\alpha 1$ is highly concentrated in skeletal muscle and brown fat, $\alpha 2$ (also called c-*erbA* $\alpha 2$) is prominent in the brain, and $\beta 1$ is high in brain, liver, and kidney. These isoforms are not regulated by TRH and are not as regulated by T_3, as are the levels of $\beta 2$ mRNA.

The ontogeny of the thyroid hormone receptor isoforms indicates that they may be important in regulating the critical effects of T_3 on brain development. In the rat, chicken, and amphibian it is the $\alpha 1$ isoform that is expressed during early development when the thyroid gland is being formed, but as development proceeds, $\beta 1$ mRNA increases considerably. The non–T_3-binding isoforms, $\alpha 2$ and $\alpha 3$, predominate in the fetal, neonatal, and adult brain (Strait et al., 1990).

18.5.6 Actions of Thyroid Hormones

Thyroid hormones are vital during fetal development for the proper development of the brain and the formation of correct connections, at the appropriate time, between neuronal synapses. Later administration of thyroid hormones to hypothyroid fetuses cannot undo the damage of dyssynchronous synaptic contacts. Concomitantly, the lack of thyroid hormones causes severe growth retardation, affecting both bone elongation and maturation, probably through a permissive action on GH. In cultures of neonatal brain cells, T_3 plays a major role in the cytoskeletal transport of tubulin and actin from their site of synthesis to that of assembly, thus facilitating axodendritic growth and synapse formation (De et al., 1994), actions that may involve thyroid hormone stimulation of nerve growth factor.

Thyroid hormones maintain normal metabolism in all tissues of the body. Although the importance of thyroid hormones in the development of the mammalian brain has long been recognized, the adult CNS was believed to be a thyroid hormone–insensitive organ. This is no longer held to be true since the adult brain contains thyroid hormones and there are high levels of nuclear T_3 receptors in brain cells. Thyroid hormones do have a role in adult brain tissue metabolism. In the brain, hypothyroidism decreases microsomal mRNA content and microsomal [^{3}H]uridine incorporation, changes that are returned to normal by T_4 treatment. Many other biochemical values are altered in the adult brain by hypothyroidism, including lysosomal dysfunction and the level and activity of several neurotransmitter and receptor enzyme systems (Sinha et al., 1994). Thyroid hormone treatment stimulates primary dehydrogenase activities in brain mitochondria and also influences mitochondrial electron transfer.

Thyroid hormones maintain body temperature in homeotherms, by increasing energy production and thus heat production through the stimulation of mitochondrial oxygen consumption, the production of ATP, and the increase in the number of plasmalemmal sodium pumps (Ismael-Beigi, 1988). Inhibition of these pumps by ouabain or other sodium pump inhibitors prevents thyroid hormone–induced thermogenesis.

Thyroid hormones have marked effects on the neuromuscular system. Hyperthyroidism produces extensive changes in the metabolic character and protein composition of muscle. Hyperactivity of the thyroid is associated with myopathy, periodic paralysis, and a decrease in muscle bulk and muscle contraction efficiency. Canine models of myasthenia gravis also are hypothyroid, with accompanying clinical evidence of polymyopathy, suggesting an association between hypothyroidism and acquired myasthenia gravis (Dewey et al., 1995), but myasthenia gravis is seen in some some patients with thyrotoxicosis (DeLong, 1996).

Perinatal hypothyroidism affects certain *behaviors* in rats, causing an increase in activity and an anxiolytic behavioral pattern and both hyperthyroidism and hypothyroidism are characterized by behavioral and cognitive changes in humans (Whybrow, 1996a and b).

18.5.7 Clinical Implications of Thyroid Hormones

18.5.7.1 Hypothyroidism

Severe hypothyroidism in preterm infants is an important cause of severe and irreversible neurological problems and mental development, accompanied by growth retardation, characteristic of cretinism. Congential hyothyroidism in young children results in a deficiency in IQ, despite early detection and treatment. In adults, hypothyroidism is characterized by symptoms resulting from the slowing of the major metabolic functions: weakness, lethargy, slow speech, memory impairment, and weight gain. Typically, there is a thickening of the features and edema of the eyelids due to an increase in the mucoprotein substances of the skin, a condition known as myxedema. Deafness is a common result of severe hypothyroidism during development in humans, indicating that children at risk of iodine deficiency, myxedema, or exposure to thyrotoxic environmental agents should be screened routinely by audiometry. The causes of hypothyroidism are varied. They include inadequate dietary intake of iodine (preventable by the addition of iodide to table salt); congenital defect in thyroid metabolism or transport of iodine; and inadequate stimulation of the thyroid by TSH, and antithyroid substances, known as goitrogens. If the thyroid is unable to secrete thyroid hormones despite stimulation by TSH, it becomes extremely enlarged, forming the disfiguring neck bulges known as goiters. This apparently paradoxical enlargement of the thyroid gland, in the absence of thyroid hormones is due to the interruption of the normal negative feedback mechanism controlling TSH secretion. The resulting high levels of TSH stimulate the formation of huge amounts of stored Tg, minus thyroid hormones.

Some natural substances, such as cabbage and yellow turnips, are goitrogens, but they are seldom eaten in sufficient amounts to cause goiter. Environmental goitrogens, such as polychlorinated biphenyls (PCBs) and dioxins, are structurally similar to thyroid hormones and their binding characteristics correspond to those of thyroid hormone. All three groups bind to the cytosolic receptor, the thyroid hormone receptor, and the serum thyroid hormone binding protein TTR. Synthetic goitrogens include propylthiouracil, which can be used to treat hyperthyroidism. Hypothyroidism, depending on the cause, may be treated with thyroid hormone, the administration of iodide, or the removal of environmental goitrogens.

18.5.7.2 Hyperthyroidism or Thyrotoxicosis

This results from an excess of thyroid hormones and may appear as Graves' disease, which is characterized by exophthalmos, weight loss, nervousness, tachycardia, hypersensitivity to heat, and sweating. Most Graves' disease patients have high levels of thyroid hormones with undetectable amounts of TSH. The hyperthyroidism may involve an autoimmune mechanism since an antibody, *long-acting thyroid stimulator (LATS)*, is sometimes found in patients with Graves' disease (McKenzie, 1974). LATS stimulates the synthesis and secretion of the thyroid hormones, induces growth of the gland, and activates adenylate cyclase. Graves' disease occurs much more frequently in women that in men. Treatment of Graves' disease may be the administration of antithyroid compounds such as propylthiouracil; focused radiotherapy through the ingestion of radioactive iodine, which is preferentially accumulated by the thyroid; or surgical ablation of part of the gland.

Thyroid abnormalities are associated with *behavioral disorders*. Children exposed to PCBs or dioxin in utero or as infants may develop varying degrees of behavioral disorders (Porterfield, 1994). Adult-onset changes in levels of thyroid hormones result in overt psychomotor and cognitive dysfunction. *Hyperthyroidism* leads to anxiety and dysphoria, emotional lability, insomnia, and, occasionally, intellectual dysfunction. Restlessness, jitteriness, and lack of concentration are also identified with hyperthyroidism (Whybrow, 1996b). The early behavioral changes associated with *hypothyroidism* are less specific and definable. The complaints include disturbances in cognition, inattentiveness, inability to calculate, and poor memory. More severe hypothyroidism may progress to lethargy, difficulty in arousal, and excessive sleep, even coma (Whybrow, 1996a). Hormones of the thyroid-pituitary axis have been used to treat patients with any of several mental illnesses, especially depression, with varying success (Jackson, 1996).

18.6 Summary

Natriuretic peptides have potent effects on water and salt homeostasis and thus also significantly affect blood pressure. ANH, BNP, and CNP are all members of the natriuretic peptide system, affecting diuresis and natriuresis with different potencies. CNP has the weakest effect on these indices as it lacks the C-terminal tail possessed by the other two peptides. ANH is found mainly in the cardiac atria but also in the CNS; BNP is found in brain and heart ventricles; and CNP in the CNS, macrophages, kidney, and endothelial cells. Each of the three natriuretic peptides is derived from a separate gene, with BNP probably being the oldest in evolutionary terms. The *ANH gene* is a single-copy gene that encodes prepro-ANH, which after cleavage of the signal peptide yields the 126–amino acid pro-ANH. Pro-ANH is processed to several peptides with different characteristics, although all have some hypotensive, diuretic, natriuretic, or kaliuretic properties. Sequence 1–18 is ANH, sequence 1–30 is long-acting natriuretic peptide (LANP), sequence 31–67 is a vasodilator, and sequence 79–98 has kaliuretic properties.

Both the human *BNP* and *ANH genes* are on chromosome 1. The *CNP gene* is on a different chromosome and has different transcription mechanisms from those of the ANH or BNP genes. Pro-CNP is processed to form CNP-53 and CNP-22: these lack the C-terminal tail required for arterial vasodilator and diuretic properties.

There are three natriuretic *receptor* types with different affinities for the three natriuretic peptides. NPR-A binds ANH preferentially, NPR-B binds CNP preferentially, and NPR-C prefers ANH. None of these receptors binds BNP preferentially, although they do bind this peptide with lower affinity. NPR-A and NPR-B activate guanylate cyclase and increase cGMP. NPR-C is a clearance receptor and does not generate cGMP but removes natriuretic peptides from the blood. NPR-C inhibits adenylate cyclase, and stimulates phosphoinositol hydrolysis. These receptors are all transmembrane proteins. *ANH receptors* are heterogeneous and are heavily distributed in smooth muscle cells of the vasculature, in the adrenal cortex, and the kidney. The receptors are also found in the

CNS, especially in the hypothalamus, the circumventricular organs, the pituitary, and cerebellum. The number of receptors varies with salt and water status.

Release of ANH from atrial myocytes occurs with increased atrial pressure, resulting in vasodilation, fluid shifts into the tissues, and increased diuresis and natriuresis through direct effects on the kidney. ANH antagonizes the renin-angiotensin system; this together with ANH's vagoexcitatory action results in a fall in cardiac output and blood pressure. ANH is present in brain areas concerned with cardiovascular function and fluid and electrolyte balance. Further inhibitory ANH actions are suppression of water intake and VP release, inhibition of POMC synthesis and ACTH release, and inhibition of glucagon release. Integration of the actions of ANH, VP, and AT II is essential to the regulation of body fluid volume. In addition, the antidiuretic actions of another peptide, *endothelin*, which has strong vasoconstrictor activity, may balance the effects of ANH on water and salt homeostasis.

BNP is derived mainly from cardiac ventricular cells and is released simultaneously with ANH in response to atrial stretch. BNP has weak vasodilator properties; its physiological role is unclear, although it is increased markedly in some pathological conditions such as essential hypertension and congestive heart failure. *CNP* is a potent relaxant of venous tissue and bronchial smooth muscle, with very weak effects on arteriolar vasodilation. CNP does not affect the renin-angiotensin system, but does inhibit LH release.

Angiotensin is a component of the renin-angiotensin system, affecting blood volume, blood pressure, water and salt balance. The presence of angiotensinogen, AT I, and AT II throughout phylogeny reflects the high degree of conservation of these neuropeptides and their importance in water and electrolyte homeostasis and volume control. The angiotensinogen gene is chiefly expressed in liver and brain, but also in many other organs. Angiotensinogen, a globulin produced by the liver and released into the circulation, is cleaved by renin, an enzyme produced by the kidney, to a decapeptide, AT I. AT I is inactive but is converted by angiotensin-converting enzyme (ACE) to the highly active octapeptide, AT II. In addition to AT II, at least two other shorter forms are produced by peptidases, including AT III and AT IV. AT III is the active form of angiotensin in the central control of cardiovascular functions and the release of VP. AT II and AT III are equally effective in evoking drinking behavior and pressor effects, but the effects of AT IV are weak. AT II is also produced locally in the brain and pituitary to form a central angiotensin system that is indispensable to the regulation of cardiovascular homeostasis, water and salt intake, and the release of pituitary hormones. *Release* of AT II is regulated by osmotic and volume changes. A fall in blood volume or hypo-osmolarity increases both central and peripheral AT II.

The *AT receptors* are characteristic members of the G protein–coupled receptor family. The receptor gene is represented as a single-copy gene, except in rodents which have two gene copies. There are four different AT receptor subtypes: AT_1, AT_2, AT_3, and AT_4. The AT_1 receptor mediates the classical effects of AT II on water balance and maintenance of blood pressure. AT_2 receptors bind both AT II and AT III and may be involved in vascular growth. The AT_3 receptor is present in cultured neuroblastoma cells, and AT_4 binds AT IV and is involved in memory acquisition and retrieval, as well as in regulation of blood flow. The second-messenger system for the AT_1 receptor is phopholipase C–induced Ca^{2+} mobilization and inhibition of adenylate cyclase; the AT_2 receptor signal transduction system involves inhibition of cGMP.

The AT receptors are differentially *expressed*. Most AT_1 receptors are in the heart and blood vessels and bind AT II. Receptors in the kidney for AT II are of the AT_2 type. The lung and reproductive organs also express mRNA for AT II receptors. In the CNS, AT_2 receptors are found in many brain areas. Specific ACE and AT II receptor antagonists have been vital in delineating the functions of the differerent AT receptors.

AT II is a potent vasoconstrictor which increases blood pressure directly, and also indirectly through activation of the sympathetic nervous system. In the kidney AT II directly decreases renal blood flow, has variable effects on glomerular filtration rate, and indirectly increases salt and water reabsorption through stimulation of aldosterone secretion, thereby restoring extracellular water and electrolyte stores. Several other factors modulate these responses, among them glucocorticoids, mineralocorticoids, catecholamines, DA, and estrogen. AT II stimulates glucocorticoid secretion and may be involved in hepatic gluconeogenesis and glycogenolysis, thereby increasing blood glucose.

These peripheral effects are integrated with central actions that increase drinking and salt appetite. AT II stimulates drinking and salt appetite when centrally administered, actions which are effectively inhibited by OT. The angiotensins also evoke central pressor responses, exciting vasomotor neurons in medullary regions that regulate blood pressure. AT II increases sympathetic activity, including the release of epinephrine at sympathetic nerve terminals and from the adrenal medulla, resulting in vasoconstriction. Centrally, AT II also causes the release of ACTH from corticotrophs, stimulates CRH and VP secretion, and the release of PRL and LH. Behavioral changes associated with AT II include changes in cognitive function, angiogenesis, and reduced male sexual behavior.

Calcitonin, together with PTH and calcitriol, a vitamin D metabolite, regulates calcium metabolism. CT is an ancient peptide, found throughout the phylogenetic scale, from unicellular organisms to humans. In mammals, CT is produced in the C cells of the thyroid but in submammalian verebrates the ultimobranchial body is its chief source. In humans, CT is also produced in the lungs, adrenals, thymus, and brain. The CT–α-CGRP gene expresses both calcitonin and CGRP, and is processed in the thyroid to CT, in neural tissue to CGRP. Transcription of the gene leads to a large RNA, which is alternatively spliced to either a CT-encoding mRNA or a CGRP-encoding mRNA. Procalcitonin is processed to the 32–amino acid CT, which has a ring of 7–amino acid residues formed by a disulfide bridge at the N-terminal The structure of the chain ends is essential to biological activity. CT, a potent hypocalcemic agent, is secreted in response to elevated serum calcium levels

The *CT receptor* is a member of the G protein–coupled receptor family, and there are several CT receptor subtypes found in bone, brain, and kidney. In bone, the CT receptors are mainly on the osteoclasts, which resorb bone, and on the osteocytes, which assist in bone synthesis. In the kidney, CT receptors are present in both cortex and medulla, especially in the ascending loop of Henle. CT receptors are widely distributed in the brain, including the pituitary, in lymphocytes, and in some tumor cells. All the receptors activate adenylate cyclase, but the various isoforms may use several different signaling pathways.

In bone, CT regulates calcium homeostasis by inhibiting osteoclast activity and decreasing osteoclast production, thus retarding bone demineralization. CT is also involved in periods of rapid bone growth, pregnancy, and lactation, all of which require high calcium levels. CT involvement is influenced by the hypercalcemic action of PTH and vitamin D metabolites, by estrogens, corticosteroids, and T_4. In the kidney, CT causes a rapid and direct increase in water and ion excretion. In the gastrointestinal tract, CT has a general inhibitory effect on secretion and on gallbladder contraction. CT stimulates the secretion of somatostatin, which may mediate the inhibitory actions of CT. Centrally, CT inhibits food intake, has antinociceptive effects, and has complex physiological roles still to be elucidated. Indirectly, through its effects on Ca^{2+} homeostasis, CT is involved in basic cellular functions such as cell permeability, enzyme activation, muscle contractility, transmitter and endocrine secretion, cardiac function, and blood coagulation.

Parathyroid hormone and *parathyroid hormone related protein* function together with calcitonin and vitamin D to maintain calcium homeostasis, a critical function essential for cellular survival. PTH and PTH-rP are present in invertebrates and primitive vertebrates on up to mammals. These two peptides are closely related but have distinct physiological roles in calcium homeostasis. PTH is secreted by the parathyroids and acts on bone and the kidney to increase plasma Ca^{2+} levels. PTH-rP is synthesized in brain and some other tissues, and is probably more important in the fetus in which it may act as a hormonal growth factor.

The *PTH gene* of different mammals shows considerable homology. Prepro-PTH probably represents four copies of a primitive gene and it is processed through pro-PTH to PTH 1–84, then released into the circulation where it is cleaved into its active form, PTH 1–34. PTH gene *expression* is limited almost completely to the parathyroids, but some is expressed in the PVN and SON. *Release* of PTH from the parathyroids and from the CNS is dependent on depletion of extracellular Ca^{2+} and suppressed by vitamin D_3. PTH is rapidly degraded in the circulation and in brain tissues.

The *PTH-rP gene* is on a different chromosome from that of PTH, but the genes are believed to be related in evolutionary terms, although the human PTH-rP gene is more complex than the PTH gene. There is considerable conservation of the primary sequence of PTH-rP up to residue 111, after which there is much species divergence. PTH-rP contains 141–amino acid residues, with 8 of the first 13 N-terminal amino acids identical to those of PTH. Like PTH, PTH-rP activity is confined to the first 34 amino acids and several PTH-rP isoforms have been isolated from different tumors. There is some homology and weak cross-reaction between PTH 15–25 and α-MSH. PTH-rP expression is mainly in the brain, especially the supramammillary nucleus of the hypothalamus, the medial superior olivary nucleus, and in meningeal cells, but it is also abundantly expressed in vascular smooth muscle. PTH-rP is much more highly expressed during ontogeny in the fetal parathyroid and the placenta. PTH-rP does not circulate in the adult but is found in milk.

There is a single *receptor* for PTH and PTH-rP, and the mRNA for this receptor is widely distributed in tissues, including the brain, with the highest concentration being in the parathyroids, indicating a possible paracrine or autocrine function for PTH. The second-messenger system for PTH is through the generation of phosphoinositol triphosphate, but the signaling pathway for PTH-rP is less certain.

The main function of PTH is to increase serum calcium through activating the bone osteoclast receptors to encourage bone resorption, and by increasing Ca^{2+} absorption in the gut through hydroxylation of vitamin D. PTH also affects the reabsorption of phosphate and bicarbonate by the kidney. Lack of PTH is life-threatening. There may be a central role for PTH as it inhibits the firing of hypothalamic neurons and counteracts hypocalcemia. Both PTH and PTH-rP antagonize vasoconstrictors in smooth muscle, causing vasorelaxation. PTH-rP has the same effect as PTH 1–34 on bone, but is also a growth factor during ontogeny, and may be an important regulator of Ca^{2+} homeostasis in the fetus and the transport of Ca^{2+} into milk during lactation. PTH-rP is found in large amounts in lung, rectal, and prostatic tumors.

Thyroid hormones are involved in almost all physiological processes and their absence causes profound deleterious effects on the CNS. They are extremely old peptides which have assumed different functions throughout phylogeny, but in all animals they increase metabolism, and in birds and mammals produce the heat necessary for the evolution from poikilothermy to homeothermy. Thyroid hormones are formed in the thyroid from iodinated amino acids, mono-, di-, tri, or tetra-iodotyrosine, and incorporated into tyrosyl groups of a glycoprotein, thyroglobulin, as T_1 or T_2. Oxidative coupling then produces T_3 and T_4, of which T_3 is the more potent. The thyroid hormones are freed from Tg by lysosomal proteolytic enzymes and secreted into the circulation. The synthesis and release of thyroid hormones is regulated by the TRH-TSH axis, which is inhibited by thyroid hormone at the hypothalamic and pituitary levels. Inadequate iodide supply interferes with thyroid hormone synthesis. Thyroid hormones are also found in the brain.

The *transport* of thyroid hormones through the circulation depends on binding with three thyroid hormone transport proteins: T_4-binding globulin, TTR, and albumin. The choroid plexus may be able to control the concentration of T_4 in the CNS through the formation of a T_4-TTR complex which is secreted into the CSF and distributed to the brain. The choroid plexus accumulates T_4, perhaps synthesizes TTR, and may be involved in the conversion of T_4 to T_3. T_3, the physiologically active form of thyroid hormone, especially in the brain, reacts with receptors in the cell nucleus, to regulate gene transcription. The placenta transfers maternal T_4 to the fetus and interference with this transport causes irreversible brain damage to the fetus. T_3 and T_4 enter the cell mainly by passive diffusion, although there may also be a transport process involving membrane binding sites and receptor-mediated internalization of the hormones. Intracellular T_4 acts as a prohormone for T_3, increasing the supply of T_3. In most cells the thyroid hormones are stored in the cytoplasm, but in pituitary cells about 50% of intracellular T_3 is in the nucleus. The thyroid hormones are *inactivated* in the thyroid, liver, kidney, muscle, and brain, by deiodination. The liberated iodide is excreted in the urine or feces, or reabsorbed and reused.

Thyroid hormone receptors are high-affinity nuclear receptors with DNA-binding properties. They share several characteristics of steroid hormone receptors, and regulate gene transcription. They are placed in the same receptor superfamily as the steroid hormones and certain oncogene receptors. The several thyroid hormone receptor isoforms are regulated in a tissue-specific manner and are synthesized in the cytoplasm and transported to the nucleus, where they interact with T_3, target genes, and other proteins. The various receptor isoforms are differentially distributed and regulated. The most highly regulated is receptor β_2 in the anterior pituitary, which is downregulated by T_3 and TRH. The thyroid receptor isoforms β_1, found in brain, liver, and kidney, and thyroid receptor α_1, present in brown fat and skeletal muscle, are not regulated by TRH, nor is regulation by T_3 as important for these receptor isoforms as it is for β_2 mRNA.

Thyroid hormones are vital for brain development, synapse formation, and proper bone growth in the fetus and neonate. Lack of thyroid hormones in these critical periods results in irrevesible damage and cretinism. The severe growth retardation affects both bone elongation and maturation. In addition, the lack of thyroid hormone prevents the normal cytoskeletal transport of tubulin and actin from their site of synthesis to the site of assembly, thus disrupting synapse formation. Thyroid hormones maintain normal metabolism in all tissues, including the adult brain, acting on several neurotransmitter and enzyme systems. Energy production is boosted by thyroid hormones through stimulation of mitochondrial oxygen consumption, increased ATP production, and an increase in the number of sodium pumps, permitting thyroid hormones to maintain body temperature in homeotherms. Thyroid hormones have marked effects on muscle metabolism, and deficiency or overproduction of thyroid hormone results in myopathies. Similarly, abnormal levels are associated with behavioral and cognitive changes. In rats, perinatal hypothyroidism causes an increase in anxiolytic behavior and in humans, changes in thyroid hormone levels are associated with behavioral and cognitive abnormalities.

Clinically, hypothyroidism in infants may result in irreversible neurological problems and poor mental development, characteristic of cretinism. In adults, hypothyroidism is characterized by weakness, lethargy, slow speech, weight gain, and memory impairment, due to the decreased metabolism. Thickening of the features and eyelid edema (myxedema) result from the accumulation of mucoproteins in the skin. Enlargement of the thyroid due to its inability to respond to TSH results in the neck bulges known as goiters. The goiters contain huge amounts of T_g which lack any thyroid hormone. Depending on the cause, hypothyroidism may be treated with thyroid hormone, iodide, or removal of any environmental goitrogen.

Hyperthyroidism is characterized by an increased metabolism, resulting in weight loss, nervousness, tachycardia, and sweating. Patients with Graves disease have high levels of thyroid hormones with little if any TSH. Treatment of hyperthyroidism may involve antithyroid compounds, radiotherapy, or surgical ablation of the thyroid.

Chapter 19 attempts to cover the vast number of invertebrate neuropeptides, many of which are also found in vertebrates. The similarities in structure and function, which often are striking, indicate the existence of a common, ancient ancestral molecule or parallel evolution of invertebrate and vertebrate neuropeptides.

Invertebrate Neuropeptides

19

19.1 Invertebrate Neuroendocrine Systems

Invertebrate hormonal systems are predominantly neurosecretory, with neurons, the only source of hormones, forming first-order systems (Scharrer, 1975; Scharrer and Scharrer, 1963). Endocrine tissues of non-nervous origin are present only in arthropods. Neurosecretory cells have been found in all metazoan invertebrates, including some coelenterates. In the lower invertebrate phyla, neurosecretions regulate growth, metabolism, water balance, and reproduction, functions that are also regulated by the neuroendocrine system in vertebrates. In addition, the invertebrate neurohormones appear to play an important role in control of visceral activities, which in vertebrates are regulated chiefly by the autonomic nervous system.

Recently, immunocytochemical studies have indicated the presence of molecules in invertebrates that are comparable to many vertebrate neuropeptides: these include CRH, CCK, insulin, glucagon, gastrin, arginine vasopressin (AVP) endorphin, and enkephalin. Some of the neuropeptides, such as vasopressin (VP) and insulin, have actions in certain insects similar to their actions in vertebrates.

The first insect neuropeptide, *proctolin*, was isolated and structurally identified in the mid-1970s from an extract of approximately 125,000 cockroaches (Brown and Starratt, 1975). The next remarkable event was the structural characterization of the first insect neuropeptide identified as a hormone, *adipokinetic hormone*, first identified as *AKH* by Stone et al. (1976), and now, with the identification of other AKHs in the same insect, known as *AKH-I*. Since then, powerful purification techniques, such as reversed-phase high-performance liquid chromatography (RP-HPLC) and high-performance size-exclusion chromatography, together with mass spectrometry, have permitted the rapid isolation and identification of a large number of invertebrate neuropeptides. These techniques, combined with immunocytochemistry, have resulted in the identification of several hundred unique invertebrate neuropeptide structures, with more being isolated and characterized yearly. Molecular biology is being applied to invertebrate neuopeptides now, as has been the case for vertebrate neuropeptides for many years, to reveal gene and precursor structures, details of peptide processing, and receptor structures and affinities, although details are still sparse for many peptides. (See the appendix, section 19.4, for a list of the neuropeptides and their abbreviations used in this chapter.)

With 20 amino acids available in biological tissues, a single peptide chain of 7 amino acids could theoretically exist in 20^7 different forms. Actually, despite the large number of biologically active, identified neuropeptides in both vertebrates and invertebrates, they represent only a small fraction of possible combinations (Agricola and Bräunig, 1995). About 200 peptide sequences have been determined so far in molluscs and arthropods (Keller, 1992; Muneoka and Kobayashi, 1992; Nässel, 1993). The task of identifying all invertebrate neuropeptides is daunting owing to the large number of different invertebrate taxa, the diversity of neuropeptides, and their proclivity to switch the expression of neuropeptide genes according to the stage of development or the type of stimulus. In addition, there is an even greater flexibility in the receptors for the peptides, so that a neuropeptide may be a potent agent in one species but ineffective in a closely related species.

19.1.1 Analogous Neurosecretory Systems of Invertebrates and Vertebrates

There are surprising analogies in the neurosecretory systems of invertebrates and vertebrates (DeLoof, 1987). In the locust, the corpora cardiaca are composed of two distinct parts, the storage and glandular lobes. There is a clear analogy with the posterior and anterior lobes of the pituitary. The storage lobe is a neurohemal gland for peptides synthesized in the pars intercerebralis region of the brain, whereas the glandular lobe is the site of synthesis and release of neuropeptides (the AKHs). Recent work has implicated locustatachykinins from the brain as releasing factors for AKHs from the glandular lobe (Nässel et al., 1993). The corpora allata, a pair of organs near the corpora cardiaca in the head, are comparable in many ways to the vertebrate anterior pituitary. Through their secretion of a neuropeptide *prothoracicotropic hormone (PTTH)* they stimulate a peripheral target organ, the prothoracic gland, to secrete the steroid, *α-ecdysone*. In turn, like the anterior pituitary, the corpora allata are regulated by neuropeptides, *allatotropic hormone (ATH)* and *allatostatin*. Some of these relationships are diagrammed in figure 19.1. The structural similarity of the mammalian hypothalamic-hypophyseal system and the pars intercerebralis-corpora cardiaca-corpora allata system in insects was observed as early as 1944 by Ernst and Berta Scharrer.

19.2 Phylogenetic Description of Invertebrate Neuropeptides

19.2.1 Cnidarians

The cnidarians are less primitive than sponges and include the diploblastic hydra, sea anenomes, corals, and jellyfishes. They have a nervous system that is basically a nerve net, from which the nervous systems of higher organisms probably evolved. Many properties of the cnidarian nervous system, including neurosecretion and neuropeptide biosynthesis, are comparable to those of higher animals. Cnidarians use chemical transmitters or hormones for signal transmission and most of these molecules appear to be peptides, indicating that peptides, not the classical transmitters ACh and the monoamines, are the evolutionarily "oldest" neurotransmitters. The neuropeptide Gly-*Arg-Phe-NH*$_2$, similar to the molluscan (and vertebrate) neuropeptide Phe-Met-*Arg-Phe-NH*$_2$ (FMRFamide, or RFamide), is found in all Cnidaria and probably was the first neurotransmitter (Grimmelikhuijzen and Graff, 1986).

Sea anemone neurons are also specialized according to their neuropeptide content and the neuropeptides

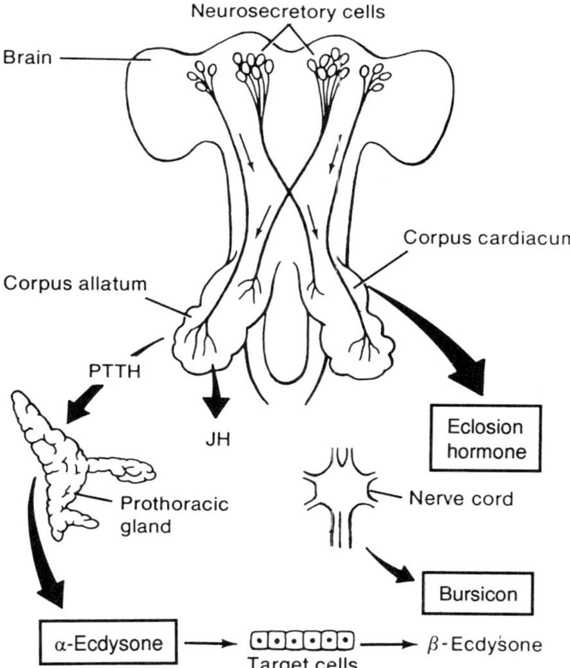

Figure 19.1
Insect endocrine system and its role in the molting process. Neurosecretory cells in the brain convey the neuropeptides, prothoracicotropic hormone (PTTH) and eclosion hormone, via axonal transport to the corpus cardiacum and corpus allatum, which are neurohemal organs. PTTH from the corpus allatum stimulates the prothoracic glands to secrete ecdysone, a steroid which causes the molting of metamorphosis. Eclosion hormone induces emergence of the adult from puparium. Other neurosecretory cells in the brain and nerve cord produce bursicon, a neuropeptide that influences the hardening and darkening (tanning) of the chitinous outer layer after each molt. JH, juvenile hormone. (From Riddiford and Truman, 1978.)

are released from dense-core vesicles from both synaptic and nonsynaptic sites. Biosynthesis of the sea anemone neuropeptides is of special interest as they are derived from large precursor proteins which may contain multiple copies of immature neuropeptides. As many as 16 different neuropeptides have been isolated from a single sea anemone species, *Anthopleura elegantissima.* These peptides are biologically active and inhibit or stimulate muscle contraction (Grimmelikhuijzen and Westfall, 1995).

19.2.2 Flatworms

The flatworms are the most primitive of the triploblastic metazoan animals. Their neurons are mostly neurosecretory, freeing their secretions into loose tissue between the internal organs and the body wall. These neuroactive messengers include a multitude of peptides, of which *neuropeptide F (NPF)* has been isolated and its primary structure determined. NPF is a 39–amino acid peptide with a C-terminal phenylalaninamide. NPF-related peptides are abundantly distributed in the nervous systems of all invertebrate taxa examined so far and they all display structural characteristics of the vertebrate NPY superfamily. Homologies between the gene structure of human NPY and molluscan NPF support the concept that the NPY-NPF gene is of ancient lineage (Maule et al., 1995) and the flatworm NPF is regarded as the phylogenetic precursor of the NPY family (Halton et al., 1992).

19.2.3 Annelids

The leech is an animal belonging to the oldest group of coelomic metazoans, the Annelida. The leech has a pro-opiomelanocortin–derivative peptide (*γ-MSH–like*) and peptides related to enkephalins and the endorphins have been purified from leech brain. A prodynorphin-derived peptide in the leech is identical to vertebrate α-neoendorphin (YGGFLRKYPK), indicating the very ancient phylogenetic origin of opiates and their conservation in the course of evolution (Salzet et al., 1996b).

Four *FMRFamide-related peptides (FaRPs)* have been purified from segmental ganglia extracts of the leech, of which two are involved in leech hydric balance, one being diuretic, the other antidiuretic (Salzet et al., 1994)

Leeches have an angiotensin I–like molecule very similar to human AT I, with a sequence homology of 78% with the N-terminal part of human angiotensinogen. In the structures of the decapeptide AT I shown below, those residues that differ from human or leech are in italics. The amino acid residue at position 5, isoleucine, is present in all leeches up to elasmobranchs, then changed in all vertebrates except humans, into valine (Laurent et al., 1995).

Human	Asp-Arg-Val-Tyr-Ile-His-Pro-Phe-His-Leu
Bird	Asp-Arg-Val-Tyr-*Val*-His-Pro-Phe-*Ser*-Leu
Bullfrog	Asp-Arg-Val-Tyr-*Val*-His-Pro-Phe-*Asn*-Leu
Goosefish	Asn-Arg-Val-Tyr-*Val*-His-Pro-Phe-His-Leu
Leech	Asp-Arg-Val-Tyr-Ile-His-Pro-Phe-His-Leu

Leech AT I also has the appropriate cleavage sites for vertebrate angiotensin metabolic enzymes and a peptide with AT II–like properties has been identified in the leech. Synthetic AT II injections have a diuretic effect in this animal. However, a purified antidiuretic molecule, *leech osmoregulatory factor (LORF)* (Ile-Pro-Glu-Pro-Tyr-Val-Trp-Asp) does not belong to the OT/VP family (Salzet et al., 1996a). It is apparent that the angiotensins are highly conserved in the course of evolution, suggesting fundamental roles for this neuropeptide family in survival and fluid homeostasis (Laurent et al., 1995).

19.2.4 Molluscs: Gastropods

The Mollusca is a large, diverse phylum that includes about 100,000 living species distributed among six classes, the major ones being the *bivalves* (clams, mussels, etc.), the *gastropods* (snails such as *Aplysia* and *Lymnaea*), and the most highly evolved molluscs, the *cephalopods* (squid, octopus, etc.). A large number of putative transmitters, including peptides, has been found in the cephalopod brain, but little is known of their specific functions (Martin and Voigt, 1987).

19.2.4.1 Aplysia Neuroendocrine System

The marine snail *Aplysia* has been used extensively for the study of neuropeptides, their genes, and their processing, since the peptides are present in easily identified, large neurons in ganglia. Neuropeptide-degrading enzymes are present in all tested tissues of *Aplysia*, the major enzymes being aminopeptidases.

Neurosecretory cells are found in the ganglia of the head and abdominal regions and are the source of all the regulatory neuropeptides. There are about 20,000 neurons separated into four pairs of symmetrical ganglia in the head region. These are the buccal, cerebral, pleural, and pedal ganglia. A single asymmetrical abdominal ganglion contains the bag cells that produce the egg-laying hormone. Figure 19.2 illustrates these structures and shows the identifiable large neurons in the abdominal ganglia.

a. Egg-laying hormone and bag cell peptides

The *bag cell neuroendocrine system* in *Aplysia* consists of a cluster of identified neurons that release multiple peptides that control egg-laying. In response to a brief stimulation, the bag cells depolarize by 15 to 20 mV and generate a prolonged afterdischarge. During this discharge, these neurons secrete a 36–amino acid peptide *egg-laying hormone (ELH)*, and three small *bag cell peptides (BCPs)* that are released simultaneously with the egg-laying hormone.

α-BCP	Ala-Pro-Arg-Leu-Arg-Phe-Tyr-Ser-Leu
β-BCP	Arg-Leu-Arg-Phe-His
γ-BCP	Arg-Leu-Arg-Phe-Asp

All three BCPs are capable of depolarizing bag cell neurons in culture. There is a seasonal variability, with the response to the peptides maximal from early summer to late fall, which parallels the frequency of egg-laying. Desensitization of the response to one peptide does not prevent the response to another peptide, which suggests that the three peptides act through separate autoreceptors on the bag cell neurons to activate a sodium-dependent inward current that depolarizes the cell membrane (Loechner and Kaczmarek, 1994).

Following the discharge and the release of the peptides, a fixed sequence of head and neck movements occurs, first a preparatory phase during which the substrate is prepared, followed by a consummatory phase when the egg string is deposited. The ELH acts directly on the smooth muscle of ovarian follicles in the ovotestes to initiate egg-laying by a mechanism analogous to the action of oxytocin on the uterus of mammals. Injection of ELH causes a similar behavioral and physiological response. Comparable control of egg-laying by specific neuroendocrine cells in the pond snail *Lymnaea stagnalis* and an opisthobranch mollusc *Achidoris montereyensis*, suggests that these neuroendocrine cells are members of a homologous group of neurons controlling egg-laying behavior in gastropods (Wiens and Brownell, 1994).

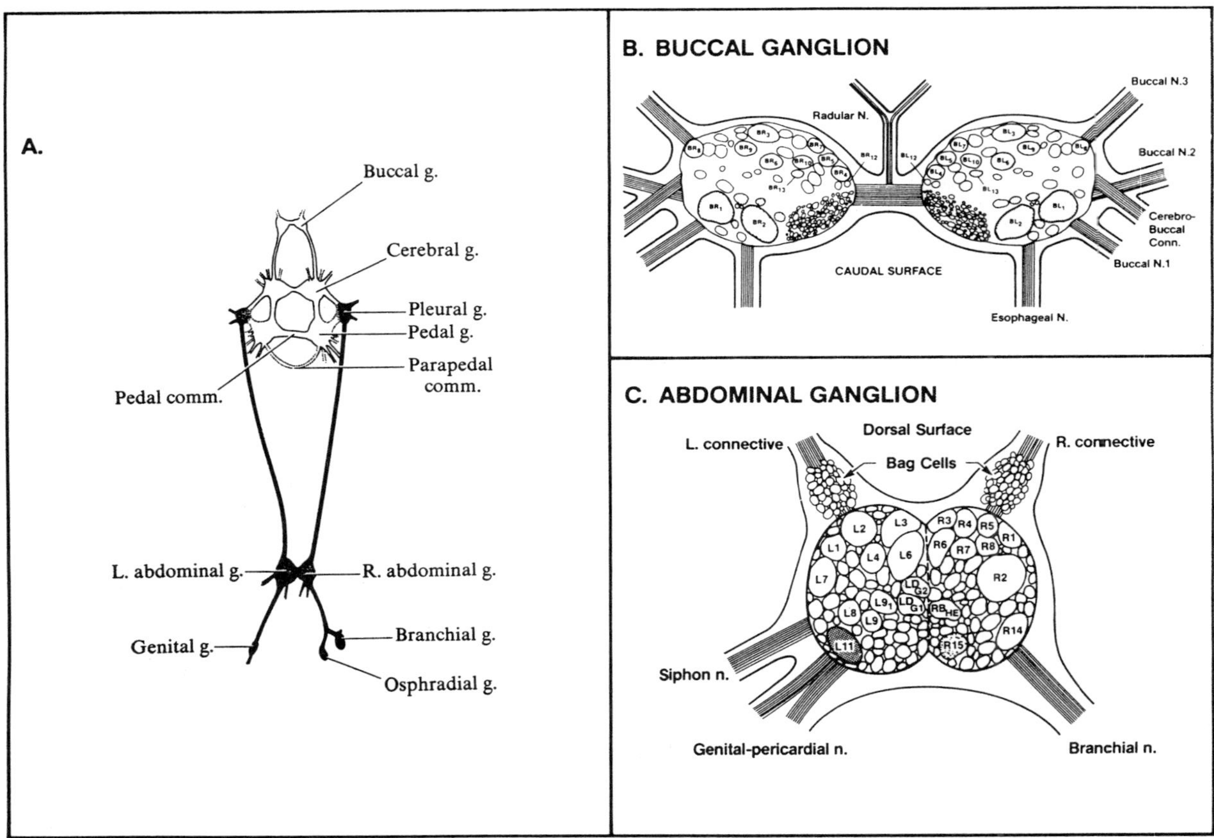

Figure 19.2
(A) Nervous system and associated secretory glands of *Aplysia.* (From Kandel, 1976.) (B) Buccal ganglion showing the large neurons BL_1 and BL_2. (C) Abdominal ganglion with the large neurons R2, R14, and R15. The bag cell neurons form two clusters of about 400 small neurosecretory cells on the pleural abdominal connectives. The bag cells express egg-laying hormone and mediate the egg-laying behavior. R3–8, and R9–13 on the ventral surface (not shown) send processes to terminate on parts of the cardiovascular system. R15 is believed to contain a peptide involved in osmoregulation. R2, the giant cell, expresses a gene encoding multiple copies of FMRFamide. (From Kreiner et al., 1986.)

b. Egg-laying hormone gene, precursor processing, and release

The ELH gene consists of three exons separated by two introns. The gene encodes a precursor molecule consisting of 271 amino acid residues. At least two distinct ELH-encoding mRNAs are found within the bag cells. The processing of the precursor to the 36–amino acid ELH follows the same procedure as in vertebrates: it is cleaved at pairs of basic residues that serve as cleavage sites separating neuroactive peptides. The three additional small BCPs are bounded by paired basic residues that serve as cleavage sites, with ELH being closer to the C-terminus than the BCPs. The peptides are packaged and stored in secretory granules, much as in vertebrate processing.

19.2.4.2 Peptide FMRFamide

Peptide FMRFamide (Phe-Met-Arg-Phe-NH_2), named after the single-letter code for its amino acids, was first identified in molluscs. FaRPs are present in both the invertebrate and vertebrate nervous systems and constitute a major class of invertebrate peptide neurotransmitters. This large, heterogeneous family includes the tetrapeptides FMRFamide and FLRFamide and N-terminally extended forms of varying lengths and structures (figure 19.3). The family of identified FaRPs is rapidly expanding as new members are discovered in almost all invertebrates studied.

a. The FMRFamide gene, precursor processing and release

The FMRFamide gene has been cloned and it consists of five exons covering at least 20 kb. The exons are alternatively spliced: exon 1 (hydrophobic leader sequence) to exon 2 (tetrapeptides) and exon 1 to exons 3 (heptapeptides), 4, and 5 (Kellett et al., 1994). The precursor protein of the FMRFamide locus also encodes two previously unknown predicted peptides, QFYRIamide and EFLRIamide (figure 19.4). Another new peptide family of RFamide peptides, Phe-Arg-Phe-amide (FRFs), related to the FaRPs, has been found in snail motor neurons in small amounts. All the peptides encoded on the FMRFamide gene of *Lymnaea* have now been shown to be expressed (Santama et al., 1996).

b. Actions of FMRFamide and related peptides

In the snail *Helix aspersa*, as well as in *Aplysia*, FMRFamide induces a fast depolarizing response due to direct activation of an amiloride-sensitive Na^+ channel. This channel has been cloned and is the first characterization of a peptide-gated ionotropic receptor (Lingueglia et al., 1995). In the leech, however, FMRFamide hyperpolarizes nephridial sensory nerve cells and decreases their firing rate in a dose-dependent manner (figures 19.5 and 19.6).

FMRFamide is involved in regulating the heartbeat of a pulmonate mollusk. FMRFamide has several effects on neural transmission: it inhibits transmitter release from presynaptic sensory neurons in the neural circuit for the siphon withdrawal reflex, and presynaptically inhibits the output of the motor neurons of the siphon withdrawal reflex. FMRFamide produces a biphasic response in these motorneurons: a fast excitatory response followed by a prolonged inhibitory response, resulting from the activation of at least two K^+ currents. FMRFamide uses the same second messenger to inhibit both sensory and motor neurons (Belkin and Abrams, 1993). A similar inhibition of motor neurons by FMRFamide is seen in the accessory radula closer (ARC) neuromuscular circuit of *Aplysia* (figure 19.7). Nerves that innervate the esophagus are heavily immunoreactive for the FMRFamide family of peptides, indicating FMRFamide's involvement in feeding behavior.

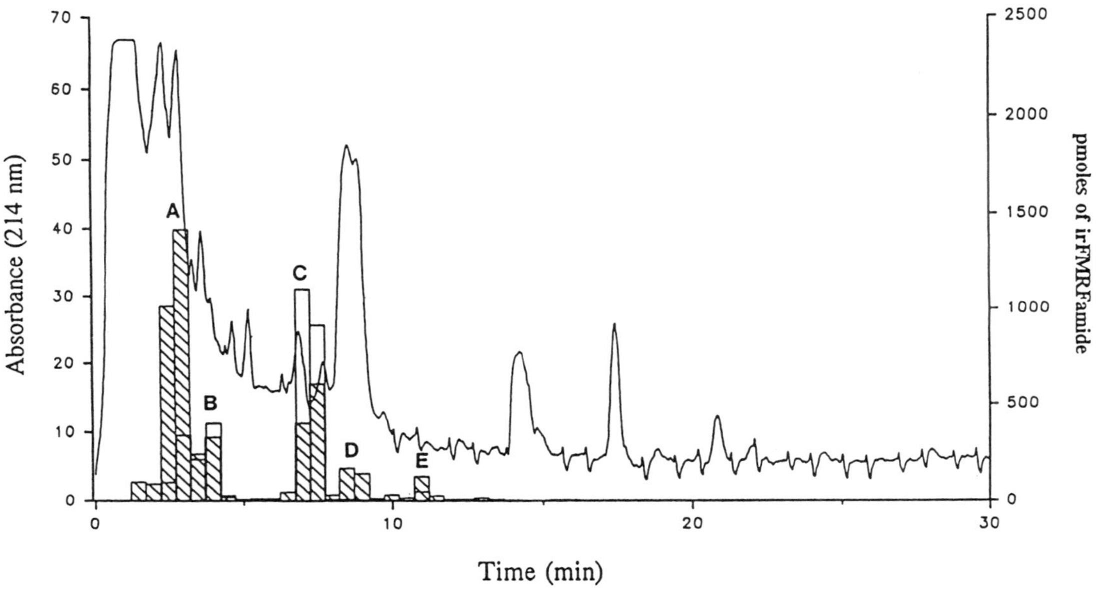

Figure 19.3
High-performance liquid chromatography (HPLC) of snail kidney extract. An extract from 800 kidneys was chromatographed using a Brownlee reversed-phase (RP) 300 (220 × 4.6 mm) column with a linear gradient of 20% to 50% of ACN-TFA solvent. HPLC fractions (2-μL aliquots) were assayed using two different radioimmunoassays (RIAs). The ultraviolet absorbency at 214 nm (solid line) and the radioimmunoreactivity (superimposed histogram) are shown. S253 antiserum is represented by the hatched histogram and Q2 antiserum is the open histogram. RIAs are expressed as picamoles of FMRFamide immunoreactivity (ir-FMRFamide). A, FMRFamide; B, FLRFamide; C, GDPFLRFamide. The two small peaks at D and E do not correspond to any known peptides. (From Madrid et al., 1994.)

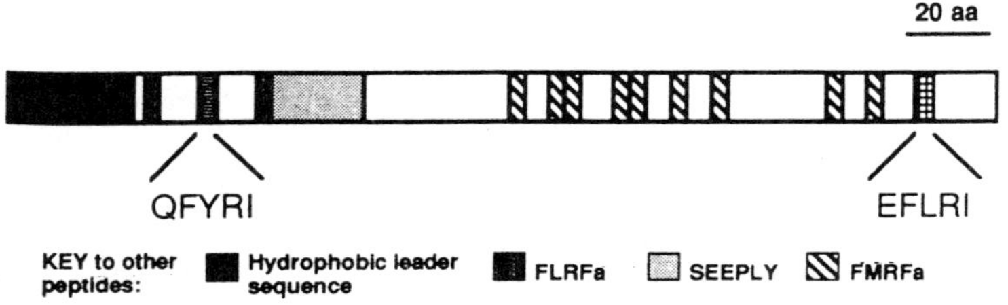

Figure 19.4
Organization of the precursor protein of the FMRFamide locus, encoding two previously unknown predicted peptides. The precursor, bearing an N-terminal hydrophobic leader sequence for post-translational targeting in the endoplasmic reticulum, encoded three types of peptides, shown at the bottom of the panel, in addition to the pentapeptides QFYRI (N-terminal) and EFLRI (C-terminal). All peptides are bound by dibasic cleavage signals and, with the exception of SEEPLY, exhibit a C-terminal signal for amidation. (From Santama et al., 1995.)

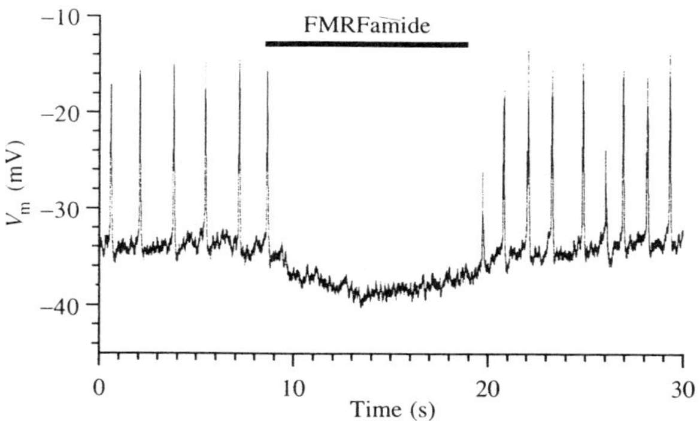

Figure 19.5
Intracellular recording of membrane potential V_m from one nephridial nerve cell in leech saline. During focal application of FMRFamide (10^{-5} mol l^{-1}) the cell hyperpolarized and stopped firing. (From Wenning and Calabrese, 1995.)

19.2.4.3 R15 Neuropeptides

These peptides have been identified in *Aplysia* and form a new family of neuropeptides acting on the cardiovascular, digestive, reproductive, and nervous systems. One member of this family, the α_2-peptide is conserved in lower mammals, such as the hedgehog, in which it is found in the PVN and accessory neurosecretory cells in the lateral hypothalamus, and in the dorsal part of the nucleus tractus solitarius. There is a high degree of coexistence of the R15 α_2-peptide and FaRP (Karagogeos and Papadopoulos, 1994).

19.2.4.4 Cerebral Peptide 1(CP1)

Neurons in the cerebral ganglia of *Aplysia* synthesize ^{35}S methionine-labeled peptides, which are trans-

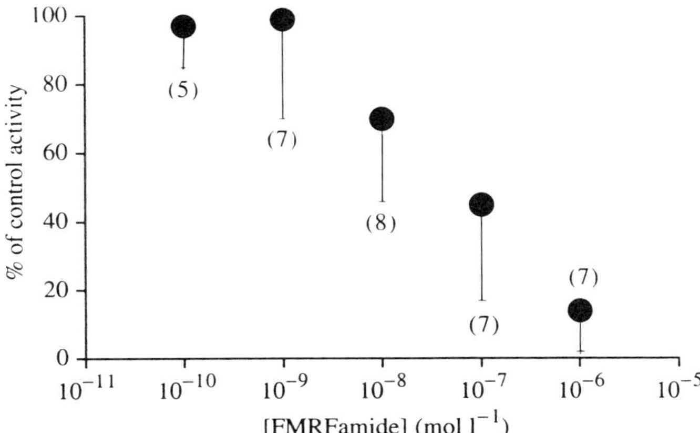

Figure 19.6
The inhibitory effects of FMRFamide on the nephridial nerve cells is dose-dependent, as seen from the extracellular recordings. Bath concentrations of FMRFamide above 10^{-8} mol l^{-1} caused inhibition of spiking when compared with the burst frequency of these cells during the previous control period of 10 minutes (taken as 100%), Data are expressed as mean burst frequency +SEM. The number of experiments is indicated in parentheses for each data point. (From Wenning and Calabrese, 1995.)

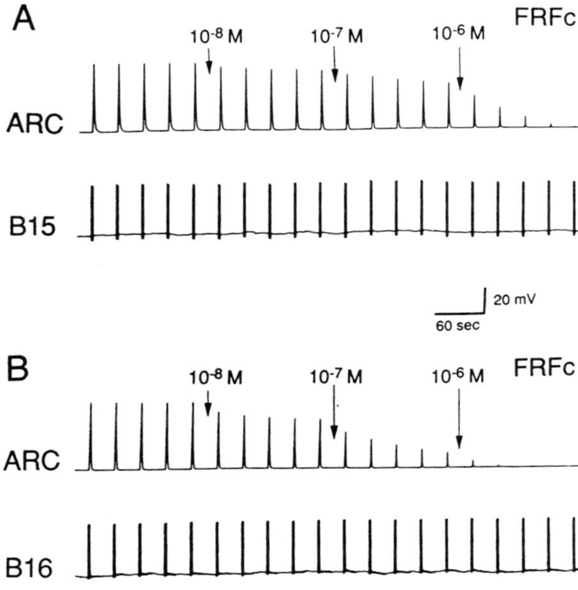

Figure 19.7
Depression of accessory radula closer (ARC) muscle contractions by the FRFs: (Phe-Arg-Phe-amide related to the FMRF-amide neuropeptide) (A). Contractions elicited by stimulation of B15 are less sensitive than B16-elicited contractions. (B). Each motor neuron was stimulated to produce bursts of action potentials (bottom traces) that produced contractions of the ARC muscle (monitored with an isotonic force transducer in the top traces). Increasing concentrations of FRF_c were applied as indicated. (From Cropper et al., 1994.)

ported to other central ganglia by fast axonal transport. One of these is CP1, a widely distributed peptide in *Aplysia* CNS (figure 19.8) and which may be a new peptide transmitter (Phares and Lloyd, 1996). The amino acid sequence of CP1 is

Phe-Ser-Gly-Leu-Met-Ser-Glu-Gly-Ser-Ser-Leu-Glu-Ala-NH_2.

19.2.4.5 Aplysia Neuromuscular Circuits in Feeding Behavior

The ARC neuromuscular circuit, which is involved in the feeding behavior of *Aplysia*, has been used extensively as a model system to study peptidergic transmission. This system displays considerable plasticity due to the modulation of the amplitude and duration of the contractions of the muscle by several neurotransmitters and peptide co-transmitters (Březina et al., 1994). ACh-induced contractions are modulated by several families of peptide co-transmitters, such as the *myomodulins* and the *small cardioactive peptides (SCPs)*. These neuropeptides are released from two motor neurons in the buccal ganglia, B15 and B16, that innervate the ARC muscle (see figure 19.2) when the motor neurons are stimulated at high frequency and over long duration. Serotonin and nitric oxide are also significant in interneuronal communication in *Aplysia*.

a. *Myomodulin structure, gene, and second messengers*

The myomodulin family of neuropeptides is a major, widely distributed group of molluscan neuropeptides that act as neuromuscular modulators and cotransmitters. Myomodulins are released from central neurons and affect the electrophysiological and contractile characteristics of muscle. The structure of myomodulin, for both *Aplysia* and *Lymnaea*, as shown by Araki et al., (1995), is

Pro-Met-Ser-Met-Leu-Arg-Leu-NH_2.

A *single gene* encodes nine structurally similar forms of myomodulin, some of which are present in multiple copies in the gene (Březina et al., 1995). The organization of the gene indicates that it is transcribed as a single spliced transcript from an upstream promoter region that contains multiple cAMP-

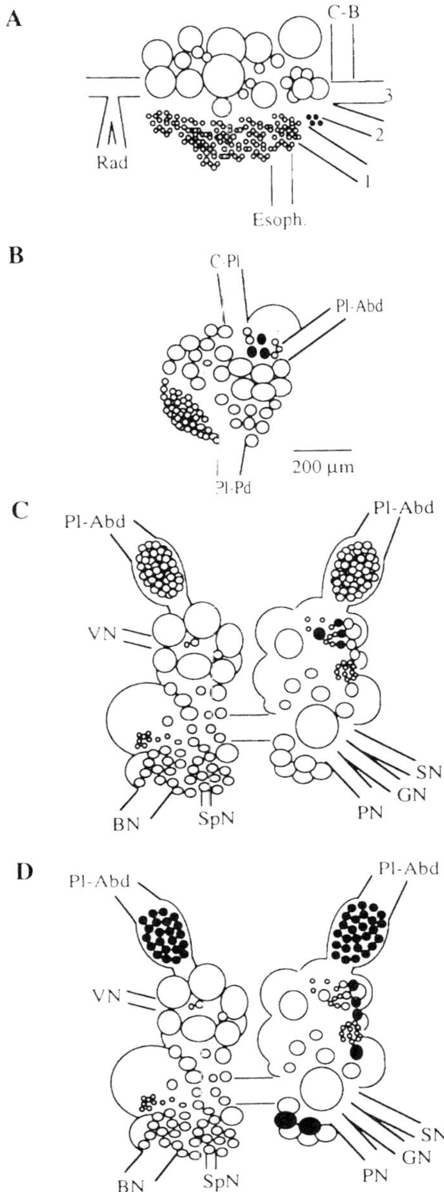

Figure 19.8
Schematic diagrams showing the location of CP1-immunoreactive neurons (black circles) in the cerebral ganglia (E and F) and other ganglia (A–D) of *Aplysia.* (A) Buccal ganglia, rostral surface. Three to five CP1-immunoreactive neurons

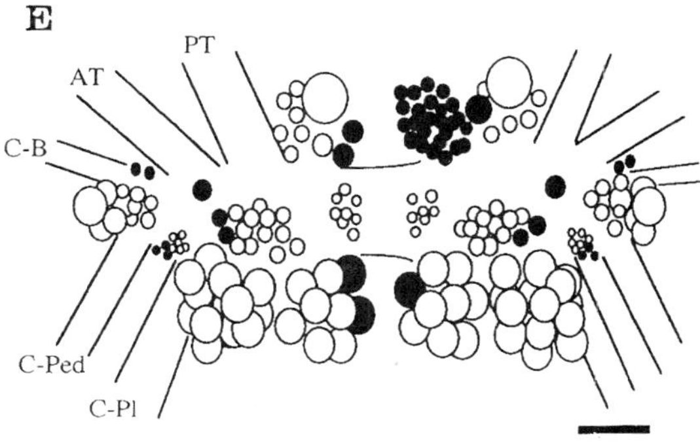

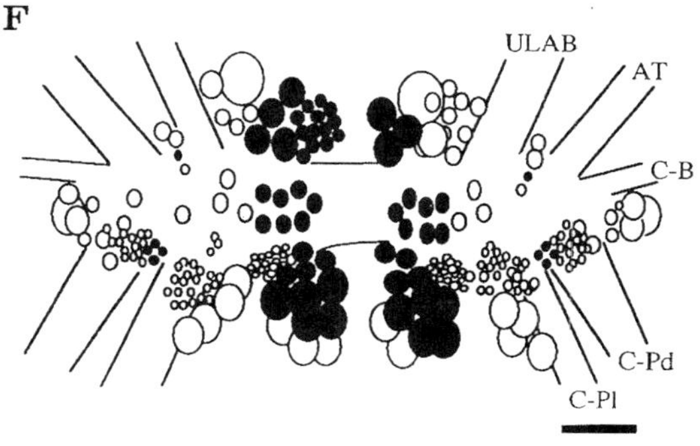

Figure 19.8 (continued)
were found in each ganglion between nerves 1 and 2. Esoph, esophagus; Rad, radular nerve; 1–3, buccal nerves 1–3. (B) Left pleural ganglion. Corresponding neurons were observed in the right pleural ganglion. Connective nerves are indicated: C-Pl, cerebral-pleural; Pl-Abd, pleural-abdominal; Pl-Pd, pleural-pedal. (C) Ventral surface of abdominal ganglion showing location of CP1 neurons. (D) Ventral surface of abdominal ganglion showing the location of neurons with CP1-immunoreactive fibers on their cell bodies. Nerves in (C) and (D) are designated after Kandel, 1976: BN, branchial nerve; GN, genital nerve; Pl-Abd, pleural-abdominal connectives; PN, pericardial nerve; SN, siphon nerve; SpN, spermathecal nerve; VN, vulvar nerve. Scale bar in B applies to all diagrams. (E) Cerebral ganglia showing the distribution of CP1 on the dosal surface. (F) Cerebral ganglia showing the distribution of CP1 on the ventral surface. Scale bar-300 μm. AT, anterior tentacular nerve; C-B, cerebral buccal connective; C-Pd, cerebral pedal connective; C-Pl, cerebral pleural connective; PT, posterior tentacular nerve; ULAB, upper labial nerve. (From Phares and Lloyd, 1996.)

responsive elements with homology to tissue-specific promoter-binding sites. The gene is expressed in single identified neurons in all ganglia of the CNS (Kellet et al., 1996).

Myomodulin increases cAMP levels and increases cAMP-dependent protein kinase levels in the ARC muscle of *Aplysia.* The similar effects of the SCPs on ARC muscle may be due to their use of the same signal transduction pathway (Hooper et al. 1994).

b. Actions of myomodulin

Myomodulins are present in the neural network, especially neurons in the buccal ganglia, that controls feeding behavior in the snails *Aplysia* and *Lymnaea.* All nine myomodulins enhance the Ca^{2+} current, potentiate the amplitude, and accelerate the relaxation rate of the contractions of the ARC neuromuscular circuit (figure 19.9). In addition, some of the myomodulins depress ARC muscle contractions by activating the K^+ current. The net potentiation or depression then depends on the balance between the relative strengths of the modulation of the two ion currents (Březina et al., 1994).

Myomodulins affect other neuromuscular circuits, for example, neurons in the right cerebral ganglion that innervate the penis complex via the penis nerve produce myomodulin, which accelerates the relaxation rate of electrically induced contractions of the penis retractor muscle (Li et al., 1994a).

c. Small cardioactive peptide

SCPs are a peptide family implicated in the control of the cardiovascular system and of the muscles involved in feeding and gut motility. The SCPs were first isolated from muscle of *Mytilus edulis* (mussel) and shown to have a primary structure of

Ala-Pro-Asn-Phe-Leu-Ala-Tyr-Pro-Arg-Leu-NH_2.

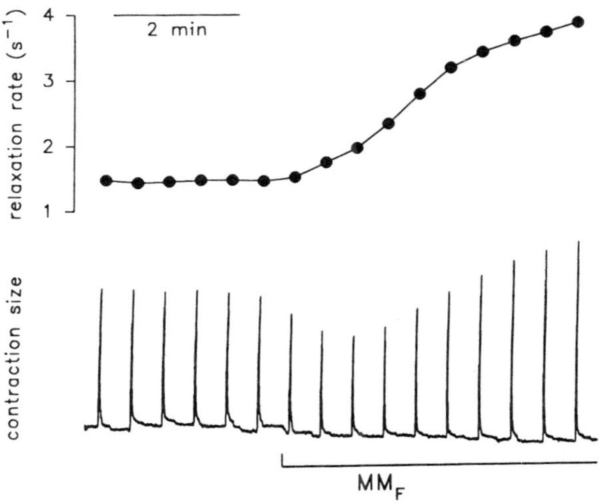

Figure 19.9
Modulation of relaxation rate (top) of the accessory radula closer muscle of *Aplysia* develops slowly, after application of 10nM myomodulin$_F$ (MM_F), paralleling potentiation of contraction amplitude, rather than the brief depression that normally precedes contraction potentiation. (From Březina et al., 1995.)

There are similar but distinctive SCPs in clams that are true homologs of the gastropod SCPs and have similar roles, controlling feeding and digestion and perhaps even cardioactivity (Candelariomartinez et al., 1993). Immunoreactive SCP-B (SCP B-ir) is found in cell bodies of buccal, cerebral, pedal, and intestinal ganglia, as well as in anterior esophagus and in buccal cones. *Aplysia* motor neurons B1, B2, and B15 synthesize the SCPs but they are released only when these neurons are stimulated at high frequency or at lower frequencies with long burst duration. The role of SCPs in feeding behavior is clearly demonstrated by their ability to activate the cerebral ganglion neurons involved in the capture of prey by the carnivorous pteropod mollusc *Clione limacina* (Norekian and Satterlie, 1994). As mentioned above, the SCPs use the same second-messenger system as the myomodulins, cAMP-dependent protein kinase.

19.2.4.6 The Insulin Superfamily of Neuropeptides

The insulin superfamily of regulatory peptides is involved in essential steps in growth, development, metabolism, and reproduction in both vertebrates and invertebrates. The members of this superfamily are quite diverse in structure and function, but they all share the basic insulin globular configuration, indicating that it must have been present in the common ancestors of these organisms, the Archaemetazoa, which date back as far as 6.10^8 years. For a detailed and engrossing description of the evolution of the insulin superfamily, see Geraerts et al. (1992).

A family of *molluscan insulin-related peptides (MIP)* is produced by the light-green cells in the cerebral ganglia of *Lymnaea.* These are giant neurons, about 90 µm in diameter, lying in two clusters in each cerebral ganglion (figure 19.10) and they are involved in the regulation of a wide variety of physiological processes asociated with growth, metabolism, and reproduction.

Four genes encode the precursors of MIPs I, II, III, IV, V, and VI. The organization of the MIP I gene is compared with that of the human insulin gene in figure 19.11. All the MIP genes show the overall structure typical of the insulin genes, with three exons interspaced with two introns. The exons code for similar domains of the precursors in both the MIP genes and the insulin genes (figure 19.12).

An insulin receptor has been identified in *Aplysia* that is similar to the vertebrate insulin receptor. Application of vertebrate insulin to clusters of bag cell neurons stimulates the phosphorylation of the receptor on tyrosine residues and produces an increase in height and decrease in duration of the action potential. This very interesting observation suggests that insulin may have quite a different function in invertebrates, regulating the excitability of the bag cell neurons (Jonas et al., 1996).

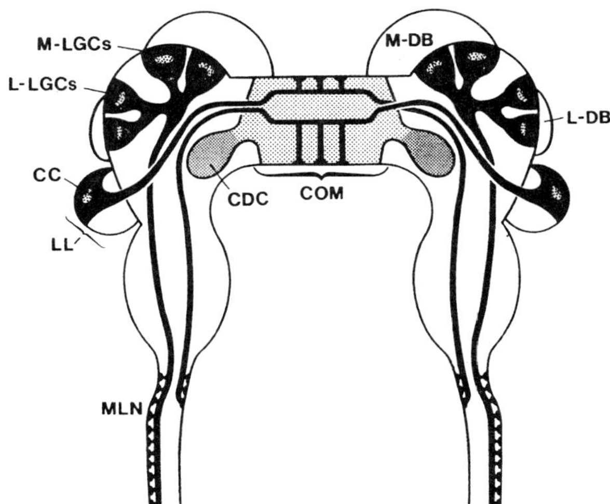

Figure 19.10
Location and anatomical organization of the light-green cell (LGC) system in the cerebral ganglia of *Lymnaea stagnalis*, based on lucifer yellow fillings and light and electron microscopy. Note the intricate axonal topology of the canopy cells (CC) in the lateral lobes, which strongly suggest that the CCs control the activities of the other LGCs, and of the female gonadotropic centers, the caudodorsal cells (CDC) and dorsal bodies (DB). M-LGC and L-LGC, medio- and laterodorsal groups of LGCs, respectively; MLN, median lip nerve, the neurohemal area of the CDCs; M-DB and L-DB, medio- and laterodorsal bodies, respectively. (From Geraerts et al., 1992.)

19.2.4.7 Neuromuscular Circuits Involved in Copulation

The neuronal network that underlies male copulatory behavior is characterized by a large diversity of peptides and a complex regulation of copulation. Conopressin which is structurally related to VP, in-

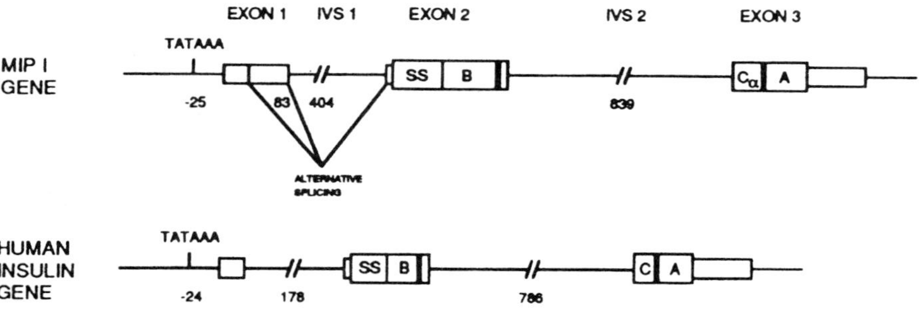

Figure 19.11
Schematic representation of the molluscan insulin–related peptide (MIP) I gene and the human insulin gene. The MIP genes II–VI have a similar organization. Indicated are the exons and the intervening sequences (IVS). SS, signal sequence: B, B chain; A, A chain; C_α, C_α peptide. Goldberg-Hogness box TATAAA. Numbers refer to nucleotide length. The alternative splicing in exon 1 of the MIP gene is also indicated. (From Geraerts et al., 1992.)

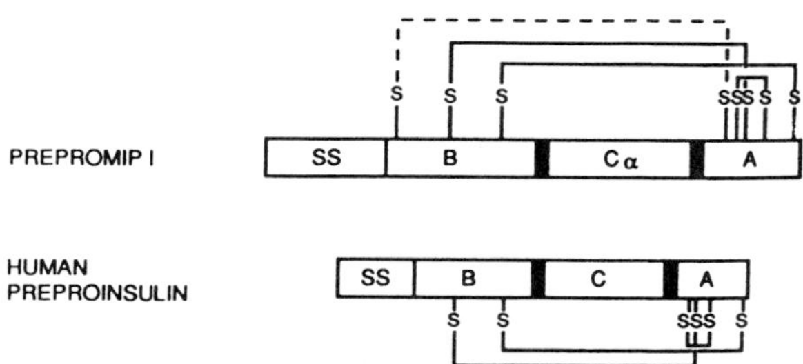

Figure 19.12
Schematic representation of the precursors of molluscan insulin–related peptide (MIP) I and human insulin. The precursors are aligned on the positions of the cysteine residues involved in the interchain disulfide bridges in the B chain domains. SS, signal sequence; B, B chain; A, A chain; C_α, C_α peptide; C, C peptide; S, position of cysteine residue. The extra putative disulfide bridge in MIP is indicated by a dotted line, others by solid lines. Vertical black bars indicate proteolytic cleavage sites. (From Geraerts et al., 1992.)

duces muscular contraction of the vas deferens in *Lymnaea*. Another peptide APGWamide, which is co-localized with conopressin, inhibits the conopressin-induced contractions. These two peptides may be balanced in regulating peristaltic movements of the vas deferens (Van Kesteren et al., 1995). Myomodulins are also implicated in the regulation of copulation, as referred to in section 19.2.4.5.

19.2.4.8 Peptides Involved in Urine Formation and Release

The light-yellow neuropeptide cell system consists of neuronal cell clusters in the ganglia of the visceral complex in many species of snails. These neurons produce three different neuropeptides: the precursor, prepro-LYCP (*l*ight-*y*ellow *c*ell *p*eptide), is processed into LYCP I, II, and III. LYCP I and II act as intermediates in a peptide-processing sequence to produce several variant peptides (Li et al., 1994a). The LYCP-containing neurons project to the muscles of the pulmonary system and to muscles of the ureter-pneumostome area, indicating that this system is probably involved in the regulation of blood pressure and urine release (Boer and Montagnewajer, 1994). Other neuropeptides involved in urine formation that are found in *Aplysia* and *Lymnaea* include AT I-, urotensin I-, and urotensin II-like peptides.

19.2.4.9 Toxic Neuropeptides

Conus peptides are conotoxins that have widespread activity on a number of voltage-sensitive calcium channels and are important pharmacological tools. They potently block sodium conductance in *Aplysia* neurons. A newly identified conotoxin, delta conotoxin GmVIA, consists of 29 amino acids, including 6 Cys residues. The peptide broadens the action potential and has an unusual specificity for molluscan sodium channels, slowing Na^+ current inactivation. Other conotoxins are Ca^{2+} channel ligands. Purified delta-conotoxin-GmVIA from the mollusc-hunting snail *Conus gloriamaris* induces convulsive-like contractions when injected into land snails but has no effects in mammals (Hasson et al., 1995).

19.2.4.10 Opiate Peptides

Opiate peptides have been found in bacteria and in almost all invertebrates, but the opiate system has been most thoroughly studied in molluscs. It has been suggested that there is a precursor in invertebrates that encodes both opiate and FMRFamide peptides. Met-enkephalin and leu-enkephalin have been isolated in some snails and octopus, as well as ACTH, α-MSH and β-endorphin (Harrison et al., 1994).

19.2.4.11 Neuropeptide F (NPF)

This peptide is widely distributed in gastropods.

19.2.5 Molluscs: Cephalopods

There is scanty information about neuropeptides in cephalopods, which have been intensively studied by electrophysiologists rather than by neuroendocrinologists. The optic glands of cephalopods are small endocrine organs lying on the optic stalks on either side of the brain. They contain no neurosecretory cells and produce a gonadotropin that induces gonadal enlargement. The production of the gonadotropin by the gland is inhibited by nerves originating in the subpedunculate lobe of the brain, which in turn are regulated by changes in photoperiod (figure 19.13).

19.2.5.1 Neuropeptide F

This peptide is absent or present only in minute amounts in the cephalopod *Loligo vulgaris* (octopus). When tested with two NPF region–specific antisera, the neural tissues of *Loligo* react only to the antiserum against the C-terminal, showing that the N-terminal region of the peptide is not conserved in cephalopods (Leung et al., 1994).

19.2.5.2 Cephalotocin

This is an OT-VP–immunoreactive peptide isolated from the nerve terminals of the "neurosecretory system of the vena cava" in the octopus. Cephalotocin has a molecular weight of 1070 and a 1–6 disulfide bond. The amino acid sequence of this neuropeptide is

Cys-Tyr-Phe-Arg-Asn-Cys-Pro-Ile-Gly-NH_2.

Cephalotocin exhibits 78% sequence homology with the vertebrate neurohypophyseal hormone mesotocin and clearly belongs to the OT-VP family of vertebrates (see chapters 1 and 11), indicating the high degree of conservation of this neuropeptide family (Reich, 1992).

19.2.6 Crustaceans

19.2.6.1 Crustacean Neuroendocrine System

Studies on crustacea have contributed substantially to

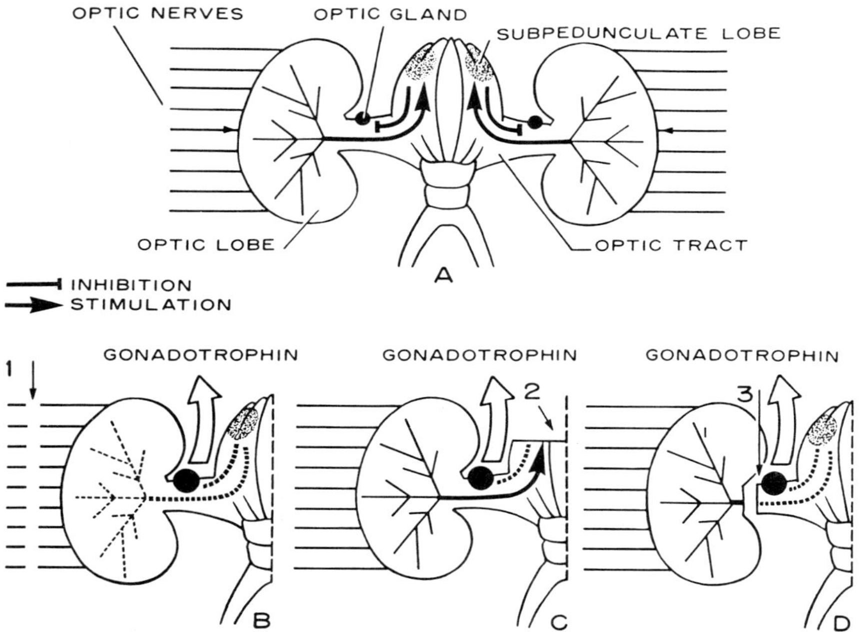

Figure 19.13
Neuroendocrine control of gonad maturation in the octopus. (A) In an immature animal the production of gonadotropin in the brain is inhibited by nerves originating in the subpedunculate lobe of the brain. (B) Section of the optic nerves (point 1) prevents activation (broken lines) of the inhibitory nerve center; the optic glands enlarge and secrete gonadotropin, which causes hypertrophy of the gonads. The same result is obtained by ablation of the subpeduncular lobes (C, point 2) or by section of the optic tract (D, point 3). (From Wells and Wells, 1959.)

the concepts of neurosecretion and neuroendocrine regulation. Many crustacean neuropeptides are concerned with color changes, and the first invertebrate neuropeptide to be isolated and sequenced was *red pigment–concentrating hormone (RPCH)*, which controls shrimp chromatophores (Fernlund and Josefsson, 1972). Since then a large number of neuropeptides has been identified in crustacea and their wide range of physiological functions examined. Many crustacean neuropeptides are found in other invertebrates, but several neuropeptides appear to be restricted to crustacea, perhaps because their different habitats (seawater, freshwater, terrestrial) require complex mechanisms of hydromineral regulation, as suggested by Keller (1992).

The neurendocrine system in crustacea consists of aggregations of neuroendocrine cells that produce neurohormones and release them from their axon terminals into neurohemal organs for storage or modification. Secondly, there are true non-neural endocrine glands that secrete their products into the circulation. The endocrine and neuroendocrine glands of a generalized crustacean are diagrammed in figure 19.14.

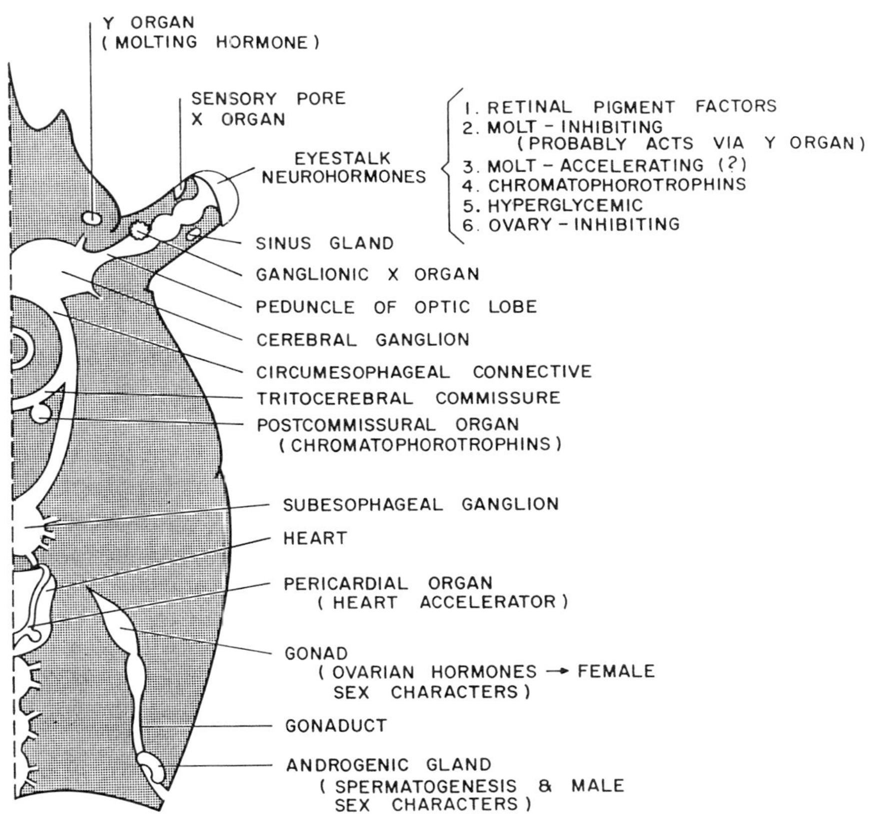

Figure 19.14
Summarizing diagram of the cephalothorax of a generalized crustacean, showing the locations of the best-known endocrine glands and neuroendocrine structures. The active principles from these structures are listed or shown in parentheses. Neurosecretory cells are present in all components of the CNS, and no attempt has been made to show them. (From Turner, 1966.)

a. *The X Organs*

These are important neuroendocrine organs present in the optic ganglia within the eyestalks. The X organs are of two types: ganglionic X organs and sensory pore X organs (see figure 19.14). In some species of crustacea, the ganglionic X organ fuses with the sensory pore X organ to form a single structure, whereas in other species they remain as separated groups of neurosecretory cells.

b. *The sinus gland*

The sinus gland is found in nearly all crustaceans. It is not a gland but rather a neurohemal organ—a storage and release site for hormones produced in neurosecretory cells. It is analogous to the neurohypophysis in vertebrates and to the corpus cardiacum of insects. The sinus gland contains axon endings of neurosecretory cells from several sources, including the X organ in the optic stalk. In its simplest form the sinus gland is a thickened disk separated from a blood sinus by a thin membrane, but invagination may result in a more complex structure in which the blood channels permeate and diffuse through the organ. Upon appropriate stimulation, the sinus releases its stored hormones into the blood. The hormones of the sinus gland are especially active in the regulation of color changes.

c. *Hormones of the X organ–sinus gland complex*

This complex is involved in the regulation of molting, color changes, and distal retinal pigment movements. Extracts from the eyestalks, from postcommissural organs, and from the CNS contain myotropic factors that influence the contraction of visceral muscles. The complex produces hormones that inhibit the ovary and some that inhibit the testis (crabs). In addition, this complex is involved in the regulation of carbohydrate metabolism, gonadal growth, and the synthesis of a crustacean form of juvenile hormone.

There are *four endocrine glands* not composed of neurosecretory cells. The *Y organs*, which produce a hormone that initiates molting and that is under the regulation of the X organ complex. An eyestalk hormone appears to inhibit production of Y organ hormone. The other two endocrine glands are the *androgenic glands*, which are usually outside the testes, along the vas deferens, and the *ovary*. The fourth gland consists of the *mandibular organs*, which in decapods are paired structures generally present near the Y organs in the mandibular region. These produce the *mandibular organ–inhibiting hormone (MOIH)*.

The *postcommissure organ* is a neurohemal organ found in higher crustaceans. It contains substances that affect color changes. The *pericardial organs* are also neurohemal structures and contain neurosecretory cells plus the axons of neurosecretory cells originating in ventral ganglia. Extracts of these organs increase the frequency and amplitude of the heartbeat.

19.2.6.2 Crustacean Neuropeptides

a. *Neuropeptides from the X organ*

This family consists of four neuropeptides synthesized by large neurons in the X organ: *crustacean hyperglycemic hormone (CHH), molt-inhibiting hormone (MIH)*, and *vitellogenesis-inhibiting hormone (VIH)* or *gonad-inhibiting hormone (GIH). MOIH* is a crustacean form of juvenile hormone (JH) analogous to the allostatins of insects (Wainwright et al., 1996). These neuropeptides are transported along axons to be stored in, then released from, the sinus gland.

CHH from three species, the crayfish, lobster, and shore crab, consists of a sequence of 72– to 73–amino acid amides with between 61% and 81% homology. The sequence differences are significant, however, as they result in striking variations on interspecific hyperglycemic activity: the shore crab CHH, for instance is ineffective in the crayfish (Keller, 1992).

Peptides belonging to the CHH family are generally polymorphic, due to changes in the amino acid sequence, and to isomerization of 1 amino acid residue (Phe^3 in lobster or crayfish CHH) from the L- to the D-configuration. This isomerization occurs in specialized neurosecretory cells and is a new method of post-translational modification.

The other two members of the X-organ neuropeptide family are 75 to 78 amino acid residue inhibitory neuropeptides involved in the regulation of molting (MIH), especially in crabs, and reproduction (VIH). Lobster and shore crab VIH are more closely related to each other (48% homology) than either is related to the CHH from the same species, indicating that these neuropeptides have diverged considerably from their common family peptide, the CHH. The precursors to the two subgroups show striking differences: in the CHH precursor, the hormone is separated from the signal peptide by a 33 to 38 amino acid peptide, which is absent in the precursor to MIH or VIH. For the latter two precursors, the signal peptide is directly next to the hormone, without a classic dibasic cleavage site (Soyez, 1997). There is no evidence that this group of neuropeptides plays a neurotransmitter or neuromodulator role.

b. Cardioactive and myotropic neuropeptides

The *pericardial organs* are large neurohemal organs in the pericardial cavity, rich in peptides that are released into the circulation, acting as classical hormones. Many of these neuropeptides are also found in the nervous system, where they probably act as transmitters or neuromodulators.

Proctolin The pentapeptide proctolin, Arg-Tyr-Leu-Pro-Thr, was first isolated and sequenced from the cockroach on the basis of its hindgut activity. Proctolin is a modulatory transmitter found throughout the crustacean nervous system and has a wide range of stimulatory actions on different types of muscles and neurons. Many of the neurons that innervate crustacean skeletal muscle directly are proctolin-immunoreactive. Proctolin stimulation of cardiac ganglion motor neurons results in the acceleration of heart rate and increased cardiac contraction amplitude. In addition, it has the unusual ability to affect the contractility of the heart valves (Kuramato and Ebara, 1989). Proctolin modulates neurons of the stomatogastric ganglia and has a potent contracting action on the crayfish hindgut (Keller, 1992). Proctolin is enzymatically degraded and thus biologically inactivated in the crab nervous system, primarily by an extracellular aminopeptidase (Coleman et al., 1994).

FMRFamide-Related Neuropeptides Five distinct FaRPs have been isolated in crustaceans, all of them unique to this family and actually belonging to the FLRFamide (Phe-Leu-Arg-Phe)amide subset of FMRFrps (Dircksen et al., 1987). These FMRFrps are mostly concentrated in the pericardial organ system, but they are also found throughout the nervous system, indicating that they may act as neurotransmitters or neuromodulators, or both. Somewhat sparse data indicate that they increase the contractile force of the heart, the hindgut, and of the deep abdominal extensor muscles of different crustacean species (Mercier et al., 1990).

Crustacean Cardioactive Peptide (CCAP) This neuropeptide has been isolated and sequenced from the pericardial organ system, in which it is most concentrated, but it is also found throughout the nervous system. Limited observations indicate that CCAP has an excitatory action on the heart, hindgut, and respiratory rhythm, but these actions vary in the different crustaceans in which CCAP has been tested (Keller, 1992). CCAP has also been identified in the insect *Locusta* (Dircksen et al., 1987).

Orcokinin This myotropic neuropeptide has been isolated from the ventral nerve cord of the crayfish and is a potent activator of the hindgut. The primary structure of orcokinin is

Asn-Phe-Asp-Glu-Ile-Glu-Arg-Ser-Gly-Phe-Gly-Phe-Asn

and it has no similarity to that of any other known neuropeptide (Bungart et al., 1994).

c. The chromatophorotropins

Red Pigment–Concentrating Hormone This neuropeptide was first isolated and sequenced from the eyestalks of the prawn (Fernland and Josefsson, 1972) and its hormonal actions on chromatophores in crustaceans have been well investigated. It is now believed to have several other physiological actions, including an excitatory action on the stomatogastric ganglion of the crab and an excitatory modulatory effect on swimmeret activity rhythms in the crayfish (Dickinson et al., 1990). RPCH is a member of the AKH-related–RPCH peptide family, which consists mostly of AKH-related insect neuropeptides. Whereas there is considerable variation in this family in insects, RPCH has been highly conserved in crustaceans. The structure of crustacean RPCH is

pGlu-Leu-Asn-Phe-Ser-Pro-Gly-Trp-NH_2.

Pigment-Dispersing Hormones This is a family of octadecapeptides, found in crustaceans and insects (Rao and Riehm, 1989). Although there are suggestions that these peptides may have local neurotransmitter or neuromodulator functions, the only demonstrated physiological effect is pigment movement in chromatophores. The structure of crab pigment-dispersing hormone is shown below, with differences in amino acid residues in the insect pigment-dispersing hormone in italic.

Crab Asn-Ser-Glu-Leu-Ile-Asn-Ser-Ile-Leu-Gly-Leu-Pro-Lys-Val-Met-Asn-Asp-Ala^{18}-NH_2

Insect Asn-Ser-Glu-*Ile*-Ile-Asn-Ser-*Leu*-Leu-Gly-Leu-Pro-Lys-Val-*Leu*-Asn-Asp-Ala^{18}-NH_2

19.2.7 Insects

19.2.7.1 Insect Neuroendocrine System

The insect neuroendocrine system is organized in a manner remarkably similar to that of vertebrates. The general pattern involves neurosecretory cells in the cerebral, subesophageal, and other ganglia. Neurosecretory cells in the protocerebrum send axons to the corpus cardiacum, which is usually a paired structure just behind the supraesophageal ganglion. The corpora cardiaca are neurohemal organs, which both store and release peptides synthesized in the brain, and have their own intrinsic peptides (AKHs), and are comparable to the neurohypophysis of vertebrates. Closely associated with the corpora cardiaca in most insects are the corpora allata, endocrine glands of non-nervous tissue origin, which are also regulated by the brain (figure 19.15).

The first experiments to demonstrate endocrine control of insect development were done by Kopě (1922), who found that removal of the brain prevents pupation and that reimplantation of the brain permits pupation to proceed. The neurons of the pars intercerebralis of the brain secrete *prothoracicotrophic hormone (PTTH)* at their nerve endings in the corpus allatum, from which PTTH is released into the blood. PTTH, a neuropeptide, stimulates the prothoracic glands to produce ecdysone, a steroid that induces molting (see figure 19.1).

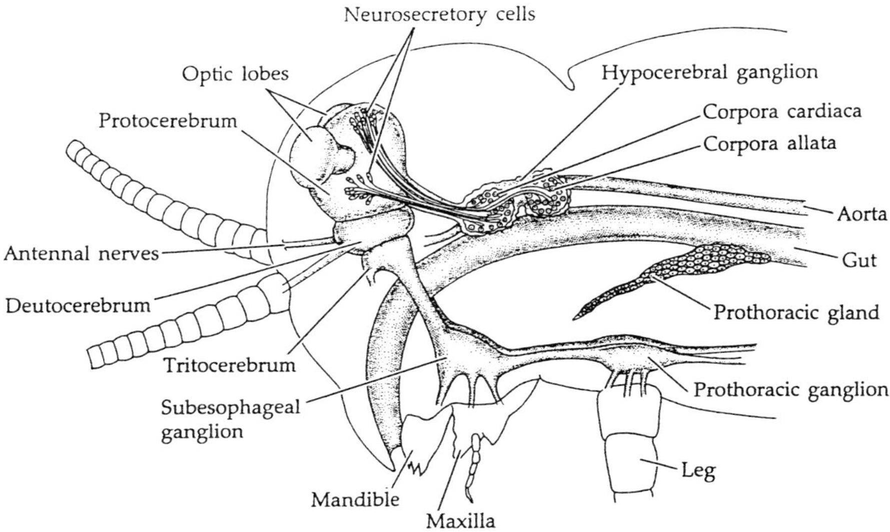

Figure 19.15
Endocrine organs and CNS in the head and thorax of a generalized insect. Hormones are produced by neurosecretory cells in the protocerebrum and subesophageal neurosecretory cells. These hormones pass in two paired nerves to the corpora cardiaca. Hormones are also secreted by two paired glands, the corpora allata, which receive axons from the corpora cardiaca. The prothoracic glands act as ecdysial glands. (From Wells, 1968.)

The accessory medulla of the cockroach has a rich assortment of neuropeptides, some of which are colocalized in secretory granules. The identified neuropeptides include allostatin 7, allatropin, gastrin-CCK, FMRFamide, leucokinin I, substance P, a peptide related to locustatachykinin I and II, and corazonin, the cockroach cardioactive peptide. It has been suggested that the accessory medulla is a circadian pacemaking center in the insect brain (Petri et al., 1995).

Insect neuropeptides may be divided into two main categories: homeostatic and behavioral neuropeptides, and developmental and reproductive neuropeptides (Menn et al., 1991). Tables 19.1 and 19.2 list some examples of these peptides, their functions, and their sequences, and table 19.3 groups together the most important of the neuropeptides involved in metamorphosis. Most of the neuropeptides so far have been isolated and sequenced from the locusts *Locusta migratoria* and *Schistocerca gregaria*, and from the cockroach *Leucophaea maderae*. The recent explosive growth in the characterization of insect neuropeptides has been facilitated by the use of a convenient bioassay, the *Leucophaea* hindgut (Holman et al., 1991), as well as physical techniques such as rP-HPLC, fast atom bombardment tandem mass spectrometry, and electrospray ionization mass spectrometry (Holman et al., 1988; Li et al., 1994a). Some of these techniques have been discussed in chapter 2, section VI, and illustrated in figures 2.7 and 2.8.

Table 19.1
Homeostatic and behavioral insect neuropeptides

General Class	Example or Abbreviation	Function	Structure
Myotropins	Leukokinin I	Muscle contraction, diuresis	DPAFNSWG-NH_2 FCX^1X^2WG-NH_2[a]
	Locustatachykinin	Muscle contraction, AKH release	GPSGFWGGVR-NH_2
Adipokinetic hormone/red pigment–concentrating hormone	AKH/RPCH	Mobilizes carbohydrate and lipid metabolism	pQLNFTPNWGT-NH_2
Diuretic hormones	Achetakinins, *Locusta*-DP	Insect diuresis	CRH-related peptide
	Myokinins	Insect diuresis	FCX^1X^2WG-NH_2[a]
Eclosion hormone	EH	Initiate ecdysis	NPAIATGYDPMEICIENCA QCKKMLGAWFEGPLCAE SCIKFKGKLIPECEDFASIA PFLNKL-OH
	Eclosion triggering hormone	Triggers EH release	
	Trypsin-modulating oostatic hormone (TMOH)	Ecdysiostasis	YDPAPPPPP-OH
Pheromone biosynthesis–activating neuropeptide	PBAN	Synthesis of sex pheromones	LSDDMPATPADQENYRQ DPEQIDSRTKYFSPRL-NH_2

Adapted from Kelley et al. (1994).
[a] X^1, H, N, F, S, or Y; X^2, A, S or P.

19.2.7.2 Myotropins

Almost half of the approximately 100 identified insect neuropeptides have myotropic effects. Most of the myotropic peptides have an amidated C-terminus, and many have a pyroglutamic acid, proline, or glycine residue at their N-terminus, which increases their resistance to degradation by aminopeptidases. Relatively simple myotropic bioassays are useful for the isolation and purification of insect neuropeptides but do not reveal much about their physiological actions, since myokinins are diuretic and pyrokinins stimulate pheromone production. Similarly, proctolin (Arg-Tyr-Leu-Pro-Thr-OH) was isolated on the basis of its ability to stimulate hindgut contraction, but it also has effects on numerous other physiological systems, acting as a neurotransmitter in visceral and somatic muscle, with effects on the CNS (O'Shea and Adams, 1986). Proctolin has been discussed in section 19.2.6.2 of this chapter. The other insect myotropins may be classified into myostimulatory and myoinhibitory peptides, first identified in the cockroach *L. maderae* and more recently in the locusts *L. migratoria* and *S. gregaria*.

The myostimulatory neuropeptides include the tachykinins, all of which share the Phe-X-Gly-Val-Arg-NH_2 terminal sequence; the myotropins and

Table 19.2
Developmental and reproductive insect neuropeptides

General Class	Example or Abbreviation	Function	Structure
Allatotropins	Allatotropin	Stimulate juvenile hormone synthesis	GFKNVEMMTA RGF-NH_2
	Allatostatin	Inhibit juvenile hormone synthesis	APSGAQRLYGF GL-NH_2
Ecdysteroidogenins	Prothoracicotropic hormone (PTTH)	Initiate molting/egg development	GNIQVENQAIP DPPCTCKYKKE IEDLGENSVPRF IETRNCNKTQQ PTCRPPYICKES LYSITILKRRET KSQESLEIPNEL KYRWVAESHP VSVACLCTRDY QLTYNNN-OH
Oostatic hormones	Trypsin-modulating oostatic factor (TMOF)	Inhibit ovarian maturation	YDPAPPPPP-OH

Adapted from Kelly et al. (1994).

Table 19.3
Insect neuropeptides involved in metamorphosis

Neuropeptide	Source	Action	Stimulus for Release
Parathoracicotropin	Pars intercerebralis	Prothoracic gland release of ecdysone	Temperature, crowding, etc.
Bursicon	Neurosecretory cells of CNS	Darkening and hardening of cuticle (tanning)	Stimuli associated with molting
Diapause hormone	Subesophageal ganglion	Diapause of egg	CNS regulation
Eclosion hormone	Neurosecretory cells of brain	Emergence of adult from pupa	Endogenous clock

pyrokinins, which share the Phe-X-Pro-Arg-Leu-NH_2 terminal sequence; sulfakinin, which is a member of the gastrin-CCK family; an allastatin with myoinhibitory properties; and a heterogeneous group of other neuropeptides, including proctolin and the myokinins, with a C-terminal sequence Phe-X-X-Trp-Gly-NH_2. *Pheromone biosynthesis activating neuropeptide (PBAN)* has the same C-terminal sequence as the pyrokinins and the latter have PBAN activity (Abernathy et al., 1995). Two of these groups are shown in table 19.1. Insect tachykinins are found in abundance in the brain and midgut of the cockroach, with relatively large amounts located in the subesophageal ganglion, esophageal nerve, and associated ganglia and intestine. This distribution signifies that the tachkinin-related peptides may be intimately involved in feeding and digestion (Muren and Nässel, 1996). Lesser amounts of the tachykinins are present in the ganglia of the ventral nerve cord, and lower levels in the corpora cardiaca, foregut, and hindgut. In the CNS, the tachykinins are present almost exclusively in interneurons, where they presumably act as neuromodulators.

The leucokinins (C-terminus Phe-X-Ser-Trp-Gly-NH_2) form a series of eight myotropins, structurally similar octomers, and named leukokinin I to VIII (Holman et al., 1990). Fragments 4 to 8 retain most or all of the myotropic activity of the octomer, but C-terminal truncation inactivates the peptide. The leucokinins also have diuretic activity (Coast et al., 1990). The locustatachykinins are 30% homologous with the substance P subfamily of vertebrates and their action on the motility of the gut is similar in vertebrates and insects. A series of at least eight isoforms of the myotropic tachykinins has been isolated from an extract of 600 midguts of the cockroach *L. maderaea*. These endogenous tachykinins increase the amplitude

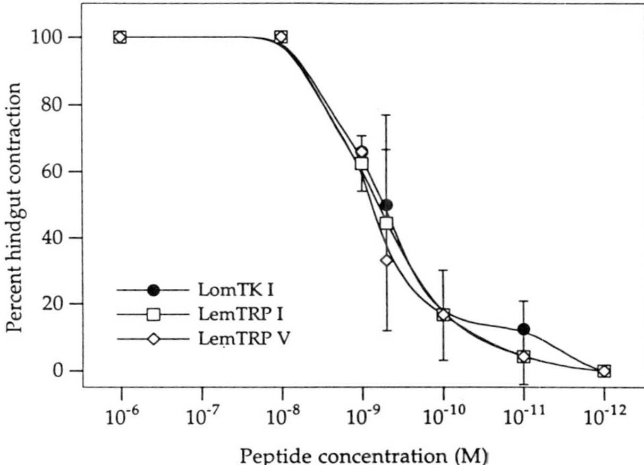

Figure 19.16
Effect of increasing doses of locustatachykinin I (LomTK I) and *Leucophaea* tachykinin-related peptides I and V (LemTRP I and V) on the isolated hindgut of *leucophaea maderae*. Maximum response is shown as 100%. Each point represents mean ± SEM of three to four preparations. (From Muren and Nässel, 1997.)

of cockroach hindgut contractions in a concentration-dependent manner (figure 19.16). The isoforms are structurally related to tachykinin-related peptides from other insect species (Muren and Nässel, 1997).

The myoinhibiting peptides or myosuppressins have C-terminal homology with the FMRFamides: they share the common C-terminal sexapeptide sequence, His-Val-Phe-Leu-Arg-Phe-NH_2, and inhibit or reduce the amplitude of cardiac and visceral muscle contractions. *Locustamyoinhibin* was one of the first myoinhibiting neuropeptides to be identified and it appears to act as a central neurotransmitter. It was isolated from an extract of 9000 brain corpora cardiaca-corpora allata-subesophageal ganglion complexes of *L. migratoria* and it suppresses the motility of the cockroach hindgut. The biologically active core lies in the C-terminal sequence but it shows no sequence similarity to other peptides from vertebrate or invertebrate sources (Schoofs et al., 1994). Other members of the insect gut myoinhibitory substances are the *callatostatins*, a cockroach allostatin homolog identified in the blowfly *Calliphora vomitoria*, but which has no allostatic effects in flies.

The myomodulins were first identified in molluscs and have been discussed in detail in section 19.2.4.5 of this chapter. They are found in the brain and retrocerebral complex of the locust and may represent another interphyletic family of neuropeptides. Myomodulin in the locust modulates the tension generated in the extensor tibiae of the locust hindleg by stimulation of the slow excitatory motor neuron. Myomodulin neuropeptides in insects may act as neurohormones and releasing agents for hormones in neurohemal areas, as well as central neurotransmitters or neuromodulators (Swales and Evans, 1995).

a. Additional actions of the myotropins

In addition to their myotropic effects, stimulating or inhibiting skeletal and visceral muscle, the myotropins affect pheromone synthesis, diapause induction, stimulation of cuticle melanization, diuresis, and allostatic activity. Obviously, these actions overlap with the functions of other insect neuropeptides, as shown in table 19.1. Some of the myotropic peptides are neurotransmitters found in nerve endings in the oviduct, the male accessory glands, and the heart, whereas others act as hormones stored in the neurohemal organs and released into the hemolymph.

b. Nonpeptide agonists of the myosuppressins

The nonpeptide benzethonium chloride mimics the actions of the myosuppressins, acting at receptors for Schisto-Phe-Leu-Arg-Phe-NH_2 (Lange et al., 1995) and inhibiting contractions of the hindgut. As the myosuppressins regulate muscle functions associated with reproduction, digestion, and locomotion, nonpeptide analogs, which are far more resistant to enzymatic degradation than the endogenous ligands, could have important potential as insect pest management agents (Nachman et al., 1996; 1977b). One such analog is an amphiphilic analog of the pyrokinin peptide family which activates pheromone synthesis in female moths (Abernathy et al., 1996). A recent discovery reveals that this pseudopheromone is effective after topical application, is able to penetrate the tough insect cuticle, extends the potential utility of such analogs in the control of insect pest populations, and reduces the environmental residues of harmful pesticides (Nachman et al., 1998).

19.2.7.3 Adipokinetic Hormone and Red Pigment–Concentrating Hormone

RPCH was discussed under chromatophorotropins (section 19.2.6.2.c) because it was first isolated from extracts of the X organ–sinus gland complex in the eyestalk of a crustacean, and named for its chromatophorotropic activity. RPCH does not seem to affect chromatophores in insects. AKH was first isolated from the corpora cardiaca in the locust, based on its ability to mobilize lipids. The peptides of this growing family (more than 20 have been isolated to date) share several common structural features. They are hydrophobic peptides, which, with few exceptions, lack acidic or basic residues. Each begins with an N-terminal residue of pyroglutamic acid and the C-terminus is amidated. Residues 4 and 8 are phenylalanine and tryptophan, respectively. The second residue may be leucine or valine, the third residue is asparagine or threonine, and the fifth residue may be serine or threonine (Holman et al., 1988). Greater variation in AKH sequences are reported by Gade et al. (1992).

RPCH pGlu-Leu-Asn-Phe-Ser-Pro-Gly-Trp-NH_2
AKH pGlu-Leu-Asn-Phe-Thr-Pro-Asn-Trp-Gly-Thr-NH_2

The AKHs range in size from octapeptides to decapeptides and are involved in lipid metabolism in some species and in proline mobilization in some flies. Processing of AKH is unusual in that the precursor is not a linear prohormone but a dimeric construct. Degradation of AKH occurs by membrane-bound endopeptidases in the fat body, muscle, and Malpighian tubules.

19.2.7.4 Diuretic Hormones

The excretory system of insects consists of the Malpighian tubules and the hindgut. The urine produced by the tubules drains into the hindgut, where most of the water, ions, and essential metabolites are reabsorbed so that insects excrete a dry feces. Water balance in insects is regulated by diuretic and antidiuretic hormones that act on the Malpighian tubules and hindgut, respectively (Spring, 1990).

A diuretic neuropeptide was first isolated and sequenced from *L. migratoria* using antibodies to vertebrate AVP. However, it has since been shown to have no effect on Malpighian tubule secretion in *Locusta* (Coast et al., 1993), but has been implicated in diurnal rhythmicity. This AVP-like hormone is a nonapeptide homodimer linked by disulfide bridges in an antiparallel manner (see table 19.1). It has 67% homology to AVP and 78% homology to arginine vasotocin (Kelly et al., 1994). Cell bodies of neurons in the subesophageal ganglion of *L. migratoria* contain a VP-like peptide, and receive synaptic input from a pair of descending brain interneurons with photosensitive cell bodies in the pars intercerebralis (Thompson and Bacon, 1991). Enzymatic conversion of the monomer to the dimer is initiated in the subesophageal ganglion.

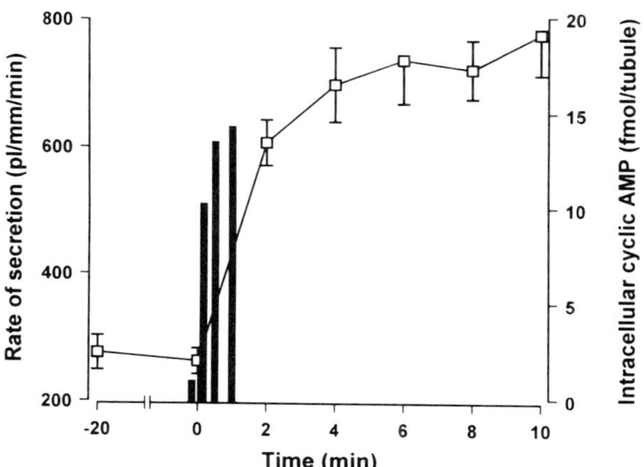

Figure 19.17
The effect of 50nM *Acheta*-diuretic hormone (*Acheta*-DP) on fluid secretion and intracellular cAMP levels in Malpighian tubules from *Acheta domesticus*. Data points or bars are the means, and vertical lines the SEs for six to eight measurements of fluid secretion and four determinations of cAMP, respectively. *Acheta*-DP was added at 0 minutes. (From Coast, 1996.)

There are at least seven neuropeptides in this family of diuretic insect neuropeptides with homology to CRH, urotensin, and sauvagine. A CRH-related diuretic hormone is present in the midgut endocrine cells of the locust, colocalized in secretory granules with substance P–like immunoreactive material. In the house cricket *Acheta domesticus* there are two distinct classes of diuretic neuropeptides (Coast and Kay, 1994). The first class (*Acheta–diuretic hormone*) belongs to the CRH-related family and stimulates maximal tubule secretion through a cAMP-dependent mechanism (figure 19.17). *Achetakinins*, which belong to the insect myokinin family, form the second class, which is much less effective in stimulating tubule secretion and which acts through a cAMP-independent mechanism (Coast et al., 1990). In locusts the two classes of peptides act synergistically to stimulate tubule secretion and the kinins may therefore have a modulatory action in the control of diuresis (Coast, 1996). In addition, a CHH-related peptide has been identified in the desert locust *S. gregaria*. It is called ion transport peptide (ITP) because it stimulates ion reabsorption in the hindgut, functioning as an antidiuretic hormone (Meredith et al., 1996).

Diuretic hormones are *released* in response to feeding or at the time of emergence (eclosion) from the pupal stage. The response to a meal is particularly marked in mosquitoes: the yellow fever mosquito voids 42% of ingested plasma within 1 to 2 hours of feeding. Several members of the insect diuretic kinin family are hydrolyzed, and thereby inactivated, by angiotensin-converting enzyme (ACE), a procedure that involves removal of the C-terminal dipeptide amide fragment (Nachman et al., 1997a). In mammals, ACE is responsible for the conversion of angiotensin I (angiotensinogen) to the active angiotensin II (see chapter 18).

19.2.7.5 Eclosion Neuropeptides

The dramatic transformation of a caterpillar into a butterfly or a moth takes several weeks and is completed when the fully formed butterfly breaks through the tough cuticle of the pupa by a series of stereotyped movements known as eclosion or ecdysis. A similar behavioral sequence occurs with each larval molt (Gammie and Truman, 1997). All stages of ecdysis behavior, in all insects, are triggered by a circulating hormone, eclosion hormone (EH) (Ewer et al., 1997), which was first isolated and identified in the tobacco hornworm, *Manduca sexta*.

EH is a 62–amino acid peptide with conserved cysteine residues which form three disulfide bonds that are necessary for biological activity (see table 19.1). EH has been cloned in several insect species and there is a high degree of cross-reactivity between them, so that extracts from one species will provoke early ecdysis behavior in another species. EH is present in two pairs of cells in the ventral midline (VM) of the brain of *Manduca*, known as the VM cells. Axons from the VM cells project to the proctodeal nerve where they form neurohemal release sites, from which EH is released at each ecdysis. This is supplemented during adult development by newly formed VM nerve processes to the corpora allata–corpora cardiaca complex (Ichikawa, 1992).

Precise coordination of two sets of endocrine cells is required for ecdysis. The VM neurons release EH, which acts on peripheral endocrine cells which secrete *ecdysis-triggering hormone (ETH)*. ETH, in turn, stimulates the further release of EH within the CNS and into the circulation. This positive feedback results in a massive surge of EH and ETH that activates peptidergic neurons, through a sharp increase in cGMP, to secrete CCAP, which rapidly induces the motor behavior that permits the insect to escape from its old cuticle (Ewer et al., 1997).

The EH gene has been isolated and sequenced. It is present as a single copy per haploid genome and contains three exons. The EH gene produces only a single translation product, pre-EH, an 88–amino acid peptide that consists of the signal peptide and one copy of the 62–amino acid EH (Horodyski, 1989).

19.2.7.6 Pheromone Biosynthesis–Activating Neuropeptide

Pheromones are chemicals produced and released by one individual and perceived by another individual of the same species, in which they evoke a behavioral or physiological response (Karlson and Luscher, 1959). Pheromones probably evolved early as a means of chemical communication, for they are used in algae, fungi, and practically all animal phyla, but the most extensive use of these pherormone systems occurs in insects.

PBAN was first isolated and sequenced from the corn earworm *Heliothis zea*. It is a 33-residue peptide (see table 19.1) with the minimal sequence necessary for biological activity being the C-terminal pentapeptide. This sequence, Phe-Ser-Pro-Arg-Leu-NH_2, is also the core sequence for the leucokinins, which were considered in section 19.2.7.2. The target organs for PBAN may vary with the species: the corpus bursae, the terminal abdominal ganglion, and the pheromone gland in the tip of the abdomen are all possibilities (Kelly et al., 1994). The regulation of photoperiod control of pheromone is at the level of release since the synthesis of pheromone is continuous. However, pheromone production is also inhibited by regulatory factors from the bursa, ovaries, and hemolymph of aging and mated females, and from the accessory glands of males during mating (Teal et al., 1990). PABN acts through cAMP and calcium.

The PBAN gene has been isolated and sequenced. It contains an intron within the region coding for amino acid 14. Two regions, 5′ and 3′, to the gene contain sequences encoding Phe-X-Pro-Arg-Leu, followed by Gly-Arg, allowing cleavage from the sequence and C-terminal amidation (Davis et al., 1992).

19.2.7.7 Allatotropins and Allatostatins

The allotropins and allatostatins are members of the class of reproductive and developmental neuropeptides (see table 19.2) that regulate the synthesis and release of *juvenile hormone* from the corpus allatum (see figures 19.1 and 19.15). JH is a terpene derivative, essential to the synthesis of larval structures and the inhibition of larval metamorphosis; metamorphosis to the adult stage occurs when JH disappears from the circulation. JH levels then rise again in the reproductively active adult, when JH stimulates yolk protein synthesis, promotes egg maturation in the ovarian follicles, and development of the accessory sexual organs in males. JH biosynthesis is regulated by both peptidergic and aminergic inputs. Depending on the species and developmental stage, these signals may be inhibitory (allatostatins) or stimulatory (allatotropins). Signal transduction within corpus allatum cells occurs by way of cyclic nucleotides, Ca^{2+}, and phosphoinositides (Rachinsky and Tobe, 1996).

Only one allatotropin has been isolated and sequenced, and tested in a bioassay in which it stimulates JH synthesis in vitro by the corpora allata from newly emerged adults. Allatotropin is a 13-residue peptide (see table 19.2) but full activity is elicited with the truncated fragment 6–13. As yet no sequence homology of allatotropin with any other known peptide has been found.

The structural and functional features of the allatostatins appear to parallel the vertebrate somatostatins and may provide one of the best examples of the parallel evolution of peptides (Scharrer, 1987; Scharrer and Scharrer, 1944). Several allatostatins have been isolated and sequenced, ranging in length from 8 to 18 amino acids, with a common C-terminal sequence of Leu/Val-Tyr-X-Phe-Gly-Leu-NH_2. The precursor molecule *preproallatostatin* for the oviparous cockroach *Periplaneta americana* has several features in common with that of the viviparous cockroach *Diploptera punctata*. The precursors are remarkably similar in size and the organization of the peptides within the precursor is conserved (figure 19.18). The *P. americana* precursor incorporates 14 allatostatin-like peptides that contain the core C-terminal sequence, in comparision to the *D. punctata* precursor which contains 13. Five of the peptides are perfectly conserved between the two

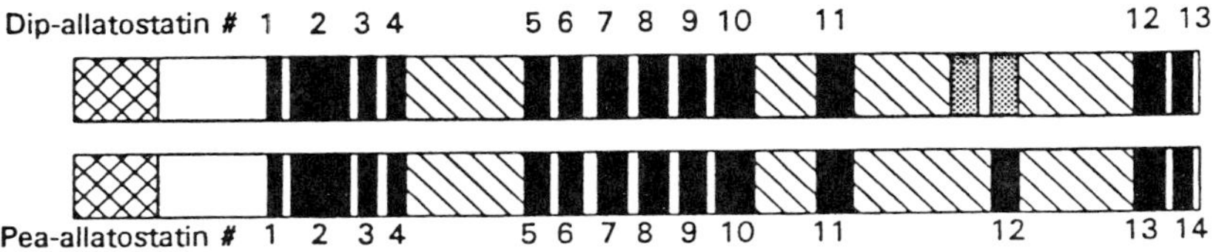

Figure 19.18
Schematic representation comparing the structure of the allatostatin polypeptide precursors of *Diploptera punctata* and *Periplanata americana*. The precursors begin with a hydrophobic leader (crosshatched boxes) that is presumably cleaved by signal endoproteases. The individual Dip-allatostatin (upper) and Pea-allatostatin (lower) peptides that are numbered according to their position relative to the N-terminus in the precursor are shown (black boxes). Acidic regions are also indicated (striped boxes). Incorporated within the third acidic spacer region of the Dip-allatostatin precursor are sequences specifying two non-amidated peptides (shaded boxes). (From Ding et al., 1995.)

species. In *P. americana* allostatin transcripts appear to be produced by numerous cells in different regions of the brain.

P. americana (Pea) has 14 allatostatins (AST), two of which are shown here:

Pea—AST 1 Ser-Pro-Ser-Gly-Met-Gln-Arg-Leu-Tyr-Gly-Phe-Gly-Leu-NH_2

Pea—AST 2 Ala-Asp-Gly-Arg-Leu-Tyr-Ala-Phe-Gly-Leu-NH_2

19.2.7.8 Ecdysiotropins and Ecdysiostatins

This class of developmental and reproductive neuropeptides includes the cerebral neuropeptide *prothoracicotropic hormone* (see figure 19.1 and table 19.2); its smaller form, *bombyxin*; noncerebral ecdysiotropins found in the hindgut, proctodeum, and certain ganglia; and the *egg development neurosecretory hormone (EDNH)*. An ecdysiostatic factor in brain and perhaps in other tissues may participate in the regulation of prothoracic gland response and insect development (Masler, 1997). *Trypsin modulating oostatic factor* (*TMOF*; see below) also has ecdysiostatic activity (Hua et al., 1997).

PTTH stimulates ecdysteroid production by the larval prothoracic gland and thereby initiates the surge of events involved in molting and metamorphosis. Cerebral ecdysiotropins are also involved in ovarian maturation in some insects. EDNH stimulates egg maturation and ecdysteroid production by adult ovaries.

The *PTTH gene* is present as a single copy per haploid genome and may be one of the earliest neuropeptides expressed in insect embryos. It is *expressed* in the group III lateral neurosecretory cells of the larva and may be co-expressed in the ventromedial cells with EH (see section 19.2.7.5). The preprohormone of 224 amino acids contains three proteolytic cleavage sites that would result in two polypeptides cleaved from the 5′-end of the preprohormone, and one PTTH unit cleaved from its 3′-end. Large PTTH (22K-PTTH) is a 109-residue peptide with a consensus sequence for glycosylation (Asn-X-Thr) at residue 41. It exists as a dimer of two identical, or nearly identical, subunits held together by disulfide bridges. Smaller forms of PTTH (4K-PTTH) are known as bombyxins but their physiological relevance is debatable.

19.2.7.9 Oostatic Hormone

One member of this class of reproductive and developmental hormones has been isolated from the ovaries of the mosquito, and sequenced. Mosquito oostatic hormone is an unusual decapeptide containing six C-terminal prolines (see table 19.2). Oostatic hormone may affect oogenesis through modulation of ovarian ecdysteroid synthesis, gut trypsin synthesis, or EDNH release. In mosquitoes, oostatic hormone affects trypsin synthesis (TMOF) preventing the breakdown of the blood meal into the amino acid components that are necessary for vitellogenesis. Another TMOF has been isolated from the fleshfly *Neobellieria bullata*, but it has no structural similarity to mosquito TMOF (Bylemans et al., 1995).

19.2.7.10 Diapause Hormone

Diapause hormone is a neuropeptide produced by neurosecretory cells in the subesophageal ganglion, and which induces diapause through its action on the developing ovary. Diapause hormone is a 24–amino acid peptide containing the C-terminal pentapeptide sequence (Phe-X-Pro-Arg-Leu-NH_2) necessary for activity (see table 19.2), and homologous to the C-terminal sequences of the PBANs (see section 19.2.7.6) and the myotropic pyrokinins (section 19.2.7.2). The common C-terminal pentapeptide is essential and sufficient to elicit myotropic and monotropic activities, but is less potent in diapause egg-inducing activity in comparison to the intact diapause hormone. Diapause hormone encodes its biological activity to induce embryonic diapause in three regions of the molecule: the C-terminal pentapeptide as a core structure—the shortest fragment that produces a response; the middle region with its duplicated amino acid structure for full potency of diapause hormone; and the N-terminal sequence, which facilitates binding of the hormone to the receptor, stabilizing the hormone-receptor interaction (Saito et al., 1994).

19.3 Summary

Invertebrate hormonal systems are basically neurosecretory, and neurosecretory cells are found in all metazoan invertebrates. These neurosecretions regulate growth, metabolism, water balance, reproduction, and visceral activities. A large number of invertebrate neuropeptides have been identified, many of which are similar in structure to vertebrate neuropeptides, and there is a remarkable similarity of the neurosecretory system of crustaceans and insects to that of the hypothalamic-hypophyseal system of mammals.

Cnidarians (hydra, sea anemones, coral, jellyfishes) contain a neuropeptide that, with modifications, is found in all animal phyla, from cnidarians to mammals. This is Phe-Met-Arg-Phe-amide (FMRF-amide) and it may have been the first neurotransmitter.

Flatworms contain neuropeptide F, which is found in all invertebrate taxa. NPF has the structural characteristics of the NPY family and homologies between the structure of human NPY and invertebrate NPF indicate that the NPY-NPF gene is of ancient lineage.

Annelids possess a neuropeptide that is identical to vertebrate α-neoendorphin as well as a γ-MSH-like peptide, both derived from a POMC precursor, The leech, a member of this group of coelomic metazoans, also secretes a peptide with AT II–like properties and which has similar diuretic effects. The precursor molecule is very similar to human AT I, with a sequence homology of 78% with human angiotensinogen, indicating that the opiates and angiotensins are also of ancient phylogenetic origin.

Molluscs consist of three main classes: the bivalves, gastropods, and cephalopods. The marine snail *Aplysia*, and the pond snail *Lymnaea* have been extensively used in the study of neuropeptides, as the peptides are easily identified in specific, large cells. Neuropeptide-degrading enzymes are also found in these gastropods. The neuroendocrine system of *Aplysia* is contained within the four symmetical pairs of head ganglia and the single abdominal ganglion, which contains the bag cells that produce the egg-laying hormone. ELH is produced in the same manner as neuropeptide synthesis occurs in vertebrates. The ELH gene, consisting of three exons separated by two introns, encodes a 271–amino acid residue precursor. The precursor is cleaved at paired basic residues to yield the 36–amino acid ELH and three additional, small bag cell peptides. All these BCPs are released together and control egg-laying behavior and the release of ova from the ovarian follicles.

FMRFamide and N-terminally extended forms of this neuropeptide form a large and heterogeneous family. The FMRFamide gene consists of five exons that are alternatively spliced to form peptides of various lengths. In *Aplysia* and *Lymnaea* FMRFamide causes a fast depolarizing response acting through a peptide-gated ionotropic receptor. The neuropeptide regulates the heartbeat and affects neural transmission in sensory neurons and in motor neurons, exciting first a brief depolarization followed by a prolonged inhibitory response. FMRFamide is involved in the feeding behavior of these molluscs.

Other neuropeptides isolated from *Aplysia* and *Lymnaea* include an FMRFamide-related family, the R15 α_2-peptide, which is also found in lower mammals such as the hedgehog, in which it is localized in the PVN, accessory neurosecretory cells in the lateral hypothalamus, and in the nucleus tractus solitarius. Cerebral peptide 1 is another neuropeptide widely distributed in *Aplysia*.

Feeding behavior in *Aplysia* has been studied using the accessory radula closer neuromuscular circuit as a model for peptidergic transmission. ACh-induced contractions are modulated by several neuropeptides such as the myomodulins and small cardioactive peptides, which are released by the two motor neurons B15 and B16 in the buccal ganglia. The myomodulin neuropeptides are a major and widely distributed group of neuropeptides that act as neuromuscular modulators and cotransmitters. A single gene encodes nine structurally similar forms of myomodulin, some of which are present in multiple copies in the gene. Myomodulin, a 7–amino acid residue peptide, increases cAMP levels and cAMP-dependent protein kinase in the ARC muscle. Some myomodulins potentiate ARC contractions by enhancing the Ca^{2+} current, whereas other myomodulins depress ARC contractions by activating the K^+ current. The net response will be a balance between these two forces. The SCPs are decapeptides that are involved in the control of the cardiovascular system and of the muscles involved in feeding and gut motility. The SCPs are found in cell bodies of all the ganglia and are released only when the neurons are stimulated at high frequency, or at lower frequencies with long burst duration. The SCPs use the same second-messenger system as the myomodulins: cAMP-dependent protein kinase. Myomodulins affect the neuromuscular circuit that innervates the penis retractor muscle.

Molluscan insulin–related peptides are produced by the light-green cells in the cerebral ganglia of *Lymnaea*, giant neurons that are involved in the regulation of physiological processes associated with growth, metabolism, and reproduction. The members of this diverse insulin superfamily share the basic insulin globular structure characteristic of vertebrate insulin, indicating that they must have shared an ancient common ancestor. Four genes encode the precursors of these peptides and they all show the structure typical of the human insulin gene. An insulin receptor has been isolated in *Aplysia* that is similar to the vertebrate insulin receptor. However, insulin may have quite a different function in invertebrates; for example, it amplifies the nerve action potential.

Conopressin, a neuropeptide structurally related to VP, is involved in male sexual behavior, inducing contraction of the vas deferens. APGWamide is colocalized with conopressin and is another neuropeptide involved in male copulation, as are the myomodulins. Three different light-yellow cell peptides are produced from a single precursor by neurons in the visceral ganglia. These neuropeptides are probably involved in regulation of blood pressure and urine release. They are aided by AT I and urotensin I and II neuropeptides. Conus peptides are potent toxins (conotoxins) that are much used as specific inhibitors of various classes of voltage-sensitive calcium channels. The POMC-derived peptides ACTH, α-MSH, and β-endorphin, and the enkephalins have all been isolated in molluscs.

Cephalopods also have NPF and an OT-VP-like peptide cephalotocin, indicating a high degree of conservation of this neuropeptide.

Crustacean neuroendocrine systems consist of aggregations of neuroendocrine cells that send their secretions along their axon terminals to neurohemal organs. In addition, there are non-neural endocrine glands. The X organs are important neuroendocrine organs in the optic ganglia within the eyestalks. The sinus gland is a neurohemal organ, a site for storage and release of hormones produced in neurosecretory cells. It is analogous to the neurohypophysis in vertebrates and the corpus cardiacum of insects. Crustaceans also have three endocrine glands not composed of neurosecretory cells: the Y organs, which produce a hormone that initiates molting under X organ regulation, the androgenic glands, and the ovary. In higher crustaceans, the postcommissure organ and the pericardial organs are neurohemal organs, extracts of which increase the frequency and amplitude of the heartbeat.

X organ neuropeptides consist of crustacean hyperglycemic hormone, molt-inhibiting hormone, vitellogenesis-inhibiting hormone, and mandibular organ–inhibiting hormone. These hormones are stored, then released from the sinus gland, and are unique to crustacea. Peptides of the CHH group are polymorphic, resulting in considerable interspecies variations in hyperglycemic activity.

Pericardial organ neuropeptides are released into the circulation as hormones but they are also found in the nervous system, where they act as neurotransmitters or neuromodulators. Proctolin is a pentapeptide first isolated from the cockroach on the basis of its ability to cause contractions of the hindgut. It has many stimulatory actions on muscle and nerve and affects the contractility of the heart valves. Proctolin modulates neurons of the stomatogastric ganglia. Five distinct FMRFamide-related peptides have been isolated, unique to crustaceans, that are concentrated in the pericardial organ system and in the nervous system. They increase muscle contractility. Crustacean cardioactive peptide is another pericardial organ neuropeptide also found in the nervous system, with variable excitatory actions on the heart, hindgut, and respiratory rhythm.

Eyestalk neuropeptides are chromatophorotropins, affecting pigment dispersal. Red pigment–concentrating hormone is an octapeptide that not only affects chromatophores but has excitatory actions on the stomatogastric ganglion of the crab and modulates swimmeret activity in crayfish. RPCH is a member of the adipokinetic family which is highly conserved in crustaceans. Pigment-dispersing hormones form a family of octapeptides found in crustaceans and insects that cause pigment movement in chromatophores.

The *insect neuroendocrine system* consists of neurosecretory cells in the cerebral, subesophageal, and other ganglia. Neurosecretory cells in the protocerebrum send axons to the corpora cardiacum, neurohemal organs comparable to the neurohypophysis of vertebrates. The corpora allata, endocrine glands of non-neural origin, are closely associated with the corpora cardiacum and directly innervated by the nervous system. Homeostatic and behavioral insect neuropeptides include the following hormones:

1. The *myotropins*, a diverse group of neuropeptides that either stimulate or inhibit contractions of visceral muscle. Most of the myotropins are stimulatory and include the tachykinins, the myotropins, pyrokinins, and sulfakinins, and a heterogeneous group of peptides including proctolin. The C-terminal sequence of myotropins and pyrokinins is Phe-X-Pro-Arg-Leu-NH_2, that for sulfakinins is Gly-His-Met-Arg-Phe-NH_2, and the myokinin sequence is Phe-X-X-Trp-Gly-NH_2. The myotropins act as neurotransmitters in muscle, but have diverse additional physiological actions. Tachykinins are found in abundance in the brain and midgut of the cockroach and appear to be associated with feeding and digestion. In the CNS they probably act as neuromodulators and have some homology with the vertebrate substance P family.

The *myoinhibitory peptides* have C-terminal homology with the FMRFamides and inhibit or reduce the amplitude of cardiac and visceral muscle contractions. The myosuppressins are FaRPs with the C-terminal sequence Phe-Leu-Arg-Phe-NH_2. Locustamyoinhibin, with a C-terminal sequence Leu-Asn-Ala-Gly-Trp-NH_2, suppresses the motility of the cockroach hindgut. The biologically active core lies in the C-terminal sequence but it shows no sequence similarity with other peptides from vertebrate or invertebrate sources. Another myoinhibitory substances is callatostatin. The myomodulins were discussed previously in *Aplysia*.

2. *Adipokinetic hormone* was first named for its red pigment–concentrating effect, but it mobilizes lipids and has no effect on insect chromatophores. There are more than 20 members of this family, each of which begins with an N-terminal residue of pyroglutamic acid and ends with an amidated C-terminal.

3. *Diuretic neuropeptides* form a group of at least seven members and have homology with several vertebrate neuropeptides: CRH, urotensin, and sauvagine. The diuretic hormones are released in response to a meal or at the time of emergence from the pupal stage (eclosion or ecdysis) They act on the Malphigian tubules and have no effect on the hindgut, with the exception of locust ITP.

4. *Eclosion hormone* is a 62–amino acid peptide with three disulfide bonds that are necessary for biological activity. EH is produced by brain cells, stored in neurohemal sites, then released at ecdysis. EH and ecdysis-triggering hormone cause the release of CCAP, which evokes ecdysis behavior.

5. Pheromone biosynthesis–activating neuropeptide is a 33–amino acid peptide, with a C-terminal peptide essential to biological activity. PBAN production is continuous, but its release is inhibited by regulatory factors from the reproductive system of males and females.

There are four main reproductive and developmental insect neuropeptides.

1. *Allatotropins* and *allatostatins* regulate the synthesis and release of juvenile hormone from the corpus allatum. JH is necesary for metamorphosis, and later for reproduction in the adult, and is regulated by pepidergic and aminergic input. Depending on the species and stage of development, the signals may be inhibitory (allatostatins) or stimulatory (allatotropins). Signal transduction within the corpus allatum is through cyclic nucleotides, Ca^{2+}, and phosphoinositides. Allatotropin is a 13-residue peptide, but full activity resides in the truncated fragment 6–13. Several allatostatins have been sequenced, ranging in length from 8 to 18 amino acids, with a common hexapeptide C-terminal sequence. The precursor to these peptides has been highly conserved and the structural and functional characteristics of these neuroeptides parallel those of the vertebrate somatostatins.

2. *Ecdysiotropins* and *ecdysiostatins* include the cerebral prothoracicotropic hormone, noncerebral ecdysiotropins, and the egg development neurosecretory hormone. The ecdysiostatic factor may be TMOF. PTTH stimulates ecdysteroid production by the larval prothoracic gland. PTTH is derived from a preprohormone that is cleaved to produce a large PTTH (109 residues), which exists as a dimer, and several smaller forms of PTTH.

3. *Oostatic hormone* is an unusual decapeptide containing six C-terminal prolines. Oostatic hormone modulates ovarian steroidogenesis, gut trypsin synthesis, or EDNH release.

4. *Diapause hormone* is a neuropeptide produced by cells in the subesophageal ganglion. It is a 24–amino acid peptide with a C-terminal pentapeptide sequence homologous to that of the PBANs and the myotropic pyrokinins. There are three regions of the molecule involved in the induction of embryonic diapause: the C-terminal pentapeptide is the shortest fragment to evoke a response; the middle region, which gives full potency; and the N-terminal sequence, which facilitates binding to the receptor.

19.4 Appendix: Abbreviations for Insect Neuropeptides

AKH	adipokinetic hormone
BCP	bag cell peptide
CHH	crustacean hyperglycemic hormone
EDNH	egg development neurosecretory hormone
EH	eclosion hormone
ELH	egg-laying hormone
ETH	ecdysis-triggering hormone
FaRP	FMRFamide-related peptide
GIH	gonad-inhibiting hormone
FMRFamide	Phe-Met-Arg-PHe-NH_2
LYCP	light yellow cell peptide
MIH	molt-inhibiting hormone
MIP	molluscan insulin-related peptide
MOIH	mandibular organ-inhibiting hormone
PBAN	pheromone biosynthesis activating neuropeptide
PTTH	prothoracicotropic hormone (prothoracicotropin)
RPCH	red pigment concentrating hormone
SCP	small cardioactive peptide
TMOF	trypsin-modulating oostatic factor
VIH	vitellogenesis-inhibiting hormone (gonad-inhibiting hormone)

References and Suggested Reading

Journals Relating to Neuropeptides and Associated Topics

Neuropeptides

Peptides

Regulatory Peptides

Regulatory Peptide Letters

Endocrine Reviews

Frontiers in Neuroendocrinology

Trends in the Neurosciences

Journal of Neuroscience

Chapter 1

Books and Literature Reviews

Beckwith, B. E., and C. A. Sandman. 1982. Central nervous system and peripheral effects of ACTH, MSH and related neuropeptides. Peptides 3: 411–420.

De Wied, D. 1987. The neuropeptide concept. Prog. Brain Res. 72: 93–108.

De Wied, D. 1997. The neuropeptide story. Front. Neuroendocrinol. 18: 101–113.

Hökfelt, T., and V. Mutt. 1987. Neuropeptides. In: The Encyclopedia of Neuroscience. Ed. G. Adelman. Boston, Birkhäuser, pp. 1–8.

Kastin, A. J., N. P. Plotnikoff, A. V. Schally, et al. 1976. Endocrine and CNS effects of hypothalamic peptides and MSH. In: Reviews of Neuroscience. Eds. S. Ehrenpreis and I. J. Kopin. New York, Raven Press, pp. 111–148.

Klavdieva, M. M. 1995/1996. The history of neuropeptides I–IV. Front. Neuroendocrinol. 16: 293–321; 17: 126–153, 155–179, 247–280.

LeRoith, D., and J. Roth. 1984. Vertebrate hormones and neuropeptides in microbes: Evolutionary origin of intercellular communication. Front. Neuroendocrinol. 8: 1–25.

Meites, J., B. T. Donovan, and S. M. McCann. 1975. Pioneers in Neuroendocrinology, Vol. 1. New York, Plenum Press.

Meites, J., B. T. Donovan, and S. M. McCann. 1978. Pioneers in Neuroendocrinology, Vol. 2. New York, Plenum Press.

References

Acher, R. 1980. Molecular evolution of biologically active polypeptides. Proc. Soc. Lond. Biol. Sci. 210: 1–43.

Acher, R., and J. Chauvet. 1995. The neurohypophyseal regulatory cascade: Precursors, mediators, receptors, and effectors. Front. Neuroendocrinol. 16: 237–289.

Acher, R., J. Chauvet, and M. T. Chauvet. 1995. Man and the chimaera. In: Oxytocin: Cellular and Molecular Approaches in Medicine and Research. Eds. R. Ivell and J. A. Russell. New York, Plenum Press, pp. 615–627.

Blomqvist, A. G., C. Söderberg, I. Lundell, et al. 1992. Strong evolutionary conservation of neuropeptide Y: Sequences of chicken, goldfish and *Torpedo marmorata* DNA clones. Proc. Natl. Acad. Sci. U.S.A. 89: 2350–2354.

Cooper, J. R., F. E. Bloom, and R. H. Roth. 1986. The Biochemical Basis of Neuropharmacology. New York, Oxford University Press, p. 371.

De Wied, D. 1969. Effects of peptide hormones on behavior. In: Frontiers in Neuroendocrinology. Eds. W. F. Ganong and L. Martini. New York, Oxford University Press, pp. 97–140.

Hökfelt. T., X. Zhang, and Z. Wiesenfeld-Hallin. 1994. Messenger plasticity in primary sensory neurons following axotomy and its functional implications. Trends Neurosi. 17: 22–30.

Kastin, A. J., R. D. Olson, A. V. Scally, et al. 1979. CNS effects of peripherally administered brain peptides. Life Sci. 25: 401–414.

Krieger, D. T., and A. S. Liotta. 1979. Pituitary hormones in brain: Where, why and how? Science 205: 366–372.

Krieger, D. T., and J. B. Martin. 1981. Brain peptides. N. Engl. J. Med. 304: 876–885.

Larhammar, D., A. Blomqvist, and C. Söderberg. 1993a. Evolution of neuropeptide Y and its related peptides. Comp. Biochem. Physiol. 106C: 743–752.

Larhammar, D., C. Söderberg, and A. G. Blomqvist. 1993b. Evolution of the neuropeptide Y family of peptides. In: The Biology of Neuropeptide Y and Related Peptides. Eds. W. F. Colmers and C. Wahlestedt. Totawa, N.J., Humana Press, pp. 1–42.

Miller, W. L., J. D. Baxter, and N. L. Eberhardt. 1983. Peptide hormone genes: Structure and evolution. In: Brain Peptides. Eds. D. T. Krieger, M. J. Brownstein, and J. B. Martin. New York, Wiley-Interscience, pp. 16–78.

Pieribone, V. A., L. Brodin, K. Friberg, et al. 1992. Differential expression of mRNAs for neuropeptide Y–related peptides in rat nervous tissue: Possible evolutionary conservation. J. Neurosci. 12: 3361–3371.

Niall, H. D. 1982. The evolution of peptide hormones. Annu. Rev. Physiol. 44: 615–624.

Scharrer, E. and B. Scharrer. 1937. Über Drüsen-Nervenzellen und Neurosekretorische Organe bei Wirbellosen und Wirbeltieren. Biol. Revs. Cambridge Phil. Soc. 12: 185–216.

Scharrer, E., and B. Scharrer. 1963. Neuroendocrinology. New York, Columbia University Press.

Simon, E. J., and J. M. Hiller. 1978. The opiate receptors. Annu. Rev. Pharmacol. Toxicol. 18: 371–394.

Stefano, G. B. 1989. Opioid peptides—comparative peripheral mechanisms. In: Comparative Physiology of Regulatory Peptides. Ed. S. Holmgren. New York, Chapman & Hall, pp. 122–129.

Strand, F. L., K. J. Rose, J. A. King, et al., 1991. ACTH modulation of nerve development and regeneration. Prog. Neurobiol. 33: 45–85.

Urano, A., S. Hyodo, and M. Suzuki. 1992. Molecular evolution of neurohypophysial hormone precursors. Prog. Brain Res. 92: 39–46.

Van Kesteren, R. E., A. B. Smit, R. P. J. De Lange, et al. 1995. Structural and functional evolution of the vasopressin/oxytocin superfamily: Vasopressin-related conopressin is the only member present in *Lymnae* and is involved in the control of sexual behavior. J. Neurosci. 15: 5989–5998.

Zuckerkandl, E., and L. Pauling. 1962. Evolving genes and proteins. In: Horizons in Biochemistry. Eds. M. Kasha, and B. Pullman. New York, Academic Press, pp. 97–166.

Chapter 2

Books and Literature Reviews

Bissette, G., and J. C. Ritchie. 1992. Radioimmunoassay methods. In: Neuroendocrinology. Ed. C. B. Nemeroff. Boca Raton, Fla., CRC Press, pp. 39–50.

Boulton, A. A., G. B. Baker, and Q. C. Pittman, Eds. 1987. Neuromethods 6: Peptides. Totawa, N.J., Humana Press.

Björklund, A., T. Hökfelt, and M. J. Kuhar, Eds. 1990. Neuropeptides in the CNS. Handbook of Chemical Neuroanatomy, Vol. 9. New York, Elsevier.

Conn, P. M., Ed. 1989. Neuroendocrine Peptide Methodology. New York, Academic Press.

Cuello, A. C., Ed. 1993. Immunohistochemistry II. IBRO Handbook Series: Methods in the Neurosciences, Vol. 14. New York, Wiley.

Davis, T. P. 1991. Methods of measuring neuropeptides and their metabolism. In: Stress, Neuropeptides and Systemic Disease. Eds. J. A. McCubbin, P. G. Kaufmann, and C. B. Nemeroff. San Diego, Academic Press, pp. 149–177.

De Wied, D., W H. Gispen, and Tj. B. van Wimersma Greidanus, Eds. 1986. Neuropeptides and Behavior, Vol 1. New York, Pergamon Press.

Grigoriadis, D. E., and E. B. De Souza. 1992. Receptor binding theory and techniques. In: Neuroendocrinology. Ed. C. B. Nemeroff. Boca Raton, Fla., CRC Press, pp. 63–86.

Grosveld, F., and G. Kollins, Eds. 1992. Transgenic Animals. San Diego, Academic Press.

Heist, E. K., and R. Poland. 1992. Bioassay methods. In: Neuroendocrinology. Ed. C. B. Nemeroff. Boca Raton, Fla., CRC Press, pp. 21–38.

Irvine, C. B., and C. H. Williams, Eds. 1997. Methods in Molecular Biology, Neuropeptide Protocols. Totowa, N.J., Humana Press.

Kilts, C. D. 1992. HPLC separation and electrochemical detection: Applications in neuroendocrinology. In: Neuroendocrinology. Ed. C. B. Nemeroff. Boca Raton, Fla., CRC Press, pp. 51–62.

Levine, J. E., Ed. 1994 Pulsatility in neuroendocrine systems. Methods Neurosci. 20, San Diego, Academic Press.

Maclean, N., Ed. 1994. Animals with Novel Genes. New York, Cambridge University Press.

Smith, A. I., Ed. 1995. Peptidases and neuropeptide processing. Methods Neurosci. 23, San Diego, Academic Press.

Spruijt, B. M., A. B. Oestreicher, and J. A. D. M. Tonnaer. 1990. Neuropeptides and brain aging. In: Neuropeptides: Basics and Perspectives. Ed. D. De Wied. Amsterdam, Elsevier, pp. 353–390.

Veldhuis, J. D., and M. Johnson. 1994. Analytical methods for evaluating episodic secretory activity within neuroendocrine axes. Neurosci. Biobehav. Rev. 18: 605–612.

Waschek, J. A. 1995. Transgenic targeting of neuroendocrine peptide genes in the hypothalamic-pituitary axis. Mol. Neurobiol. 10: 205–217.

References

Baldino, F., Jr., M.-F. Chesselet, and M. E. Lewis. 1989. High resolution in in situ hybridization histochemistry. In: Neuroendocrine Peptide Methodology. Ed. P. M. Conn. New York, Academic Press, pp. 79–95.

Bangham, D. R. 1983. What's in a bioassay? In: Cytochemical Bioassays: Techniques and Clinical Applications. Eds. J. Chayen and L. Bitensky. New York, Marcel Dekker, p. 7.

Banks, W. A., and A. J. Kastin. 1994. Brain-to-blood transport systems and the alcohol-withdrawal syndrome. Ann. N.Y. Acad. Sci. 739: 108–118.

Bissette, G., and J. C. Ritchie. 1992. Radioimmunoassay methods. In: Neuroendocrinology. Ed. C. B. Nemeroff, Boca Raton, Fla., CRC Press, pp. 39–50.

Blanchard, S. G., K.-J. Chang, and P. Cuatrecasas. 1989. Visualization of enkephalin receptors by image-intensified fluorescence microscopy. In: Neuroendocrine Peptide Methodology. Ed. P. M. Conn. New York, Academic Press, pp. 777–785.

Boden, P. 1995. Neuropeptide receptor-ion channel coupling in the mammalian brain. In: Metabolism of Brain Peptides. Ed. G. O'Cuinn. Boca Raton, Fla., CRC Press, pp. 69–97.

Bohus, B. 1986. Opiomelanocortins and behavioral adaptation. In: Neuropeptides and Behavior, Vol. 1. Eds. D. De Wied, W. H. Gispen, and Tj. B. van Wimersma Greidanus. New York, Pergamon Press, pp. 313–348.

Campenot, R. B. 1977. Local control of neurite outgrowth by nerve growth factor. Proc. Natl. Acad. Sci. U.S.A. 74: 4516–4519.

Castano, J. P., R. D. Kineman, W. J. Faught, et al. 1994. Real-time measurement of prolactin secretion from individual lactotropes. Neuroprotocols 5: 216–220.

Chan Palay, V. 1987. Somatostatin immunoreactive neurons in the human hippocampus and cortex shown by immunogold-silver intensification on vibratome sections: Coexistence with neuropeptide Y neurons and effects in Alzheimer-type dementia. J. Comp. Neurol. 260: 201–223.

Chayen, J., and L. Bitensky. 1983. General introduction to cytochemical bioassays. In: Cytochemical Bioassays: Techniques and Clinical Applications. Eds. J. Chayen and L. Bitensky. New York, Marcel Dekker.

Coy, D. H., and A. J. Kastin. 1986. Structure-CNS activity studies with the enkephalins. In: Neuropeptides and Behavior, Vol 1. Eds. D. De Wied, W. H. Gispen, and Tj. B. van Wimersma Greidanus. New York, Pergamon Press, pp. 349–384.

Critchley, G., and B. Worster. 1997. Identification of peptides by matrix-assisted laser desorption ionization time of flight mass spectrometry (MALDI-TOF-MS) and direct analysis of the laterobuccal nerve from the pond snail *Lymnaea stagnalis*. In: Methods in Molecular Biology, Neuropeptide Protocols. Eds. G. B. Irvine and C. H. Williams. Totawa, N.J., Humana Press, pp. 141–152.

Crow, T. J., I. N. Ferrier, E. C. Johnstone, et al. 1982. Neuroendocrine aspects of schizophrenia. In: Neuropeptides: Basic and Clinical Aspects. Eds. G. Fink and L. J. Whaley. Edinburgh, Churchill Livingstone, pp. 227–238.

Dahlstrom, A., and K. Fuxe. 1965. Evidence for the existence of monoamine neurons in the central nervous system. Acta Physiol. Scand. Suppl. 64: 1–85.

Davis, T. P. 1991. Methods of measuring neuropeptides and their metabolism. In: Stress, Neuropeptides and Systemic Disease. Eds. J. A. McCubbin, P. G. Kaufmann, and C. B. Nemeroff. New York, Academic Press, pp. 149–177.

De Wied, D. 1964. Influence of anterior pituitary on avoidance learning and escape behavior. Am. J. Physiol. 207: 255–259.

De Wied, D. 1990. Effects of peptide hormones on behavior. In: Neuropeptides: Basics and Perspectives. Ed. D. De Wied. Amsterdam, Elsevier, pp. 1–44.

De Wied, D., M. Diamant, and M. Fodor. 1993. Central nervous system effects of the neurohypophyseal hormones and related peptides. Front. Neuroendocrinol. 14: 251–302.

Evans, M. J., D. T. Gilmour, and W. H. Colledge. 1994. Transgenic rodents. In: Animals with Novel Genes. Ed. N. Maclean. New York, Cambridge University Press, pp. 138–178.

Falck, B., N.-Å. Hillarp, G. Thieme, et al. 1962. Fluorescence of catecholamines and related compounds condensed with formaldehyde. J. Histochem. Cytochem. 10: 348–354.

Ferguson, A. V., and L. P. Renaud. 1987. In vivo electrophysiological techniques in the study of peptidergic neurons and actions. In: Neuromethods 6: Peptides. Eds. A. A. Boulton, G. B. Baker, and Q. C. Pittman. Totawa, N.J., Humana Press, pp. 379–408.

Flynn, F. W. 1994. Bombesin-like peptides in the regulation of ingestive behavior. Ann. N.Y. Acad. Sci. 739: 120–134.

Fuxe, K., L. Agnati, M. Kalia, et al. 1985. In: The Dopaminergic System. Eds. E. Flückiger, E. E. Müller, and M. O. Thorner. Berlin, Springer-Verlag, pp. 11–25.

Gispen, W. H., and R. L. Isaacson. 1986. Excessive grooming in response to ACTH. In: Neuropeptides and Behavior, Vol 1. Eds. D. De Wied, W. H. Gispen, and Tj. B. van Wimersma Greidanus. New York, Pergamon Press, pp. 273–312.

Grigoriadis, D. E., and E. B. De Souza. 1992. Receptor binding theory and techniques. In: Neuroendocrinology. Ed. C. B. Nemeroff. Boca Raton, Fla., CRC Press, pp. 63–83.

Hol, E. M., P. Sodaar, and P. R. Bär. 1994. Dorsal root ganglia as an in vitro mode for melanocortin-induced neuritogenesis. Ann. N.Y. Acad. Sci. 739: 74–86.

Jaspan, J. B., W. A. Banks, and A. J. Kastin. 1994. Study of peptides across the blood-brain barrier: Biological effects of cyclo (His-Pro) after intravenous and oral administration. Ann. N.Y. Acad. Sci. 739: 101–107.

Jennes, L., P. M. Conn, and W. E. Stumpf. 1989. Synthesis and use of colloidal gold–coupled receptor ligands. In: Neuroendocrine Peptide Methodology. Ed. P. M. Conn. New York, Academic Press, pp. 429–440.

Kastin, A. J., R. H. Ehrensing, C. Hara, et al. 1986. Parallel behavioral and EEG studies of the CNS effects of MSH in animals and humans. In: Central Actions of ACTH and Related Peptides. Eds. D. De Wied and W. Ferrari. Fidia Research Series, Symposia in Neuroscience IV Padova, Italy, Liviana Press, pp. 147–152.

Kastin, A. J., N. P. Plotnikoff, A. V. Schally, et al. 1976. Endocrine and CNS effects of hypothalamic peptides and MSH. In: Reviews of Neuroscience. Eds. S. Ehrenpreis and I. J. Kopin. New York, Raven Press, pp. 111–148.

Kendall, M. E., and W. C. Hymer. 1989. Measurement of hormone secretion from individual cells by bioassay. In: Neuroendocrine Peptide Methodology. Ed. P. M. Conn. New York, Academic Press, pp. 193–204.

Kilts, C. D. 1992. Electrochemical detection: Applications in neuroendocrinology. In: Neuroendocrinology. Ed. C. B. Nemeroff. Boca Raton, Fla., CRC Press, pp. 51–61.

Kuhar, M. J. 1987. Imaging receptors for drugs in neural tissue. Neuropharmacology 26(7B): 911–916.

Kuypers, H. G. J. M., and G. Ugolini. 1990. Viruses as transneuronal tracers. Trends Neurosci. 13: 71–75.

Grigoriadis, D. E., and E. B. De Souza. 1992. Receptor binding theory and techniques. In: Neuroendocrinology. Ed. C. B. Nemeroff. Boca Raton, Fla., CRC Press, pp. 63–83.

Lee, S. J. 1995. The Neurotropic Role of Adrenocorticotropic Hormone (ACTH) 4–10 in the Developing and Regenerating Rat Central Nervous System: In vitro and in vivo Studies. Ph.D. thesis, New York University.

Leibowitz, S. F. 1994. Specificity of hypothalamic peptides in the control of behavioral and physiological processes. Ann. N.Y. Acad. Sci. 739: 12–35.

Levine, J. E., J. M. Meredith, K. M. Vogelsong, et al. 1991. Microdialysis for the study of hypothalamic and pituitary function. In: Microdialysis in the Neurosciences. Eds. T. E. Robinson and Justice. New York, Elsevier, p. 308.

Levine, J. E., A. M. Wolfe, T. Porkka-Heiskanen, et al. 1994. In vivo sampling and administration of hormone pulses in rodents. Methods Neurosci. 20: 129–161.

Maggi, C. A., R. Patacchini, M. Astolfi, et al. 1991. NK-2 receptor agonists and antagonists. Ann. N.Y. Acad. Sci. 632: 184–191.

Mandys, V., R. van der Neut, P. R. Bär, et al. 1991. Cultivation of rat fetal spinal cord slices in a semi-solid medium: A new approach to studying axonal outgrowth and regeneration. J. Neurosci. Methods 38: 63–69.

Mocchetti, I., and E. Costa. 1987. In vivo studies of the regulation of neuropeptide stores in structures of the rat brain. Neuropharmacology 26(7B): 855–862.

Muglia, L., N. A. Jenkins, D. J. Gilbert, et al. 1994. Expression of the mouse corticotropin-releasing hormone gene in vivo and targeted inactivation in embryonic stem cells. J. Clin. Invest. 93: 2066–2072

Muglia, L., L. Jacobson, and J. A. Majzoub. 1996. Production of corticotropin-releasing hormone deficient mice by targeted mutation in embryonic stem cells. Ann. N.Y. Acad. Sci. 780: 49–59.

Neil, J. D., and L. S. Frawley. 1983. Detection of hormone release from individual cells in mixed populations using a reverse hemolytic plaque assay. Endocrinology 112: 1135–1137.

Palkowits, M. 1973. Isolated removal of hypothalamic or other brain nuclei of the rat. Brain Res. 59: 449–450.

Renaud, L. P., C. W. Bourque, T. A. Day, et al. 1985. Electrophysiology of mammalian hypothalamic supraoptic and paraventricular neurosecretory cells. In: The Electrophysiology of the Secretory Cell. Eds. A. N. Poisner and J. Trifaro. Amsterdam, Elsevier, pp. 89–99.

Sagar, S. M., and F. R. Sharp. 1992. Early response genes as markers of neuronal activity and growth factor action. In: Neural Regeneration. Ed. F. J. Seil. New York, Raven Press. pp. 273–284.

Saint-Come, C., and F. L. Strand. 1985. ACTH/MSH 4–10 improves motor unit reorganization during peripheral nerve regeneration in the rat. Peptides 6 (Suppl. 1): 77–83.

Sandman, C. A., and J. P. O'Halloran. 1986 Pro-opiomelanocortin, learning, memory and attention. In: Neuropeptides and Behavior, Vol 1. Eds. D. De Wied, W. H. Gispen, and Tj. B. van Wimersma Greidanus. New York, Pergamon Press, pp. 397–420.

Sar, M., and W. E. Stumpf. 1989. Simultaneous localization of steroid hormones and neuropeptides in the brain by combined autoradiography and immunocytochemistry. In: Neuroendocrine Peptide Methodology. Ed. P. M. Conn. New York, Academic Press, pp. 907–915.

Silberring, J. 1997a. Characterization of neuropeptide processing by fast atom bombardment mass spectrometry. In: Methods in Molecular Biology, Neuropeptide Protocols. Eds. G. B. Irvine and C. H. Williams. Totawa, N.J., Humana Press, pp. 113–128, 141–152.

Silberring, J. 1997b. Analysis of neuropeptides by size-exclusion HPLC linked to electrospray ionization mass spectrometry. In: Methods in Molecular Biology, Neuropeptide Protocols. Eds. G. B. Irvine and C. H. Williams. Totawa, N.J., Humana Press, pp. 129–140.

Smith, D., and A. M. Hanley. 1997. Purification of synthetic peptides by high performance liquid chromatography. In: Neuropeptide Protocols. Eds. C. B. Irvine and C. H. Williams. Totawa, N.J., Humana Press, pp. 75–87.

Spruijt, B. M., A. B. Destreicher, and J. A. D. M. Tonnaer. 1990. Neuropeptides and brain aging. In: Neuropeptides: Basics and Perspectives. Ed. D. De Wied. Amsterdam, Elsevier, pp. 353–390.

Stenzel-Poore, M. P., J. E. Duncan, M. B. Rittenberg, et al. 1996. CRH overproduction in transgenic mice: Behavioral and immune system modulation. Ann. N.Y. Acad. Sci. 780: 36–48.

Strand, F. L., C. Saint-Come, T. S. Lee, et al. 1993. ACTH/MSH 4–10 analog BIM 22015 aids regeneration via neurotrophic and myotrophic attributes. Peptides 14: 287–296.

Urban, I. J. A. 1986. Electrophysiological effects of peptides derived from pro-opiomelanocortin. In: Neuropeptides and Behavior, Vol. 1. Eds. D. De Wied, W. H. Gispen, and Tj. B. van Wimersma Greidanus. New York, Pergamon Press, pp. 211–244.

Van der Neut, R., P. R. Bär, P. Sodar, et al. 1988. Trophic influences of alpha-MSH and ACTH 4–10 on neuronal outgrowth in vitro. Peptides 9: 1015–1020.

Van Nispen, J. W., and H. M. Greven. 1986. Structure-activity relationships of peptides derived from ACTH, β-LPH and MSH with regard to avoidance behavior in rats. In: Neuropeptides and Behavior, Vol. 1. Eds. D. De Wied, W. H. Gispen, and Tj. B. van Wimersma Greidanus. New York, Pergamon Press, pp. 349–384.

Varndell, I. M., and J. M. Polak. 1984. The use of double immunogold-staining procedures at the ultrastructural level for demonstrating neurochemical coexistence. In: Coexistence of Neuroactive Substances in Neurons. Eds. V. Chan-Palay and S. L. Palay. New York, Wiley, pp. 279–303.

Viville, S. 1994. Site-directed mutagenesis using a double-stranded DNA template. Methods Mol. Biol. 31: 57–66.

Waschek, J. A. 1995. Transgenic targeting of neuroendocrine peptide genes in the hypothalamic-pituitary axis. Mol. Neurobiol. 10: 205–217.

Waterfall, A. H., R. W. Clarke, and G. W. Bennett. 1994. Novel methods for the preparation of antibody microprobes. J. Neurosci. Methods 55: 41–45.

Yang, X. F., H. Fournier, N. Dion, et al. 1994. Site-directed mutagenesis and transfection methods in the study of prohormone processing. Neuroprotocols 5: 157–168.

Chapter 3

Books and Literature Reviews

Fricker, L. D., Ed. 1991. Peptide Biosynthesis and Processing. Boca Raton, Fla., CRC Press.

Loh, Y. P., Ed. 1993. Mechanisms of Intracellular Trafficking and Processing of Proproteins. Boca Raton, Fla., CRC Press.

Nicholls, D. G. 1994. Proteins, Transmitters and Synapses. London, Blackwell.

Siegel, G., Ed. 1994. Basic Neurochemistry: Molecular, Cellular and Medical Aspects, 5th Ed. New York, Raven Press.

References

Acher, R., and J. Chauvet. 1995. The neurohypophyseal endocrine regulatory cascade: Precursors, mediators, receptors and effectors. Front. Endocrinol. 16: 237–289.

Alberts, B., D. Bray, J. Lewis, et al. 1983. Molecular Biology of the Cell. New York, Garland Press.

Ashcroft, F. M., and P. Rorsman. 1995. Electrophysiology of pancreatic islet cells. In: The Electrophysiology of Neuroendocrine Cells. Eds. H. Scherübl and J. Hescheler. Boca Raton, Fla., CRC Press, pp. 207–256.

Beinfeld, M. C., J. Bourdais, P. Kuks, et al. 1989. Characterization of an endoprotease from rat small intestinal mucosal secretory granules which generates somatostatin-28 from prosomatostatin by cleavage after a single arginine residue. J. Biol. Chem. 264: 4460–4465.

Bennett, H. P. J., A. F. Bradbury, W. B. Huttner, et al. 1993. Processing of pro-peptides: Glycosylation, phosphorylation, sulfation, acetylation and amidation. In: Mechanisms of Intracellular Trafficking and Processing of Prohormones. Ed. Y. P. Loh. Boca Raton, Fla., CRC Press, pp. 251–288.

Blobel G., and B. Dobberstein, 1975. Transfer of proteins across membranes. J. Cell Biol. 67: 835–851.

Blondel, O., G. I. Bell, and S. Seino. 1995. Inositol 1,4,5-triphosphate receptors, secretory granules and secretion in endocrine and neuroendocrine cells. Trends Neurosci. 18: 157–161.

Boileau, G., N. G. Seidah, and M. Chretien. 1981. Biosynthesis of β-endorphin from proopiomelancortin. In: Hormonal Proteins and Peptides, Vol. 10. Ed. C. H. Li. New York, Academic Press, pp. 65–87.

Brakch, N., H. Boussetta, M. Rholam, et al. 1989. Processing endoprotease recognizes a structural feature at the cleavage site of peptide prohormones. J. Biol. Chem. 264: 15912–15916.

Burgoyne R. D., and A. Morgan. 1995. Ca^{2+} and secretory-vesicle dynamics. Trends Neurosci. 18: 191–196.

Castro, M. G., and E. Morrison. 1997. Posttranslational processing of proopiomelanocortin in the pituitary and in the brain. Critical Rev. Neurobiol. 11: 35–57.

Conlon, J. M. 1989. Biosynthesis of regulatory peptides—Evolutionary aspects. In: The Comparative Physiology of Regulatory Peptides. Ed. S. Holmgren. New York, Chapman & Hall, pp. 345–369.

Cool, D. R., M. Fenger, C. R. Snell, et al. 1995. Identification of the sorting signal motif within proopiomelanocortin for the regulated secretory pathway. J. Biol. Chem. 270: 8723–8729.

Cool, D. R., E. Normant, F. Shen, et al. 1997. Carboxypeptidase E is a regulated secretory pathway sorting receptor: Genetic obliteration leads to endocrine disorders in Cpe^{fat} mice. Cell 88: 73–83.

De Bie, I., M. Marcinkiewicz, D. Malide, et al. 1996. The isoforms of the proprotein convertase 5 are sorted to different subcellular compartments. J. Cell Biol. 135: 1261–1275.

De Wied, D. 1987. The neuropeptide concept. In: Prog. Brain Res. 72. Eds. E. R. de Kloet, V. M. Wiegant and D. De Wied. Amsterdam, Elsevier, pp. 93–108.

Dong, W., B. Seidel, M. Mieczyslaw, et al. 1997. Cellular localization of the prohormone convertases in the hypothalamic paraventricular and supraoptic nuclei: Selective regulation of PC1 in corticotropin-releasing hormone parvocellular neurons mediated by glucocorticoids. J. Neurosci. 17: 563–575.

Dores, R. M. 1988. Pituitary melanotropin biosynthesis. In: The Melanocortins, Vol. 1. Ed. M. E. Hadley. Boca Raton, Fla., CRC Press, pp. 26–38.

Fricker, L. D. 1992. Peptide processing exopeptidases: Amino- and carboxypeptidase involved with peptide biosynthesis. In: Peptide Biosynthesis and Processing. Ed. L. D. Fricker. Boca Raton, Fla., CRC Press, pp. 199–229.

Häkinson, R., R. Ekman, F. Sundler, et al. 1982. The life cycle of the gastrin granule. Cell Tissue Res. 222: 479–491.

Hardie, D. G. 1991. Biochemical Messengers. London, Chapman & Hall.

Hook, V. Y. H., A. V. Azaryan, S.-R. Hwang, et al. 1994. Proteases and the emerging role of protease inhibitors in prohormone processing. FASEB J. 8: 1269–1278.

Lemke, G. 1992. Gene regulation in the nervous system. In: An Introduction to Molecular Biology. Ed. Z. W. Hall. Sunderland, Mass., Sinauer Associates, pp. 313–354.

Littelton, J. T., and H. J. Bellen. 1995. Synaptotagmin controls and modulates synaptic-vesicle fusion in a Ca^{2+} dependent manner. Trends Neurosci. 18: 177–183.

Loh, Y. P. 1987. Peptide precursor processing enzymes within secretory vesicles. Ann. N.Y. Acad. Sci. 493: 292–307.

Loh, Y. P., M. C. Beinfeld, and N. P. Birch. 1993. Proteolytic processing of prohormones and proneuropeptides. In:

Mechanisms of Intracellular Trafficking and Processing of Prohormones. Ed. Y. P. Loh. Boca Raton, Fla., CRC Press, pp. 179–224.

Mains, R. E., E. I. Cullen, V. May, et al. 1987. The role of secretory granules in peptide biosynthesis. Ann. N.Y. Acad. Sci. 493: 279–291.

Mains, R. E., I. M. Dickerson, V. May, et al. 1990. Cellular and molecular aspects of peptide hormone biosynthesis. Front. Neuroendocrinol. 11: 52–89.

May, V., C. A. Brandenburg, and K. M. Braas. 1995. Differential regulation of sympathetic neuron neuropeptide Y and catecholamine content and secretion. J. Neurosci. 15: 4580–4591.

May, V., and B. A. Eipper. 1986. Long term culture of primary rat pituitary adrenocorticotropin/endorphin-producing cells in serum-free medium. Endocrinology 118: 1284–1295.

Mizuno, K., and H. Matsuo. 1994. Processing of peptide hormone precursors. In: The Pituitary Gland, 2nd Ed. Ed. H. Imura. New York, Raven Press, pp. 153–178.

Nakanishi, S. Y., A. Inoue, T. Kita, et al. 1979. Nucleotide sequence of cloned DNA for bovine corticotropin/β-lipotropin precursor. Nature 278: 423–429.

Nakanishi, S. Y. Teranishi, Y. Watanabe, et al. 1981. Isolation and characterization of the bovine corticotropin/β-lipotropin precursor gene. Eur. J. Biochem. 115: 429–438.

Nicholls, D. G. 1994. Proteins, Transmitters and Synapses. Oxford, Blackwell, pp. 142–152.

Orci, L., and A. Perrelet. 1975. Freeze-Etch Histology. Heidelberg, Springer-Verlag, pl. 36.

Petersen. O. H. 1996. New aspects of cytosolic calcium signaling. News Physiol. Sci. 11: 13–17.

Plevrakis, I., C. Clamagirand, C. Créminon, et al. 1989. Prooxcytocin/neurophysin convertase from bovine neurohypophysis and corpus luteum secretory granules: Complete purification, structure-function relationships and competitive inhibitor. Biochemistry 28: 2705–2710.

Rothman J. E., and L. Orci. 1996. Budding vesicles in living cells. Sci. Am., 274(3) 70–75.

Rouille, Y., S. J. Duguay, K. Lund, et al. 1995. Proteolytic processing mechanisms in the biosynthesis of neuroendocrine peptides: The subtilisin-like proprotein convertases. Front. Neuroendocrinol. 16: 322–361.

Schlegel, W., and P. Mollard. 1995. Electrical activity and stimulus-secretion coupling in neuroendocrine cells. In: The Electrophysiology of Neuroendocrine Cells. Eds. H. Scherübl and J. Hescheler. Boca Raton, Fla., CRC Press, pp. 23–38.

Seidah, N. G. 1995. The mammalian family of subtilisin/kexin-like pro-protein convertases. In: Intramolecular Chaperones and Protein Folding. Eds. U. Shinde and M. Inouye. Austin, Tex., Landes, pp. 181–203.

Seidah, N. G., and M. Chrétien. 1997. Eucaryotic protein processing: Endoproteolysis of precursor proteins is an obligatory process common to the synthesis of many biologically active proteins and peptides in yeast, invertebrates and mammalian cells. Curr. Opin. Biotechnol., 8: 602–606.

Sherman, T. G., H. Akil, and S. J. Watson. 1989. The Molecular Biology of Neuropeptides. Discussions in Neuroscience, Vol. 6. Amsterdam, Elsevier, pp. 1–58.

Uhler, M., E. Herbert, P. D'Eustachio, et al. 1983. The mouse genome contains two nonallelic pro-opiomelanocortin genes. J. Biol. Chem. 258: 9444–9453.

Vaudry, H., B. G. Jenks, L. Verburg-van-Kemenade, et al. 1986. Effect of tunimycin on biosynthesis, processing and release of proopiomelanocortin-derived peptides in the intermediate lobe of the frog *Rana ridibunda*. Peptides 7: 163–169.

Wilcox, J. N., and J. L. Roberts. 1985. Estrogen decreases rat hypothalamic proopiomelanocortin messenger ribonucleic acid levels. Endocrinology 117: 2392–2395.

Zheng, M., R. D. Streck, R. E. M. Scott, et al. 1994. The developmental expression in rat of proteases furin, PC1, PC2 and carboxypeptidase E: Implications for early maturation of proteolytic processing capacity. J. Neurosci. 4: 4656–4673.

Zhou, Z., and S. Misler. 1995. Action potential-induced quantal secretion of catecholamines from rat adrenal chromaffin cells. J. Biol. Chem. 270: 3498–3505.

Chapter 4

Books and Literature Reviews

Björkland, A., T. Hökfelt, and M. J. Kuhar. 1990. Neuropeptides in the CNS. Handbook of Chemical Neuroanatomy, Vol. 9. New York, Elsevier.

Chan-Palay, V., and S. L. Palay. 1984. Coexistence of Neuroactive Substances in Neurons. New York, Wiley.

Guillemin, R. 1978. Peptides in the brain: The new endocrinology of the neuron. Science 202: 390–402.

Krieger, D. T. 1983. Brain peptides: What, where and why? Science 222: 975–985.

Krieger, D. T., and A. S. Liotta. 1979. Pituitary hormones in brain: Where, how and why? Science 205: 366–372.

Strand, F. L., A. E. Segarra, L. A. Zuccarelli, et al. 1990. Neuropeptides: Fail-safe, redundant or special? In: Neuroendocrinology: New Frontiers. Ed. D. Gupta. Tübingen, Brain Research Promotion, pp. 19–28.

References

Belin, M. F., D. Nanopoulos, M. Didier, et al. 1983. Immunohistochemical evidence for the presence of gamma-aminobutyric acid and serotonin in one nerve cell. A study on the raphe nuclei with antibodies to glutamate decarboxylase and serotonin. Brain Res. 275: 329–332.

Eccles, J. C. 1957. The Physiology of Nerve Cells. Baltimore, Johns Hopkins Press, p. 212.

Fuxe, K., and L. F. Agnati. 1991. Two principal models of electrochemical communication in the brain: Volume versus wiring transmission. In: Advances in Neuroscience, Vol. 1, Volume Transmission in the Brain, Novel Mechanisms for Neural Transmission. Eds. K. Fuxe and L. Agnati. New York, Raven Press, pp. 1–9.

Fuxe, K., X.-M. Li, B. Bjelke, et al. 1994. Possible mechanisms for the powerful actions of neuropeptides. Ann. N.Y. Acad. Sci. 739: 42–59.

Gibbins, I. L. 1989. Co-existence and co-function. In: The Comparative Physiology of Regulatory Peptides. Ed. S. Holmgren. New York, Chapman & Hall, pp. 308–343.

Gibbins, I. L., and J. L. Morris. 1987. Co-existence of neuropeptides in sympathetic cranial autonomic and sensory neurones innervating the iris of the guinea-pig. J. Auton. Nerv. Syst. 21: 67–82.

Helke, C. J., and L. Yang. 1996. Interactions and coexistence of neuropeptides and serotonin in spinal autonomic systems. Ann. N.Y. Acad. Sci. 780: 185–192.

Hökfelt, T., V. R. Holets, W. Staines, et al. 1986. Coexistence of neuronal messengers—an overview. Prog. Brain Res. 68: 33–70.

Hökfelt, T., O. Johansson, and M. Goldstein. 1984. Chemical anatomy of the brain. Science 225: 1326–1334.

Lundberg, J. M., and T. Hökfelt. 1985. Coexistence of peptides and classical neurotransmitters. In: Neurotransmitters in Action. Ed. D. Bousfield. New York, Elsevier, pp. 104–118.

Palkowits, M. 1980. Functional anatomy of the "endocrine" brain. In: The Endocrine Functions of the Brain. Ed. M. Motta. New York, Raven Press, pp. 1–19.

Peng, Y., and J. P. Horn. 1991. Continuous repetitive stimuli are more effective than bursts for evoking LHRH release in bullfrog sympathetic ganglia. J. Neurosci. 11: 85–95.

Sawchenko, P. E., T. Imaki, and W. Vale. 1992. Colocalization of neuroactive substances in the endocrine hypothalamus. Ciba Found. Symp. 168: 16–42.

Strand, F. L., A. E. Segarra, L. A. Zuccarelli, et al. 1990. Neuropeptides: Fail-safe, redundant or special? In: Neuroendocrinology: New Frontiers. Eds. D. Gupta, H. A. Wollman, and M. B. Ranke. Tübingen, Brain Research Promotion, pp. 19–28.

Whittaker, V. P. 1984. What is Dale's principle? In: Coexistence of Neuroactive Substances in Neurons. Eds. V. Chan-Palay and S. L. Palay. New York, Wiley, pp. 137–140.

Chapter 5

Books and Literature Reviews

Banks, W. A., and A. J. Kastin. 1995. Permeability of the blood-brain barrier to melanocortins. Peptides 16: 1157–1161.

Davson. H., and M. B. Segal. 1995. Physiology of the CSF and Blood-Brain Barriers. Boca Raton, Fla., CRC Press.

Greenwood, J., D. J. Begley, and M. B. Segal. 1995. New Concepts of a Blood-Brain Barrier. New York, Plenum Press.

Halász, B. 1994. Hypothalamo-Anterior Pituitary System and Pituitary Portal Vessels. In: The Pituitary Gland, 2nd Ed. Ed. H. Imura. New York, Raven Press, pp. 1–28.

Moody, T. W., Ed. 1986. Neural and Endocrine Peptides and Receptors. New York, Plenum Press.

Nemeroff, C. B., Ed. 1992. Neuroendocrinology. Boca Raton, Fla., CRC Press.

Pardridge, W. M. 1983. Brain metabolism: A perspective from the blood-brain barrier. Physiol. Rev. 63: 1481–1535.

References

Banks, W. A., and A. J. Kastin. 1984. A brain-to-blood carrier–mediated transport system for small N-tyrosinated peptides. Pharmacol. Biochem. Behav. 21: 943–946.

Banks, W. A., and A. J. Kastin. 1985. Permeability of the blood-brain barrier to neuropeptides: The case for penetration. Psychoneuroendocrinolog 10: 385–399.

Banks, W. A., and A. J. Kastin. 1988. Review: Interactions between the blood-brain barrier and endogenous peptides: Emerging clinical implications. Am. J. Med. Sci. 31(5): 459–465.

Banks, W. A., and A. J. Kastin. 1995a. Review: Permeability of the blood-brain barrier to melanocortins. Peptides 16: 1157–1161.

Banks, W. A., and A. J. Kastin. 1995b. Peptide transport system—1. In: New Concepts of a Blood-Brain Barrier. Eds. J. Greenwood, D. J. Begley, and M. B. Segal. New York, Plenum Press, pp. 111–117.

Banks, W. A., A. J. Kastin, A. Horvath, et al. 1987a. Carrier-mediated transport of vasopressin across the blood-brain barrier of the mouse. Neurosci. Res. 18: 326–332.

Banks, W. A,. A. J. Kastin, and E. A. Michals. 1987b. Tyr-MIF-I and met–enkephalin share a saturable blood-brain-barrier transport system. Peptides 8: 899–903.

Baura, G. D., D. M. Foster, D. Porte, et al. 1993. Saturable transport of insulin from plasma into the central nervous system of dogs in vivo: a mechanism for regulated insulin delivery into the brain. J. Clin. Invest. 92: 1824–1830.

Begley, D. J. 1994. Peptides and the blood-brain barrier: The status of our understanding. Ann. N.Y. Acad. Sci. 739: 89–100.

Bergland, R. M., and R. B. Page. 1979. Pituitary-brain vascular relations: A new paradigm. Science 104: 18–20.

Brightman, M. W. 1977. Morphology of the blood-brain barrier. Exp. Eye Res. (Suppl): 1–25.

Bouldin, T. W., and M. R. Krigman. 1975. Differential permeability of cerebral capillary and choroid plexus to lanthanum ion. Brain Res. 99: 444–448.

Brownson, E. A., T. J. Abbruscato, T. J. Gillespie, et al. 1994. Effect of peptidases at the blood brain barrier on the permeability of enkephalin. J. Pharmacol. Exp. Ther. 270: 675–680.

Coomber, B. L., and P. A. Stewart. 1985. Morphometric analysis of CNS microvascular endothelium. Microvasc. Res. 30: 99–115.

Cserr, H. F., and M. Bundgaard. 1984. Blood-brain interfaces in vertebrates: A comparative approach. Am. J. Physiol 84: R277–288.

Davson, H., and M. B. Segal. 1995. Physiology of the CSF and Blood-Brain Barriers. Boca Raton, Fla., CRC Press, pp. 174–188.

Davson, H., K. Welch, and M. B. Segal. 1987. Some special aspects of the blood-brain barrier. In: Physiology and

Pathophysiology of the Cerebrospinal Fluid. Edinburgh, Churchill Livingstone, pp. 247–374.

De Wied, D. 1969. Effects of peptide hormones on behavior. In: Frontiers in Neuroendocrinology. Eds. W. F. Ganong and L. Martini. New York, Oxford University Press, pp. 97–140.

De Wied, D., A. Witter, and H. M. Greven. 1975. Behaviorally active ACTH analogues. Biochem. Pharmacol. 24: 1463–1468.

Dingledine, R., and G. Somjen. 1981. Calcium dependence of synaptic transmission in the hippocampal slice. Brain Res. 207: 218–222.

Dogtorom, J., Tj. van W. Greidanus, and D. F. Swaab. 1977. Evidence for the release of vasopressin and oxytocin into cerebrospinal fluid: Measurements in plasma and CSF of intact and hypophysectomized rats. Neuroendocrinology 24: 108–118.

Ermisch, A., P. Brust, R. Kretzschmar, et al. 1993. Peptides and blood-brain barrier transport. Physiol. Rev. 73: 489–527.

Everitt, B. J., B. Meister, and T. Hökfelt. 1992. The organization of monoaminergic neurons in the hypothalamus in relation to neuroendocrine integration. In: Neuroendocrinology. Ed. C. B. Nemeroff. Boca Raton, Fla., CRC Press, pp. 87–128.

Frank, H. J. L., and W. M. Pardridge. 1987. A direct in vivo demonstration of insulin binding in isolated brain microvessels. Diabetes 30: 757–761.

Fuxe, K., X.-M. Li, B. Bjelke, et al. 1994. Possible mechanisms for the powerful actions of neuropeptides. Ann. N.Y. Acad. Sci. 739: 42–59.

Goldmann, E. E. 1909. Die äussere und innere Sekretion des gesundes und kranken Organismus im Lichte der "vitalen Färbung." Beitr. Klin. Chir. 64: 192–198.

Goldstein, G. W. 1988. Endothelial cell–astrocyte interactions: A cellular model of the blood-brain barrier. Ann. N.Y. Acad. Sci. 529: 31–39.

Green, J. D., and G. W. Harris. 1947. The neurovascular link between the neurohypophysis and the adenohypophysis. J. Endocrinol. 5: 136–146.

Gross, P. M., and A. Weindl. 1987. Peering through the windows of the brain. J. Cereb. Blood Flow Metab. 7: 663–672.

Halász, B. 1994. Hypothalamo-anterior pituitary system and pituitary portal vessels. In: The Pituitary Gland, 2nd Ed. Ed. H. Imura. New York, Raven Press, pp. 1–28.

Harris, G. W. 1955. Neural Control of the Pituitary Gland. London, Edward Arnold.

Jaspan, J. B., W. A. Banks, and A. J. Kastin. 1994. Study of passage of peptides across the blood-brain barrier: Biological effects of cyclo(His-Pro) after intravenous and oral administration. Ann. N.Y. Acad. Sci. 739: 101–107.

Joó, F. 1987. Current aspects of the development of the blood-brain barrier. Int. J. Dev. Neurosci. 5: 369–372.

Kastin, A. J., J. E. Zadina, R. D. Olson, et al. 1996. The history of neuropeptide research: Version 5.a. Ann. N.Y. Acad. Sci. 780: 1–18.

Kastin, A. K., J. E. Zadina, W. A. Banks, et al. 1984. Misleading concepts in the field of brain peptides. Peptides 5(Suppl. 1): 249–253.

Müller, E. E., and G. Nisticò. 1989. Neurotransmitter regulation of the anterior pituitary. In: Brain Messengers and the Pituitary. New York, Academic Press, pp. 404–537.

Noback, C. R., and R. J. Demarest. 1975. The Human Nervous System: Basic Principles of Neurobiology, 2nd Ed. New York, McGraw-Hill.

Palkowits, M. 1980. Functional anatomy of the "endocrine" brain. In: The Endocrine Functions of the Brain. Ed. M. Motta. New York, Raven Press, pp. 1–19.

Pardridge, W. M. 1986. Receptor-mediated peptide transport through the blood-brain barrier. Endocr. Rev. 7: 314–330.

Pardridge, W. M. 1988. New directions in blood-brain barrier research: Studies with isolated human brain capillaries. Ann. N.Y. Acad. Sci. 529: 50–60.

Pardridge, W. M. 1990. Receptor-mediated transport of peptides through the blood-brain barrier. In: Fernström Foundation Series. Pathophysiology of the Blood-Brain Barrier. Long-Term Consequences of Barrier Dysfunction for the Brain, Vol. 14. Eds. B. B. Johansson, C. Owman, and H. Widner. Amsterdam, Elsevier, pp. 61–69.

Patlak, C. S., R. G. Blasberg, and J. D. Fenstermacher. 1983. Graphical evaluation of blood to brain transfer constants from multiple time uptake data. J. Cereb. Blood Flow Metab. 3: 1–7.

Popa, G. T., and U. Fielding. 1930. A portal circulation from the pituitary to the hypothalamic region. J. Anat. 65: 88–91.

Scharrer, E., and B. Scharrer. 1937. Über Drüsen-Nervenzellen und Neurosekretorische Organe bei Wirbellosen und Wirbeltieren. Biol. Revs. Cambridge Phil. Soc. 12: 185–216.

Simpkins, J. W., X. Ouyang, L. Prokai, et al. 1994. Delivery of peptides into the central nervous system by molecular packaging and sequential metabolism as a method of altering neuropeptide activity during aging. Neuroprotocols 4: 225–234.

Strand, F. L. 1983. Physiology: A Regulatory Systems Approach, 2nd Ed. New York, Macmillan.

Swanson, L. W. 1993. Patterns of transcriptional regulation in the neuroendocrine system. In: Brain Functions of Neuropeptides. Eds. J. P. H. Burbach and D. de Wied. New York, Parthenon, pp. 41–64.

Wislocki, G. B., and L. S. King. 1936. The permeability of the hypophysis and the hypothalamus to vital dyes, with a study of the hypophysial vascular supply. Am. J. Anat. 58: 421–472.

Chapter 6

Books and Literature Reviews

Bolander, F. F. 1989. Molecular Endocrinology. San Diego, Academic Press.

Brann, M. R., Ed. 1992. Molecular Biology of G-Protein–Coupled Receptors. Boston, Birkhäuser.

Dawson, T. M., and V. L. Dawson, 1994. Nitric oxide: Actions and pathological roles. Neuroscientist, preview issue, pp. 9–20.

Dawson, T. M., and S. H. Snyder. 1994. Gases as biological messengers: Nitric oxide and carbon monoxide. J. Neurosci. 14: 5147–5159.

Gantz, I., H. Miwa, Y. Konda, et al. 1993. Molecular cloning, expression and gene localization of a fourth melanocortin receptor. J. Biol. Chem. 268: 15174–15479.

Hall, Z. W. 1992. An Introduction to Molecular Neurobiology. Sunderland, Mass., Sinauer.

Lolait, S. J., A-M. O'Carroll, and M. J. Brownstein. 1995. Molecular biology of vasopressin receptors. Ann. N.Y. Acad. Sci. 771: 273–292.

Spiegel, A. M., T. L. Z. Jones, W. F. Simonds, et al. 1994. G Proteins. Austin, Tex., Landes.

References

Adan, R. A. H., R. D. Cone, J. P. H. Burbach, et al. 1994. Differential effects of melanocortin peptides on neural melanocortin receptors. Mol. Pharmacol. 46: 1182–1190.

Bolander, F. F. 1989. Molecular Endocrinology. San Diego, Academic Press.

Boyd, N. D., R. Kage, J. J. Dumas, et al. 1995 Localization of the peptide binding domain of the NK-1 tachykinin receptor using photoreactive analogues of substance P. Ann. N.Y. Acad. Sci. 757: 405–409.

Bult, H., G. R. Boeckxstaens, P. A. Pelckmans, et al. 1990. Nitric oxide as an inhibitory non-adrenergic non-cholinergic neurotransmitter. Nature 345: 346–347.

Burnett, A. L., C. J. Lowenstein, D. S. Bredt, et al. 1992. Nitric oxide: A physiologic mediator of penile erection. Science 257: 401–403.

Ceccatelli, S., J. M. Lundberg, J. Fahrenkrug, et al. 1992. Evidence for involvement of nitric oxide in the regulation of hypothalamic portal blood flow. Neuroscience 51: 769–772.

Cone, R. D., K. G. Mountjoy, L. S. Robbins, et al. 1993. Cloning and functional characterization of a family of receptors for the melanotropic peptides. Ann. N.Y. Acad. Sci. 680: 342–363.

Dale, H. H. 1914. The actions of certain esters and ethers of choline, and their relation to muscarine. J. Pharmacol. Exp. Ther. 6: 147–190.

De Meyts, P., B. Ursø, C. T. Christoffersen, et al. 1995. Mechanism of insulin and IGF-I receptor activation and signal transduction specificity. Ann. N.Y. Acad. Sci. 766: 388–401.

Elde, R., U. Arvidsson, M. Riedl, et al. 1995. Distribution of neuropeptide receptors. Ann. N.Y. Acad. Sci. 757: 390–404.

Faraci, F. M. 1992. Regulation of the cerebral circulation by endothelium. Pharmacol. Ther. 56: 1–22.

Fuxe, K., X.-M. Li, S. Tanganelli, et al. 1995. Receptor-receptor interactions and their relevance for receptor diversity. Ann. N.Y. Acad. Sci. 757: 365–376.

Garthwaite, J., S. L. Charles, and R. Chess-Williams. 1988. Endothelium-derived relaxing factor release on activation of NMDA receptors suggests role as intercellular messenger in the brain. Nature 336: 385–388.

Huang, P. L., T. M. Dawson, D. S. Bredt, et al. 1993. Targeted disruption of the neuronal nitric oxide synthase gene. Cell 75: 1273–1286.

Ignarro, L. J., B. M. Buga, K. S. Wood, et al. 1987. Endothelium-derived relaxing factor produced and released from artery and vein is nitric oxide. Proc. Natl. Acad. Sci. U.S.A. 84: 9265–9269.

Jinnah, H. A., and P. M. Conn. 1988. GnRH action at the pituitary: Basic research and clinical applications. In: Peptide Hormones: Effects and Mechanisms of Action, Vol. 3. Eds. A. Negro-Vilar and P. M. Conn. Boca Raton, Fla., CRC Press. pp. 120–142.

Kennedy, M. B. 1992. Second messengers and neuronal function. In: An Introduction to Molecular Neurobiology. Ed. Z. W. Hall. Sunderland, Mass., Sinauer, pp. 207–246.

Krause, J. E., A. D. Hershey, P. E. Dykema, et al. 1990. Molecular biological studies on the diversity of chemical signalling in tachykinin peptidergic neurons. Ann. N.Y. Acad. Sci. 579: 254–272.

Lipton, S. A., Y. B. Choi, Z.-H. Pan, et al. 1993. A redox-based mechanism for the neuroprotective and neurodestructive effects of nitric oxide and related nitroso-compounds. Nature 364: 626–623.

Lolait, S. J., A-M. O'Carroll, and M. J. Brownstein, 1995. Molecular biology of vasopressin receptors. Ann. N.Y. Acad. Sci. 771: 273–292.

Mani, S. K., J. M. C. Allen, V. Rettori, et al. 1994. Nitric oxide mediates sexual behavior in female rats. Proc. Soc. Natl. Acad. Sci. U.S.A. 91: 6468–6472.

Mons, N., and D. M. F. Cooper. 1995. Adenylate cyclases: Critical foci in neuronal signaling. Trends Neurosci. 18: 536–542.

Nelson, R. J., G. E. Demas, P. L. Huang, et al. 1995. Behavioral abnormalities in male mice lacking neuronal nitric oxide. Nature 378: 383–386.

O'Dell, T. J., P. L. Huang, T. M. Dawson, et al. 1994. Endothelial NOS and the blockade of LTP by NOS inhibitors in mice lacking neuronal NOS. Science 265: 542–546.

Poyner, D. R., and M. R. Hanley. 1992. Molecular biology of peptide and glycoprotein hormone receptors. In: Molecular Biology of G Protein–Coupled Receptors. Ed. M. R. Brann. Boston, Birkhäuser, pp. 198–232.

Rettori, V., N. Belova, Y.-WH. Gimeno, et al. 1994. Role of nitric oxide in control of growth hormone release in the rat. Neuroimmunomodulation 1: 195–200.

Ross, E. M. 1992. G proteins and receptors in neuronal signalling. In: An Introduction to Molecular Neurobiology. Ed. Z. W. Hall. Sunderland, Mass., Sinauer, pp. 181–206.

Siderovski, D. P., A. Hessel, S. Chung, et al. 1996. A new family of regulators of G protein–coupled receptors. Curr. Biol. 6: 211–212.

Simon, M. I., M. P. Strathmann, and N. Gautam. 1991. Diversity of G proteins in signal transduction. Science 252: 802–808.

Sutherland, E. W. 1972. Studies on the mechanism of hormone action. Science 177: 401–408.

Toda, N., K. Ayajiki, and T. Okamura. 1993. Cerebroarterial relaxations mediated by nitric oxide derived from endothelium and vasodilator nerve. J. Vasc. Res. 30: 61–67.

Ullrich, A., A. Grau, A. W. Tam, et al. 1986. Schematic comparison of IGF-1 receptor with other cell surface receptors and oncogenes. EMBO J. 5: 2503–2512.

Vanderwinden, J. M., P. Mailleux, S. N. Schiffmann, et al. 1992. Nitric oxide synthase activity in infantile hypertrophic pyloric stenosis. N. Engl. J. Med. 327: 511–515.

Chapter 7

Books and Literature Reviews

Aidley, D. J. 1989. The Physiology of Excitable Cells, 3rd Ed. New York, Cambridge University Press.

Bousfield, D., Ed. 1985. Neurotransmitters in Action. Amsterdam, Elsevier.

Leeman, S. E., J. E. Krause, and F. Lemcke, Eds. 1991. Substance P and Related Peptides. Ann. N.Y. Acad. Sci. 632.

Levitan, I. B., and L. K. Kaczmarek. 1996. The Neuron: Cell and Molecular Biology, 2nd Ed. New York, Oxford University Press.

Moncada, S., R. M. J. Palmer, and E. A. Higgs. 1991. Nitric oxide: Physiology, pathophysiology and pharmacology. Pharmacol. Rev. 43: 109–143.

Nicholls, D. G. 1994. Proteins, Transmitters and Synapses. London, Blackwell.

Otsuka, M., and S. Konishi. 1985. Substance P—the first peptide neurotransmitter? In: Neurotransmitters in Action. Ed. D. Bousfield. New York, Elsevier, pp. 163–169.

Powis, D. A., and S. J. Bunn, Eds. 1995. Neurotransmitter Release and Its Modulation. Cambridge U.K., University Press.

Siegel, G. B. Agranoff, R. W. Albers, et al. 1993. Basic Neurochemistry, 5th Ed. New York, Raven Press.

References

Barker, J. L., B. Dufy, N. L. Harrison, et al. 1987. Signal transduction mechanisms in cultured CNS neurons and clonal pituitary cells. Neuropharmacology 26: 941–955.

Beckwith, B. E., and C. A. Sandman. 1982. Central nervous system and peripheral effects of ACTH, MSH and related neuropeptides. Peptides 3: 414–420.

Carraway, R., and S. E. Leeman. 1973. The isoloation of a new hypotensive peptide, neurotensin, from bovine hypothalami. J. Biol Chem 248: 6854–6861.

Clarke, G., and L. P. Merrick. 1985. Electrophysiological studies of the magnocellular neurons. In: Curr. Top. Neuroendocrinol. 4: 35–59.

Colmers, W. F., and D. Bleakman. 1994. Effects of neuropeptide Y on the electrical properties of neurons. Trends Neurosci. 17: 373–379.

Cuello, A. C. 1983. Central distribution of opioid peptides. Br. Med. Bull. 39: 11–16.

De Graan, P. N. E., P. Schotman, and D. H. G Versteeg. 1990. Neural mechanisms of action of neuropeptides: Macromolecules and neurotransmitters. In: Neuropeptides, Basics and Perspectives. Ed. D. De Wied. Amsterdam, Elsevier, pp. 139–174.

Dekin, M. S., G. B. Richerson, and P. A. Getting, 1985. Thyrotropin releasing hormone induces rhythmic bursting in neurons of the tractus solitarius. Science 229: 67–69.

De Kloet, E. R., M. Joëls, and I. J. A. Urban. 1990. Central neurohypophyseal hormone receptors and receptor mediated cellular responses.

Dreifuss, J. J., M. Dubois-Dauphin, H. Widmer, et al. 1992. Ann. N.Y. Acad. Sci. 652: 46–57.

Fahrenkrug, J., B. Ottesen, and C. Palle. 1988. Vasoactive intestinal polypeptide and the reproductive system. Ann. N.Y. Acad. Sci. 527: 393–404.

Gold, M. R. 1984. The action of vasoactive intestinal peptide at the frog's neuromuscular junction. In: Coexistence of Neuroactive Substances in Neurons. Eds. V. Chan-Palay and S. L. Palay. New York, Wiley, pp. 161–170.

Gonzalez, E. R., and F. L. Strand. 1981. Neurotropic action of MSH/ACTH 4–10 on neuromuscular function in hypophysectomized rats. Peptides 2 (Suppl. 1): 107–113.

Jan, L. Y., and Y. N. Jan. 1982. Peptidergic transmission in sympathetic ganglia of the frog. J. Physiol. (Lond.) 327: 219–246.

Jan, Y. N., and L. Y. Jan. 1985. A LHRH-like peptidergic neurotransmitter capable of "action at a distance" in autonomic ganglia. In: Neurotransmitters in Action. Ed. D. Bousfield. New York, Elsevier, pp. 94–103.

Johnston, M. F., E. A. Kravitz, H. Meiri, et al. 1983. Adrenocorticotropic hormone causes long-lasting potentiation of transmitter release from frog motor nerve terminals. Science 220: 1071–1072.

Kitagabi, P. C. 1982. Effects of neurotensin on intestinal smooth muscle: Application to the study of structure-activity relationships. Ann. N.Y. Acad. Sci. 400: 37–55.

Krivoy, W. A., and E. Zimmermann. 1977. An effect of β-melanocyte stimulating hormone (β-MSH) on α-motoneurons of cat spinal cord. Eur. J. Pharmacol. 46: 315–322.

Love, J. A., V. L. W. Go, and J. H. Szurszewski. 1988. Vasoactive intestinal peptide and other peptides as neuromodulators of colonic motility in the guinea pig. Ann. N.Y. Acad. Sci. 527: 360–368.

Lundberg, J. M., and T. Hökfelt. 1985. Coexistence of peptides and classical neurotransmitters. In: Neurotransmitters in Action. Ed. D. Bousfield. Amsterdam, Elsevier, pp. 104–118.

Mayer, E. A. 1994. Signal transduction and intercellular communication. In: Gut Peptides: Biochemistry and Physiology. Eds. J. H. Walsh and G. J. Dockray. New York, Raven Press, pp. 33–73.

Morris, B. J., and H. M. Johnston. 1995. A role for hippocampal opioids in long-term functional plasticity. Trends Neurosci. 18: 350–355.

Olson, G. A., R. D. Olson, and A. J. Kastin. 1994. Endogenous opiates: 1993. Peptides 15: 1513–1556.

Olson, G. A., R. D. Olson, and A. J. Kastin. 1995. Endogenous opiates: 1994. Peptides 16: 1517–1555.

Otsuka, M., and S. Konishi, 1976. Substance P—an excitatory transmitter of primary sensory neurons. Cold Spring Harbor Symp. Quant. Biol. 40: 135–143.

Potter, E. K., and L. G. Ulman. 1994. Neuropeptides in sympathetic nerves affect vagal regulation of the heart. News Physiol. Sci. 9: 174–177.

Reid, J. J., Z. Khalil, and P. D. Marley. 1995. Modulation of neurotransmitter release by hormones and local tissue factors. In: Neurotransmitter Release and Its Modulation. Eds. D. A. Powis and S. J. Bunn. Cambridge, U.K., Cambridge University Press, pp. 122–142.

Renaud, L. P., and C. W. Bourque. 1991. Neurophysiology and neuropharmacology of hypothalamic magnocellular neurons secreting vasopressin and oxytocin. Prog. Neurobiol. 36: 131–169.

Renaud, L. P., and B. Hu. 1995. Electrical activity, osmosensitivity, and neuromodulation of hypothalamic supraoptic and paraventricular neurosecretory cells. In: Electrophysiology of Neuroendocrine Cells. Eds. H. Scherübl and J. Hescheler. Boca Raton, Fla., CRC Press, pp. 89–99.

Ryall, R. W., and G. Belcher. 1977. Substance P selectively blocks nicotinic receptors on Renshaw cells: A possible synaptic inhibitory mechanism. Brain Res. 137: 376–380.

Sandman, C. A., P. Denman, L. H. Miller, et al. 1971. Electroencephalographic measures of melanocyte-stimulating hormone activity. J. Comp. Physiol. Psychol. 76: 303–310.

Sandman, C. A., and A. J. Kastin. 1987. Behavioral actions of ACTH and related peptides. In: Hormonal Proteins and Peptides. Ed. C. H. Li. 13: 147–171.

Scharfman, H. E. 1993. Presynaptic and postsynaptic actions of somatostatin in area CA1 and the dentate gyrus of rat and rabbit hippocampal slices. In: Presynaptic Receptors in the Mammalian Brain. Eds. T. V. Dunwiddie and D. M. Lovinger. Boston, Birkhäuser, pp. 42–70.

Scharfman, H. E., and P. A. Schwartzkroin. 1988. Further studies on the effects of somatostatin and related peptides in area CA1 of rabbit hippocampus. Cell. Mol. Neurobiol. 8: 411–429.

Scheller, R. H., and Z. W. Hall. 1992. Chemical messengers at synapses. In: An Introduction to Molecular Neurobiology. Ed. Z. W. Hall. Sunderland, Mass., Sinauer, pp. 119–147.

Shi, W.-X., and B. S. Bunney. 1992. Actions of neurotensin: A review of the electrophysiological studies. Ann. N.Y. Acad. Sci. 668: 129–145.

Smith, C. M., and F. L. Strand. 1981. Neuromuscular response of the immature rat to ACTH/MSH (4–10). Peptides 2: 197–206.

Spigelman, I., and E. Puil. 1991. Substance P actions on sensory neurons. Ann. N.Y. Acad. Sci. 632: 220–228.

Strand, F. L., S. J. Lee, T. S. Lee, et al. 1993. Non-corticotropic ACTH peptides modulate nerve development and regeneration. Rev. Neurosci. 4: 321–364.

Strand, F. L., and C. M. Smith. 1986. LPH, ACTH, MSH and motor systems. In: Neuropeptides and Behavior, Vol. 1. Eds. D. de Wied, W. H. Gispen, and Tj. B. van Wimersma Greidanus. New York, Pergamon Press, pp. 245–272.

Zeiler, R. H., F. L. Strand, and N. El-Sherif. 1982. Electrophysiological and contractile responses of canine atrial tissues to adrenocorticotropin. Peptides 3: 815–822.

Chapter 8

Books and Literature Reviews

Ader, R., N. Cohen, and D. L. Felter, Eds. 1991. Psychoneuroimmunology, 2nd Ed. New York, Academic Press.

Bateman, A., A. Singh, T. Kral, et al. 1989. The immune-hypothalamic-pituitary-adrenal axis. Endocrinol. Rev. 10: 9–112.

Blalock, J. E. Ed. 1992. Neuroimmunoendocrinology. 2nd Ed. Basel, Karger.

Chrousos, G. P. R. McCarty, K. Pacák, et al. 1995. Stress: Basic Mechanism and Clinical Implications, Ann. N.Y. Acad. Sci. 771.

Davey, B. 1990. Immunology: A Foundation. Englewood Ciffs, N.J., Prentice Hall.

De Wied, D. 1993. From stress hormones to neuropeptides. In: Brain Functions of Neuropeptides. Eds. J. P. H. Burbach and D. De Wied. New York, Parthenon, pp. 65–84.

Endröczi, E. 1991. Stress and Adaptation. Budapest, Akadémiai Kiadó.

Golub, E., and D. R. Green. Eds. 1991. Immunology: A Synthesis, 2nd Ed. Sunderland, Mass., Sinauer.

Kuby, J. 1992. Immunology. New York, Freeman.

McCann, S. M., J. M. Lipton, E. M. Sternberg et al. Eds. 1998. Neuroimmunomodulation: Molecular, integrative systems, and clinical advances. Ann. N.Y. Acad. Sci. 840.

McCubbin, J. A., P. G. Kaufmann, and C. B. Nemeroff, Eds. 1991. Stress, Neuropeptides and Systemic Disease. San Diego, Academic Press.

Scharrer, B., E. M. Smith, and G. B. Stefano, Eds. 1994. Neuropeptides and Immunoregulation. Berlin, Springer-Verlag.

Schneider. D. M., M. Cohn, and K. Bulloch. 1987. Overview of the immune system. In: The Neuro-Immune-Endocrine Connection. Eds. C. W. Cotman, R. E. Brinton, A. Galaburda, et al. New York, Raven Press, pp. 1–14.

Weiner, H., I. Florin, R. Murison, et al., Eds. 1987. Frontiers of Stress Research. Toronto, Huber.

References

Ader, R., N. Cohen, and D. L. Felter, Eds. 1991. Psychoneuroimmunology, 2nd Ed. New York, Academic Press.

Alves, S. E., H. M. Akbari, E. C. Azmitia, et al. 1993. Neonatal ACTH and corticosterone alter hypothalamic monoamine innervation and reproductive parameters in the female rat. Peptides 14: 379–384.

Banks, W. A., and A. J. Kastin. 1994. Brain-to-blood transport of peptides and the alcohol withdrawal syndrome. Ann. N.Y. Acad. Sci. 739: 108–118.

Beckwith, B. E., C. A. Sandman, D. Hotherstall, et al. 1977. The influence of neonatal injections of α-MSH on learning, memory and attention in rats. Physiol. Behav. 18: 63–71.

Berczi, I. 1994. Hormonal interactions between the pituitary and immune systems. In: Bilateral Communication Between the Endocrine and Immune Systems. Ed. C. J. Grossman. New York, Springer-Verlag, pp. 96–157.

Blalock, J. E. 1992. Production of peptide hormones and neurotransmitters by the immune system. In: Neuroimmunoendocrinology, 2nd Ed. Ed. J. E. Blalock. Basel, Karger, pp. 1–24.

Blalock, J. E. 1994. The syntax of immune-neuroendocrine communication. Immunol. Today 15: 503–511.

Cannon, W. B., and D. de la Paz. 1911. Emotional stimulation of adrenal secretion. Am. J. Physiol. 27: 64–70.

Cannon, J. G., J. B. Tatro, S. Reichlin, et al. 1986. Alpha melanocyte stimulating hormone inhibits immunostimulatory and inflammatory actions of interleukin I. J. Immunol. 137: 2232–2236.

Carr, D. J. J. 1991. The role of endogenous opioids and their receptors in the immune system. Proc. Soc. Exp. Biol. Med. 198: 710–720.

Chrousos, G. P., and P. W. Gold. 1992. The concepts of stress and stress system disorders. Overview of physical and behavioral homeostasis. JAMA 267: 1244–1252.

Clarke, B. L., and K. L. Bost. 1989. Differential expression of functional adrenocorticotropic hormone receptors by subpopulation of lymphocytes. J. Immunol.143: 464–469.

Dardenne, M., and W. Savino. 1994. Control of thymus physiology by peptidic hormones and neuropeptides. Immunol. Today 15: 518–523.

DeRijk, R., and F. Berkenbosch. 1994. Suppressive and permissive actions of glucocorticoids: A way to control innate immunity and to facilitate specificity of adaptive immunity? In: Bilateral Communication Between the Endocrine and Immune Systems. Ed. C. J. Grossman. New York, Springer-Verlag, pp. 73–95.

Fabris, N., E. Moccheiani, M. Muzzioli, et al. 1988. Immune-neuroendocrine interactions during aging. Prog. Neuroendocrinimmunol. 1: 49.

Gold, P. W. 1992. The stress-response, depression, and inflammatory disease. Ann. Intern. Med. 117: 854–866.

Jacobson, J. D., B. C. Nisula, and A. D. Steinberg. 1994. Modulation of the expression of murine lupus by gonadotropin-releasing hormone analogs. Endocrinology 134: 2516–2523.

Jain, R., D. Zwickler, C. S. Hollander, et al. 1991. Corticotropin-releasing factor modulates the immune respnse to stress in the rat. Endocrinology 128: 1329–1336.

Johnson, H. W., M. O. Downs, and C. H. Pontzer. 1992. Neuroendocrine peptide hormone regulation of immunity. In: Neuroimmunoendocrinology, 2nd Ed. Chemical Immunology. Ed. J. E. Blalock. Basel, Karger, pp. 49–83.

Lee, S., and C. Rivier. 1994. Hypophysiotrophic role and hypothalamic gene expression of corticotropin-releasing factor and vasopressin in rats injected with interleukin-1β systemically or into the brain ventricles. J. Neuroendocrinol. 6: 217–224.

Long, N. C. 1996. Evolution of infectious disease: How evolutionary forces shape physiological responses to pathogens. News Physiol Sci. 11: 83–89.

Majde, J. 1994. An overview of cytokines and their associations with the brain. Ann. N.Y. Acad. Sci. 739: 262–269.

Marchetti, B., M. C. Morale, N. Batticane, et al. 1991. Aging of the reproductive-neuroimmune axis. A crucial role for the hypothalamic neuropeptide luteinizing hormone–releasing hormone. Ann. N.Y. Acad. Sci. 621: 169–173.

Mastorakos, G., G. P. Chrousos, and J. S. Weber. 1993. Recombinant interleukin-6 activates the hypothalamic-pituitary-adrenal axis in humans. J. Clin. Endocrinol. Metab. 77: 1690–1694.

Munck, A., P. Guyre, and N. Holbrook. 1984. Physiological functions of glucocorticoids in stress and their relation to pharmacological actions. Endocr. Rev. 5: 25–44.

Munck, A., and A. Náray-Fejes-Tóth. 1994. Glucocorticoids and stress: Permissive and suppressive actions. Ann. N.Y. Acad. Sci. 746: 155–130.

Nyakis, C., G. Levay, J. Viltsek, et al. 1981. Effects of ACTH 4–10 administration on adult adaptive behavior and brain tyrosine hydroxylase activity. Dev. Neurosci. 4: 225–232.

Plotnikoff, N. P., R. E. Faith, A. J. Murgo, et al., Eds. 1986. Enkephalins and Endorphins: Stress and the Immune System. New York, Plenum Press.

Rivest, S. 1995. Molecular mechanisms and neural pathways mediating the influence of interleukin-1 on the activity of neuroendocrine CRF motoneurons in the rat. Int. J. Dev. Neurosci. 13: 135–146.

Sapolsky, R. M. 1994. The physiological relevance of glucocorticoid endangerment of the hippocampus. Ann. N.Y. Acad. Sci. 746: 294–304.

Sapolsky, R. M., L. C. Krey, and B. S. McEwen. 1984. Glucocorticoid-sensitive hippocampal neurons are involved in terminating the adrenocortical stress response. Proc. Natl. Acad. Sci. U.S.A. 81: 6174–6177.

Segarra, A. C., V. N. Luine, and F. L. Strand. 1991. Sexual behavior of male rats is differentially affected by timing of perinatal ACTH administration. Physiol. Behav. 50: 689–697.

Selye, H. 1936. A syndrome produced by diverse nocuous agents. Nature 138: 32.

Sherrington, C. S. 1906. Integrative Action of the Nervous System. New Haven, Conn., Yale University Press.

Smith, E. M., T. K. Hughes, F. Hashemi, et al. 1992. Immunosuppressive effects of ACTH and MSH and their possible significance in human immunodeficiency virus infection. Proc. Natl. Acad. Sci. USA. 89: 782–786.

Spangelo, B. L., and W. C. Gorospe. 1995. Role of the cytokines in the neuroendocrine-immune system axis. Front. Neuroendocrinol. 16: 1–22.

Stenzel-Poore, M. P., J. E. Duncan, M. B. Rittenberg, et al. 1996. CRH overproduction in transgenic mice: Behavioral and immune system modulation. Ann. N.Y. Acad. Sci. 780: 36–48.

Sternberg, E. M., and J. Licinio. 1995. Overview of neuroimmune stress interactions: Implications for susceptibility to inflammatory disease. Ann. N.Y. Acad. Sci. 771: 364–371.

Stratakis, C. A., and G. P. Chrousos. 1995. Neuroendocrinology and pathophysiology of the stress system. Ann. N.Y. Acad. Sci. 771: 1–18.

Stratakis, C. A., P. W. Gold, and G. P. Chrousos. 1995. Neuroendocrinology of stress—Implications for growth and development. Horm. Res. 43: 162–167.

Wang, J., M. Whetsell, and J. R. Klein. 1997. Local hormone networks and intestinal T cell homeostasis. Science 275: 1937–1939.

Weigent, D. A., and J. E. Blalock. 1995. Associations between the neuroendocrine and immune systems. J. Leukocyte Biol. 58: 137–150.

Wilder, R. 1995. Neuroendocrine-immune system interactions and autoimmunity. Annu. Rev. Immunol. 13: 307–338.

Chapter 9

Books and Literature Reviews

Alves, S. E., and F. L. Strand. 1993. Stress hormones and the sexual differentiation of the brain. Neuroendocrinol. Lett. 15: 14–31.

Gorski, R. A. 1971. Gonadal hormones and the development of neuroendocrine function. In: Frontiers of Neuroendocrinology. Eds. L. Martini and W. F. Ganong. London, Oxford University Press, pp. 237–290.

Goy, E., and B. S. McEwen. 1980. Sexual Differentiation of the Brain. Cambridge, Mass., MIT Press.

Harlan, R. E. 1988. Regulation of neuropeptide gene expression by steroid hormones. Mol. Neurobiol. 2: 183–200.

McCann, S. M. 1992. An introduction to neuroendocrinology: Basic principles and historical considerations. In: Neuroendocrinology. Ed. C. B. Nemeroff. Boca Raton, Fla., CRC Press pp. 1–18.

McEwen, B. S. 1994. How do sex and stress hormones affect nerve cells? Ann. N.Y. Acad. Sci. 743: 1–18.

Motta, M., Ed. 1991. Brain Endocrinology, 2nd Ed. New York, Raven Press.

Müller, E. E., and G. Nisticò. 1989. In: Brain Messengers and the Pituitary. San Diego, Academic Press, pp. 336–371.

Swaab, D. F., and M. A. Hofman. 1995. Sexual differentiation of the human hypothalamus in relation to gender and sexual orientation. Trends Neurosci. 18: 264–270.

Vaudry, H., M.-C. Tonon, E. W. Roubos, et al. Eds. 1998. Trends in comparative endocrinology and neurobiology. Ann. N.Y. Acad. Sci. 839.

References

Alves, S. E., H. M. Akbari, E. C. Azmitia, et al. 1993. Neonatal ACTH and corticosterone alter hypothalamic monoamine innervation and reproductive parameters in the female rat. Peptides 14: 379–384.

Arnold, A. P., and R. A. Gorski. 1984. Gonadal steroid induction of structural sex differences in the CNS. Annu. Rev. Neurosci. 7: 413–442.

Brazeau, P., W. Vale, R. Burgus, et al. 1973. Hypothalamic polypeptide that inhibits the secretion of immunoreactive pituitary growth hormone. Science 179: 77–79.

Breier, A. 1989. Experimental approaches to human stress research: Assessment of neurobiological mechanisms of stress in volunteers and psychiatric patients. Biol. Psychiatry 26: 438–462.

Clarke, A. S., D. J. Wittwer, D. H. Abbott, et al. 1994. Long-term effects of prenatal stress on HPA axis activity in juvenile rhesus monkeys. Dev. Psychobiol. 27: 257–269.

Corini, H., and B. S. McEwen. 1990. Progestin receptor induction and sexual behavior by estradiol treatment in male and female rats. J. Neuroendocrinol. 2: 467–472.

Ferris, C. F. The rage of innocents. The Sciences, March/April 1996, pp. 22–26.

Goy, E., and B. S. McEwen. 1980. Sexual Differentiation of the Brain. Cambridge, Mass., MIT Press.

Grady, K. L., C. H. Phoenix, and W. C. Young. 1965. Role of the developing rat testis in differentiation of the neural tissues mediating mating behavior. J. Comp. Physiol. Psychol. 59: 176–182.

Guillemin, R., and B. Rosenberg. 1955. Humoral hypothalamic control of anterior pituitary: Study with combined tissue cultures. Endocrinology 57: 599–607.

Harlow, C. M., Ed. 1986. From Learning to Love—The Selected Papers of H. F. Harlow. New York, Praeger.

Kalra, S. P., and P. S. Kalra. 1994. Regulation of gonadotropin secretion: Emerging new concepts. In: The Pituitary Gland, 2nd Ed. Ed. H. Imura. New York, Raven Press, pp. 285–308.

Levine, S. 1966. Sex differences in the brain. Sci. Am. 214: 84–90.

McCann, S. M. 1991. Neuroregulatory peptides. In: Brain Endocrinology, 2nd Ed. Ed. M. Motta. New York, Raven Press, pp. 1–30.

McCann, S. M., and J. R. Brobeck. 1954. Evidence for the role of the supraopticohypophyseal system in the regulation of adrenocorticotrophin secretion. Proc. Soc. Exp. Biol. Med. 87: 318–324.

McCann, S. M., and L. Krulich. 1989. Role of transmitters in control of anterior pituitary hormone release. In: Endocrinology, 2nd Ed., Vol. 1. Ed. L. K. DeGroot. Philadelphia, W. B. Saunders, pp. 117–130.

McEwen, B. S. 1978. Sexual maturation and differentiation: The role of the gonadal steroids. Prog. Brain Res. 48: 291–307.

McEwen, B. S. 1983. Gonadal steroids influences on brain development and sexual differentiation. In: Int. Rev. Physiol. 27: 99–145.

McEwen, B. S. 1991. Steroids affect neural activity by acting on the membrane and the genome. Trends Pharmacol. Sci. 12: 141–147.

McEwen, B. S., I. Lieberburgh, C. Chantal, et al. 1977. Aromatization: Important for sexual differentiation of the neonatal rat brain. Horm. Behav. 9: 249–263.

Majzoub, J. A., R. Emanuel, G. Adler, et al. 1993. Second messenger regulation of CRF mRNA. In: Ciba Found. Symp. 172: 30–58.

Merchenthaler, I. 1991. Current status of brain hypophysiotropic factors: Morphological aspects. Trends Endocrinol. Metab. 2: 219–226.

Motta, M., G. Mangili, and L. Martini. 1965. A "short" feedback loop in the control of ACTH secretion. Endocrinology 77: 392–395.

Petrusz, P., and I. Merchenthaler. 1992. The corticotropin-releasing factor. In: Neuroendocrinology. Ed. C. B. Nemeroff. Boca Raton, Fla., CRC Press. pp. 129–183.

Plotsky, P. M., K. V. Thrivikraman, and M. J. Meany. 1993. Central and feedback regulation of hypothalamic corticotropin-releasing factor secretion. In: Ciba Found. Symp. 172: 59–84.

Price, D. 1975. Feedback control of gonadal and hypophyseal hormones: Evolution of the concept. In: Pioneers in Neuroendocrinology. Eds. J. Meites, B. T. Donovan, and S. M. McCann. New York, Plenum Press, pp. 218–238.

Rhees, R. W., and D. E. Fleming. 1981. Effects of malnutrition, maternal stress or ACTH injections during pregnancy on sexual behavior of male offspring. Physiol. Behav. 27: 879–882.

Saffran, M., and A. V. Schally. 1955. Release of corticotropin by anterior pituitary tissue in vitro. Can. J. Biochem. Physiol. 33: 408–415.

Sandman, C. A., P. D. Wadhwa, A. Chicz-DeMet, et al. 1997. Maternal stress, HPA activity and fetal/infant outcome. Ann. N.Y. Acad. Sci. 814: 266–275.

Sayers, G., and M. A. Sayers. 1947. Regulation of pituitary adrenocorticotrophic activity during the response of the rat to acute stress. Endocrinology 40: 265–273.

Segarra, A. C., and F. L. Strand. 1989. Perinatal administration of nicotine alters subsequent sexual behavior and testosterone levels of male rats. Brain Res. 480: 151–159.

Segarra, A. C., V. N. Luine, and F. L. Strand. 1991. Sexual behavior of male rats is differentially affected by timing of perinatal ACTH administration. Physiol. Behav. 50: 689–697.

Swaab, D. F., and M. A. Hofman. 1995. Sexual differentiation of the human hypothalamus in relation to gender and sexual orientation. Trends Neurosci. 18: 264–270.

Toran-Allerand, C. D. 1984. On the genesis of sexual differentiation of the central nervous system: Morphogenetic consequences of steroidal exposure and possible role of α-fetoprotein. Prog. Brain Res. 61: 63–98.

Vale, W., J. Spiess, C. Rivier, et al. 1981. Characterization of a 41-residue ovine hypothalamic peptide that stimulates secretion of corticotropin and β-endorphin. Science 213: 1394–1397.

Ward, I. L. 1972. Prenatal stress feminizes and demasculinizes the behavior of males. Science 143: 212–218.

Chapter 10

Books and Literature Reviews

Arimura, A., and S. I. Said, Eds. 1996. VIP, PACAP and Related Peptides. Second International Symposium. Ann. N.Y. Acad. Sci. 805.

Bertherat, J., M. T. Bluet-Pajot, and J. Epelbaum. 1995. Neuroendocrine regulation of growth hormone. Eur. J. Endocrinol. 132: 12–24.

Chadwick, D., and G. Cardew, Eds. 1995. Somatostatin and its receptors. CIBA Foundation Symposium 196 Chichester, New York, Wiley.

Clarke, I. J. 1995. The preovulatory LH surge—A case of an endocrine switch. Trends. Endocrinol. Metab. 6: 241–247.

Forssmann, W.-G. Ed. 1998. VIP, PACAP, and related peptides: Third International Symposium. Ann. N.Y. Acad. Sci. 805.

Frohman, L. A., T. R. Downs, and P. Chomczynski. 1992. Regulation of growth hormone secretion. Front. Neuroendocrinol. 13: 344–405.

Graf, M. V., and A. J. Kastin. 1986. Delta-sleep-inducing peptide (DSIP): An update. Peptides 7: 1165–1187.

Koob, G. F. 1992. The behavioral neuroendocrinology of corticotropin–releasing factor, growth hormone–releasing factor, somatostatin and gonadotropin–releasing hormone. In: Neuroendocrinology. Ed. C. B. Nemeroff. Boca Raton, Fla., CRC Press, pp. 353–364.

Lightman, S. L. 1994. How does the hypothalamus respond to stress? Semin. Neurosci. 6: 215–219.

Rawlings, S. R., and M. Hezareh. 1996. Pituitary adenylate cyclase–activating polypeptide (PACAP) and PACAP/vasoactive intestinal polypeptide receptors: Actions on the pituitary gland. Endocr. Rev. 17: 24–46.

Sherwood, N. M., D. A. Lovejoy, and I. R. Coe. 1993. Origin of mammalian gonadotropin-releasing hormones. Endocr. Rev. 14: 241–254.

Stout, S. C., and C. B. Nemeroff. 1994. Stress and psychiatric disturbances. Semin. Neurosci. 6: 271–280.

Whitnall, M. H. 1992. Regulation of the hypothalamic corticotropin-releasing hormone neurosecretory system. Prog. Neurobiol. 40: 573–629.

References

Adelman, J. P., A. J. Mason, and P. H. Seeburg. 1986. Isolation of the gene and hypothalamic cDNA for the common precursor of gonadotropin-releasing hormone and prolactin release inhibiting factor in human and rat. Proc. Natl. Acad. Sci. U.S.A. 83: 179–183.

Amoss, M., R. Burgus, R. Blackwell, et al. 1971. Purification, amino acid composition and N-terminus of the hypothalamic luteinizing hormone releasing factor (LRF) of bovine origin. Biochem. Biophys. Res. Commun. 44: 205–210.

Anderson, S. T., K. Sawangjaroen, and J. D. Curlewis. 1996. Pituitary adenylate cyclase activating polypeptide acts within the medial basal hypothalamus to inhibit prolactin and luteinizing hormone secretion. Endocrinology 137: 3424–3429.

Argente, J., J. A. Chowen, P. Zeitler, et al. 1991. Sexual dimorphism of growth hormone releasing hormone and somatostatin gene expression in the hypothalamus of the rat during development. Endocrinology 128: 2369–2375.

Arimura, A., and S. Shioda. 1995. Pituitary adenylate cyclase activating polypeptide (PACAP) and its receptors: Neuroendocrine and endocrine interaction. Front. Neuroendocrinol. 16: 53–88.

Arimura, A., A. Somagyvari-Vigh, A. Miyata, et al. 1991. Tissue distribution of PACAP as determined by RIA: Highly abundant in rat brain and testis. Endocrinology 129: 2787–2789.

Arimura, A., A. Somagyvari-Vigh, C. Weill, et al. 1994. PACAP functions as a neurotrophic factor. Ann. N.Y. Acad. Sci. 739: 228–243.

Arvidsson, U., B. Ulfhake, S. Cullheim, et al. 1992. Thyrotropin-releasing hormone (TRH)–like immunoreactivity in the gray monkey (*Macaca fuseata*) spinal cord and medulla oblongata with special emphasis on the bulbospinal tract. J. Comp. Neurol. 322: 293–310.

Bauer, K. 1995. Inactivation of thyrotropin releasing hormone (TRH). The TRH-degrading enzyme as a regulator and/or terminator of TRH signals? In: Metabolism of Brain Peptides. Ed. G. O'Cuinn. Boca Raton, Fla., CRC Press, pp. 201–213.

Bayliss, D. A., F. Viana, and A. J. Berger. 1994. Effects of thyrotropin-releasing hormone on rat motoneurons are mediated by G proteins. Brain Res. 668: 220–229.

Beaudet, A., D. Greenspun, J. Raelson, et al. 1995. Patterns of expression of SSR1 and SSR2 somatostatin receptor subtypes in the hypothalamus of the adult rat—relationship to neuroendocrine function. Neuroscience 65: 551–561.

Beck-Peccoz, P. S. Amir, M. M. Menendez-Ferreira, et al. 1985. Decreased receptor binding of biologically inactive thyrotropin in central hypothyroidism: Effect of treatment with thyrotropin-releasing hormone. N. Engl. J. Med. 312: 1085–1090.

Behan, D. P., E. B. De Souza, E. Potter, et al. 1996. Modulatory actions of corticotropin-releasing factor-binding protein. Ann. N.Y. Acad. Sci. 780: 81–95.

Belchetz, P. E., T. M. Plant, Y. Nakai, et al. 1978. Hypophyseal responses to continuous and intermittent delivery of hypothalamic gonadotropin-releasing hormone. Science 202: 631–633.

Ben-Jonathan, N. 1990. Prolactin releasing and inhibiting factors in the posterior pituitary. In: Neuroendocrine Perspectives, Vol. 8. New York, Springer-Verlag, pp. 1–38.

Ben-Jonathan, N., M. Laudon, and P. A. Garris. 1991. Novel aspects of posterior pituitary function: Regulation of prolactin secretion. Front. Neuroendocrinol. 10: 231–277.

Bertherat, J., M. T. Bluet-Pajot, and J. Epelbaum. 1995. Neuroendocrine regulation of growth hormone. Eur. J. Endocrinol. 132: 12–24.

Bjartell, A., F. Sundler, and R. Ekman. 1991. Immunoreactive delta sleep–inducing peptide in the rat hypothalamus, pituitary and adrenal gland—Effects of adrenalectomy. Horm. Res. 36: 52–62.

Bonavera, J. J., P. S. Kalra, and S. P. Kalra. 1996. L-arginine nitric oxide amplifies the magnitude and duration of the luteinizing hormone surge induced by estrogen—Involvement of neuropeptide Y. Endocrinology 137: 1956–1962.

Brazelau, P., W. Vale, R. Burgus, et al. 1973. Hypothalamic polypeptide that inhibits the secretion of immunoreactive pituitary growth hormone. Science 179: 77–79.

Brown, M. R., and L. A. Fisher. 1990. Regulation of the autonomic nervous system by corticotropin-releasing factor. In: Corticotropin-releasing factor: Basic and Clinical Studies of a Neuropeptide. Eds. E. B. De Souza and C. B. Nemeroff. Boca Raton, Fla., CRC Press, pp. 292–298.

Bruhn, T. O., J. M. M. Rondeel, T. G. Bolduc, et al. 1994. Thyrotropin-releasing hormone (TRH) gene expression in the anterior pituitary. 1. Presence of pro-TRH messenger ribonucleic acid and pro-TRH derived peptide in a subpopulation of somatotrophs. Endocrinology 134: 815–820

Burbach, J. P. H., R. A. H. Adan and F. M. de Bree. 1995. Regulation of oxytocin gene expression and forms of oxytocin in the brain. Ann. N.Y. Acad. Sci. 652: 1–13.

Burgus, R., T. F. Dunn, D. DeSiderio, et al. 1970. Characterization of ovine hypothalamic hypophysiotropic TSH-releasing factor. Nature 226: 321–325.

Ceccatelli, S., M. Eriksson, and T. Hökfelt. 1989. Distribution and existence of corticotropin-releasing factor-, neurotensin-, enkephalin-, cholecystokinin-, galanin- and vasoactive intestinal polypeptide/peptide histidine isoleucine-like peptides in the parvocellular part of the paraventricular nucleus. Neuroendocrinology 49: 309–323.

Conn, P. M. and C. Y. Bowers. 1996. A new receptor for growth hormone-release peptide. Science 273: 923.

Conn, P. M. and J. C. Venter. 1985. Radiation activation (target size analysis) of the gonadotropin-releasing hormone receptor: Evidence for a high molecular weight complex. Endocrinology 116: 1324–1326.

Culler, M. D., and C. S. Paschall. 1992. Pituitary adenylate cyclase activating polypeptide (PACAP) potentiates the gonadotropin-releasing activity of luteinizing hormone–releasing hormone. Endocrinology 129: 2260–2261.

Delecea, L., J. R. Criado, O. Prosperogarcia, et al. 1996. A cortical neuropeptide with neuronal depressent and sleep-modulating properties. Nature: 381: 242–245.

De Souza, E. B. 1995. Corticotropin-releasing factor receptors: Physiology, pharmacology, biochemistry and role in central nervous system and immune disorders. Psychoneuroendocrinology 20: 789–819.

De Souza, E. B., C. Tinajero, and A. Fabbri. 1993. Corticotropin-releasing factor: An antireproductive hormone of the testis. FASEB J. 7: 299–307.

Devesa, J., M.. Barros, M. Gondar, et al. 1995. Regulation of hypothalamic somatostatin by glucocorticoids. J. Steroid Biochem. Mol. Biol. 53: 277–282.

Diamant, M., and D. De Wied. 1993. Structure-related effects of CRF and CRF-derived peptides: Dissociation of behavioral, endocrine and autonomic activity. Neuroendocrinology 57: 1071–1081.

Diedrich, K., and K. Schmutzler. 1991. Indication for GnRH agonists in an in vitro fertilization program. Ann. N.Y. Acad. Sci. 626: 228–237.

Dudley, C. A., and R. L. Moss. 1988. Facilitation of lordosis in female rats by CNS-site specific infusions of an LH-RH fragment AC-LH-RH-(5–10). Brain Res. 441: 161–167.

Dufau, M. L., J. Endröczi, E., K. Lissak, et al. 1959. The inhibitory influence of archicortical structures on pituitary-adrenal function. Acta Physiol. Hung. 16: 17–24.

Dufy, L., J. D. Dufy-Barbe, and E. Knobil. 1979. Etude électrophysiologique des neurones hypothalamiques et régulation gonadotrope chez le single rhésus. J. Physiol. Paris. 75: 105–108.

Elde, R., and T. Hökfelt, 1979. Localization of hypophysiotropic peptides and other biologically active peptides within the brain. Annu. Rev. Physiol. 41: 587–602.

Endröczi, E., K. Lissak, and B. Bohus. 1959. The inhibitory influence of archicortical structures on pituitary-adrenal function. Acta Physiol. Hung. 16: 17–24.

Eppelbaum, J. 1986. Somatostatin in the central nervous system: Physiology and pathophysiological modifications. Prog. Neurobiol. 27: 63–89.

Eppelbaum, J. P. Douurnaud, M. Fodor, et al. 1994. The neurobiology of somatostatin. Crit. Rev. Neurobiol. 8: 25–44.

Feldman, S. C., M. R. Harris, and L. K. Laemle. 1990. The maturation of the somatostatin systems in the rat visual cortex. Peptides 11: 1055–1064.

Fink, G. 1988. Gonadotropin secretion and its control. In: The Physiology of Reproduction. Eds. E. Knobil and J. Neill. New York, Raven Press, pp. 1349–1377.

Frawley, L. S. 1994. Role of the hypophyseal neurointermediate lobe in the dynamic release of prolactin. Trends Endocrinol. Metab. 5: 107–112.

Frieboes, R. M., H. Murck, P. Maier, et al. 1995. Growth hormone releasing peptide-6 stimulates sleep, growth hormone, ACTH and cortisol release in normal man. Neuroendocrinology 61: 584–589.

Friedman, T. C., D. Garciaborreguero, D. Hardwick, et al. 1994. Diurnal rhythm of plasma delta sleep–inducing peptide in humans—Evidence for a positive correlation with body temperature and negative correlation with rapid eye movements and slow wave sleep. J. Clin. Endocrinol. Metab. 78: 1085–1089.

Frohman, L. A., T. R. Downs, E. P. Heimer, et al. 1989. Dipeptidylpeptidase IV and trypsin-like enzymatic degradation of human growth hormone-releasing hormone in plasma. J. Clin. Invest. 83: 1533–1540.

Gershengorn, M. C., and C. Thaw. 1985. TRH stimulates biphasic elevation of cytoplasmic free calcium in GH_3 cells: Further evidence that TRH mobilizes cellular and extracellular Ca^{2+}. Endocrinology 116: 591–596.

Giri, M., C. Q. Gag, and J. M. Kaufman. 1996. The *N*-methyl-D-aspartate–mediated inhibitory control of gonadotropin-releasing hormone release in the hypothalamus of the adult male guinea pig is expressed through opioidergic systems. Endocrinology 137: 1468–1473.

Graf, M. V., and A. J. Kastin. 1986. Delta sleep-inducing peptide (DSIP): An update. Peptides 6: 1165–1187.

Grigoriadis, D. E., J. A. Heroux, and E. B. De Souza. 1993. Characterization and regulation of corticotropin-releasing factor receptors in the central nervous, endocrine and immune systems. Ciba Found. Symp. 172: 85–107.

Grigoriadis, D. E., T. W. Lovenberg, D. T. Chalmers, et al. 1996. Characterization of corticotropin-releasing factor subtypes. Ann. N.Y. Acad. Sci. 780: 60–80.

Guillemin, R., P. Brazeau, P. Bholen, et al. 1982. Growth hormone releasing factor from a human pancreatic tumor that caused acromegaly. Science 218: 585–587.

Guilloff, R. J., and D. J. Eckland. 1987. Observation of the clinical assessment of patients with motor neuron disease. Experience with a TRH analogue. Neurol. Clin. 5: 171–192.

Harvey, S. 1995. Growth hormone release: mechanisms. In: Growth Hormone. Eds. S. Harvey, C. G. Scanes, and W. H. Daughaday. Boca Raton, Fla., CRC Press, pp. 87–95.

Heindel, J. J., J. Sneeden, C. J. Powell, et al. 1996. A novel hypothalamic peptide, pituitary adenylate cyclase–activating peptide, regulates the function of rat granulosa cells in vitro. Biol. Reproduction 54: 523–530.

Hinkle, P. 1989. Pituitary TRH receptors. Ann. N.Y. Acad. Sci. 553: 176–187.

Hoffman, G., W.-S. Lee, and S. Wray. 1992. Gonadotropin releasing hormone (GnRH). In: Neuroendocrinology. Ed. C. B. Nemeroff. Boca Raton, Fla., CRC Press, pp. 185–217.

Hulse, G. K., G. J. Coleman, D. L. Copolov, et al. 1984. Relationship between endogenous opioids and the oestrous cycle in the rat. J. Endocrinol. 100: 271–275.

Inagaki, N., H. Kuromi, and S. Seino. 1996. PACAP/VIP receptors in pancreatic β-cells: Their role in insulin secretion. Ann. N.Y. Acad. Sci. 805: 44–53.

Ishibashi, H., and N. Akaike. 1995. Somatostatin modulates high-voltage-activated Ca^{2+} channels in freshly dissociated rat hippocampal neurons. J. Neurophysiol. 74: 1028–1036.

Jacobs, H. S., J. Adams, S. Franks, et al. 1984. Induction of ovulation with LHRH—Problems, indications and contraindications. In: LHRH and Its Analogues. Eds. F. Labrie, A. Belanger, and A. Dupont. New York, Elsevier, pp. 464–473.

Jan, L. Y., and Y. N. Jan. 1982. Peptidergic transmission in sympathetic ganglia of the frog. J. Physiol. (Lond.) 327: 219–246.

Jarry, H., S. Leonhardt, T. Schwarze, et al. 1995. Preoptic rather than mediobasal hypothalamic amino acid neurotransmitter release regulates GnRH secretion during the estrogen-induced LH surge in the ovariectomized rat. Neuroendocrinology 62: 479–486.

Jennes, L., and S. Woolums. 1994. Localization of gonadotropin-releasing hormone receptor messenger RNA in rat brain. Endocrinologist 2: 521–528.

Jinnah, H. A., and P. M. Conn. 1988. GnRH action at the pituitary: Basic research and clinical applications. In: Peptide Hormones: Effects and Mechanisms of Action, Vol 3. Eds. A. Negro-Vilar and P. M. Conn. Boca Raton, Fla., CRC Press, pp. 120–142.

Kalra, S. P., and P. S. Kalra. 1994. Regulation of gonadotropin secretion: Emerging new concepts. In: The Pituitary Gland, 2nd Ed. Ed. H. Imura. New York, Raven Press, pp. 285–308.

Kastin, A. J., G. A. Olson, A. V. Schally, et al. 1980. DSIP—more than a sleep peptide? Trends Neurosci. 3: 163–165.

Kastin, A. J., J. E. Zadina, W. A. Banks, et al. 1984. Misleading concepts in the field of brain peptides. Peptides 5 (Suppl. 1): 249–253.

Katsoulis, S., and W. E. Schmidt. 1996. Role of PACAP in the regulation of gastrointestinal motility. Ann. N.Y. Acad. Sci. 805: 364–378

Kitajima, N., K. Chihara, H. Abe, et al. 1989. Effects of dopamine on immunoreactive growth hormone releasing hormone and somatostatin secretion from hypothalamic slices perifused in vitro. Endocrinology 124: 69–76.

Knobil, E. 1989. The electrophysiology of the GnRH pulse generator. J. Steroid Biochem. Mol. Biol. 33: 669–671.

Koob, G. F. 1992. The behavioral neuroendocrinology of corticotropin-releasing factor, growth hormone-releasing factor, somatostatin and gonadotropin-releasing hormone. In: Neuroendocrinology. Ed. C. B. Nemeroff. Boca Raton, CRC Press, pp. 353–364.

Kow, L. M., and D. W. Pfaff. 1996. Thyrotropin-releasing hormone (TRH) has independent excitatory and modulatory actions on lamina-IX neurons of lumbosacral spinal cord slices from adult rats. Peptides 17: 131–138.

Krulich, L., A. P. S. Dhariwai, and S. M. McCann. 1968. Stimulatory and inhibitory effects of purified hypothalamic extracts on growth hormone release from rat pituitary in vitro. Endocrinology 83: 783–790.

Ladram, A., M. Bulant, A. Delfour, et al. 1994. Modulation of the biological activity of thyrotropin-releasing hormone by alternate processing of pro-TRH. Biochemie 76: 320–328.

Lam, K. S. L., M. F. Lee, S. P. Tam, et al. 1996. Gene expression of the receptor for growth hormone releasing hormone is physiologically regulated by glucocorticoids and estrogen. Neuroendocrinology 63: 475–480.

Lechan, R. M., Y. P. Qi, I. M. D. Jackson, et al. 1994. Identification of thyroid hormone receptor isoforms in thyrotropin-releasing hormone neurons of the hypothalamic paraventricular nucleus. Endocrinology 135: 92–100.

Lechan, R. M., and R. Toni. 1992. Thyrotropin-releasing hormone neuronal systems in the central nervous system. In: Neuroendocrinology. Ed. C. B. Nemeroff. Boca Raton, Fla., CRC Press, pp. 279–330.

Lechan, R. M., P. W. Wu, I. M. D. Jackson, et al. 1986. Thyrotropin-releasing hormone precursor: Characterization in rat brain. Science 231: 159–161.

Lee, S. L., K. Sevarion, B. A. Roos, et al. 1989. Characterization and expression of the gene-encoding rat thyrotropin-releasing hormone (TRH). Ann. N.Y. Acad. Sci. 553: 14–28.

Leonhardt, S., P. Arias, C. Feleder, et al. 1995. Pituitary adenylate cyclase activating polypeptide (PACAP) stimulates LH release by direct action in the pituitary without affecting GnRH release. Neuroendocr. Lett. 17: 13–19.

Leshin, L. S., C. R. Barb, T. E. Kiser, et al. 1994. Growth hormone releasing hormone and somatostatin neurons within the porcine and bovine hypothalamus. Neuroendocrinology 59: 251–264.

Lightman, S. L. 1994. How does the hypothalamus respond to stress? Semin. Neurosci. 6: 215–219.

Lightman, S., and M. S. Harbuz. 1993. Expression of corticotropin-releasing factor mRNA in response to stress. Ciba Found. Symp. 172: 173–198.

Luo, L. G., T. Bruhn, and I. M. D. Jackson. 1995. Glucocorticoids stimulate thyrotropin-releasing hormone gene expression in cultured hypothalamic neurons. Endocrinology 136: 4945–4950.

Lyson, K., and S. M. McCann. 1994. Alpha-melanocyte–stimulating hormone inhibits corticotropin-releasing factor by blocking protein kinase C. Neuroimmunomodulation 1: 153–158.

McCann, S. M., S. Taleisnik, and H. M. Friedman. 1960. LH releasing activity in hypothalamic extracts. Proc. Soc. Exp. Biol. Med. 82: 432–434.

Maeda, K., H. Tsukamura, S. Ohkura, et al. 1995. The LHRH pulse generator: A mediobasal hypothalamic location. Neurosci. Biobehav. Rev. 19: 427–437.

Maggi, R., F. Pimpinelli, L. Martini, et al. 1995. Inhibition of luteinizing hormone releasing hormone secretion by delta-opioid agonists in GT1-1 neuronal cells. Endocrinology 136: 5177–5181.

Makino, S., P. Gold, and J. Schulkin. 1994. Corticosterone effects on corticotropin-releasing hormone messenger RNA in the central nucleus of the amygdala and the parvocellular region of the paraventricular nucleus of the hypothalamus. Brain Res. 640: 105–112.

Marchetti, B., M. C. Morale, N. Batticane, et al. 1991. Aging of the reproductive-neuroendocrine axis. A crucial role for the hypothalamic neuropeptide luteinizing hormone–releasing hormone. Ann. N.Y. Acad. Sci. 621: 159–173.

Mason, A. J., S. L. Pitts, K. Nikolics, et al. 1986. The hypogonadal mouse: Reproductive functions restored by gene therapy. Science 234: 1372–1378.

Meister, B., and T. Hökfelt. 1992. The somatostatin and growth hormone-releasing factor systems. In: Neuroendocrinology. Ed. C. B. Nemeroff. Boca Raton, Fla., CRC Press. pp. 219–278.

Millar, R. P., and J. A. King. 1988. Evolution of a gonadotropin-releasing hormone: Multiple usage of a peptide. News Physiol. Sci. 3: 49–53.

Miyamoto, K., Y. Hasegawa, M. Nomura, et al. 1984. Identification of the second gonadotropin-releasing hormone in the chicken hypothalamus: Evidence that gonadotropin secretion is probably controlled by two distinct gonadotropin-releasing hormones in avian species. Proc. Natl. Acad. Sci. U.S.A. 81: 3874–3878.

Morrison, E., P. Tomasec, E. A. Linton, et al. 1995. Expression of biologically active procorticotropin-releasing hormone (ProCRH) in stably transfected CHO-K1 cells: Characterization of nuclear ProCRH. J. Neuroendocrinology 7: 263–272.

Müller, E. E., S. G. Cella, and C. V. de Gennaro Colonna. 1988. Central nervous system control of growth hormone secretion. In: Progress in Endocrinology, Vol 2. Amsterdam, Excerpta Medica, pp. 811–817.

Müller, E. E., and G. Nisticò. 1989. The role of brain peptides in the control of anterior pituitary hormone secretion. In: Brain Messengers and the Pituitary. Academic Press, San Diego. pp. 336–371.

Munsat, T. L., R. Lechan, J. M. Taft, et al. 1989. TRH and diseases of the motor system. Ann. N.Y. Acad. Sci. 553: 388–398.

Nair, R. M. G., J. F. Barrett, C. Y. Bowers, et al. 1970. Structure of porcine thyrotropin releasing hormone. Biochemistry 9: 1103–1106.

Nikolics, K., A. J. Mason, E. Szonyi, et al. 1985. A prolactin-inhibiting factor within the precursor for human gonadotropin–releasing hormone prohormone. Nature 316: 511–517.

Numa, S. 1985. Precursors of opioid peptides and the corticotropin-releasing factor and their genes. In: Biogenetics of Neurohormonal Peptides. London, Academic Press, pp. 29–45.

Ono, N., Bedan de Castro, J., and S. M. McCann. 1985. Ultrashort-loop positive feedback of corticotropin-releasing factor (CRF) to enhance ACTH release in stress. Proc. Soc. Natl. Acad. Sci. U.S.A. 82: 3528–3531.

Patel, Y. C. 1987. Somatostatin. In: Growth Hormone, Growth Factors and Acromegaly. Eds. D. K. Lüdecke and G. Tolis. New York, Raven Press, pp. 21–36.

Paulmeyerlacroix, O., V. Guillaume, G. Anglade, et al. 1995. Regulation of corticotropic function in stress situations. Ann. Endocrinol. (Paris) 56: 245–251.

Perrone, M. H., T. L. Greer, and P. M. Hinkle. 1980. Relationships between thyroid hormone and glucocorticoid effects in GH3 pituitary cells. Endocrinology 106: 600–604.

Peterfreund, R. A., and W. Vale. 1983. Muscarinic cholinergic stimulation of somatostatin secretion from long term dispersed cell cultures of fetal rat hypothalamus: Inhibition by gamma-aminobutyric acid and serotonin. Endocrinology 112: 526–534.

Plant, T. M., V. L. Gay, G. R. Marshall, et al. 1989. Puberty in monkeys is triggered by chemical stimulation of the hypothalamus. Proc. Natl. Acad. Sci. U.S.A. 86: 2506–2510.

Plotsky, P. M. 1989. Regulation of the adrenocortical axis: Hypophysiotropic coding, catecholamines and glucocorticoids. In: The Control of the Hypothalamo-Pituitary-Adrenocortical Axis. Ed. F. C. Rose. Madison, CT., International University Press, pp. 131–146.

Quinonesjenab, V., S. Jenab, S. Ogawa, et al. 1996. Estrogen regulation of gonadotropin-releasing hormone receptor messenger RNA in female rat pituitary tissue. Mol. Brain Res. 38: 243–250.

Raber, J., G. F. Koob, and F. E. Bloom. 1995. Interleukin-2 (IL-2) induces corticotropin-releasing factor (CRF) from the amygdala and involves a nitric oxide–mediated signaling—Comparison with the hypothalamic response. J. Pharmacol Exper. Ther. 272: 815–824.

Reichlin, S. 1989. TRH: Historical aspects. Ann. N.Y. Acad. Sci. 553: 1–6.

René, F., D. Monnier, C. Gaiddon, et al. 1996. Pituitary adenylate cyclase–activating polypeptide transduces through cAMP/PKA and PKC pathways and stimulates proopiomelanocortin gene transcription in mouse melanatropes. Neuroendocrinology 64: 2–13.

Richardson, S. B., C. S. Hollander, R. D'Eletto, et al. 1980. Acetylcholine inhibits the release of somatostatin from rat hypothalamus in vitro. Endocrinology 107: 122–129.

Rivier, J., C. Rivier, and W. Vale. 1984. Synthetic competitive antagonists of corticotropin-releasing factor: Effect on ACTH secretion in the rat. Science 224: 889–891.

Rivier, J., J. Spiess, M. Thorner, et al. 1982. Characterization of a growth hormone releasing factor from a human pancreatic islet tumor. Nature 300: 276–278.

Root, A. W., A. M. Bongiovanni, and W. R. Eberlein. 1970. Inhibition of thyroidal radioiodine uptake by human growth hormone. J. Pediatr. 76: 422–429.

Samson, W. K., C. Aquila, M. D. Lumpkin, et al. 1988. Somatostatin: Recent studies on hypothalamic secretion and local bioaction. In: Peptide Hormones: Effects and Mechanisms of Action, Vol. 3. Eds. A. Negro-Vilar and P. M. Conn. pp. 65–77.

Saphier, D., and S. Feldman. 1988. Iontophoretic application of glucocorticoids inhibits identified neurones in the rat paraventricular nucleus. Brain Res. 453: 183–190.

Sapolsky, R. M., S. Zola-Morgan, and L. R. Squire. 1991. Inhibition of glucocorticoid secretion by the hippocampal formation in the primate. J. Neurosci. 11: 3695–3704.

Sarkar, D. K., S. A. Chiappa, G. Fink, et al. 1976. Gonadotropin releasing hormone surge in pro-oestrous rats. Nature 264: 461–463.

Sawchenko, P. E., T. Imaki, E. Potter, et al. 1993. The functional anatomy of corticotropin-releasing factor. Ciba Found. Symp. 172: 5–29.

Schally, A. V., A. Arimura, Y. Baba, et al. 1971. Isolation and properties of the FSH- and LH- releasing hormone. Biochem. Biophys. Res. Commun. 43: 393–399.

Segerson, T. P., J. Kauer, H. C. Wolfe, et al. 1987. Thyroid hormone regulates TRH biosynthesis in the paraventricular nucleus of the rat hypothalamus. Science 238: 78–80.

Senaris, R. M., M. Schindler, P. P. A. Humphrey, et al. 1995. Expression of somatostatin receptor 3 messenger RNA in the motor neurons of the rat spinal cord and the sensory neurons of the spinal ganglia. Mol. Brain Res. 29: 185–190.

Sevarino, K. A., R. H. Goodman, J. Spiess, et al. 1989. Thyrotropin-releasing hormone (TRH) precursor processing. Characterization of mature TRH and non-TRH peptide synthesized by transfected mammalian cells. J. Biol. Chem. 264: 21529–21535.

Sherwood, N. M., D. A. Lovejoy, and I. R. Coe. 1993. Origin of mammalian gonadotropin-releasing hormones. Endocr. Rev. 14: 241–254.

Shibahara, S., Y. Morimoto, Y. Furutani, et al. 1983. Isolation and sequence analysis of the human corticotropin-releasing factor precursor gene. EMBO J. 2: 775–779.

Shivers, B. D., R. Harlan, J. Morrell, et al. 1984. Absence of oestradiol concentration in cell nuclei of LHRH-immunoreactive neurons. Nature 304: 345–347.

Silverman, A.-J. 1988. The gonadotropin-releasing hormone (GnRH) neuronal systems: Immunocytochemistry. In: The Physiology of Reproduction. Eds. E. Knobil and J. D. Neill. New York, Raven Press, pp. 1283–1304.

Steiger, A. 1995. Sleep—Physiology and pathophysiology. Schweiz. Medi. Wochenschr. 125: 2338–2345.

Stenzel-Poore, M. P, S. C. Heinrichs, S. Rivest, et al. 1994. Overproduction of corticotropic-releasing factor in transgenic mice—a genetic model of anxiogenic behavior. J. Neurosci. 14: 2579–2584.

Suda, T., M. Iwashita, T. Ushiyama, et al. 1989. Responses to corticotropin-releasing hormone and its free and bound forms in pregnant and nonpregnant women. J. Clin. Endocrinol. Metab. 69: 38–42.

Swaab, D. F. 1995. Aging of the human hypothalamus. Horm. Res. 43: 8–11.

Szabo, M., M. R. Butz, S. A. Banarjee, et al. 1995. Autofeedback suppression of growth hormone (GH) secretion in transgenic mice expressing a human GH reporter targeted by tyrosine hydroxylase 5′-flanking sequences to the hypothalamus. Endocrinology 136: 4044–4048.

Tannenbaum, G. S., and N. Ling. 1984. The interrelationship of growth hormone (GH)–releasing factor and somatostatin in generation of the ultradian rhythm of GH secretion. Endocrinology 115: 1952–1957.

Terasawa, E. 1995. Control of luteinizing-hormone–releasing hormone pulse generation in non-human primates. Cell. Mol. Neurobiol. 15: 141–164.

Thomas, G. B., J. T. Cummins, B. W. Doughton, et al. 1988. Gonadotropin-releasing hormone associated peptide (GAP) and putative processed GAP peptides do not release luteinizing hormone or follicle stimulating hormone or inhibit prolactin secretion in the sheep. Neuroendocrinology 48: 342–350.

Thompson, R. C., A. F. Seascholtz, and E. Herbert, 1987. Rat corticotropin-releasing hormone gene: Sequence and tissue specific expression. Mol. Endocrinol. 1: 363–370.

Turner, J. P., and G. S. Tannenbaum. 1995. In vivo evidence for a positive role for somatostatin to optimize pulsatile growth hormone secretion. Am. J. Physiol. Endocrinol. Metab. 32: E683–690.

Vaccarino, F. J., P. Sovaran, J. P. Baird, et al. 1995. Growth hormone–releasing hormone mediates feeding-specific feedback to the suprachiasmatic circadian clock. Peptides 16: 595–598.

Vale, W. J. Spiess, C. Rivier, et al. 1981. Characterization of a 41-residue ovine hypothalamic peptide that stimulates secretion of corticotropin and β-endorphin. Science 213: 1394–1397.

Valentino, R. J., L. A. Pavcovich, and H. Hirata. 1995. Evidence for corticotropin-releasing hormone projections from Barrington's nucleus to the periaqueductal gray and dorsal motor nucleus of the vagus in the rat. J. Comp. Neurol. 363: 402–422.

Vallarino, M., M. Feuilloley, L. Yon, et al. 1992. Immunohistochemical localization of delta sleep–inducing peptide (DSIP) in the brain and pituitary of the cartilaginous fish *Scyliorhinus canicula*. Peptides 13: 645–652.

Vanbockstaele, E. J., E. E. O. Colago, and R. J. Valentino. 1996. Corticotropin releasing factor–containing axon terminals synapse onto catecholamine dendrites and may presynaptically modulate other afferents in the rostral pole of the nucleus locus coeruleus in the rat brain. J. Comp. Neurol. 364: 523–534.

Vance, M. L., and M. O. Thorner. 1988. Some clinical considerations of growth hormone and growth hormone releasing hormone. Front. Neuroendocrinol. 10: 279–294.

Vanecek, J., and D. C. Klein. 1995. Melatonin inhibition of GnRH-induced LH release from neonatal rat gonadotroph—Involvement of Ca^{2+} not cAMP. Am. J. Physiol. Endocrinol. Metab. 32: E85–E90.

Vaughan, J., C. Donaldson, J. Bittencourt, et al. 1995. Urocortin, a mammalian neuropeptide related to fish urotensin-I and to corticotropin-releasing factor. Nature 378: 287–292.

Wang, P. S., S. W. Huang, Y. F. Tung, et al. 1994. Interrelationship between thyroxine and estradiol on the secretion of thyrotropin-releasing hormone and dopamine into hypophyseal portal blood in ovariectomized-thyroidectomized rats. Neuroendocrinology 59: 202–207.

Waschek, J. A., D. T. Bravo, and M. L. Richards. 1995. High levels of vasoactive intestinal peptide/pituitary adenylate cyclase–activating peptide receptor mRNA expression in primary and tumor lymphoid cells. Regul. Peptides 60: 149–157.

Wiesenfeld-Hallin, Z. 1995. Neuropeptides and spinal cord reflexes. Prog. Brain Res. 104: 271–282.

Chapter 11

Books and Literature Reviews

Acher, R., and J. Chauvet. 1995. The neurohypophyseal regulatory cascade: Precursors, mediators and effectors. Front. Neuroendocrinol. 16: 237–289.

Burbach, J. D. H., R. A. H. Adan, S. J. Lolait, et al. 1995. Molecular neurobiology and pharmacology of the vasopressin oxytocin receptor family. Cell. Mol. Neurobiol. 15: 573–595.

De Wied, D., M. Diamant, and M. Fodor. 1993. Central nervous effects of the neurohypophyseal hormones and related peptides. Front. Neuroendocrinol. 14: 251–302.

Engelmann, M., C. T. Wotjak, I. Neumann, et al. 1996. Behavioral consequences of intracerebral vasopressin and oxytocin: Focus on learning and memory. Neurosci. Biobehav. Rev. 20: 341–358.

Ivell, R., and J. Russell., Eds. 1995. Oxytocin. New York, Plenum Press.

North, W. G., A. M. Moses, and L. Share, Eds. 1993. The neurohypophysis: A window on brain function. Ann. N.Y. Acad. Sci. 689.

Pedersen, C. A., J. D. Caldwell, G. F. Jirikowski et al., Eds. 1992. Oxytocin in maternal, sexual and social behaviors. Ann. N.Y. Acad. Sci. 652.

Sokol, H. W., and H. Valtin. Eds. 1982. The Brattleboro rat. Ann. N.Y. Acad. Sci. 394.

References

Acher, R., and J. Chauvet, 1995. The neurohypophyseal regulatory cascade: Precursors, mediators, and effectors. Front. Neuroendocrinol. 16: 237–289.

Acher, R., J. Chauvet, and M. T. Chauvet. 1995. Man and the chimera: Selective versus neutral oxytocin evolution. In: Oxytocin. Eds. R. Ivell and J. Russell. New York, Plenum Press, pp. 615–627.

Acher, R., and C. Fromageot. 1957. The relationship of oxytocin and vasopressin to active proteins of posterior pituitary origin. In: The Neurophysis, Vol. 8. Ed. H. Heller. London, Butterworth, pp. 39–50.

Anderson-Hunt, M., and Dennerstein, L. 1995. Oxytocin and female sexuality. Gynecol. Obstet. Invest. 40: 217–221.

Andersson, B. 1971. Thirst and central control of water balance. Am. Sci. 59: 408–415.

Antoni, F. A. 1993. Vasopressinergic control of pituitary adrenocorticotropin secretion comes of age. In: Front. Neuroendocrinol. 14: 76–122.

Badoer, E. 1996. Cardiovascular role of parvocellular neurons in the paraventricular nucleus of the hypothalamus. News Physiol. Sci. 11: 43–47.

Bargmann, W., and E. Scharrer. 1951. The site of origin of the hormones of the posterior pituitary. Am. Sci. 39: 25–106.

Beckwith, B. E., R. E. Till, and V. Schneider. 1984. Vasopressin analog (DDAVP) improves memory in human males. Peptides 5: 819–822.

Bohus, B. 1993. Physiological functions of vasopressin in behavioral and autonomic responses to stress. In: Brain Functions of Neuropeptides. Eds. J. P. H. Burdoch and D. de Wied. New York, Parthenon, pp. 15–40.

Bohus, B., J. Borrell, J. M. Koolhaas, et al. 1993. The neurohypophyseal peptides, learning and memory processing. Ann. N.Y. Acad. Sci. 689: 285–299.

Bohus, B., G. L. Kovacs, and D. De Wied. 1978. Oxytocin, vasopressin and memory processes: Opposite effects on consolidation and retrieval processes. Brain Res. 157: 414–417.

Bourque, C. W., and L. P. Renaud. 1990. Electrophysiology of mammalian magnocellular vasopressin and oxytocin neurons. Front. Neuroendocrinol. 11: 183–212.

Brown, J. R., H. Ye, R. T. Bronson, et al. 1996. A defect in nurturing mice lacking the immediate early gene *fos*B. Cell 86: 297–309.

Buijs, R. M. 1987. Vasopressin localization and putative functions in the brain. In: Vasopressin: Principles and Properties. Eds. D. M. Gash and G. J. Boer. New York, Plenum Press, pp. 91–115.

Burbach, J. P. H., R. A. H. Adan, and F. M. de Bree. 1992. Regulation of oxytocin gene expression and forms of oxytocin in the brain. Ann. N.Y. Acad. Sci. 652: 1–13.

Burbach, J. P. H., B. Liu, M. A. Seger, et al. 1988. Vasopressin gene regulation and gene products in the brain. In: Vasopressin: Cellular and Integrative Functions. Eds. A. W. Cowley, Jr., J-F. Liard, and D. A. Ausiello. New York, Raven Press, pp. 295–300.

Caldwell, J. D. 1992. Central oxytocin and female sexual behavior. Ann. N.Y. Acad. Sci. 652: 166–179.

Carter, C. S., J. R. Williams, D. M. Witt, et al. 1992. Oxytocin and social bonding. Ann. N.Y. Acad. Sci. 652: 204–211.

Carter, D. A., and S. l. Lightman. 1985. Neuroendocrine control of vasopressin secretion. In: The Posterior Pituitary: Hormone Secretion in Health and Disease. Eds. P. H. Baylis and P. L. Padfield. New York, Marcel Dekker, pp. 53–118.

Carter, D. A., and D. Murphy. 1991. Rapid changes in poly (A) tail length of vasopressin and oxytocin mRNAs form a common early component of neurohypophyseal peptide gene activation following physiological stimulation. Neuroendocrinology 53: 1–6.

Chauvet, J. Y. Rouille, C. Chauveau, et al. 1994. Special evolution of neurohypophyseal hormones in cartilaginous fishes—asvatocin and phasvatocin, 2 oxytocin-like peptides isolated from the spotted dogfish (*Scylirhinus caniculus*). Proc. Natl. Acad. Sci. U.S.A. 91: 11266–11270.

Chini, B., Y. Mouillac, Y. Ala, et al. 1995. Molecular basis for agonist selectivity in the vasopressin/oxytocin receptor family. In: Oxytocin. Eds. R. Ivell and J. Russell. New York, Plenum Press, pp. 321–328.

Claybaugh, J. R., and C. F. T. Uyehara. 1993. Metabolism of neurohypophyseal hormones. Ann. N.Y. Acad. Sci. 698: 250–268.

Condés Lara, M., P. Veinante, M. Rabai, et al. 1994. Correlation between oxytocin neuronal sensitivity and oxytocin-binding sites in the amygdala of the rat—Electrophysiological and histoautoradiographic study. Brain Res. 637: 277–286.

Csiffary, A., Z. Ruttner, Z. Toth, et al. 1992. Oxytocin nerve fibers innervate beta-endorphin neurons in the arcuate nucleus of the rat hypothalamus. Neuroendocrinology 56: 429–435.

Dawood, M. Y. 1995. Novel approach to oxytocin induction-augmentation of labor: Application of oxytocin physiology during pregnancy. In: Oxytocin: Cellular and Molecular Approaches in Medicine and Research. Eds. R. Ivell and J. Russell. New York, Plenum Press, pp. 585–594.

De Kloet, E. R., M. Jöels, and I. J. A. Urban. 1990. Central neurohypophyseal hormone receptors and receptor mediated cellular responses. In: Neuropeptides: Basics and Perspectives. Ed. D. De Wied. Amsterdam, Elsevier, pp. 105–138.

De Vries, G. J., H. A. Al-Shamma, and L. Zhou. 1994. The sexually dimorphic vasopressin innervation of the brain as a model for steroid modulation of neuropeptide transmission. Ann. N.Y. Acad. Sci. 743: 95–120.

De Vries, G. R., R. M. Buijs, F. W. Van Leeuwen, et al. 1985. The vasopressinergic innervation of the brain in normal and castratėd rats. J. Comp. Neurol. 223: 236–254.

De Wied, D. 1965. The influence of the posterior and intermediate lobe of the pituitary and pituitary peptides on the maintenance of a conditioned avoidance response in rats. Int. J. Neuropharmacol. 4: 157–167.

De Wied, D. 1983. Central actions of neurohypophyseal hormones. Prog. Brain Res. 60: 155–167.

De Wied, D., O. Gaffori, P. Burbach, et al. 1987. Structure activity relationship studies with C-terminal fragments of vasopressin an oxytocin on avoidance behaviors of rats. J. Pharmacol. Exp. Ther. 242: 268–274.

Douglas, A. J., R. J. Bicknell and J. A. Russell. 1995. Pathways to parturition. In: Oxytocin. Eds. R. Ivell and J. Russell. New York, Plenum Press, pp. 381–394.

Dreifuss, J. J., M. Dubois-Dauphin, H. Widmer, et al. 1992. Electrophysiology of oxytocin actions on central neurons. Ann. N.Y. Acad. Sci. 652: 46–57.

Du Vignaud, V., C. Ressler, J. M. Swan, et al. 1953. The synthesis of an octapeptide amide with the hormonal activity of oxytocin. J. Am. Chem. Soc. 75: 4879–4880.

Freund-Mercier, M. J., and M. E. Stoekel. 1995, Somatodendritic autoreceptors on oxytocin neurons. In: Oxytocin. Eds. R. Ivell and J. Russell. New York, Plenum Press, pp. 185–194.

Gainer, H., S.-W. Jeong, D. M. Witt, et al. 1995. Strategies for cell biological studies in oxytocinergic neurons. In: Oxytocin. Eds. R. Ivell and J. Russell. New York, Plenum Press, pp. 1–8.

Gainer, H., and S. Wray. 1992. Oxytocin and vasopressin: From genes to peptides. Ann. N.Y. Acad. Sci. 652: 14–28.

Gauer, O. H. 1968. Osmocontrol versus volume control. Fed. Proc. 27: 1132–1136.

Ghosh, R., and C. D. Sladek. 1995. Prolactin modulates oxytocin messenger RNA during lactation by its action of the hypothalamic-neurohypophyseal axis. Brain Res. 672: 24–28.

Ginsberg, S. D., P. R. Hof, W. G. Wise, et al. 1994. Noradrenergic innervation of vasopressin-containing and oxytocin-containing neurons in the hypothalamic paraventricular nucleus of the macaque monkey—Quantitative analysis using double-label immunohistochemistry and confocal laser microscopy. J. Comp. Neurol. 341: 476–491.

Greidanus, T. B. V., and C. Maigret. 1996. The role of limbic vasopressin and oxytocin in social recognition. Brain Res. 713: 153–159.

Guldenaar, S. E. F., and D. F. Swaab. 1995. Estimation of oxytocin messenger RNA in the human paraventricular nucleus in AIDS by means of quantitative in-situ hybridization. Brain Res. 700: 107–114.

Haberich, F. J. 1968. Osmoreceptors in the portal circulation. Fed. Proc. 27: 1137–1141.

Hara, Y., J. Battey, and H. Gainer. 1990. Structure of mouse vasopressin and oxytocin genes. Mol. Brain Res. 8: 319–324.

Hatton, G. I., B. K. Modney, and A. K. Salm. 1992. Increases in dendritic bundling and dye coupling of supraoptic neurons after the induction of maternal behavior. Ann. N.Y. Acad. Sci. 652: 142–155.

Hruby, V. J., and M. S. Chow. 1990. Conformational and structural considerations in oxytocin-receptor binding and biological activity. Annu. Rev. Pharmacol. Toxicol. 30: 501–534.

Insel, T. R., J. T. Winslow, Z.-X. Wang, et al. 1995. Oxytocin and the molecular basis of monogamy. In: Oxytocin. Eds. R. Ivell and J. Russell. New York, Plenum Press, pp. 227–234.

Joëls, M. 1987. Electrophysiological actions of vasopressin in extrahypothalamic regions of the central nervous system. In: Vasopressin: Principles and Properties. Eds. D. M. Gash and G. J. Boer. New York, Plenum Press, pp. 257–274.

Jolles, J. 1987. Vasopressin and human behavior. In: Vasopressin: Principles and Properties. Eds. D. M. Gash and G. J. Boer. New York, Plenum Press, pp. 549–578.

Kendrick, K. M., and E. B. Keverne. 1992. Control of synthesis and release of oxytocin in the sheep brain. Ann. N.Y. Acad. Sci. 652: 102–121.

Kiss, J. Z., M. Palkovits, L. Záborsky, et al. 1983. Quantitative histological studies on the hypothalamic paraventricular nucleus in rats. II. Number of local and central afferent nerve terminals. Brain Res. 265: 11–20.

Landgraf, R. I. Neumann, F. Holsboer, et al. 1995. Interleukin-1-beta stimulates both central and peripheral release of oxytocin and vasopressin. Eur. J. Neurosci. 7: 592–598.

Landgraf, R., I. Neumann, J. A. Russell, et al. 1992. Push-pull perfusion and microdialysis studies of central oxytocin and vasopressin release in freely moving rats during pregnancy, parturition and lactation. Ann. N.Y. Acad. Sci. 652: 326–339.

Legros, J. J., and V. Geenen. 1996. Neurophysins in central diabetes insipidus. Horm. Res. 45: 182–186.

Leng, G., S. M. Luckman, R. E. J. Dyball, M., et al. 1993. Induction of *c-fos* in magnocellular neurosecretory neurons. Ann. N.Y. Acad. Sci. 689: 133–145.

Lenkei, Z., P. Corvol, and C. Llorenscortes. 1995. Comparative expression of vasopressin and angiotensin type-1 receptor messenger RNA in rat hypothalamic nuclei—A double in situ hybridization study. Mol. Brain Res. 34: 135–142.

Lolait, S. J., A.-M. O'Carroll, L. C. Mahan, et al. 1995. Extrapituitary expression of the rat V1b vasopressin receptor gene. Proc. Natl. Acad. Sci. U.S.A. 92: 6783–6787.

Luckman, S. M. 1995. *Fos* expression within regions of the preoptic area, hypothalamus and brain-stem during pregnancy and parturition. Brain Res. 669: 115–124.

Ludwig, M., M. F. Callahan, I. Neumann, et al. 1994. Systemic osmotic stimulation increases vasopressin and oxytocin release within the supraoptic nucleus. J. Neuroendocrinol. 6: 369–373.

Ma, R. C. and N. J. Dun. 1985. Vasopressin depolarizes lateral horn cells of the neonatal rat spinal cord in vitro. Brain Res. 348: 36–43.

McCarthy, M. M., S. P. Kleopoulos, C. V. Mobbs, et al. 1994. Infusion of antisense oligodeoxynucleotides to the oxytocin receptor in the ventromedial hypothalamus reduces estrogen-induced sexual receptivity and oxytocin receptor-binding in the female rat. Neuroendocrinology 59: 432–440.

McKinley, M. J. 1985. Volume regulation of antidiuretic hormone secretion. Curr. Top. Neuroendocrinol. 4: 61–100.

Margolis, B., J. Angel, S. Kremer, et al. 1988. Vasopressin action in the kidney—Overview and glomerular actions. In: Vasopressin: Cellular and Integrative functions. Eds. A. W. Cowley, J-F. Liard, and D. A. Ausiello. New York, Raven Press, pp. 97–106.

Melis, M. R., and A. Argiolas. 1995. Nitric oxide donors induce penile erection and yawning when injected into the central nervous system of male rats. Eur. J. Phrmacol. 294: 1–9.

Mizuno, K., and H. Matsuo. 1994. Processing of peptide hormone precursors. In: The Pituitary Gland, 2nd Ed. Ed. H. Imura. New York, Raven Press, pp. 153–178.

Morris, J. F., and D. V. Pow. 1993. New anatomical insights into the inputs and outputs from hypothalamic magnocellular neurons. Ann. N.Y. Acad. Sci. 689: 16–33.

Oliver, G., and E. A. Schaefer 1895. On the physiological actions of extracts of the pituitary body and certain other glandular organs. J. Physiol. (Lond.) 18: 277–279.

Pedersen, C. A. 1992. Preface. In: Oxytocin in maternal, sexual and social behaviors. Ann. N.Y. Acad. Sci. 652: ix–xi.

Pedersen, C. A., J. D. Caldwell, F. Drago, et al. 1988. Grooming behavioral effects of oxytocin: Pharmacology, ontogeny and comparisons with other nonapeptides. Ann. N.Y. Acad. Sci. 525: 245–256.

Pedersen, C. A., J. D. Caldwell, M. F. Johnson, et al. 1985. Oxytocin antiserum delays onset of ovarian steroid-induced maternal behavior. Neuropeptides 6: 175–182.

Pietrowsky, R., C. Struben, M. Molle, et al. 1996. Brain potential changes after intranasal vs intravenous administration of vasopressin—evidence for a direct nose-brain pathway for peptide effects in humans. Biol. Psychiatry 39: 332–340.

Purba, J. S., M. A. Hofman, and D. F. Swaab. 1994. Decreased number of oxytocin-immunoreactive neurons in the paraventricular nucleus of the hypothalamus in Parkinson's disease. Neurology 44: 84–89.

Richter, D. 1985. The neurohypophyseal hormones vasopressin and oxytocin: Gene structure, biosynthesis and processing. In: The Posterior Pituitary: Hormone Secretion in Health and Disease. Eds. P. H. Baylis and P. L. Padfield. New York, Marcel Dekker, pp. 37–51.

Rouille, Y., Y. Ouedraogo, J. Chauvet, et al. 1995. Distinct hydro-osmotic receptors for the neurohypophyseal peptides vasotocin and hydrins in the frog *Rana esculenta.* Neuropeptides 29: 301–307.

Schmale, H., U. Bahnsen, and D. Richter. 1993. Structure and expression of the vasopressin precursor gene in central diabetes insipidus. Ann. N.Y. Acad. Sci. 689: 74–82.

Schmale, H., S. Fehr, and D. Richter. 1987. Vasopressin biosynthesis: From gene to peptide hormone. Kidney Int. 32 (Suppl. 21): S8–S13.

Sharp, F. R., S. M. Sagar, K. Hicks, et al. 1991. *C-fos* mRNA, *fos* and *fos*-related induction by hypertonic saline and stress. J. Neurosci. 11: 3221–2331.

Smith, H. 1952. Renal excretion of sodium and water. Fed. Proc. 11: 701–705.

Swaab, D. F., B. Roozendaal, D. Rauid, et al. 1987. Suprachiasmatic nucleus in aging, Alzheimer's disease, transsexuality and Prader-Willi syndrome. Prog. Brain Res. 72: 301–310.

Thrasher, T. N. 1985. Circumventricular organs, thirst and vasopressin secretion. In: Vasopressin. Ed. R. W. Schrier. New York, Raven Press, pp. 311–318.

Tribollet, E., M. Dubois-Dauphin, and J. J. Dreifuss. 1992. Oxytocin receptors in the central nervous system: Distribution, development and species differences. Ann. N.Y. Acad. Sci. 652: 29–38.

Van den Hooff, P., I. J. A. Urban, and D. de Wied. 1989. Vasopressin maintains long-term potentiation in rat lateral septum slices. Brain Res. 505: 181–186.

Vanerp, A. M. M., M. R. Kruk, J. G. Veening, et al. 1995. Neuronal substrate of electrically-induced grooming in the PVN of the rat—Involvement of oxytocinergic systems. Physiol. Behav. 57: 881–885.

Vankesteren, R. E., A. B. Smit, R. P. J. Delange, et al. 1995. Structural and functional evolution of the vasopressin-oxytocin family—Vasopressin-related conopressin is the only member present in *Lymnaea* and is involved in the control of sexual behavior. J. Neurosci. 15: 5989–5998.

Van Ree, J. M., R. Hijman, J. Jolles, et al. 1985. Vasopressin and related peptides: Animal and human studies. Prog. Neuropsychopharmacol. Biol. Psychiatry 9: 551–559.

Verney, E. B. 1947. The antidiuretic hormone and the factors which determine its release. Proc. Soc. Lond. B. Biol. Sci. 135: 25–106.

Wang, H., A. R. Ward, and J. F. Morris. 1995. Estradiol acutely stimulates exocytosis of oxytocin and vasopressin from dendrites and somata of hypothalamic magnocellular neurons. Neuroscience 68: 1179–1188.

Winslow, J. T., N. Hastings, C. S. Carter, et al. 1993. A role for central vasopressin in pair bonding in monogamous prairie voles. Nature 365: 545–548.

Witt, D. M. 1995. Oxytocin and rodent sociosexual responses—from behavior to gene expression. Neurosci. Biobehav. Rev. 19: 315–324.

Xu, X. J., and Z. Wiesenfeldhallin. 1994. Intrathecal oxytocin facilitates the spinal nociceptive flexor reflex in the rat. Neuroreport 5: 750–752

Zingg, H. H., F. Rozen, C. Breton, et al. 1995. Gonadal steroid regulation of oxytocin and oxytocin receptor gene expression. In: Oxytocin. Eds. R. Ivell and J. Russell. New York, Plenum Press, pp. 395–404.

Chapter 12

Books and Literature Reivews

Beckwith, B. E., and A. J. Kastin. 1988. Central actions of melanocyte-stimulating hormone (MSH). In: Peptide Hormones: Effects and Mechanisms of Action. Eds. A. Negro-Vilar and P. M. Conn. Boca Raton, Fla., CRC Press, pp. 195–218.

De Graan, P. N. E., P. Schoman, and D. H. G. Versteeg. 1990. Neural mechanisms of action of neuropeptides: Macromolecules and neurotransmitters. In: Neuropeptides: Basics and Perspectives. Ed. D. De Wied. Amsterdam, Elsevier, pp. 139–174.

De Wied D. 1969. Effects of peptide hormones on behavior. In: Frontiers in Neuroendocrinology. Eds. W. F. Ganong and L. Martini. New York, Oxford University Press, pp. 97–140.

De Wied, D., W. H. Gispen, and Tj. van Wimersma Greidanus. 1986. Neuropeptides and Behavior: CNS Effects of ACTH, MSH and Opioid Peptides, Vol. 1. Oxford, Pergamon Press.

De Wied, D., and J. Jolles. 1982. Neuropeptides derived from pro-opiocortin: Behavioral, physiological and neurochemical effects. Physiol. Rev. 62: 976–1059.

De Wied, D., and G. Wolterink. 1989. Structure-activity studies on the neuroactive and neurotropic effects of neuropeptides related to ACTH. Ann. N.Y. Acad. Sci. 525: 130–140.

Eberle, A. N. 1988. The Melanotrophins: Chemistry, Physiology and Mechanism of Action. Basel, Karger.

Fan, W., B. A. Boston, R. A. Kesterson, et al. 1997. Role of melanocortinergic neurons in feeding and the agouti obesity syndrome. Nature 385: 165–168.

Gispen, W. H., J. Verhaagen, and D. Bär. 1994. ACTH/MSH-derived peptides and peripheral nerve plasticity: Neuropathies, neuroprotection and repair. Prog. Brain Res. 100: 223–229.

Hol, E. M., W. H. Gispen, and P. R. Bär. 1995. ACTH-related peptides: Receptors and signal transduction systems involved in their neurotrophic and neuroprotective actions. Peptides 16: 979–993.

Houben, H., and C. Denef. 1994. Bioactive peptides in anterior pituitary cells. Peptides 15: 547–582.

McDaniel, W. F. 1993. The influences of fragments and analogs of ACTH/MSH upon recovery from nervous system injury. Behav. Brain Res. 56: 11–22.

Sandman, C. A., and J. P. O'Halloran. 1986. Proopiomelanocortin, learning, memory and attention. In: Neuropeptides and Behavior. Vol 1, CNS Effects of ACTH, MSH and Opioid Peptides. Eds. D. de Wied, W. H. Gispen, and Tj. van Wimersma Greidanus. Oxford, Pergamon Press, pp. 397–420.

Strand, F. L., S. J. Lee, T. S. Lee, et al. 1993. Non-corticotropic ACTH peptides modulate nerve development and regeneration. Rev. Neurosci. 4: 321–364.

Strand, F. L., K. J. Rose, J. A. King, et al. 1989. ACTH modulation of nerve development and regeneration. Prog. Neurobiol. 33: 45–85.

Strand, F. L., K. A. Williams, S. E. Alves, et al. 1996. Melanocortins as factors in somatic neuromuscular growth and regrowth. In: International Encyclopedia of Pharmacology and Therapeutics: Chemical Factors in Neural Growth. Ed. C. Bell. Amsterdam, Elsevier. pp. 311–337.

Tatro, J. E. 1996. Receptor biology of the melanocortins, a family of neuroimmunomodulatory peptides. Neuroimmunomodulation 3: 259–284.

Verhaagen, J., and W. H. Gispen. 1988. Peripheral nerve regeneration, neurotrophic factors and neuropeptides. In: Recovery of Function in the Nervous System. Eds. F. Cohadon and J. L. Antunes. Fidia Research Series 1. Padova, Italy; Liviana Press. pp. 21–44.

References

Adan R. A. H., R. D. Cone, J. P. H. Burbach, et al. 1994. Differential effects of melanocortin peptides on neural melanocortin receptors. Mol. Pharmacol. 46: 1182–1190.

Adan, R. A. H., and E. H. Gispen. 1997. Brain melanocortin receptors: From cloning to function. Peptides 18: 1279–1287.

Alves S. E., H. M. Akbari, E. C. Azmitia, et al. 1993. Neonatal ACTH and corticosterone alter hypothalamic monoamine innervation and reproductive parameters in the female rat. Peptides 14: 379–384.

Amir A., Z. H. Galina, R. Blair, et al. 1980. Opiate receptors may mediate the suppressive but not the excitatory action of ACTH on motor activity in the rat. Eur. J. Pharmacol. 66: 307–313.

Antonawich F. J., E. C. Azmitia, H. K. Kramer, et al. 1994. Specificity versus redundancy of melanocortins in nerve regeneration. Ann. N.Y. Acad. Sci. 739: 60–73.

Antonawich F. J., E. C. Azmitia, and F. L. Strand. 1993. Rapid neurotrophic actions of an ACTH/MSH(4–9) analogue after nigrostriatal 6-OHDA lesioning. Peptides 14: 1317–1324.

Atella M. J., S. W. Hoffman, M. P. Pilotte, et al. 1992. Effects of BIM 22015, an analog of ACTH (4–10), on functional recovery after frontal cortex injury. Behav. Neurol. Biol. 57: 157–166.

Azmitia E. C., and E. de Kloet. 1987. ACTH neuropeptide stimulation of serotonergic neuronal maturation in tissue culture: Modulation by hippocampal cells. Prog. Brain Res. 72: 311–318.

Baker, B. I. 1994. Melanin-concentrating hormone updated: Functional considerations. Trends Endocrinol. Meta. 5: 120–126.

Banks, W. A., and A. J. Kastin. 1988. Review: Interactions between the blood-brain barrier and endogenous peptides: Emerging clinical implications. Am. J. Med. Sci. 295: 459–465.

Bär, P. R. D., L. H. Schrama, and W. H. Gispen. 1990. Neurotrophic effects of the ACTH/MSH-like peptides in the peripheral nervous system. In: Neuropeptide Concept. Ed. D. de Wied. Amsterdam, Elsevier, pp. 175–211.

Beckwith B. E. 1988. The melanotropins: Learning and memory. In: The Melanotropic Peptides, Vol 2. Ed. M. E. Hadley. Boca Raton, Fla., CRC Press, pp. 43–85.

Beckwith B. E., and A. J. Kastin. 1988. Central actions of melanocyte-stimulating hormone (MSH). In: Peptide Hormones: Effects and Mechanisms of Action. Eds. A. Negro-Vilar and P. M. Conn. Boca Raton, Fla., CRC Press, pp. 195–218.

Beckwith B. E., C. A. Sandman, D. Hothersall, et al. 1977. The influence of neonatal injections of α-MSH on learning, memory and attention in rats. Physiol. Behav. 18: 63–71.

Beckwith, B. E., T. P. Tinius, V. J. Hruby, et al. 1989. The effects of structure-conformation modifications of melanotropin analogs on learning and memory: D-amino acid substituted linear and cyclic analogs. Peptides 10: 361–368.

Berkenbosch, F., F. J. H. Tilders, and I. Vermes. 1983. β-Adrenoceptor activation mediates stress-induced secretion of β-endorphin related peptides from intermediate but not from anterior pituitary. Nature 305: 237–239.

Bertolini A., G. L. Gessa, and W. Ferrari. 1975. Penile erection and ejaculation: A central effect of ACTH-like peptides in mammals. In: Sexual Behavior, Pharmacology and Biochemistry. Eds. M. Sandler and G. L. Gessa. New York, Raven Press, pp. 247–257.

Bijlsma W. A., F. G. I. Jennekens, P. Schotman, et al. 1981. Effects of corticotropin (ACTH) on recovery of sensorimotor function in the rat: Structure activity study. Eur. J. Pharmacol. 76: 73–79.

Bohus. B. 1993. Physiological functions of vasopressin in behavioral and autonomic responses to stress. In: Brain Functions of Neuropeptides. Eds. J. P. H. Burdoch and D. De Wied. The Parthenon Publishing Group, New York. pp. 15–40.

Bohus B., G. A. Cottrell, C. Nyakis, et al. 1986. Melanocortin-related peptides and behavioral inhibition. In: Central Actions of ACTH and Related Peptides. Eds. D. De Wied and W. Ferrari. Fidia Research Series, Symposia in Neuroscience 4, Padova, Italy, Liviana Press, pp. 189–198.

Bohus, B., and D. De Wied. 1966. Inhibitory and facilitatory effect of two related peptides on extinction of avoidance behavior. Science 153: 318–320.

Calvet, M.-C., M.-J. Drian, and J. Calvet. 1992. Neuronal firing patterns of organotypic rat spinal cord cultures in normal and in ACTH/alpha MSH(4–10) analog(BIM 22015)–supplemented medium. Brain Res. 571: 218–229.

Champney T. F., T. C. Shaley, and C. A. Sandman. 1976. Effects of neonatal cerebral ventricular injections of ACTH4–9 and subsequent adult injections on learning in male and female albino rats. Pharmacol. Biochem. Behav. 5: 3–10.

Chhajlani, V., R. Muceniece, and J. E. S. Wikberg. 1993. Molecular cloning of a novel human melanocortin receptor. Biochem. Biophys. Res. Commun. 195: 866–873.

Chronwall, B. 1985. Anatomy and physiology of the neuroendocrine arcuate nucleus. Peptides 6 (Suppl. 2): 1–9.

Civelli, O., N. Birnberg, and E. Herbert. 1982. Detection and quantification of pro-opiomelanocortin mRNA in pituitary and brain tissues from different species. J. Biol. Chem. 257: 6783–6787.

Cone, R. D., K. G. Mountjoy, L. S. Robbins, et al. 1993. Cloning and functional characterization of a family of receptors for the melanotropic peptides. Ann. N.Y. Acad. Sci. 680: 342–363.

Cushing, H. 1909. The hypophysis cerebri. JAMA. 53: 250–255.

Croiset, G., and D. De Wied. 1992. A structure-activity study on pilocarpine-induced epilepsy. Eur. J. Pharmacol. 229: 211–216.

De Graan, P. N. E., P. Schoman, and D. H. Versteeg. 1990. Neural mechanisms of action of neuropeptides: Macromolecules and neurotransmitters. In: Neuropeptides: Basics and Perspectives. Ed. D. De Wied. Amsterdam, Elsevier, pp. 139–174.

Dekker A. J. A. M., M. M. Princen, H. De Nijs, et al. 1987. Acceleration of recovery from sciatic nerve damage by the ACTH(4–9) analog Org 2766: Different routes of administration. Peptides 8: 1057–1059.

De Koning P, J. P. Neijt, F. G. I. Jennekens, et al. 1988. Org 2766 protects from cisplatin-induced neurotoxicity in rats. Exp. Neurol. 97: 746–750.

De Wied, D. 1969. Effects of peptide hormones on behavior. In: Frontiers in Endocrinology. Eds. W. F. Ganong and L. Martini. New York, Oxford University Press, pp. 97–140.

De Wied, D. 1976. Hormonal influences on motivation, learning and memory processes. Hosp. Pract. (January) 123–131.

De Wied, D., and J. J. Jolles. 1982. Neuropeptides derived from pro-opiocortin; Behavioral, physiological and neurochemical effects. Physiol. Rev. 62: 976–1059.

De Wied, D., and G. Wolterink, 1989. Structure-activity studies on the neuroactive and neurotropic effects of neuropeptides related to ACTH. Ann. N.Y. Acad. Sci. 525: 130–140.

Dores, R. M., T. C. Steveson, and M. L. Price. 1993. A view of the *N*-acetylation of α-melanococyte-stimulating hormone and β-endorphin from a phylogenetic perspective. Ann. N.Y. Acad. Sci. 680: 161–174

Duckers H. J., J. Verhaagen, E. de Bruijn, et al. 1994. Effective use of a neurotrophic ACTH (4–9) analogue in the treatment of a peripheral demyelinating syndrome (experimental allergic neuritis)—an intervention study. Brain 117: 365–374.

Dunn, A. J. 1988. Studies on the neurochemical mechanisms and significance of ACTH-induced grooming. Ann. N.Y. Acad. Sci. 525: 150–168.

Dyer, J. K., A. R. H. Ahmed, G. W. J. Oliver, et al. 1993. Solubilization and partial characterization of the alpha-MSH receptor on primary rat Schwann cells. FEBS Lett. 336: 103–106.

Eberle, A. N. 1988. The Melanotropins. Chemistry, Physiology and Mechanisms of Action. Basel, Karger, pp. 210–252.

Fan, W., B. A. Boston, R. A. Kesterson, et al. 1997. Role of melanocortinergic neurons in feeding and the agouti obesity syndrome. Nature 385: 165–168.

Ferrari, W. 1958. Behavioral changes in animals after intracisternal injection with adrenocorticotrophic hormone and melanocyte stimulating hormone. Nature 181: 925–926.

File S. E., and S. Vellucci. 1978. Studies on the role of ACTH and 5-HT in anxiety, using an animal model. J. Pharmacol. Exp. Ther. 30: 105–110.

Flohr, H., and U. Lüneburg. 1989. Influence of melanocortin fragments on vestibular compensation. In: Vestibular Compensation: Facts, Theories and Clinical Perspectives. Eds. M. Lacour, M. Toupet, P. Denise, et al. Paris, Elsevier, pp. 161–174.

Frischer, R. E., and F. L. Strand, 1988. ACTH peptides stimulate motor nerve sprouting in development. Exp. Neurol. 100: 531–541.

Gantz, I., H. Miwa, Y. Konda, et al. 1993. Molecular cloning, expression, and gene localization of a fourth melanocortin receptor. J. Biol. Chem. 268: 15174–15179.

Gantz, I., Y. Shimoto, Y. Konda, et al. 1994. Molecular cloning, expression, and characterization of a fifth melanocortin receptor. Biochem. Biophys. Res. Commun. 200: 1214–1220.

Gerritsen van der Hoop, R., C. J. Vecht, M. E. L. Van der Burg, et al. 1990. Prevention of cisplatin neurotoxicity with an ACTH (4–9) analogue in patients with ovarian cancer. N. Engl. J. Med. 322: 89–94.

Gispen, W. H., V. J. Aloyo, P. R. Bär, et al. 1983. Neuromodulation by ACTH: A role for membrane phosphorylation. In: Integrative Neurohumoral Mechanisms. Eds. E. Endröczi, D. De Wied, L. Angelucci, et al. Developments in Neuroscience, Vol. 16. Amsterdam, Elsevier, pp. 129–144.

Gispen, W. H., J. Verhaagen, and D. Bär. 1994. ACTH/MSH-derived peptides and peripheral nerve plasticity: Neuropathies, neuroprotection and repair. Prog. Brain Res. 100: 223–229.

Gold, P. E., and R. L. Delanoy. 1981. ACTH modulation of memory storage processing. In: Endogenous Peptides and Learning and Memory Processes. Eds. J. L. Martinez, Jr., R. A. Jensen, R. B. Messing, et al. New York, Academic Press, pp. 79–98.

Greep, R. O. 1974. History of research on anterior pituitary hormones. In: Handbook of Physiology, Sec. 7, Vol. 4, Pt. 2. American Physiological Society, Washington, D.C., pp. 1–27.

Greven, H. M., and D. De Wied. 1973. The influence of peptides derived from corticotropin (ACTH) on performance: Structure activity studies. Prog. Brain Res. 39: 429–441.

Griffon, N., V. Mignon, P. Facchinetti et al. 1994. Molecular cloning and characterization of the rat fifth melanocortin receptor. Biochem. Biophys. Res. Commun. 200: 1007–1014.

Hadley, M. E., C. Zechel, B. C. Wilkes, et al. 1987. Differential structural requirements for the MSH and MCH activities of melanin concentrating hormone. Life Sci. 40: 1139–1145.

Hamers, F. P. T., C. Pette, B. Bravenboer, et al. 1993. Cisplatin-induced neuropathy in mature rats. Effects of the melanocortin-derived peptide ORG 2766. Cancer Chemother. Pharmacol. 32: 162–166.

Hannigan J., and R. Isaacson. 1985. The effects of ORG 2766 on the performance of sham, neocortical and hippocampal-lesioned rats in a food search task. Pharmacol. Biochem. Behav. 23: 1019–1027.

Haynes, L. W., and M. E., Smith. 1985. Presence of immunoreactive α-melanotropin and β-endorphin in spinal motoneurons of the dystrophic mouse. Neurosci. Lett. 58: 13–18.

Hökfelt, T., X. Zhang, and Z. Wiesenfeld-Hallin. 1994. Messenger plasticity in primary sensory neurons following axotomy and its functional implications. Trends Neurosci. 17: 22–30.

Hol, E. M., P. Sodaar, and P. R. Bär. 1994. Dorsal root ganglia as an in vitro model for melanocortin-induced neuritogenesis. Ann. N.Y. Acad. Sci. 739: 74–86.

Hughes, S., and M. E. Smith. 1994. Up-regulation of the proopiomelanocortin gene in motoneurons after nerve section in mice. Mol. Brain Res. 25: 41–49.

Johnson, H. M., E. M. Smith, B. A. Torres, et al. 1982. Regulation of the in vitro antibody response by neuroendocrine hormones. Proc. Natl. Acad. Sci. U.S.A. 79: 4171–4174.

Kastin, A. J., R. H. Ehrensing, W. A. Banks, et al. 1987. Possible therapeutic implications of the effects of some peptides on the brain. Prog. Brain Res. 72: 223–234.

Kastin, A. J., G. Gennser, A. Arimura, et al. 1968. Melanocyte-stimulating and corticotrophic activities in human foetal pituitary glands. Acta Endocrinol. 58: 6–10.

Kastin, A. J., L. H. Miller, D. Gonzalez-Barcena, et al. 1971. Psycho-physiologic correlates of MSH activity in man. Physiol. Behav. 7: 893–896.

Kawauchi, H. 1988. The melanotropic peptides: Structure and chemistry. In: The Melanotropic Peptides, Vol. 1. Ed. M. E. Hadley. Boca Raton, Fla., CRC Press, pp. 39–53.

Kiss, J. Z., E. Mezey, M. D. Cassell, et al. 1985. Topographical distribution of proopiomelanocortin-derived peptides (ACTH/β-endorphin/α-MSH) in the rat median eminence. Brain Res. 329: 169–176.

Knigge, K. M., D. Baxter-Grillo, J. Speciale, et al. 1996. Melanotropic peptides in the mammalian brain: The melanin-concentrating hormone. Peptides 17: 1063–1073.

Krieger, D. T., A. S. Liotta, M. J. Brownstein, et al. 1980. β-Lipotropin and related peptides in brain, pituitary and blood. Recent Prog. Horm. Res. 36: 277–344.

Krivoy W., and R. Guillemin. 1961. On a possible role of β-melanocyte stimulating hormone (β-MSH) in the central nervous system of Mammalia. Endocrinology 69: 170–175.

Labbe, O., F. Desarnaud, D. Eggerickx, et al. 1994. Molecular cloning of a mouse melanocortin-5 receptor gene widely expressed in peripheral tissues. Biochemistry 33: 4543–4549.

Larsson, L. I. 1977. Corticotropin-like peptides in central nerves and in endocrine cells of the gut and pancreas. Lancet 2: 1321–1323.

Lauder, J. M. 1990. Ontogeny of the serotonergic system in the rat: Serotonin as a developmental signal. Ann. N.Y. Acad. Sci. 600: 297–314.

Lee S. J., T. S. Lee, S. E. Alves, et al. 1994. Immunocytochemical localization of ACTH-(4–10) in the rat spinal cord following peripheral nerve trauma. Ann. N.Y. Acad. Sci. 739: 320–323.

Lee, S. J., T. S. Lee, and F. L. Strand. 1991. Local control of neurite outgrowth of dorsal root ganglia and spinal cord neurons by ACTH analog Org 2766, BIM 22015 and NGF. Soc. Neurosci. Abstract 598: 12.

Lee, T. H., and A. B. Lerner. 1956. Isolation of melanocyte-stimulating hormoen from hog pituitary gland. J. Biol. Chem. 221: 943–948.

Leiba, H., N. B. Garty, J. Schmidt-Sole, et al. 1990. The melanocortin receptor in the rat lacrimal gland: A model system for the study of MSH (melanocyte stimulating hormone) as a potential neurotransmitter. Eur. J. Pharmacol. 181: 71–82.

Levin, N., and J. L. Roberts. 1991. Positive regulation of proopiomelanocortin gene expression in corticotropes and melanotropes. Fronti. Neuroendocrinol. 12: 1–22.

Li, C. H. 1981. β-endorphin: Synthetic analogs and structure-activity relationship. In: Hormonal Proteins and Peptides. Ed. C. H. Li. New York, Academic Press, pp. 4–34.

Li, C. H., and D. Chung. 1976. Isolation and structure of an untriakontapeptide with opiate activity from camel pituitary glands. Proc. Natl. Acad. Sci. U.S.A. 73: 1145–1148.

Li, C. H., I. I. Geschwind, J. S. Dixon, et al. 1955. Corticotropins (ACTH): Isolation of α-corticotropin from sheep pituitary glands. J. Biol. Chem. 213: 171–185.

Lichtensteiger, W., B. Hanimann, W. Siegrist, et al. 1996. Region-specific and stage-specific patterns of melanocortin receptor onotgeny in rat central nervous system, cranial nerve ganglia and sympathetic ganglia. Dev. Brain Res. 91: 93–110.

Loh, Y. Peng., S. Elkabes, and B. Myers. 1988. Regulation of pro-opiomelanocortin (POMC) biosynthesis in the amphibian and mouse pituitary intermediate lobe. In: The Melanotropic Peptides, Vol. 1. Ed. M. E. Hadley. Boca Raton, Fla., CRC Press, pp. 85–101.

Lolait, S. J., J. A. Clements, A. J. Marwick, et al. 1986. Proopiomelanocortin, messenger ribonucleic acid and post-translational processing of beta endorphin in spleen macrophages. J. Clin. Invest. 77: 1776–1779.

Lüneburg, U., and H. Flohr. 1988. Effects of melanocortins on vestibular compensation. Prog. Brain Res. 76: 421–429.

Luger, T. A. 1997. The skin immune system: Role of α-melanocyte stimulating hormone. Int. J. Immunopath. Pharm. 10: 47–48.

Macaluso A., D. McCoy, G. Ceriani, et al. 1994. Anti-inflammatory influences of α-MSH molecules: Central neurogenic and peripheral actions. J. Neurosci. 14: 2377–2382.

McBride, R. B., B. E. Beckwith, R. R. Swenson, et al. 1994. The actions of melanin concentrating hormone (MCH) on passive avoidance in rats: A preliminary study. Peptides 15: 757–759.

Mains, R. E., B. A. Eipper, and N. Ling. 1977. Common precursor to corticotropins and endorphins. Proc. Natl. Acad. Sci. U.S.A. 74: 3014–3018.

Martens, G. J. M. 1988. The pro-opiomelanocortin gene in *Xenopus laevis*: Structure, expression, and evolutionary aspects. In: The Melanotropic Peptides, Vol. 1. Ed. M. E. Hadley. Boca Raton, Fla., CRC Press, pp. 67–83.

Martin, L. W., and J. M. Lipton. 1990. Acute phase response to endotoxin: Rise in plasma α-MSH and effects of α-MSH injections. Am. J. Physiol. 259: R768–772.

Mountjoy, K. G., M. T. Mortrud, M. J. Low, et al. 1994. Localization of the melanocortin-4 receptor (MC4-R) in neuroendocrine and autonomic control circuits in the brain. Mol. Endocrinol. 8: 1298–1308.

Miachon S., B. Claustrat, and R. Cespuglio R: 1995. Induction of muricidal behavior by ACTH or adrenalectomy in young male Wistar rats. Brain Res. Bull. 36: 119–123.

Mountjoy, K. G., L. S. Robbins, M. T. Mortud et al. 1992. The cloning of a family of genes that encode the melanocortin receptors. Science 257: 1248–1251.

Nakanishi, S., A. Inoue, S. Taii, et al. 1977. Cell-free translation product containing corticotropin and β-endorphin encoded by messenger RNA from anterior lobe and intermediate lobe of bovine pituitary. FEBS Lett. 84: 105–109.

Nelson, C., V. R. Albert, H. P. Elsholtz, et al. 1988. Activation of rat growth hormone and prolactin genes by a common transcription factor. Science 239: 1400–1405.

O'Donohue, T. L., and D. M. Dorsa. 1982. The opiomelanotropinergic neuronal and endocrine system. Peptides 3: 353–395.

Pitsikas N., B. Spruijt, S. Algeri, et al. 1990. The ACTH/MSH (4–9) analog Org 2766 improves retrieval of information after a fimbria fornix transection. Peptides 11: 911–914.

Plotnikoff N. P., and A. J. Kastin. 1976. Neuropharmacological tests with α-melanocyte stimulating hormone. Life Sci. 18: 1217–1222.

Rees, H. D., J. Verhoef, A. Witter, et al. 1980. Autoradiographic studies with a behaviorally potent ^{3}G-ACTH 4–9 analog in the brain after intraventricular injection in rats. Brain Res. Bull. 5: 509–514.

Rittenhouse, P. A., E. A. Bakkum, A. D. Levy, et al. 1994. Evidence that ACTH secretion is regulated by serotonin $_{2A/2C}$(5-HT$_{2A/2C}$) receptors. J. Pharmacol. Exp. Ther. 271: 1647–1655.

Roberts, J. L., and E. Herbert. 1977. Characterization of a common precursor to corticotropin and β-endorphin: Cell-free synthesis of the precursor and identification of corticotropin peptides in the molecule. Proc. Natl. Acad. Sci. U.S.A. 74: 4826–4830.

Rose, K. J., R. E. Frischer, J. A. King, et al. 1988. Neonatal neuromuscular parameters vary in susceptibility to ACTH/MSH 4–10 administration. Peptides 9: 151–156.

Rose, K. J., and F. L. Strand. 1988. Mammalian neuromuscular development accelerated with early but slowed with late gestational administration of ACTH peptides. Synapse 2: 200–204.

Roselli-Rehfuss, L., K. G. Mountjoy, L. S. Robbins, et al. 1993. Identification of a receptor for γ melanotropin and other proopiomelanocortin peptides in the hypothalamus and limbic system. Proc. Natl. Acad. Sci. U.S.A. 90: 8856–8860.

Saint-Come, C., G. R. Acker, and F. L. Strand. 1982. Peptide influences on the development and regeneration of motor performance. Peptides 3: 439–449.

Saint-Come, C., and F. L. Strand. 1985. ACTH/MSH improves motor unit reorganization during periphereal nerve regeneration in the rat. Peptides 6: 77–83.

Saint-Come, C., and F. L. Strand. 1988. ACTH 4–9 analogue (Org 2766) improves qualitative and quantitative aspects of motor nerve regneration. Peptides 8: 215–221.

Salomon, Y. 1990. Melanocortin receptors: Targets for control by extracellular calcium. Mol. Cell. Endocrinol. 70: 139–145.

Sandman, C. A., and A. J. Kastin. 1977. Pituitary peptide influences on attention and memory. In: Neurobiology of Sleep and Memory. Eds. R. Drucker-Colin and J. L. McGaugh. New York, Academic Press, pp. 347–360.

Sandman, C. A., L. H. Miller, A. J. Kastin, et al. 1972. A neuroendocrine influence on attention and memory. J. Comp. Physiol. Psychol. 80: 54–58.

Sandman, C. A., and J. P. O'Halloran. 1986. Proopiomelanocortin, learning, memory and attention. In: Neuropeptides and Behavior. Vol. 1, CNS Effects of ACTH, MSH and Opioid Peptides. Eds. D. De Wied, W. H. Gispen, and Tj. van Wimersma Greidanus. Oxford, Pergamon Press, pp. 397–420.

Sawchenko, P. E., T. Imaki, E. Potter, et al. 1993. The functional anatomy of corticotropin-releasing factor. Ciba Found. Symp. 172: 5–29.

Segarra A. C., V. N. Luine, and F. L. Strand. 1991. Sexual behavior of male rats is differentially affected by timing of perinatal ACTH administration. Physiol. Behav. 50: 689–697.

Seldenrijk, R., D. R. W. Hup, P. N. E. de Graan, et al. 1979. Morphological and physiological aspects of melanophores in primary culture from tadpoles of *Xenopus laevis*. Cell Tissue Res. 198: 397–409.

Smith, C. M., and F. L. Strand. 1981. Neuromuscular response of the immature rat to ACTH/MSH 4–10. Peptides 2: 197–206.

Smith, E. M., T. K. Hughes, F. Hashemi, and G. B. Stefano. 1992. Immunosuppressive effects of corticotropin and melanotropin and their possible significance in human immunodeficiency virus infection. Proc. Natl. Acad. Sci. U.S.A. 89: 782–786.

Smith, M. E., and S. Hughes. 1993. POMC neuropeptides and their receptors in the neuromuscular system of wobbler mice. J. Neurol. Sci. 124 (Suppl. S): 56–58.

Smith, P. E. 1916. The effect of hypophysectomy in the early embryo upon the growth and development of the frog. Anat. Rec. 11: 57–64.

Smith, P. E. 1930. Hypophysectomy and replacement therapy in the rat. Am. J. Anat. 45: 205–274

Smyth, D. G., Zakarian, S. J. W. F. Deakin, et al. 1979. Endorphins are stored in biologically active and inactive forms: Isolation of α-*N*-acetyl peptides. Nature 279: 252–254.

Spruijt, B., N. Pitsikas, S. Algeri, et al. 1990. Org 2766 improves performance of rats with unilateral lesions in the fimbrai fornix in a spatial learning task. Brain Res. 527: 192–197.

Strand, F. L., and T. T. Kung. 1980. ACTH accelerates recovery of neuromuscular function following crushing of peripheral nerve. Peptides 1: 135–138.

Strand, F. L., S. J. Lee, T. S. Lee, et al. 1993a. Non-corticotropic ACTH peptides modulate nerve development and regeneration. Rev. Neurosci. 4: 321–364.

Strand, F. L., K. J. Rose, J. A. King, et al. 1989. ACTH modulation of nerve development and regeneration. Prog. Neurobiol. 33: 45–48.

Strand, F. L., C. Saint-Come, T. S. Lee, et al. 1993b. An ACTH 4–10 analog BIM 22015 has neurotrophic and myotrophic attributes during peripheral nerve regeneration. Peptides 14: 287–296.

Strand, F. L., H. Stoboy, G. Friedebold, et al. 1977. Changes in muscle action potentials of patients with diseases of motor units following the infusion of a peptide fragment of ACTH. Drug Res. 27: 681–683.

Strand, F. L., L. Zuccarelli, B. Kirschenbaum, et al. 1988. Sprouting pattern and B-50 phosphorylation in regenerating sciatic nerve respond to ACTH peptides. In: Post-Lesion Neural Plasticity. Ed. H. Flohr. Berlin, Springer-Verlag, pp. 605–614.

Strand, F. L., L. A. Zuccarelli, K. A. Williams, et al. 1993c. Melanotropins as growth factors. Ann. N.Y. Acad. Sci. 680: 29–50.

Sundler, F., E. Ekblad, G. Böttcher, et al. 1985. Coexistence of peptides in the neuroendocrine system. In: Biogenetics of Neurohormonal Peptides. Eds. R. Håkanson and J. Thorell. London, Academic Press, pp. 29–45.

Swaab, D. F., M. Visser, and J. Dogterom. 1977. A function for α-MSH in fetal development and the presence of an α-MSH compound in nervous tissue. Front. Horm Res. 4: 170–178.

Swanson, L. W. 1993. Patterns of transcriptional regulation in the neuroendocrine system. In: Brain Functions of Neuropeptides: A Current View. Eds. J. P. H. Burbach and D. de Wied. New York, Parthenon, pp. 41–64.

Tatro, J. B. 1990. Melanotropin receptors in the brain are differentially distributed and recognize both corticotropin and α-melanocyte stimulating hormone. Brain Res. 536: 124–132.

Tatro, J. B., and M. L. Entwistle. 1993. Identification of a specific mammalian melanocortin receptor antagonist. Ann. N.Y. Acad. Sci. 680: 315–319.

Thody, A. J., M. E. Celis, and C. Fisher. 1979. Changes in plasma, pituitary and brain α-MSH content in rats from birth to sexual maturity. Peptides 1: 125–129.

Thody, A. J., G. Hunt, P. D. Donatien, et al. 1993. Human melanocytes express functional melanocyte-stimulating hormone receptors. Ann. N.Y. Acad. Sci. 680: 381–390.

Tilders, J. H., F. Berkenbosch, and P. G. Smelik. 1985. Control of secretion of peptides related to adrenocorticotropin, melanocyte-stimulating hormone and endorphin. Horm. Res. 14: 161–196.

Tonon, M.-C., J.-M. Danger, M. Lamacz, et al. 1988. Multihormonal control of melanotropin secretion in cold-blooded vertebrates. In: The Melanotropic Peptides, Vol. 1. Ed. M. E. Hadley. Boca Raton, Fla., CRC Press, pp. 127–170.

Torda, C., and H. G. Wolff. 1952. Effects of pituitary hormones, cortisone and adrenalectomy on some aspects of neuromuscular function and acetylcholine synthesis. Am. J. Physiol. 169: 133–141.

Valentijn, J. A., H. Vaudry, W. Kloas, et al. 1994. Melanostatin (NPY) inhibited electrical activity in frog melanotrophs through modulation of K^+, Ma^+ and Ca^{2+} currents. J. Physiol. (Lond.). 475: 185–195.

Van der Helm-Hykema H., and D. De Wied. 1976. Effect of neonatally injected ACTH and ACTH analogues on eye-opening of the rat. Life Sci. 18: 1099–1104.

Van der Neut, R., E. M. Hol, W. H. Gispen, et al. 1992. Stimulation by melanocortins of neurite outgrowth from spinal and sensory neurons in vitro. Peptides 13: 1109–1115.

Van der Zee, C. E. E. M., J. H. Brakkee, and W. H. Gispen. 1991. Putative neurotrophic factors and functional recovery from peripheral nerve damage in the rat. Br. J. Pharmacol. 103: 1941–1046.

Van der Zee, C. E. E. M., H. B. Nielander, J. P. Vos, et al. 1989. Expression of growth-associated protein B-50 (GAP 43) in dorsal root ganglia and sciatic nerve during regenerative sprouting. J. Neurosci 9: 3505–3512.

Van Ree, J. M., B. Bohus, K. M. Csontos, et al. 1981. Behavioral profile of γ-MSH: Relationship with ACTH and β-endorphin action. Life Sci. 28: 2875–2888.

Veals, J. 1979. Effects of Adrenocorticotropic Hormone on ^{14}C-Choline Accumulation and ^{14}C-Radioactivity Release by Brain Synaptosomes. Ph.D. thesis, New York University.

Verhaagen, J., P. M. Edwards, F. G. I. Jennekens, et al. 1987a. Alpha-melanocyte stimulating hormone stimulates the outgrowth of myelinated nerve fibers after peripheral nerve crush. Exp. Neurol. 92: 451–454.

Verhaagen, J., P. M. Edwards, F. G. I. Jennekens, 1987b. Pharmacological aspects of the influence of melanocortins on the formation of regenerative peripheral nerve sprouts. Peptides 8: 581–584.

Whitaker-Azmitia, P. M. 1991. Role of serotonin and other neurotransmitter receptors in brain development: Basis for developmental pharmacology. Pharmacol. Rev. 43: 553–561.

Wiemer, G., H. J. Gerhards, F. J. Hock, et al. 1988. Neurochemical effects of the synthetic ACTH 4–9 analog Hoe 427 (Ebiratide) in rat brain. Peptides 9: 1081–1087.

Wolterink, G., and J. M. van Ree. 1988. Stress-induced hypokinesia is facilitated by ACTH-(7–10). Peptides 9: 277–282.

Wolterink G., E. Van Zanten, K. Kamsteeg, et al. 1990. Functional recovery after destruction of dopamine systems in the nucleus accumbens of rats. II Facilitation by the ACTH (4–9) analog ORG 2766. Brain Res. 507: 101–108.

Yalow, R. S., and S. A. Berson. 1973. Characteristics of "big ACTH" in human plasma and pituitary extracts. J. Clin. Endocrinol. Metab. 36: 415–423.

Chapter 13

Books and Literature Reviews

Ackland, J. F., N. B. Schwartz, K. E. Mayo, et al. 1992. Nonsteroidal signals originating in the gonads. Physiol. Rev. 72: 731–787.

Clapp, C., and G. Martínez de la Escalera. 1997. Prolactins: Novel regulators of angiogenesis. News Physiol. Sci. 12: 231–237.

Hadley, M. E. 1992. Endocrinology, 3rd Ed. Englewood Cliffs, N.J., Prentice Hall.

Harvey, S., C. G. Scanes, and W. H. Daughaday. 1995. Growth Hormone Boca. Raton, Fla., CRC Press, pp. 407–413.

Imura, H., Ed. 1994. The Pituitary Gland, 2nd Ed. New York, Raven Press.

Leung, P. C. K., A. J. W. Hseuh, and H. G. Friesen, Eds. 1993. Molecular Basis of Reproductive Endocrinology. New York, Springer-Verlag.

Martin, J. B., and S. Reichlin. 1987. Clinical Neuroendocrinology, 2nd Ed. Philadelphia, F. A. Davis.

References

Aguilar, E., M. Tenasempere, R. Aguilar, et al. 1997. Interactions between *N*-methyl-D-aspartate, nitric oxide and serotonin in the control of prolactin secretion in prepubertal male rats. Eur. J. Endocrinol. 137: 99–106.

Andries, M., G. F. M. Jacobs, D. Tilemans, et al. 1996. In vitro immunoneutralization of a cleaved prolactin variant: Evidence for a local paracrine action of cleaved prolactin in the development of gonadotrophs and thyrotrophs in rat pituitary. J. Neuroendocrinol. 8: 123–127.

Arbogast, L. A., and J. L. Voogt. 1997. Prolactin (PRL) receptors are colocalized in dopaminergic neurons in fetal hypothalamic cell cultures: Effect of PRL on tyrosine hydroxylase activity. Endocrinology 138: 3016–3023.

Asa, S. L., K. Kovacs, L. Stefaneanu, et al. 1990. Pituitary mammosomatotroph adenomas develop in old mice transgenic for growth hormone. Proc. Soc. Exp. Biol. Med. 193: 232–235.

Attie, K. A., N. R. Ramirez, F. Conte, et al. 1990. The pubertal growth spurt in eight patients with true precocious puberty and growth hormone deficiency: Evidence for a direct role of sex steroids. J. Clin. Endocrinol. Metab. 71: 975–983.

Bakowska, J. C., and J. I. Morrell. 1997. Atlas of the neurons that express messenger RNA for the long form of the prolactin receptor in the forebrain of the female rat. J. Comp. Neurol. 386: 161–177.

Barinaga, M., L. M. Bilezikjian, W. W. Vale, et al. 1985. Independent effects of growth hormone releasing factor on growth hormone release and gene transcription. Nature 314: 279–281.

Ben-Jonathan, N., M. Laudon, and P. A. Garris. 1991. Novel aspects of posterior pituitary function: Regulation of prolactin secretion. Front. Neuroendocrinol. 12: 231–277.

Blackford, S. P., P. J. Little, and C. M. Kuhn. 1992. Mu-opiate and kappa-opiate receptor control of prolactin secretion in rats: Ontogeny and interaction with serotonin. Endocrinology 131: 2891–2897.

Boulton, T. J. C., R. Smith, and T. Single. 1992. Psychosocial growth failure: A positive response to growth hormone and placebo. Acta Pediatr. Scand. 81: 322–325.

Braden, T. D., and P. M. Conn. 1992. Activin stimulates the synthesis of gonadotropin releasing hormone receptors. Endocrinology 130: 2101–2105.

Bremner W. J., and A. M. Matsumoto. 1990. Follicle stimulating hormone and the control of spermatogenesis and inhibin secretion in men. In: Follicle Stimulating Hormone: Regulation of Secretion and Molecular Mechanisms of Action. Eds. M. Hunzicker-Dunn and N. B. Schwartz. New York, Springer-Verlag, pp. 257–261.

Brent, G. A., P. R. Larsen, J. W. Harney, et al. 1989. Functional characterization of the rat growth hormone promoter elements required for induction by thyroid hormone with and without a co-transfected b type thyroid hormone receptor. J. Biol. Chem. 264: 178–182.

Bruhn, T. O., T. G. Bolduc, J. E. Deckey, et al. 1992. Analysis of pulsatile secretion of thyrotropin and growth hormone in the hypothyroid rat. Endocrinology 13: 2615–2621.

Burger, H. G. 1989. Regulation of gonadotropin secretion. In: Neuroendocrine Perspectives, Vol 6. Eds. J. A. H. Wass and M. F. Scanlon. New York, Springer-Verlag, pp. 107–118.

Castrillo, J. L., L. E. Theill, and M. Karin. 1991. Function of the homeodomain protein GHF1 in pituitary cell proliferation. Science 253: 197–199.

Chen, E. Y., Y. C. Liao, D. H. Smith, et al. 1989. The human growth hormone locus nucleotide sequence, biology, evolution. Genomics 4: 479–497.

Chen, W. Y., D. C. Wight, B. V. Mehta, et al. 1991. Glycine 119 of bovine growth hormone is critical for growth-promoting activity. Mol. Endocrinol. 5: 1845–1852.

Clapp, C., and G. Martínez de la Escalera. 1997. Prolactins: Novel regulators of angiogenesis. News Physiol. Sci. 12: 231–237.

Corpas, E., S. M. Harman, and M. R. Blackman. 1993. Human growth hormone and human aging. Endocr. Rev. 14: 20–39.

Cunningham, B. C., M. Ultsch, A. M. de Vos, et al. 1991. Dimerization of the extracellular domain of the human growth hormone receptor by a single hormone molecule. Science 254: 821–825.

Daughaday, W. H., and B. Trivedi. 1987. Absence of serum growth hormone binding protein in patients with growth hormone receptor deficiency (Laron dwarfism). Proc. Natl. Acad. Sci. U.S.A. 84: 4636–4640.

Denef, C., E. Hautekeete, R. Dewals, et al. 1980. Differential control of luteinizing hormone and follicle-stimulating hormone secretion by androgens in rat pituitary cells in culture: Functional diversity of of subpopulations separated by unit gravity sedimentation. Endocrinology 106: 724–729.

Doneen, B. A., T. A. Bewley, and C. H. Li. 1979. Studies on prolactin. Selective reduction of the disulfide bonds of the ovine hormone. Biochemistry 18: 4851–4860.

Drago, F., B. Bohus, R. Bitetti, et al. 1986. Intracerebroventricular injection of anti-prolactin serum suppresses excessive grooming of pituitary homografted rats. Behav. Neural Biol. 46: 99–105.

Drago, F., B. Bohus, J. M. Van Ree, et al. 1982. Behavioral responses of long-term hyperprolatinaemic rats. Eur. J. Pharmacol. 79: 323–327.

Edery, M., C. Jolicoeur, C. Levi, et al. 1989. Identification and sequence analysis of a second form of prolactin receptor by molecular cloning of complementary DNA from rabbit mammary gland. Proc. Natl. Acad. Sci. U.S.A. 86: 2112–2116.

Evans, R. M. 1988. The steroid and thyroid hormone receptor family. Science 240: 889–895.

Frawley, L. S. 1989. Mammosomatotropes: current status and possible functions. Trends Endocr. Metabol. 1: 31–34.

Freemark, M., P. Driscoll, J. Andrews, et al. 1996. Ontogeny of prolactin gene expression in the rat olfactory system: potential roles for lactogenic hormones in olfactory development. Endocrinology 137: 934–942.

Frischer-Colbrie, A. Laslop, and R. Kirchmair. 1995. Secretogranin II: Molecular properties, regulation of biosynthesis and processing to the neuropeptide secretoneurin. Prog. Neurobiol. 46: 49–70.

Fukuhara, K., R. Kvetnancsky, G. Cizza, et al. 1996. Interrelationships between sympathoadrenal system and hypothalamo-pituitary-adrenocortical/thyroid system in rats exposed to cold stress. J. Neuroendocrinol. 8: 533–541.

Gharib, S. D., M. E. Wierman, M. A. Shupnik, et al. 1990. Molecular biology of the pituitary gonadotropins. Endocr. Rev. 11: 177–199.

Gibori, G., and J. S. Richards. 1978. Dissociation of two distinct luteotropic effects of prolactin: Regulation of luteinizing hormone receptor content and progesterone secretion during pregnancy. Endocrinology 102: 767–774.

Golde, D. W., N. Bersch, S. A. Kaplan, et al. 1980. Peripheral unresponsiveness to human growth hormone in Laron dwarfism. N. Engl. J. Med. 303: 1156–1158.

Gonzalezparra, S., J. A. Chowen, L. M. G. Segura, et al. 1996. Ontogeny of pituitary transcription factor-I (Pit-1), growth hormone (GH) and prolactin (PRL) messenger RNA levels in male and female rats and the differential expression of Pit-1 in lactotrophs and somatotrophs. J. Neuroendocrinol. 8: 211–225.

Gore-Langton, R. E., and D. T. Armstrong. 1988. Follicular steroidogenesis and its control. In: The Physiology of Reproduction. Eds. E. Knobil and J. Neill. New York, Raven Press, pp. 331–385.

Gustafson, T. A., B. E. Markham, J. J. Bahl, et al. 1987. Thyroid hormone regulates expression of a transfected α-myosin heavy chain fusion gene in fetal heart cells. Proc. Natl. Acad. Sci. U.S.A. 84: 3122–3126.

Harvey, S., C. G. Scanes, and W. H. Daughaday. 1995. Growth Hormone. Boca Raton, Fla., CRC Press.

Harvey, S., W. R. Baumbach, H. Sadeghi, et al. 1993. Endocrinology 133: 1125–1130.

Hirt, H., J. Kimelman, M. J. Birnbaum, et al. 1987. The human growth hormone gene locus, structure, evolution, allelic variations. DNA 5: 59–70.

Horrobin, D. F. 1981. Cellular basis of prolactin action: involvement of cyclic nucleotides, polyamines, prostaglandins, steroids, thyroid hormones, Na/K ATPases and calcium: Relevance to breast cancer and the nenstrual cycle. Med. Hypotheses 1979: 599–620.

Hurley, D. L., B. E. F. Wee, and C. J. Phelps. 1997. Hypophysiotropic somatostatin expression during postnatal development in growth hormone deficient Ames dwarf mice—messenger RNA in situ hybridization. Neuroendocrinology 65: 98–106.

Igarashi, M., K. Miyamoto, Y. Hasegawa, et al. 1993. Role of inhibins and activins in reproduction. In: Molecular Basis of Reproductive Endocrinology. Eds. P. C. K. Leung, A. J. W. Hseuh, and H. G. Friesen. New York, Springer-Verlag, pp. 50–62.

Jackson, I. M. D. 1994. Regulation of thyrotropin secretion. In: The Pituitary Gland, 2nd Ed. Ed. H. Imura. New York, Raven Press, pp. 179–216.

Jameson. J. L., R. C. Jaffee, S. L. Gleason, et al. 1986. Transcriptional regulation of chorionic gonadotropin alpha- and beta-subunit gene expression by 8-bromo-adenosine 3′,5′-monophosphate. Endocrinology 119: 2560–2567.

Jorgensen, H., U. Knigge, A. Kjaer, et al. 1996. Interactions of histaminergic and serotonergic neurons in the hypothalamic regulation of prolactin and ACTH. Neuroendocrinology 64: 329–336.

Juszczak, M., and B. Stempniak. 1997. Effect of melatonin on suckling-induced oxytocin and prolactin release in the rat. Brain Res. Bull. 44: 253–258.

Kastin, A. J., R. H. Ehrensing, D. S. Schalch, et al. 1972. Improvement in mental depression with decreased thyrotropin response after administration of thyrotropin-releasing hormone. Lancet 2: 740–742.

Kelly, P. A., M. Edery, J. Finidori, et al. 1994. Receptor domains involved in signal transduction of prolactin and growth hormone. Proc. Soc. Exp. Biol. Med. 206: 280–283.

Kirchmair, R., R. Hogue-Angeletti, J. Gutierrez, et al. 1993. Secretoneurin—A neuropeptide generated in brain, adrenal medulla and other endocrine tissues by proteolytic processing of secretogranin (chomogranin C). Neuroscience 53: 359–365.

Kleinberg, D. L., J. Todd, and G. Babitsky. 1983. Inhibition by estradiol of the lactogenic effect of prolactin in primary mammary tissue: Reversal by antiestrogens LY 156758 and tamoxifen. Proc. Natl. Acad. Sci. U.S.A. 80: 4144–4148.

Kumar, T. R., and M. J. Low. 1995. Hormonal regulation of human follicle stimulating hormone-beta subunit gene expression: GnRH stimulation and GnRH-independent androgen inhibition. Neuroendocrinology 61: 628–637.

Lash, R. W., R. K. Desai, and C. A. Zimmerman. 1992. Mutation of the human thyrotropin-beta subunit glycosylation site reduces thyrotropin synthesis independent of changes in glycosylation status. Endocr. Invest. 15: 255–263.

Lechan, R. M., Y. P. Qi, I. M. D. Jackson, et al. 1994. Identification of thyroid hormone receptor isoforms in thyrotropin-rleasing hormone neurons of the hypothalamic paraventricular nucleus. Endocrinology 135: 92–100.

Magner, J. A. 1990. Thyroid-stimulating hormone: Biosynthesis, cell biology and bioactivity. Endocr. Rev. 11: 354–385.

Mann, D. R., G. G. Jackson, and M. S. Blank. 1982. Influence of adrenocorticotropin and adrenalectomy on gonadotropin secretion in immature rats. Neuroendocrinology 34: 20–26.

Mansfield, M. J., D. E. Beardsworth, J. S. Loughlin, et al. 1983. Long-term treatment of central precocious puberty with a long-acting analogue of luteinizing horone releasing hormone. N. Engl. J. Med. 309: 1286–1290.

Markoff, E., M. B. Siegel, N. Lacour, et al. 1988. Glycosylation selectively alters the biological activity of prolactin. Endocrinology 123: 1303–1306.

Martin, J. B., and S. Reichlin. 1987. Clinical Neuroendocrinology, 2nd Ed. Philadelphia, F. A. Davis, pp. 509–527.

Martínez de la Escalera, G., and R. I. Weiner. 1992. Dissociation of dopamine from its receptor as a signal in the pleitropic hypothalamic regulation of prolactin secretion. Endocr. Rev. 13: 241–255.

McNeilly, A. S. 1979. Effects of lactation on fertility. Brit. Med. Bull. 35: 151–154.

Merrimee, T. J., G. Baumann, and W. H. Daughaday. 1990. Growth hormone–binding protein II: Studies in pygmies and normal statured subjects. J. Clin. Endocrinol. Metab. 71: 1183–1188.

Mick, C. C., and C. S. Nicoll. 1985. Prolactin directly stimulates the liver in vivo to secrete a factor (synlactin) which acts synergistically with the hormone. Endocrinology 116: 2049–2053.

Miller, W. L., and N. L. Eberhardt. 1983. Structure and evolution of the growth hormone gene family. Endocr. Rev 4: 97–130.

Nagaya, T., and J. L. Jameson. 1994. Structural features of the glycoprotein hormone genes and their encoded proteins. In: The Pituitary Gland, 2nd Ed. Ed. H. Imura. New York, Raven Press, pp. 63–89.

Niall, H. D. 1982. The evolution of peptide hormones. Ann. Rev. Physiol. 44: 615–624.

Owerbach, D., W. Rutter, J. Martial, et al. 1980. Genes for growth hormone, somatomammotropin, and growth hormone-like genes on chromosome 17 in humans. Science 209: 289–292.

Postel-Vinay, M. C., L. Belair, C. Kayser, et al. 1991. Identification of prolactin and growth hormone binding proteins in rabbit milk. Proc. Natl. Acad. Sci. U.S.A. 88: 6687–6690.

Reichert, L. E., Jr., and B. Dattatreyamurty. 1989. The follicle-stimulating hormone (FSH) receptor in testis: Interaction with FSH, mechanism of signal transduction, and properties of the purified receptor. Biol. Reprod. 40: 13–26.

Reinisch N., R. Kirchmair, C. M. Kähler, et al. 1993. Attraction of human monocytes by the neuropeptide secretoneurin. FEBS Lett. 334: 41–44.

Reyroldan, E. B., V. Luxlantos, A. Chamsonreig, et al. 1997. In vivo interaction of baclofen, TRH and serotonin on PRL and TSH secretion in developing and adult male and female rats. Life Sci. 61: 2283–2290.

Richards, J. S., and L. Hedin. 1988. Molecular aspects of hormone action in ovarian follicular development, ovulation, and luteinization. Annu. Rev. Physiol. 50: 441–463.

Roth, J., S. M. Glick, R. S. Yalow, et al. 1963. Hyperglycemia: A potent stimulus to secretion of growth hormone. Science 140: 987–988.

Sakaguchi, K., M. Tanaka, T. Ohkubo, et al. 1996. Induction of brain prolactin receptor long-form messenger-RNA expression and maternal behavior in pup-contacted male rats—Promotion by prolactin administration and suppression by female contact. Neuroendocrinology 63: 559–568.

Sakuma, Y., and D. W. Pfaff. 1980. LH-RH in the mesencephalic central gray can potentiate lordosis reflex of female rats. Nature 283: 566–567.

Salvador, J., C. Dieguez, and M. F. Scanlon. 1988. The circadian rhythms of thyrotropin and prolactin secretion. Chronobiol. Int. 5: 85–93.

Samuels, M. H., D. Wilson, and G. Sexton. 1994. Effects of naloxone infusions on pulsatile thyrotropin secretion. J. Clin. Endocrinol. Metab. 78: 1249–1252.

Saria, A., W. A. Kaufmann, J. Marksteiner, et al. 1997. Distribution and processing of secretoneurin in the developing rat brain. Ann. N.Y. Acad. Sci. 814: 90–96.

Saria, A, J. Troger, R. Kirchmair, et al. 1993. Secretoneurin releases dopamine from rat striatal slices: A biological effect of a peptide derived from secretogranin II (chromagranin C). Neuroscience 54: 1–4.

Sato, F., H. Aoki, K. Nakamura, et al. 1997. Suppressive effects of chronic hyperprolactinemia on penile erection and yawning following administration of apomorphine to pituitary-transplanted rats.

Sauve, D., and B. Woodside. 1996. The effect of central administration of prolactin on food intake in virgin female rats is dose-dependent, occurs in the absence of ovarian hormones and the latency to onset varies with feeding regimen. Brain Res. 729: 75–81.

Shamgochian, M. D., C. Avakian, N. H. Truong et al. 1995. Regulation of prolactin receptor by estradiol in the female rat brain. Neuroreport 6: 2537–2541.

Shieh, K. R., and J. T. Pan. 1997. Nicotinic control of tuberoinfundibular dopaminergic neuron activity and prolactin secretion: Diurnal rhythm and involvement of endogenous opioidergic system. Brain Res. 756: 266–272.

Shiu, R. P., and H. G. Friesen. 1980. Mechanism of action of prolactin in the control of mammary gland function. Annu. Rev. Physiol. 42: 83–96.

Shupnik, M. A., and P. C. Fallest. 1994. Pulsatile GnRH regulation of gonadotropin subunit gene transcription. Neurosci. Biobehav. Rev. 18: 597–599.

Shupnik, M. A., E. C. Ridgway, and W. W. Chin. 1989. Molecular biology of thyrotropin. Endocr. Rev. 10: 459–475.

Silva, J. D. B., and M. T. Nunes. 1996. Facilitatory role of serotonin (5-HT) in the control of thyrotropin-releasing hormone/thyrotropin (TRH/TSH) secretion in rats. Braz. J. Med. Biol. Res. 29: 677–683.

Smith, P. E. 1916. The effect of hypophysectomy in the early embryo upon the growth and development of the frog. Anat. Rec. 11: 57–74.

Stolar, M. W., and G. Baumann. 1986. Secretory patterns of growth hormone during basal periods in man. Metabolism 35: 883–888.

Struthers, R. S., D. Gaddy-Kurten, and W. W. Vale. 1992. Activin inhibits binding of the transcription factor Pit-1 to the growth hormone promoter. Proc. Natl. Acad. Sci. U.S.A. 89: 11451–11455.

Subramanian, M. G. 1997. Evaluation of lactational parameters after alcohol administration for 4 days during early or midlactation in the rat. Alcohol. Clin. Exp. Res. 21: 799–803.

Sugiyama, T., H. Minoura, N. Toyoda, et al. 1996. Pup contact induces the expression of long form prolactin receptor messenger-RNA in the brain of female rats—Effects of ovariectomy and hypophysectomy on receptor gene expression. J. Endocrinol. 149: 335–340.

Syms, A. J., M. E. Harper, and K. Griffiths. 1985. The effect of prolactin on human BPH epithelial cell proliferation. Prostate 6: 145–153.

Vancauter, E., and L. Plat. 1996. Physiology of growth hormone secretion during sleep. J. Pediatr. 128 (Pt. 2, Suppl. S): S32–S37.

Vaudry, H., and J. M. Conlon. 1991. Identification of a peptide arising from specific post-translational processing of secretogranin II. Fed. Eur. Biochem. Soc. Lett. 284: 31–33.

Waldstreicher, J. J. F. Duffy, E. N. Brown, et al. 1996. Gender differences in the temporal organization of prolactin (PRL) secretion—Evidence for a sleep-independent circadian rhythm of circulating PRL levels—A clinical research center study. J. Clin. Endocrinol. Metab. 81: 1483–1487.

Walker, W. H., S. L. Fitzpatrick, H. A. Barrera-Saldana, et al. 1991. The human placental lactogen genes: Structure, function, evolution and transcriptional regulation. Endocr. Rev. 12: 316–336.

Wells, J. A., B. C. Cunningham, G. Fuh, et al. 1993. The molecular basis for growth hormone-receptor interactions. Recent Prog. Horm. Res. 48: 253–275.

Wiedermann, K., L. Herzog, and M. Kellner. 1995. Atrial natriuretic hormone inhibits corticortropin-releasing hormone-induced prolactin release in man. J. Psychia. Res. 29: 51–58.

Ying, S.-Y. 1988. Inhibins and activins. In: Frontiers in Neuroendocrinology, Vol 10. Eds. L. Martini and W. F. Ganong. New York, Raven Press, pp. 167–184.

Yu-Lee, L. Y. 1997. Molecular actions of prolactin in the immune system. Proc. Soc. Biol. Med. 215: 35–52.

Chapter 14

Books and Literature Reviews

Besson, J. M., and Chaouch. 1987. Peripheral and spinal mechanism of nociception. Physiol Rev. 67: 67–186.

Cox, B. M., and E. R. Baizman. 1982. Physiological functions of endorphins. In: Endorphins: Chemistry, Physiology, Pharmacology and Clinical Relevance. Eds. J. B. Malick and B. M. S. Bell. New York, Marcel Dekker, pp. 113–196.

De Wied, D. 1987. The neuropeptide concept. Prog. Brain Res. 72: 93–108.

Kieffer, B. L. 1995. Recent advances in molecular recognition and signal transduction of active peptides: Receptors for opioid peptides. Cell. Mol. Neurobiol. 15: 615–635.

Kreek, M. J. 1996. Opioid receptors: Some perspectives from early studies of their role in normal physiology, stress responsivity, and in specific addictive diseases. Neurochem. Res. 21: 1469–1488.

Negri, N. M., G. Lotti, and A. Grossman, Eds. 1992. Clinical Perspectives in Endogenous Opioid Peptides. Chichester, U.K. Wiley.

Olson, G. A. Olson, R. D., and A. J. Kastin. 1991. Review: Endogenous Opiates 1990. Peptides 13: 1247–1287. [Also see subsequent years, 1992–1998, *Peptides* Vols. 14–20, for annual reviews of endogenous opiates.]

Satoh, M., and M. Minami. 1995. Molecular pharmacology of the opioid receptors. Pharmacol. Ther. 68: 343–364.

Simon, E. J. 1982. History. In: Endorphins: Chemistry, Physiology, Pharmacology and Clinical Relevance. Eds. J. B. Malick and R. M. S. Bell. New York, Marcel Dekker, pp. 1–8.

Simon, E. 1991. Opioid receptors and endogenous opioid peptides. Med. Res. Rev. 357–374.

Snyder, S. H. 1989. Brainstorming: The Science and Politics of Opiate Research. Cambridge, Mass., Harvard University Press.

Van Nispen, J. W., and Tj. B. Van Wimersma Greidanus. 1990. Neuropeptides and behavioral adaptation: Structure-activity relationships. In: Neuropeptides: Basics and Perspectives. Ed. D. De Wied. Amsterdam, Elsevier, pp. 213–254.

References

Abboud, T. K. 1988. Maternal and fetal β-endorphin: Effects of pregnancy and labour. Arch. Dis. Child. 63: 707–709.

Agmo, A., M. Gomez, and Y. Irazabal. 1994. Enkephalinase inhibition facilitates sexual behavior in the male rat but does not produce conditioned place preference. Pharmacol. Biochem. Behav. 47: 771–778.

Almay, B. G. L., F. Johannsson, L. Terenius, et al. 1978. Pain perception and endorphin levels in cerebrospinal fluid. Pain 5: 153.

Alvaro, J. D., J. B. Tatro, and R. S. Duman. 1997. Melanocortins and opiate addiction. Life Sci. 61: 1–9.

Atweh, S. F., and M. J. Kuhar. 1983. Regional distribution of opioid receptor binding in the brain. Med. Bull. 39: 47–52.

Berzeteigurske, I. P., R. W. Schwartz, and L. Toll. 1996. Determination of activity for nociceptin in the mouse vas deferens. Eur. J. Pharmacol. 302: R1–R2.

Bloom, F., D. Segal, N. Ling, et al. 1976. Endorphins: Profound behavioral effects in rats suggest new etiological factors in mental illness. Science 194: 630–632.

Borsodi, A., and G. Tóth. 1995. Characterization of opioid receptor types and subtypes with new ligands. Ann. N.Y. Acad. Sci. 757: 339–361.

Brady, L. S. 1993. Opiate receptor regulation by opiate agonists and antagonists. In: The Neurobiology of Opiates.

Ed. R. P. Hammer. Boca Raton, Fla., CRC Press, pp. 125–145.

Butour, J. L., C. Moisand, H. Mazarguil, et al. 1997. Recognition and activation of the opioid receptor-like ORL_1 receptor by nociceptin, nociceptin analogs and opioids. Eur. J. Pharmacol. 321: 97–103.

Chichara, K., A. Arimura, D. H. Coy, et al. 1978. Studies on the interaction of endorphins, substance P and endogenous somatostatin in growth hormone and prolactin release in rats. Endocrinology 102: 281–290.

Cohen, M. L., L. G. Mendelsohn, C. H. Mitch, et al. 1994. Use of the mouse vas deferens to determine μ, δ, and κ receptor affinities of opioid antagonists. Receptor 4: 43–53.

Cox, B. M. 1994. Opiate drug tolerance: An introduction. Regul. Peptides 54: 71–72.

Cox, B. M., and E. R. Baizman. 1982. Physiological functions of endorphins. In: Endorphins: Chemistry, Physiology, Pharmacology, and Clinical Relevance. Eds. J. B. Malick and B. M. S. Bell. New York, Marcel Dekker, pp. 113–196.

Cuello, A. C. 1983. Central distribution of opioid peptides. Br. Med. Bull. 39: 11–16.

Delitala, G. 1991. Opioid peptides and pituitary function. In: Brain Endocrinology, 2nd Ed. Ed. M. Motta. New York, Raven Press, pp. 217–244.

De Wied, D., G. L. Kovács, B. Bohus, et al. 1987. Neuroleptic activity of the neuropeptide β-LPH_{62-77} ([Des-Tyr_1]) γ-endorphin: DTγE). Eur. J. Pharmacol. 49: 427–436.

Ding, Y.-Q., T. Kaneko, S. Momura, et al. 1996. Immunohistochemical localization of μ-opioid receptors in the central nervous system of the rat. J. Comp. Neurol. 367: 375–402.

Drake, C. T., G. W. Terman, M. L. Simmons, et al. 1994. Dynorphin opioids present in dentate granule cells may function as as retrograde inhibitory transmitters. J. Neurosci. 14: 3736–3750.

Erchegyi, J., A. J. Kastin, and J. E. Zadina. 1992. Isolation of a novel tetrapeptide with opiate and antiopiate activity from human brain cortex: Tyr-Pro-Trp-Gly-NH_2 (Tyr-W-MIF-1). Peptides 13: 623–631.

Evans, C. J., D. E. Keith Jr., H. Morrison, et al. 1992. Cloning of a delta opioid receptor by functional expression. Science 258: 1952–1955.

Frederickson, R. C. A. 1984. Endogenous opioids and related derivatives. In: Analgesics: Neurochemical, Behavioral and Clinical Perspectives. Eds. M. J. Kuhar and G. W. Pasternak. New York, Raven Press, pp. 69–96.

Galina, Z. H., and A. J. Kastin. 1986. Existence of antiopiate systems as illustrated by MIF-1/Tyr-MIF-1 (minireview). Life Sci. 39: 2153–2159.

Gergen, K. A., J. E. Zadina, and D. Paul. 1997. Analgesic effects of Tyr-W-MIF-1—a mixed μ_2 opioid receptor antagonist. Eur. J. Pharmacol. 316: 33–38.

Giuliani, S., and C. A. Maggi. 1996. Inhibition of tachykinin release from peripheral endings of sensory nerves by nociceptin, a novel opioid peptide. Br. J. Pharmacol. 118: 1567–1569.

Goldstein, A., W. Fischli, L. I. Lowney, et al. 1979. Dynorphin (1–13), an extraordinarily potent opioid peptide. Proc. Natl. Acad. Sci. U.S.A. 76: 6666–6670.

Grossman, A., W. A. Stubbs, R. C. Gaillard, et al. 1981. Studies of the opiate control of GH and TSH. Clin. Endocrinol. 14: 381–386.

Hackler, L., A. J. Kastin, J. Erchegyi, et al. 1993. Isolation of Tyr-W-MIF-1 from bovine hypothalami. Neuropeptides 24: 159–164.

Hackler, L., A. J. Kastin, and J. E. Zadina. 1994. Isolation of a novel peptide with a unique binding profile from human brain cortex: Tyr-K-MIF-1 (Tyr-Pro-Lys-Gly-NH_2). Peptides 15: 945–950.

Han, J. S., and L. Terenius. 1982. Neurochemical basis of acupuncture analgesia. Annu. Rev. Pharmacol. Toxicol. 22: 193–220.

Han, J. S., and G.-X. Xi. 1984. Dynorphin: Important mediator of electroacupuncture analgesia in the spinal cord of the rabbit. Pain 18: 367–376.

Henderson, G., J. Hughes, and H. W. Kosterlitz. 1978. In vitro release of [Leu^5] and [Met^5]-enkephalins from the corpus striatum. Nature 271: 677–679.

Herz, A. 1997. Endogenous opioid systems and alcohol addiction. Psychopharmacology 129: 99–111.

Hoffmann, P., I. H. Jonsdottir, and P. Thorén. 1996. Activation of different opioid systems by muscle activity and exercise. News Physiol. Sci. 11: 223–228.

Hughes, J. S. 1975. Isolation of an endogenous compound from the brain with pharmacological properties similar to morphine. Brain Res. 88: 295–308.

Hughes, S., and M. E. Smith. 1994. Upregulation of the pro-opiomelanocortin gene in motoneurons after nerve section in mice. Mol. Brain. Res. 25: 41–49.

Itzhak, Y., J. M. Hiller, and E. J. Simon. 1984. Solubilization and characterization of μ, δ and κ opioid binding sites from guinea pig brain: Physical separation of κ receptors. Proc. Natl. Acad. Sci. U.S.A. 81: 4217–4221.

Iverson, L. L., S. D. Iverson, F. E. Bloom, et al. 1978. Release of enkephalin from rat globus pallidus in vitro. Nature 271: 679–681.

Kaneko, S., S. Nakamura, K. Adachi, et al. 1994. Mobilization of intracellular Ca^{2+} and stimulation of cyclic AMP production by kappa opioid receptors expressed in *Xenopus* oocytes. Mol. Brain Res. 27: 258–264.

Khachaturian, H., M. E. Lewis, M. K.-H. Schäfer, et al. 1985. Anatomy of the CNS opioid systems. Trends Neurosci. 111–119.

Kieffer, B. L. 1995. Recent advances in molecular recognition and signal transduction of active peptides: Receptors for opioid peptides. Cell. Mol. Neurobiol. 15: 615–635.

Koob, G. F., and F. E. Bloom. 1988. Cellular and molecular mechanisms of drug dependence. Science 242: 715–723.

Koob, G. F., and N. E. Goeders. 1989. Neuroanatomical substrates of drug self-administration. In: The Neuropharmacological Basis of Reward. Eds. J. M. Liebman and S. J. Cooper. Oxford Science Foundation, pp. 214–263.

Koob, G. F., L. Stinus, M. Le Moal, et al. 1989. Opponent process theory of motivation: Neurobiological evidence from studies of opiate dependence. Neurosci. Behav. Rev. 13: 135–140.

Krahn, D. D., B. A. Gosnell, R. J. Davidson, et al. 1994. EEG responses to ice cream and pain: Opioid and preference effects. Soc. Neurosci. Abstr. 20: 1225.

Kreek, M. J. 1996. Opioid receptors: Some perspectives from early studies of their role in normal physiology, stress responsivity, and in specific addictive diseases. Neurochem. Res. 21: 1469–1488.

Lambert, P. D., J. P. H. Wilding, A. A. M. Al-Dokhayel, et al. 1994. Naloxone-induced anorexia increases neuropeptide Y concentrations in the dorsomedial hypothalamus: Evidence for neuropeptide Y–opioid interactions in the control of food intake. Peptides 15: 657–660.

Leng, G., S. Mansfield, R. J. Bicknell, et al. 1985. Central opioids: A possible role in parturition. J. Endocrinol. 106: 219–224.

Lewis, R. V., A. S. Stern, S. Kimura, et al. 1980. An about 50,000-dalton protein in adrenal medulla: A common precursor of [Met]- and [Leu]-enkephalin. Science 208: 1459–1461.

Lin, J.-Y., and J.-T. Pan. 1994. Effects of endogenous opioid peptides and their analogs on the activities of hypothalamic arcuate neurons in brain slices from diestrous and ovariectomized rats. Brain Res. Bull. 36: 225–233.

Lord, J. A. H., A. A. Waterfield, J. Hughes, et al. 1977. Endogenous opioid peptides: Multiple agonists and receptors. Nature 267: 495–499.

Mansour, A., S. Burke, R. J. Pavlic, et al. 1996. Immunohistochemical localization of the cloned κ_1 receptor in the rat CNS and pituitary. Neuroscience 71: 671–690.

Mansour, A., C. A. Fox, H. Akil, et al. 1995. Opioid-receptor mRNA expression in the rat CNS: Anatomical and functional implications. Trends Neurosci. 18: 22–29.

Mansour, A., M. E. Lewis, H. Khachaturian, et al. 1987. Autoradiographic distribution of mu, delta and kappa opioid receptors in the rat forebrain and midbrain. J. Neurosci. 7: 2445–2464.

Margules, D. L., B. Moisset, M. J. Lewis, et al. 1978. Beta-endorphin is associated with over-eating in genetically obese mice (*ob/ob*) and rats (*fa/fa*). Science 202: 988–991.

Meites, J. 1984. Effects of opiates on neuroendocrine functions in animals. Overview. In: Opioid Modulation of Endocrine Function. Eds. G. Delitalia and M. Motta. Series M. New York, Raven Press, pp. 58–63.

Mollereau, C., M.-J. Simons, P. Soularue, et al. 1996. Structure, tissue distribution, and chromosomal localization of the prepronociceptin gene. Proc. Natl. Acad. Sci. U.S.A. 93: 8666–8670.

Nakasawa, T., M. Ikeda, T. Kaneko, et al. 1985. Analgesic effects of dynorphin-A and morphine in mice. Peptides 6: 75–78.

Nightingale, S. L. 1995. Naltrexone approved as adjunct in alcoholism treatment. JAMA 273: 613.

Olson, G. A., R. D. Olson, and A. J. Kastin. 1991. Review: Endogenous opiates 1991. Peptides 13: 1247–1287.

O'Malley, S. S. 1995. Current strategies for the treatment of alcohol dependence in the United States. Drug Alcohol Depend. 39: S3–S7.

Oyama, J. T. Jin, R. Yamaya, et al. 1980. Profound analgesic effects of β-endorphin in man. Lancet 1: 122–125.

Papadouka, V., and K. D. Carr. 1994. The role of multiple opioid receptors in the maintenance of stimulus-induced feeding. Brain Res. 639: 42–48.

Pasternak, G. W. 1988. Multiple morphine and enkephalin receptors and the relief of pain. JAMA 259: 1362–1367.

Pelton, J., K. Gulya, V. Hruby, et al. 1985. Conformationally restricted analogs of somatostatin with high μ opiate receptor specificity. Proc. Natl. Acad. Sci. U.S.A. 82: 236–239.

Pert, C. B., and S. H. Snyder. 1973. Opiate receptor: Demonstration in nervous tissue. Science 179: 1011–1014.

Phillips, R. L., R. Herning, and E. D. London. 1994. Morphine effects on the spontaneous electroencephalogram in polydrug abusers: Correlation with subjective self-reports. Neuropsychopharmacology 10: 171–181.

Qu, Z.-X., and L. Isaac. 1993. Dynorphin A (1–13) potentiates dynorphin A (1–17) on loss of the tail-flick reflex after intrathecal injection in the rat. Brain Res. 610: 340–343.

Ramirez, V. D., H. H. Feder, and C. H. Sawyer. 1984. The role of brain catecholamines in the regulation of LH secretion: A critical inquiry. Front. Neuroendocrinol. 8: 27–83.

Reinscheid, R. K., A. Ardati, F. J. Monsma, et al. 1996. Structure-activity relationship studies on the novel neuropeptide orphanin FQ. J. Biol. Chem. 271: 14163–14168.

Reisine, T., and G. I. Bell. 1993. Molecular biology of opioid receptors. Trends Neurosci. 16: 506–510.

Reisine, T., J. Heerding, and K. Raynor. 1994. The third intracellular loop of the delta receptor is necessary for coupling to adenyl cyclase and receptor desensitization. Regul. Peptides 54: 241–242.

Ristic, H., and L. Isaac. 1994. Pharmacological characterization of dynorphin A (1–17)–induced effects on spinal cord-evoked potentials. J. Pharmacol. Exp. Ther. 270: 534–539.

Roby, A., J.-C. Willer, and B. Bussel. 1983. Effect of a synthetic enkephalin analogue on spinal nociceptive messages in humans. Neuropharmacology 22: 1121–1125.

Sarnyai, Z., and G. L. Kovacs. 1994. Role of oxytocin in the neuroadaptation of drugs of abuse. Psychoneuroendocrinology 19: 85–117.

Schafer, M. K.-H. Day, S. J. Watson, et al. 1991. Distribution of opioids in brain and peripheral tissues. In: Neurobiology of Opioids. Eds. O. F. X. Almeida and T. S. Shippenberg. Berlin, Springer-Verlag, pp. 53–62.

Schmauss, C., and T. L. Yaksh. 1984. In vivo studies on spinal opiate receptor systems mediating antinociception. II. Pharmacological profiles suggesting a differential association of mu, delta and kappa receptors with visceral chemical and cutaneous thermal stimuli in the rat. J. Pharmacol. Exp. Ther. 228: 1–12.

Schwyzer, R. 1977. ACTH: A short introductory review. Ann. N.Y. Acad. Sci. 247: 3–26.

Simon, E. J., and J. M. Hiller. 1978. The opiate receptors. Annu. Rev. Pharmacol. 18: 371–394.

Simon, E. J., and J. M. Hiller. 1988. Solubilization and purification of opioid binding sites. In: The Opiate Receptors. Ed. G. W. Pasternak. Totawa, N.J., Humana Press, pp. 165–194.

Simon, E. J., and J. M. Hiller. 1994. Opioid peptides and opioid receptors. In: Basic Neurochemistry: Molecular, Cellular and Medical Aspects. Ed. G. J. Siegel. 5th Ed. New York, Raven Press, pp. 321–339.

Simon, E. J., J. M. Hiller, and I. Edelman. 1973. Stereospecific binding of the potent narcotic analgesic ^{3}H-etorphine to rat brain homogenate. Proc. Soc. Natl. Acad. Sci. U.S.A. 70: 1947–1949.

Smith, E. M., and J. E. Blalock. 1981. Human lymphocyte production of ACTH and endorphin-like substances: Association with leucocyte interferon. Proc. Natl. Acad. Sci. U.S.A.: 78: 7530–7534.

Stefano, G. 1989. Opioid peptides—Comparative peripheral mechanisms. In: The Comparative Physiology of Regulatory Peptides. Ed. S. Holmgren. New York, Chapman & Hall, pp. 112–129.

Stinus, L., D. Nadaud, J. Jauregui, et al. 1986. Chronic treatment with five different narcoleptics elicits behavioral sensitivity to opiate infusion into the nucleus accumbens. Biol. Psychiatry 21: 34–38.

Swift, R. M. 1995. Effect of naltrexone on human alcohol consumption. J. Clin. Psychiatry 56 (Suppl. 7): 24–29.

Tallent, M., M. Dichter, G. I. Bell, et al. 1994. The cloned κ opioid receptors to an N-type Ca^{2+} current in undifferentiated PC-12 cells. Neuroscience 63: 1033–1040.

Terenius, L. 1973. Stereospecific interaction between narcotic analgesics and a synaptic plasma membrane fraction of rat cerebral cortex. Acta Pharmacol. Toxicol. (Copenhagen) 32: 317–320.

Teschenmacher, H., K. E. Ophim, B. M. Cox, et al. 1975. A peptide-like substance that acts like morphine. Life Sci. 16: 1771–1776.

Tsou, K., H. Khachaturian, H. Akil, et al. 1986. Immunocytochemical localization of proopiomelanocortin-derived peptides in the adult spinal cord. Brain Res. 378: 28–35.

Uhl, G. R., S. Childers, and G. Pasternak. 1994. An opiate-receptor gene family reunion. Trends Neurosci. 17: 89–93.

Ulm, R. R., J. R. Volpicelli, and L. A. Volpicelli. 1995. Opiates and self-administration of alcohol in animals. J. Clin. Psychiatry 56 (Suppl. 7): 5–14.

Van Nispen, J. W., and Tj. B. Van Wimersma Greidanus. 1990. Neuropeptides and behavioral adaptation: Structure-activity relationships. In: Neuropeptides: Basics and Perspectives. Ed. D. De Wied. Amsterdam, Elsevier, pp. 213–254.

Vaughan, C. W., and M. J. Christie. 1996. Increase by the ORL_1 receptor (opioid receptor-like$_1$) ligand, nociceptin, of inwardly rectifying K^+ conductance in dorsal raphe nucleus neurons. Br. J. Pharmacol. 117: 1609–1611.

Vaughan, C. W., S. L. Ingram, and M. J. Christie. 1997. Actions of the ORL_1 receptor ligand nociceptin on membrane properties of rat periaqueductal gray neurons in vitro. J. Neurosci. 17: 996–1003.

Volpicelli, J. R., L. A. Volpicelli, and C. P. O'Brien. 1995. The medical management of alcohol dependence—clinical use and limitations of naltrexone treatment. Alcohol Alcohol 30: 789–798.

Wang, J. B., Y. Imai, C. M. Eppler, et al. 1993. μ opiate receptor: cDNA cloning and expression. Proc. Natl. Acad. Sci. U.S.A. 90: 10230–10234.

Wang, J. B., P. S. Johnson, A. M. Persico, et al. 1994. Human mu-opiate receptor—cDNA and genomic clones, pharmacological characterization and chromosomal assignment. FEBS Lett. 338: 217–222.

Wang, X. M., K. M. Zhang, and S. S. Mokha. 1996. Nociceptin (Orphanin FQ), an endogenous ligand for the ORL-1 (opioid receptor–like 1) receptor, modulates responses of trigeminal neurons evoked by excitatory amino acids and somatosensory stimuli. J. Neurophysiol. 76: 3568–3572.

Watson, B., F. Meng, and H. Akil. 1996. A chimeric analysis of the opioid receptor domains critical for the binding selectivity of μ-opioid ligands. Neurobiol Dis. 3: 87–96.

Watson, S. J., H. Akil, W. Fischli, et al. 1982. Dynorphin and vasopressin: Common localization in magnocellular neurons. Science 216: 85–87.

Yasuda K., K. Raynor, H. Kong, et al. 1993. Cloning and functional comparison of κ and δ opioid receptors. Proc. Natl. Acad. Sci. U.S.A. 90: 6736–6740.

Zadina, J. E., L. Hackler, L.-J. Ge, et al. 1997. A potent and selective endogenous agonist for the μ-opiate receptor. Nature 386: 499–502.

Zadina, J. E., A. J. Kastin, L. Hackler, et al. 1994b. Cyclic analogs of Tyr-W-MIF-1 with prolonged analgesic activity and potency comparable to DAMGO and morphine. Peptides 15: 1567–1569.

Zadina, J. E., A. J. Kastin, L. Hackler, et al. 1994a. Opiate receptor binding, guinea pig ileum activity, and prolonged analgesia induced by the brain peptide Tyr-W-MIF-1 and two potent analogs. Regul. Peptides 54: 341–342.

Zadina, J. E., D. Paul, K. A. Gergen, et al. 1996. Binding of Tyr-W-MIF-1 (Tyr-Pro-Trp-Gly-NH_2) and related peptides to $\mu(1)$ and $\mu(2)$ opiate receptors. Neurosci. Lett. 215: 65–69.

Zhang, X., V. M. Verge, Z. Wiesenfeld-Hallin, et al. 1993. Expression of neuropeptide mRNAs in spinal cord after axotomy in the rat, with special reference to motoneurons and galanin. Exp. Brain Res. 93: 450–461.

Chapter 15

Books and Literature Reviews

Buck, S. H. 1994. The Tachykinin Receptors. Totowa, N.J., Humana Press.

Khawaja, A. M., and D. F. Rogers. 1996. Tachykinins—receptor to effector. Int. J. Biochem. Cell Biol. 28: 721–738.

Klavdieva, M. M. 1996. The history of neuropeptides. 3. Behavioral effects of neuropeptides, tachykinins, opiate receptors and other discoveries. Neuroendocrinology 17 (2): 155–179.

Leeman, S. E., J. E. Krause, and F. Lembeck, Eds. 1991. Substance P and Related Peptides: Cellular and Molecular Physiology. Ann. N.Y. Acad. Sci. 632.

Maggi, C. A. 1995. The mammalian tachykinin receptors. Gen. Pharmacol. 26: 911–944.

Maggi, C. A. 1995. Neuropeptides as regulators of airway function: Vasoactive intestinal peptide and the tachykinins. Physiol. Rev. 75: 277–322.

Maggi, C. A. 1996. Tachykinins in the autonomic nervous system. Pharmacol. Res. 33: 161–170.

Sluka, K. A. 1996. Pain mechanisms involved in musculoskeletal disorders. J. Orthop. Sports Phys. Ther. 24: 240–254.

References

Abbadie, C., J. L. Brown, P. W. Mantyh, et al. 1996. Spinal cord substance P receptor immunoreactivity increases in both inflammatory and nerve injury models of persistent pain. Neuroscience 70: 201–209.

Alblas, J., I. Vanetten, A. Khanum, et al. 1995. C-terminal truncation of the neurokinin-2 receptor causes enhanced and sustained agonist-induced signaling—Role of receptor phosphorylation in signal attenuation. J. Biol. Chem. 270: 8944–8951.

Bai, T. R., D. Y. Zhou, T. Weir, et al. 1995. Substance P (NK1)-receptor and neurokinin-A (NK2)-receptor gene expression in inflammatory airway diseases. Am. J. Physiol. Lung, Cell. Mol. Physiol. 13: L309–317.

Bannon, M. J., D. M. Haverstick, K. Shibata, et al. 1991. Preprotachykinin gene expression in the forebrain: Regulation by dopamine. Ann. N.Y. Acad. Sci. 632: 31–37.

Barbut, D. J. M. Polak, and P. D. Wall. 1981. Substance P in spinal cord dorsal horn decreases following peripheral nerve injury. Brain Res. 205: 289–298.

Brown, J. L., H. T. Liu, J. E. Maggio, et al. 1995. Morphological characterization of SP receptor immunoreactive neurons in the rat spinal cord and trigeminal nucleus caudalis. J. Comp. Neurol. 356: 327–344.

Burcher, E., C. J. Mussap, and J. A. Stephenson. 1994. Autoradiographic localization of receptors in peripheral tissues. In: The Tachykinin Receptors. Ed. S. H. Buck. Totowa, N.J., Humana Press.

Chang, M. M., and S. E. Leeman. 1970. Isolation of a sialogogic pepide from bovine hypothalamic tissue and its characterization as substance P. J. Biol. Chem. 245: 4784–4790.

Chang, M. M., S. E. Leeman, and H. D. Niall. 1971. Amino acid sequence of substance P. Nature New Biol. 232: 86–87.

Chawla, M. K., G. M. Gutierrez, W. S. Young, et al. 1997. Localization of neurons expressing substance P and neurokinin B gene transcripts in the human hypothalamus and basal forebrain. J. Comp. Neurol. 384: 429–442.

Cooper, P. E., M. H. Fernstrom, O. P. Rorstad, et al. 1981. The regional distribution of somatostatin, substance P and neurotensin in human brain. Brain Res. 218: 219–232.

Costa, M. Jb. Furness, I. J. Llewellyn-Smith, and A. C. Cuello. 1981. The projections of substance P–containing neurons within the guinea pig small intestine. Neuroscience 6: 411–424.

Cuello, A. C. 1987. Peptides as neurotransmitters in primary sensory neurons. Neuropharmacology 26: 971–979.

Culman, J., and T. Unger. 1995. Central tachykinins—Mediators of defense reaction and stress reactions. Can. J. Physiol. Pharmacol. 73: 885–891.

Dam. T.-V., and R. Quirion. 1994. Comparative distribution of receptor types in the mammalian brain. In: The Tachykinin Receptors. Ed. S. H. Buck. Totowa, N.J., Humana Press, pp. 101–123.

Dockray, G. J. 1994. Substance P and other tachykinins. In: Gut Peptides: Biochemistry and Physiology. Eds. J. H. Walsh and G. J. Dockray. New York, Raven Press, pp. 401–422.

Duval, P., V. Lenoir, S. Moussaoui, et al. 1996. Substance P and neurokinin A variations throughout the rat estrous cycle—Comparison with ovariectomized and male rats. 1. Plasma, hypothalamus, anterior and posterior pituitary. J. Neurosci. Res. 45: 598–609.

Erspamer, V. 1949. Ricerche preliminaria sulla moschatina. Experientia 5: 79–81.

Erspamer, V., and A. Anastasi. 1962. Structure and pharmacological actions of eledoisin, the active endecapeptide of the posterior salivary glands of *Eledone*. Experientia 18: 58–59.

Euler, U. S. von, and J. H. Gaddum. 1931. An unidentified depressor substance in certain tissue extracts. J. Physiol. (Lond.) 72: 74–87.

Euler, U. S. von, and B. Pernow. 1956. Neurotropic actions of substance P. Acta Physiol. Scand. 36: 265–275.

Gates, T. S., R. P. Zimmerman, C. R. Mantyh, et al. 1988. Substance P and substance K receptor binding sites in the human gastrointestinal tract: Localization by autoradiography. Peptides 9: 1207–1219.

Helke, C. J., J. E. Krause, P. W. Mantyh, et al. 1990. Diversity in mammalian tachykinin peptidergic neurons: Multiple peptides, receptors, and regulatory mechanism. FASEB J. 4: 1606–1615.

Helke, C. J., C. A. Sasek, A. J. Niederer, et al. 1991. Tachykinins in autonomic control systems. Ann. N.Y. Acad. Sci. 632: 154–169.

Hershey, A. D., L. Polenzani, R. M. Woodward, et al. 1991. Molecular and genetic characterization, functional expression, and mRNA expression patterns of a rat substance P receptor. Ann. N.Y. Acad. Sci. 632: 63–78.

Hökfelt, T., J. O. Kellerth, G. Nilsson, et al. 1975. Substance P: Localization in the central nervous system and in some primary sensory neurons. Science 190: 889–890.

Holzer, P. 1988. Local effector functions of capsaicin-sensitive sensory nerve endings: Involvement of tachykinins, calcitonin gene-related peptide, and other neuropeptides. Neuroscience 24: 739–768.

Holzer, P., W. Schluet, and C. A. Maggi. 1995. Substance P stimulates and inhibits intestinal peristalsis via distinct receptors. J. Pharmacol. Exp. Ther. 274: 322–328.

Huang, R. R. C., D. Huang, C. D. Strader, et al. 1995. Conformational compatability as a basis of differentail affinities of tachykinins for the neurokinin 1 receptor. Biochemistry 34: 16467–16472.

Hunter, J. C., and J. E. Maggio. 1984. Pharmacological characterization of a novel tachykinin isolated from mammalian spinal cord. Eur. J. Pharmacol. 97: 159–160.

Huston, J. P., and R. U. Hasenohrl. 1995. The role of neuropeptides in learning—Focus on the neurokinin substance P. Behav. Brain Res. 66: 117–127.

Ishikawa, K., and T. Ozaki. 1997. Central tachykinins: Mediators of defense reaction and stress reactions. Can. J. Physiol. Pharmacol. 73: 91–100.

Jonassen, J. A., and S. E. Leeman. 1991. Developmental and hormonal regulation of the sex difference in preprotachykinin gene expression in rat anterior pituitaries. Ann. N.Y. Acad. Sci. 632: 1–18.

Kawanga, K., N. Minamino, A. Fukada, et al. 1983. A novel mammalian tachikinin identified in porcine spinal cord. Biochem. Biophys. Res. Comm. 114: 533–540.

Keast, J. R. 1987. Mucosal innervation and control of water and ion transport in the intestine. Rev. Physiol. Biochem. Pharmacol. 109: 1–59.

Kessler, J. A., and M. Freidin. 1991. Regulation of substance P expression in sympathetic neurons. Ann. N.Y. Acad. Sci. 632: 10–18.

Khawaja, A. M., and D. F. Rogers. 1996. Tachykinins—receptor to effector. Int. J. Biochem. Cell Biol. 28: 721–738.

Killingsworth, C. R., and S. A. Shore. 1995. Tachykinin receptors mediating contraction of guinea-pig lung strips. Regul. Peptides 57: 149–161.

Kimura, S., M. Okada, Y. Sugita, et al. 1983. Novel neuropeptides, neurokinins α and β, isolated from porcine spinal cord. Proc. Jpn. Acad. Sci. Ser. B. Phys. Biol. Sci. 59: 101–104.

Krause, J. E., J. E. Chirgwin, M. S. Carter, et al. 1987. Three rat preprotachykinin mRNAs encode the neuropeptides substance P and neurokinin A. Proc. Natl. Acad. Sci. U.S.A. 84: 881–885.

Kurihara, T., K. Yoshioka, and M. Otsuka. 1995. Tachykinergic slow depolarization of motoneurons evoked by descending fibers in the neonatal rat spinal cord. J. Physiol. (Lond.) 485: 787–796.

Lang, S., and G. Sperk. 1995. Neurochemical characterization of preprotachykinin B (50–79) immunoreactivity in the rat. Regul. Peptides 57: 183–192.

Lecci, A., and C. A. Maggi. 1995. Spinal cord tachykinins in the micturition reflex. Prog. Brain Res. 104: 145–159.

Leeman, S. E., and R. Hammerschlag. 1967. Stimulation of salivary secretion by a factor from hypothalamic tissue. Endocrinology 81: 803–810.

Lembeck, F. 1953. Zur Frage der zentralen Übertragung afferenter Impulse. III. Mitteilung. Das Vorkommen und die Bedeutung der Substanz P in den dorsalen Wurzeln des Rückenmarks. Naunyn Schmiedebergs Arch. Pharmacol. 219: 197–213.

Li, Y. Q., Z. M. Wang, H. X. Zheng, et al. 1996. Central origins of substance P–like immunoreactive fibers and terminals in the spinal trigeminal caudal subnucleus in the rat. Brain Res. 719: 219–224.

Lindefors, N., Y. Yamamoto, T. Pantaleo, et al. 1986. In vivo release of substance P in the nucleus tractus solitarii increased during hypoxia. Neurosci. Lett. 69: 94–97.

Lucas, L. R., and R. E. Harlan. 1995. Cholinergic regulation of tachykinin gene- and enkephalin-gene expression in the rat striatum. Mol. Brain Res. 30: 181–195.

Lucas, L. R., D. L. Hurley, J. E. Krause, et al. 1992. Localization of tachykinin neurokinin B precursor peptide in rat brain by immunocytochemistry and in situ hybridization. J. Comp. Neurol. 317: 341–356.

Lundberg, J. M. 1995. Tachykinins, sensory nerves and asthma—An overview. Can. J. Physiol. Pharmacol. 73: 908–914.

McCormack, R. J., R. P. Hart, and D. Ganea. 1996. Expression of NK1 receptor messenger RNA in murine T-lymphocytes. Neuroimmunomodulation 3: 35–46.

McMahon, S. B. 1996. NGF as a mediator of inflammatory pain. Philos. Trans. R. Soc. Lond. [Biol.]. 351: 431–440.

Maggi, C. A. 1995. Neuropeptides as regulators of airway function: Vasoactive intestinal peptide and the tachykinins. Physiol. Rev. 75: 277–322.

Maggi, C. A., R. Patacchini, D. Mei Feng, et al. 1991. Activity of spantide I and II at various tachykinin receptors and NK-2 tachykinin receptor subtypes. Eur. J. Pharmacol. 199: 127–129.

Maggio, J. E., B. E. B. Sandberg, C. V. Bradley, et al. 1983. Substance K: A novel tachykinin in mammalian spinal cord. In: International Substance P Symposium, Eds. P. Skrabanek and D. Powell. Irish J. Med. Sci. 152 (Supplement): 20–21.

Mantyh, P. W., S. D. Rogers, P. Horn, et al. 1997. Inhibition of hyperalgesia by ablation of lamina I spinal neurons expressing substance P receptor. Science 278: 275–279.

Mao, Y. K., Y. F. Wang, and E. E. Daniel. 1996. Characterization of neurokinin type-1 receptor in canine small intestinal muscle. Peptides 17: 839–843.

Mizuta, A., Y. Takano, K. Honda, et al. 1995. Nitric oxide is a mediator of tachykinin NK3 receptor–induced relaxation in rat mesenteric artery. Br. J. Pharmacol. 116: 2919–2922.

Nakajima, Y., S. Nakajima, and M. Inoue. 1991. Sunstance P induced inhibition of potassium channels via a pertussis toxin–insensitive G protein. Ann. N.Y. Acad. Sci. 632: 103–111.

Neugebauer, V., P. Rumenapp, and H. G. Schaible. 1996. The role of spinal neurokinin-2 receptors in the processing of nociceptive information from the joint and in the generation and maintenance of inflammation-evoked hyperexcitability of dorsal horn neurons in the rat. Eur. J. Neurosci. 8: 249–260.

Nicoll, R. A., C. Schenker, and S. E. Leeman. 1980. Substance P as a transmitter candidate. Annu. Rev. Neurosci. 3: 227–268.

Ohkubo, H., and S. Nakanoshi. 1991. Molecular characterization of the three tachykinin receptors. Ann. N.Y. Acad. Sci. 632: 53–62.

Otsuka, M., S. Konishi, M. Yanagisawa, et al. 1982. Role of substance P as a sensory transmitter in spinal cord and sympathetic ganglia. Ciba Found. Symp. 91: 13–43.

Otsuka, M., K. Yoshioka, M. Yanagisawa, et al. 1995. Use of NK1 receptor antagonists in the exploration of physiological functions of substance P and neurokinin A. Can. J. Physiol. Pharmacol. 73: 903–907.

Piggins, H. D., D. J. Cutler, and B. Rusak. 1995. Iontophoretically applied substance P activates hamster suprachiasmatic nucleus neurons. Brain Res. Bull. 37: 475–479.

Polidori, C., G. Staffiniti, M. C. Perfumi, et al. 1995. Neuropeptide gamma—A mammalian tachykinin endowed with potent antidipsogenic action in the rat. Physiol. Behav. 58: 595–602.

Regoli, D., G. Drapeau, S. Dion, et al. 1987. Pharmacological receptors for substance P and neurokinins. Life Sci. 40: 109–117.

Reid, J. J., Z. Khalil, and P. D. Marley. 1995. Modulation of neurotransmitter release by hormones and local tissue factors. In: Neurotransmitter Release and Its Modulation. Eds. D. A. Powis and S. J. Bunn. Cambridge, U.K., Cambridge University Press, pp. 123–142.

Reid, M. S., M. Herrera-Marschitz, T. Hökfelt, et al. 1990. Effects of intranigral substance P and neurokinin A on striatal dopamine release I. Interactions with substance P antagonists. Neuroscience 36: 643–658.

Ryall, R. W., and G. Belcher. 1977. Substance P selectively blocks nicotinic receptors on Renshaw cells: A possible synaptic inhibitory mechanism. Brain Res. 137: 476–380.

Schmidt, P., S. S. Poulsen, L. Hilsted, et al. 1996. Tachykinins mediate vagal inhibition of gastrin secretion in pigs. Gastroenterology 111: 925–935.

Sheldrick, R. L. G., K. F. Rabe, A. Fischer, et al. 1995. Further evidence that tachykinin-induced contraction of human isolated brochus is mediated only by NK2 receptors. Neuropeptides 29: 281–292.

Sivam, S. P. 1996. Dopamine, serotonin and tachykinin in self-injurious behavior. Life Sci. 58: 2367–2375.

Sluka, K. A. 1996. Pain mechanisms involved in musculoskeletal disorders. J. Orthop. Sports Phys. Ther. 24: 240–254.

Stoessl, A. J., M. Brackstone, N. Rajakumar, et al. 1995. Pharmacological characterization of grooming induced by a selective NK1 tachykinin receptor agonist. Brain Res. 700: 115–120.

Stoessl, A. J., E. Szczutkowski, B. Glenn, et al. 1991. Behavioral effects of selective tachykinin agonists in midbrain dopamine regions. Brain Res. 565: 254–262.

Strigas, J., and E. Burcher. 1993. Autoradiographic localization of tachykinin binding sites in guinea-pig and human airways, using selective radioligands (abstract). Clin. Exp. Pharmacol. Physiol. (Suppl. 1): 705.

Tregear, G. W., H. D. Niall, J. T. Potts, et al. 1971. Synthesis of substance P. Nature New Biol. 232: 87–89.

Tschope, C., N. Jost, T. Unger, et al. 1995. Central cardiovascular and behavioral effects of carboxy-terminal fragments of substance P in conscious rats. Brain Res. 690: 15–24.

Virta, E., S. Kangas, R. Tolonen, et al. 1991. Neurokinin A in the parotid and submandibular glands of the rat: Immunohistochemical localization and effect on protein and peroxidase secretion. Acta Physiol Scand. 142: 157–163.

Wagner, U., H. C. Fehmann, D. Bredenbroker, et al. 1995. Galanin and somatostatin inhibition of neurokinin-A and neurokinin-B induced mucus secretion in the rat. Life Sci. 57: 283–289.

Waugh, D., V. Bondareva, Y. Rusakov, et al. 1995. Tachykinins with unusual structural features from a urodele, the amphiuma, an elasmobranch, the hammerhead shark and an agnathan, the river lamprey. Peptides 16: 615–621.

Wiesenfeld-Hallin, Z., X.-J. Xu, R. Håkinson, et al. 1990. The specific antagonistic effect of intrathecal spantide II on substance P- and C-fiber conditioning stimulation-induced facilitation of the nociceptive flexor response in rat. Brain Res. 526: 284–290.

Wiesenfeld-Hallin, Z., X.-J. Xu, R. Håkinson, et al. 1991. On the role of substance P, galanin, vasoactive intestinal peptide, and calcitonin-gene–related peptide in mediation of spinal reflex excitability in rats with intact and sectioned peripheral nerves. Ann. N.Y. Acad, Sci. 632: 198–211.

Yang, L., N. D. Thomas, and C. J. Helke. 1996. Characterization of substance P release from the intermediate area of rat thoracic spinal cord. Synapse 23: 265–273.

Chapter 16

Books and Literature Reviews

Allen, J. M., and J. I. Koenig. (Eds.) 1990. Central and Peripheral Significance of Neuropeptide Y and Its Related Peptides. Ann. N.Y. Acad. Sci. 611.

Arimura, A., and S. I. Said, Eds. 1996. VIP, PACAP and Related Peptides. Second International Symposium. Ann. N.Y. Acad. Sci. 805.

Colmers, W. F., and C. Wahlestedt, Eds.. 1993. The Biology of Neuropeptide Y and Related Peptides. Totowa. N.J., Humana Press.

Crawley, J. N. 1991. Cholecystokinin-dopamine interactions. Trends Pharmacol. Sci. 12: 232–236.

Crawley, J. N., and R. L. Corwin. 1994. Biological actions of cholecystokinin. Peptides 15: 731–755.

Cuatrecasas, P., and S. Jacobs, Eds. 1990. Insulin. Berlin, Springer-Verlag.

Grundemar, L., Ed. 1997. Neuropeptide Y and Drug Development. San Diego, Academic Press.

Johnson, L. R., Ed. 1986. Physiology of the Gastrointestinal Tract. N.Y., Raven Press.

Hökfelt, T., T. Bartfai, D. Jacobowitz, et al., Eds. 1991. Galanin: A New Multifunctional Peptide in the Neuroendocrine System. New York, Macmillan.

Holzer, P. 1988. Local effector functions of capsaicin-sensitive nerve endings: Involvement of tachykinins, calcitonin gene–related peptide and other neuropeptides. Neuroscience 24: 739–768.

Ishida-Yamamoto, A., and M. Tohyama. 1989. CGRP in the nervous tissue. Prog. Neurobiol. 33: 335–386.

Ito, Z. 1984. Hormones, peptides, opioids, and prostaglandins in normal gastric contractions. In: Gastric and Gastroduodenal Motility. Eds. L. M. A. Akkermans, A. G. Johnson, and N. W. Read. New York, Praeger, pp. 41–59.

Kahn, C. R., and G. C. Weir, Eds. 1994. Joslin's Diabetes Mellitus, 13th Ed. Philadelphia, Lea & Febiger, pp. 163–176.

Kalra, S. P., and W. R. Crowley. 1992. Neuropeptide Y: A novel neuroendocrine peptide in the control of pituitary hormone secretion and its relation to luteinizing hormone. Front. Neuroendocrinol. 13: 1–46.

Mutt, V., Ed. 1988. Gastrointestinal Hormones. Advances in Metabolic Disorders, Vol. 11. San Diego, Academic Press.

Mutt, V., Ed. Neuropeptide Y. New York, Raven Press.

Reeve, J. R., Jr., V. Eysselin, T. E. Solomon, et al., Eds. 1994. Cholecystokinin. Ann. N.Y. Acad. Sci. 713.

Rostene, W. H. 1984. Neurobiological and neuroendocrine functions of the vasoactive intestinal peptide (VIP). Prog. Neurobiol. 22: 13–29.

Samols, E., Ed. 1991. The Endocrine Pancreas. New York, Raven Press.

Spindel, E. R., E. Giladi, T. P. Segerson, et al. 1993. Bombesin-like peptides: Of ligands and receptors. Recent Prog. Horm. Res. 48: 365–391.

Taché, Y., P. Melchiorri, and L. Negri. 1988. Bombesin-like Peptides in Health and Disease. Ann. N.Y. Acad. Sci. 547.

Walsh, J. H., and G. J. Dockray, Eds. 1994. Gut Peptides: Biochemistry and Physiology. New York, Raven Press.

References

Akabayashi, A., C. T. B. V. Zaia, S. M. Gabriel, et al. 1994. Intracerebroventricular injection of dibutyryl cyclic adenosine 3′5′-monophosphate increases hypothalamic levels of neuropeptide Y. Brain Res. 660: 323–328.

Alvarez, E., I. Roncero, J. A. Chowen, et al. 1996. Expression of the glucagon-like peptide-1 receptor gene in rat brain. J. Neurochem. 66: 920–927.

Amiranoff, B., N. Vauclin-Jacques, and M.Laburthe. 1985. Interaction of gastric inhibitory polypeptide (GIP) with the insulin-secreting beta-cell line In 111: Characteristics of GIP binding sites. Life Sci. 36: 805–813.

Aoki, C., and V. M. Pickel. 1990. Neuropeptide Y in cortex and striatum. Ann. N.Y. Acad. Sci. 611: 186–205.

Baldino, F., S. Fitzpatrick-McElligott, I. Gozes, et al. 1989. Localization of VIP and PHI-27 messenger RNA in rat thalamic and cortical neurons. J. Mol. Neurosci. 1: 199–207.

Bardram, L., L. Hilsted, and J. F. Rehfeld. 1989. Cholecystokinin, gastrin and their precursors in pheochromocytomas. Acta Endocrinol. (Copenhagen) 120: 479–484.

Bataille, D., P. Blache, and F. Bergeron. 1996. Endoprotease regulation of miniglucagon production. Ann. N.Y. Acad. Sci. 805: 1–9.

Battey, J., and E. Wada. 1991. Two distinct receptor subtypes for mammalian bombesin-like peptides. Trends Neurosci. 14: 524–528.

Bayliss, W. M., and E. H. Starling. 1902. The mechanism of pancreatic secretion. J. Physiol. 28: 325–353.

Beglinger, C., P. Hildebrand, R. Meier, et al. 1992. A physiological role for cholecystokinin as a regulator of gastrin. secretion. Gastroenterology 103: 490–495.

Besson, J. 1988. Distribution and pharmacology of vasoactive intestinal peptide receptors in brain and pituitary. Ann. N.Y. Acad. Sci. 527: 204–219.

Bishop, A. E., S. R. Bloom, and J. M. Polak. 1988. Cytochemical techniques in work with gastrointestinal hormones. In: Advances in Metabolic Disorders. Vol. 11, Gastrointestinal Hormones. Ed. V. Mutt. San Diego, Academic Press.

Bissonnette, B. M., M. J. Collen, H. Adachi, et al. 1984. Receptors for vasoactive intestinal peptide and secretin on rat pancreatic acini. Am. J. Physiol. 246: G710–G717.

Bloom, S. R. 1978. Vasoactive intestinal peptide, the major mediator of the WDHA (pancreatic cholera) syndrome: Value of measurement in diagnosis and treatment. Am. J. Dig. Dis. 23: 373–376.

Bloom, S. R., and A. V. Edwards. 1984. Characteristics of the neuroendocrine responses to stimulation of the splanchnic nerves in bursts in the conscious calf. J. Physiol. 346: 533–545.

Brenneman, D. E., and L. E. Eiden 1986. Vasoactive intestinal peptide and electrical activity influence neuronal survival. Proc. Natl. Acad. Sci. U.S.A. 83: 1159–1162.

Brenner, L. A., and R. C. Ritter. 1996. Type A CCK receptors mediate satiety effects of intestinal nutrients. Pharmacol. Biochem. Behav. 54: 625–631.

Buchan, A. M. J., J. M. Polak, C. Capella, et al. 1978a. Electron immunocytochemical evidence for K cell localization of gastric inhibitory polypeptide (GIP) in man. Histochemistry 546: 37–44.

Buchan, A. M. J., J. M. Polak, E. Solcia, et al. 1978b. Electron immunohistochemical evidence for the human intestinal I cell as the source of CCK. Gut 19: 403–407.

Christophe, J. 1996. Glucagon and its receptor in various tissues. Ann. N.Y. Acad. Sci. 805: 31–43.

Colmers, W. F. 1990. Modulation of synaptic transmission in hippocampus by neuropeptide Y: Presynaptic actions. Ann. N.Y. Acad. Sci. 611: 206–218.

Considine, R. V., M. K. Sinha, M. L. Heiman, et al. 1996. Serum immunoreactive leptin concentrations in normal and obese humans. N. Engl. J. Med. 334: 292–295.

Conter, R. L., M. T. Hughes, and G. L. Kaufmann. 1996. Intracerebroventricular secretin enhances pancreatic volume and bicarbonate response in rats. Surgery 119: 208–213.

Costa, M., J. B. Furness, and I. L. Gibbins. 1986a. Chemical coding of enteric neurons. Prog. Brain Res. 68: 217–239.

Costa, M., J. B. Furness, and I. J. Llewllyn-Smith. 1986b. Histochemistry of the enteric nervous system. In: Physiology of the Gastrointestinal Tract. Ed. L. R. Johnson. New York, Raven Press, p. 140.

Coy, D. H., P. Heinz-Erian, N-Y. Jiang, et al. 1988. Progress in the development of competitive bombesin antagonists. Ann. N.Y. Acad. Sci. 547: 150–157.

Crawley, J. 1985. Comparative distribution of cholecystokinin and other neuropeptides: Why is this peptide different from all other peptides? Ann. N.Y. Acad. Sci. 448: 1–8.

Crawley, J. N. 1991. Cholecystokinin-dopamine interactions. Trends Pharamacol. Sci. 12: 232–236.

Danger, J. M., M. C. Tonon, L. Cazin, et al. 1990. Regulation of MSH secretion by neuropeptide Y in amphibians. Ann. N.Y. Acad. Sci. 611: 302–315.

Deschenes, R. J., R. S. Haun, C. L. Funckes, et al. 1985. A gene encoding rat cholecystokinin. J. Biol. Chem. 260: 1280–1286.

Dockray, G. J. 1994. Vasoactive intestinal polypeptide and related peptides. In: Gut Peptides: Biochemistry and Physiology. Eds. J. H. Walsh and G. J. Dockray. New York, Raven Press, pp. 447–472.

Dougherty, D., and T. Yamada. 1989. Posttranslational processing of gastrin. Physiol. Rev. 69: 482–502.

Drucker, D. J., and S. Asa. 1988. Glucagon gene expression in vertebrate brain. J. Biol. Chem. 263: 13475–13478.

Ebert, R. and W. Creutzfeldt. 1987. Metabolic effects of gastric inhibitory polypeptide. Front. Horm. Res. 16: 175–185.

Edwards, G. L., and R. C. Ritter. 1981. Ablation of area postrema causes exaggerated consumption of preferred foods in the rat. Brain Res. 216: 265–276.

Ekblad, E. R. Hakanson, and F. Sundler. 1984. VIP and PHI coexist with NPY-like peptide in intramural neurons of the small intestine. Regul. Peptides 10: 47–55.

Eng, J. H.-R. Li, and R. S. Yalow. 1990. Purification of bovine cholecystokinin-58 and sequencing of its N-terminus. Regul. Peptides 30: 15–19.

Erickson, J. C., G. Hollopeter, and R. D. Palmiter. 1996. Attenuation of obesity syndrome of *ob/ob* mice by the loss of neuropeptide Y. Science 274: 1704–1707.

Erspamer, V., G. Falconieri Erspamer, M. Inselvini, et al. 1972. Occurrence of bombesin and alytesin in extracts of the skin of three European discoglossid frogs and pharmacological actions of bombesin on extravascular smooth muscle. Br. J. Pharmacol. 45: 333–348.

Erusalimsky, J. D., I. Friedberg, and E. Rozengurt. 1988. Bombesin, diacylglycerols and phorbol esters rapidly stimulate the phosphorylation of an $M_r = 80{,}000$ protein kinase C substrate in permeabilized 3T3 cells; effects of gunanine nucleotides. J. Biol. Chem. 263: 19188–19194.

Fahrenkrug, J., J. Holst Pedersen, Y. Yamashita, et al. 1987. Occurrence of VIP and peptide HM in human pancreas and their influence on pancreatic endocrine secretion in man. Regul. Peptides 18: 51–61.

Fahrenkrug, F., B. Ottesen, and C. Palle. 1988. Vasoactive intestinal polypeptide and the reproductive system. Ann. N.Y. Acad. Sci. 527: 393–404.

Fan, W., B. A. Boston, R. A. Kesterson, et al. 1997. Role of melanocortinergic neurons in feeding and the *agouti* obesity syndrome. Naure 385: 165–168.

Fehmann, H. C., and J. F. Habener. 1991. Functional receptors for the insulinotropic hormone glucagon-like peptide-1 (7–36) amide on a somatostatin-secreting cell line. FEBBS Lett. 279: 335–340.

Flood, J. F., and J. E. Morley. 1989. Dissociation of the effects of neuropeptide Y on feeding and memory: Evidence for pre- and postsynaptic mediation. Peptides 10: 963–966.

Flynn, F. W. 1996. Mammalian bombesin-like peptides suppress sham drinking of salt by sodium-deficient rats. Peptides 17: 951–956.

Fuxe, K., L. F. Agnati, A. Harfstrand, et al. 1989. Studies on the neurochemical mechanisms underlying the neuroendocrine actions of neuropeptide Y. In: Neuropeptide Y. Eds. Y. V. Mutt, T. Hökfelt, K. Fuxe, et al. New York, Raven Press, pp. 115–136.

Fuxe, K., J. A. Aguirre, L. F. Agnati, et al. 1990. Neuropeptide Y and central cardiovascular regulation. Ann. N.Y. Acad. Sci. 611: 111–132.

Gardner, J. D., and R. T. Jensen. 1984. Cholecystokinin receptor antagonists. Am. J. Physiol. 246: G471–G476.

Gardner, J. D., and R. T. Jensen. 1990. Role of receptors in expression of gastrointestinal hormone functions. In: Gastrointestinal Endocrinology: Receptors and Post-Receptor Mechanisms. Ed. J. C. Thompson. San Diego, Academic Press, pp. 1–12.

Gibbs, J., R. C. Young, and G. P. Smith. 1978. Cholecystokinin decreases food intake in rats. J. Comp. Physiol. Psychol. 84: 488–495.

Glazer, R., and I. Gozes. 1994. Diurnal oscillation in vasoactive intestinal peptide gene expression independent of environmental light entraining. Brain Res. 644: 164–168.

Gozes, I. 1988. Biosynthesis and regulation of expression: The vasoactive intestinal peptide gene. Ann. N.Y. Acad. Sci. 527: 77–86.

Gozes, I., A. Bardea, M. Bechar, et al. 1997. Neuropeptides and neuronal survival: Neuroprotective strategy for Alzheimer's disease. Ann. N.Y. Acad. Sci. 814: 161–166.

Gozes, I., and D. E. Brenneman. 1993. Neuropeptides as growth and differentiation factors in general and VIP in particular. J. Mol. Neurosci. 4: 1–9.

Gozes, I., M. Fridkin, and D. E. Brenneman. 1995. A VIP hybrid antagonist: From developmental neurobiology to clinical applications. Cell Mol. Neurobiol. 15: 675–687.

Gozes, I., G. Lilling, A. Davidson, et al. 1996. Development of VIP agonists and antagonists with tissue and receptor specificity: Effects on behavioral maturation, sexual function and the biologic clock. Ann. N.Y. Acad. Sci. 805: 159–171.

Gressens, P., J. M. Hill, I. Gozes, et al. 1993. Growth factor function of vasoactive intestinal peptide in whole cultured mouse embryos. Nature 362: 155–158.

Gressens, P., J. M. Hill, B. Paindaveine, et al. 1994. Severe microencephaly induced by blockade of vasoactive intestinal peptide function in the primitive neuroepithelium of the mouse. J. Clin. Invest. 94: 2020–2027.

Grider, J. R. 1994. Role of neuropeptides in peristalsis. In: Gut Peptides: Biochemistry and Physiology. Eds. J. H. Walsh and G. J. Dockray. New York, Raven Press, pp. 701–713.

Grider, J. R., and G. M. Makhlouf. 1986. Colonic peristaltic reflex: Identification of vasoactive intestinal peptide as mediator of descending relaxation. Am. J. Physiol. 251: G40–G45.

Gubler, U., A. O. Chua, B. J. Hoffman, et al. 1984. Cloned cDNA to cholecystokinin mRNA prohormones cholecystokinin and gastrin. Proc. Natl. Acad. Sci. U.S.A. 81: 4307–4310.

Gutniak, M., J. J. Holst, C. Ørskov, et al. 1992. Antidiabetogenic effect of glucagon-like peptide-1 (7–36)amide in normal subjects and patients with diabetes mellitus. N. Engl. J. Med. 236: 1316–1322.

Han, J. S., X. Z. Ding, and S. G. Fan. 1986. Cholecystokinin octapeptide (CCK-8): Antagonism to electroacupuncture analgesia and a possible role in electroacupuncture tolerance. Pain 27: 101–115.

Hansen, L. H., N. Abrahamsen, and E. Nishimura. 1995. Glucagon receptor mRNA distribution in rat tissues. Peptides 16: 1163–1166.

Haun, R. S., C. D. Minth, P. C. Andrews, et al. 1989. Molecular biology of gut peptides. In: Handbook of

Physiology; the Gastrointestinal System. Vol. 2, Neural and Endocrine Biology. Ed. G. M. Makhlouf. New York, Oxford University Press, pp. 1–43.

Heinemann, A., M. Jocic, B. M. Peskar, et al. 1996. CCK-evoked hyperemia in rat gastric mucosa involves neural mechanisms and nitric oxide. Am. J. Physiol. 33: G253–G258.

Heinz-Erian, P., and S. I. Said. 1988. Vasoactive intestinal peptide as a regulator of exocrine function and a possible factor in cystic fibrosis. Ann. N.Y. Acad. Sci. 527: 568–573.

Hill, J. M., D. V. Agoston, P. Gressens, et al. 1994. Distribution of VIP mRNA and two distinct VIP binding sites in the developing rat brain: Relation to ontogenic events. J. Comp. Neurol. 342: 186–205.

Hill, J. M., P. Gressens, and D. E. Brenneman. 1997. Growth of the early postimplantation embryo. Ann. N.Y. Acad. Sci. 814: 174–180.

Hill, J. M., R. F. Mervis, J. Politi, et al. 1994. Blockade of VIP during neonatal development induces neuronal damage and increases VIP and VIP receptors in brain. Ann. N.Y. Acad. Sci. 527: 211–225.

Hökfelt, T., X. Zhang, and Z. Wiesenfeld-Hallin. 1994. Messenger plasticity in primary sensory neurons following axotomy and its functional implications. Trends Neurosci. 17: 22–30.

Holzer, P., I. T. Lippe, L. Bartho, et al. 1987. Neuropeptide Y inhibits excitatory enteric neurons supplying the circular muscle of the guinea pig small intestine. Gastroenterology 92: 1944–1950.

Huszar, D., C. A. Lynch, V. Fairchild Huntress, et al. 1997. Targeted disruption of the melanocortin 4 receptor results in obesity in mice. Cell 88: 131–141.

Inagaki, N., Y. Seino, J. Takeda, et al. 1989. Gastric inhibitory polypeptide: Structure and chromosomal localization of the human gene. Mol. Endocrinol. 3: 1014–1021.

Ishihara, T., S. Nakamura, Y. Kaziro, et al. 1991. Molecular cloning and expression of a cDNA encoding the secretin receptor, EMBO J. 10: 1635–1641.

Ito, Z., K. Sato, T. Helmer, G. Jay and K. Agarwal. 1984. Structural analysis of the gene encoding human gastrin: the large intron contains an Alu sequence. Proc. Natl. Acad. Sci. U.S.A. 81: 4662–4666.

Jarhult, J., L. O. Farnebo, and F. Hamberger. 1981. The relation between catechoamines, glucagon, and pancreatic polypeptide during hypoglycemia in man. Acta Endocrinol. 98: 402–406.

Jörnvall, H., M. Carlquist, S. Kwauk, et al. 1981. Amino acid sequence and heterogeneity of gastric inhibitory peptide (GIP). FEBS Lett. 123: 205–210.

Karnik, P. S., S. J. Monahan, and M. M. Wolfe. 1989. Inhibition of gastrin gene expression by somatostatin. J. Clin. Invest. 83: 367–372.

Katchinski, M., J. Schirra, C. Beglinger, et al. 1996. Intestinal phase of human anteropyloroduodenal motility: Cholinergic and CCK-mediated regulation. Eur. J. Clin. Invest. 26: 574–583.

Kentroti, S., and S. M. McCann. 1996. Role of dopamine in the inhibitory control of growth hormone and prolactin release by gastrin-releasing peptide. Brain Res. Bull. 39: 201–204.

Kirby, D. A., K. T. Britton, M. L. Aubert, et al. 1997. Identification of high potency neuropeptide Y analogs through systemic lactamization. J. Med. Chem. 40: 210–215.

Knuhtsen, S., J. J. Holst, S. L. Jensen, et al. 1985. Gastrin-releasing peptide: Effect on exocrine secretion and release from isolated perfused porcine pancreas. Am. J. Physiol. 248: G281–G286.

Kopin, A. 1992. Expression, cloning and characterization of the canine parietal cell gastrin receptor. Proc. Natl. Acad. Sci. U.S.A. 89: 3605–3609.

Kopin, A., M. B. Wheeler, J. Nishitani, et al. 1991. The secretin gene: Evolutionary history, alternative splicing and developmental regulation. Proc. Natl. Acad. Sci. U.S.A. 88: 5335–5339.

Kopin, A. S., M. B. Wheeler, and A. B. Leiter. 1990. Secretin: Structure of the precursor and tissue distribution of the mRNA. Proc. Natl. Acad. Sci. U.S.A. 87: 2299–2303.

Krasinski, S. D., M. S. Wheeler, and A. S. Kopin. 1990. Pancreatic and peptide YY gene expression. Ann. N.Y. Acad. Sci. 611: 73–88.

Larhammar, D., A. Ericsson, and H. Persson. 1987. Structure and expression of the rat neuropeptide Y gene. Proc. Natl. Acad. Sci. U.S.A. 84: 2068–2072.

Lee, Y., S. Shiosaka, P. E. Emson, et al. 1985. Neuropeptide Y–like immunoreactive structures in the rat stomach with special reference to the noradrenaline neurons system. Gastroenterology 89: 118–126.

Leiter, A. B., W. Y Chey, and A. S. Kopin. 1994. Secretin. In: Gut Peptides: Biochemistry and Physiology. Eds. J. H. Walsh and G. J. Dockray. New York, Raven Press, pp. 147–173.

Leiter, A. B., M. R. Montminy, and E. Jamieson. 1985. Exons of the human pancreatic polypeptide gene define functional domains of the precursor. J. Biol. Chem. 260: 14702–14705.

Li, P., K. Y. Lee, T.-M. Chang, et al. 1990. Mechanism of acid-induced release of secretin in rats: Presence of a secretin releasing factor. J. Clin. Invest. 86: 1474–1479.

Liddle, R. A. 1994a. Regulation of cholecystokinin gene expression in rat intestine. Ann. N.Y. Acad. Sci. 713: 22–31.

Liddle, R. A. 1994b. Cholecystokinin. In: Gut Peptides: Biochemistry and Physiology. Ed. J. H. Walsh and G. J. Dockray. New York, Raven Press, pp. 175–216.

Liddle, R. A., B. J. Gertz, S. Kanayama, et al. 1989. Effects of a novel cholecystokinin (CCK) receptor antagonist, MK-329, on gallbladder contraction and gastric emptying in humans: Implications for the physiology of CCK. J. Clin. Invest. 84: 1220–1225.

Love, J. A., V. L. G. Go, and J. H. Szurszewski. 1988. Vasoactive intestinal peptide and other peptides as neuromodulators of colonic motility in the guinea pig. Ann. N.Y. Acad. Sci. 527: 360–368.

Lu, L. D. Louie, and C. Owyang. 1989. A cholecystokinin releasing peptide mediates feedback regulation of pancreatic secretion. Am. J. Physiol. 256: G175–G181.

Lund, P. K., R. H. Goodman, P. C. Dee, et al. 1982. Pancreatic preproglucagon cDNA contains two glucagon-related coding sequences arranged in tandem. Proc. Natl. Acad. Sci. U.S.A. 79: 345–349.

McDonald, J. K. 1988. NPY and related substances. Crit. Rev. Neurobiol. 4: 97–135.

Magistretti, P. J., O. Sorg, N. Yu, et al. 1993. Neurotransmitters regulate energy metabolism in astrocytes: Implications for the metabolic trafficking between neural cells. Dev. Neurosci. 15: 306–312.

Maggi, C. A., A. Giachetti, R. D. Dey, et al. 1995. Neuropeptides as regulators of airway function: Vasoactive intestinal peptide and the tachykinins. Physiol Rev. 75: 277–322.

Makhlouf, G. M., and M. L. Schubert. 1988. Antral bombesin: Physiological regulator of gastrin secretion. Ann. N.Y. Acad. Sci. 547: 225–233.

Manela, F. D., J. Ren, J. Gao, et al. 1985. Calcitonin gene–related peptide modulates acid-mediated regulation of somatostatin and gastrin release from rat antrum. Gastroenterology 109: 701–706.

Mangel, A. W. 1984. Potentiation of colonic contractility to cholecystokinin and other peptides. Eur. J. Pharmacol. 100: 285–290.

Maruyama, H. A. Histatomi, L. Orci, et al. 1994. Insulin within islets is a physiological glucagon release inhibitor. J. Clin. Invest. 74: 2296–2299.

Merchanthaler, I., F. J. Lopez, and A. Negro-Vilar. 1993. Anatomy and physiology of central galanin-containing pathways. Prog. Neurobiol. 40: 711–769.

Miholic, J. C. Ørskov, J. J. Holst, et al. 1991. Emptying of the gastric substitute, glucagon-like peptide-1 (GLP-1) and reactive hypoglycemia after total gastrectomy. Dig. Dis. Sci. 36: 1361–1370.

Minamino, N., K. Kangawa, and H. Matsuo. 1988. Neuromedin B and neuromedin C: Two mammalian bombesin-like peptides identified in porcine spinal cord and brain. Ann. N.Y. Acad. Sci. 547: 373–390.

Mitchell, J. E., D. E. Laine, J. E. Morley, et al. 1986. Naloxone but not CCK-8 may attenuate binge-eating behavior in patients with the bulimia syndrome. Biol. Psychol. 21: 1399–1406.

Miyasaka, K., R. A. Liddle, and G. M. Green. 1989. Feedback regulation by trypsin: Evidence for intraluminal CCK-releasing peptide. Am. J. Physiol. 257: G175–G181.

Moghimazadeh, E. R. Ekman, R. Håkanson, et al. 1983. Neuronal gastrin-releasing peptide in the mammalian gut and pancreas. Neuroscience 10: 553–563.

Mojsov, S., G. Heinrich, and I. B. Wilson. 1986. Preproglucagon gene expression in pancreas and intestine diversifies at the level of post-translational processing. J. Biol. Chem. 261: 11880–11889.

Moody, A. J., L. Thim, and I. Valverde. 1984. The isolation and sequencing of human gastric inhibitory peptide (GIP). FEBS Lett. 172: 142–148.

Moody, T. W., R. Getz, T. L. O'Donohue, et al. 1988. Localization of receptors for bombesin-like peptides in the rat brain. Ann. N.Y. Acad. Sci. 547: 114–130.

Moriarty, K. J., J. E. Hegarty, K. Tatemoto, et al. 1984. Effect of peptide histidine isoleucine on water and electrolyte transport in the human jejunum. Gut 25: 624–628.

Morley, J. S., H. J. Tracy, and R. A. Gregory. 1965. Structure-function relationships in the active C-terminal tetrapeptide sequence of gastrin. Nature 207: 1356–1359.

Mutt, V., and J. E. Jorpes. 1968. Structure of porcine cholecystokinin-pancrezymin. Cleavage with thrombin and with trypsin. Eur. J. Biochem. 6: 156–162.

Namba, M., M. A. Ghatei, A. E. Bishop, et al. 1985. Presence of neuromedin B–like immunoreactivity in the brain and gut of rat and guinea pig. Peptides 6 (Suppl. 3): 257–163.

Nicolodi, M., and E. Del Bianco. 1990. Sensory neuropeptides (substance P, calcitonin gene–related peptide) and vasoactive intestinal polypeptide in human saliva: Their pattern in migraine and cluster headache. Cephalalgia 10: 39–50.

Niederau, C., R. A. Liddle, K. A. Williams, et al. 1987. Pancreatic growth: Interaction of exogenous cholecystokinin, a protease inhibitor, and a cholecystokinin receptor antagonist in mice. Gut 28: (Suppl. 1). 63–69.

O'Hare, M. M. T., S. Tenmoku, L. Aakerland, et al. 1988. Neuropeptide Y in guinea pig, rabbit, rat and man. Identical amino acid sequence and oxidation of methionine-17. Regul. Peptides 20: 293–304.

Orci, L., and A. Perrelet. 1981. The morphology of the A-cell. In: Glucagon: Physiology, Pathophysiology and Morphology of the Pancreatic A-cells. Eds. R. H. Unger and L. Orci. New York, Elsevier, pp. 3–36.

Ørskov, C., M. Bersani, A. H. Johnson, et al. 1989. Complete sequences of glucagon-like peptide-1 from human and pig small intestine. J. Biol. Chem. 264: 12826–12829.

Ørskov, C., J. J. Holst, and S. Knuhtsen. 1986. Glucagon-like peptides GLP-1 and GLP-2, predicted products of the glucagon gene, are secreted separately from the pig small intestine but not pancreas. Endocrinology 119: 1467–1475.

Oshea, D., I. Gunn, X. H. Chen, et al. 1996. A role for central glucagon-like peptide-1 in temperature regulation. Neuroreport 7: 830–832.

Ottoway, C. A. 1988. Vasoactive intestinal peptide as a modulator of lymphocyte and immune function. Ann. N.Y. Acad. Sci. 527: 486–500.

Owyang, C. 1996. Physiological mechanisms of cholecystokinin action on pancreatic secretion. Am. J. Physiol. 34: G1–G7.

Owyang, C., D. S. Louie, and D. Tatum. 1986. Feedback regulation of pancreatic enzyme secretion—suppression of cholecystokinin release by trypsin. J. Clin. Invest. 84: 1220–1225.

Pederson, R. A., H. E. Schubert, and J. C. Brown. 1975. Gastric inhibitory polypeptide, its physiological release and insulinotropic action in the dog. Diabetes 24: 1050–1056.

Pert, C. B., J. M. Hill, M. R. Ruff, et al. 1986. Octapeptides deduced from the neuropeptide receptor-like pattern of antigen T4 in brain potently inhibit human immunodeficiency virus receptor binding and T-cell infectivity. Proc. Natl. Acad. Sci. U.S.A. 83: 9254–9258.

Pert, C. B., C. C. Smith, M. R. Ruff, et al. 1988. AIDS and its dementia as a neuropeptide disorder: Role of VIP receptor blockade by human immunodeficiency virus envelope. Ann. Neurol. 23 (Suppl.): S71–S73.

Pincus, D. W., E. M. Dicicco-Bloom, and I. B. Black. 1990. Vasoactive intestinal peptide regulates mitosis, differentiation and survival of cultured sympathetic neuroblasts. Nature 343: 564–567.

Ponsalle, P., L. Srivastava, R. Unt, et al. 1992. Glucocorticoids are required for food-deprivation-induced increases in hypothalamic neuropeptide Y expression. J. Neuroendocrinol. 4: 586–591.

Power, R. F., A. E. Bishop, J. Wharton, et al. 1988. Anatomical distribution of vasoactive intestinal polypeptide binding sites in peripheral tissues investigated by in vitro autoradiography. Ann. N.Y. Acad. Sci. 527: 314–325.

Presse, F., I. Sorokovsky, J. P. Max, et al. 1996. Melanin-concentrating hormone is a potent anorectic peptide regulated by food deprivation and glucopenia in the rat. Neuroscience 71: 735–745.

Qu, D., D. S. Ludwig, S. Gammeltoft, et al. 1996. A role for melanin-concentrating hormone in the central regulation of feeding behavior. Nature 380: 243–247.

Rao, R. K., Y. Lopez. J. Lai, et al. 1996. Attenuation of gastrin induced gastric acid secretion by antisense oligonucleotide to the CCK B/gastrin receptor. Neuroreport 6: 2373–2377.

Rehfeld, J. F., L. I. Larsson, K. Stengaard-Pedersen, et al. 1984. Gastrin and cholecystokinin in pituitary neurons. Proc. Natl. Acad. Sci. U.S.A. 81: 1902–1905.

Reeve, J. R., Jr., V. Eysselein, F. J. Ho, et al. 1994. Natural and synthetic cholecystokinin. Ann. N.Y. Acad. Sci. 713: 11–31.

Reeve, J. R., Jr., V. Eysselein, J. H. Walsh, et al. 1986. New molecular forms of cholecystokinin—microsequence analysis of forms previously characterized by chromatographic methods. J. Biol. Chem. 261: 16392–16397.

Rosselin, G. 1994. Vasoactive Intestinal Peptide, Pituitary Adenylate Cyclase Activating Polypeptide and Related Peptides: From Molecular Biology to Clinical Applications. Singapore, World Scientific Publishers.

Rostene, W. H. 1984. Neurobiological and neuroendocrine functions of the vasoactive intestinal peptide (VIP). Prog. Neurobiol. 22: 1–129.

Rovere, C., A. Viale, J. H. Nahon, et al. 1996. Impaired processing of brain proneurotensin and promelanin-concentrating hormone in obese fat/fat mice. Endocrinology 137: 2954–2958.

Ruff, M. R., P. L. Hallberg, J. M. Hill, et al. 1988. Peptide T_{4-8} is core envelope sequence required for CD4 receptor attachment. Lancet 8561: 751.

Said, S. I. 1988. Vasoactive intestinal peptide in the lung. Ann. N.Y. Acad. Sci. 527: 450–464.

Said, S. I., and V. Mutt. 1970. Potent peripheral and splanchnic vasodilator peptide from normal gut. Nature 225: 863–864.

Saito, A., H. Sankaran, I. D. Goldfine, et al. 1980. Cholecystokinin receptors in the brain: Characterization and distribution. Science 208: 1155–1156.

Sakuri, T., A. Amemiya, M. Ishii, et al. 1998. Orexins and orexin receptors: A family of hypothalamic neuropeptides and G protein-coupled receptors that regulate feeding behavior. Cell 92: 573–585.

Sandvick, A. K., and H. L. Waldum. 1991. CCK-B (gastrin) receptor regulates gastric histamine release and acid secretion. Am. J. Physiol. 260: G925–G928.

Saria, A., and E. Beubler. 1985. Neuropeptide Y (NPY) and peptide YY (PYY) inhibit prostaglandin E2–induced intestinal fluid and electrolyte secretion in the rat jejunum in vivo. Eur. J. Pharmacol. 119: 47–52.

Sarson, D. L., N. Scopinari and S. R. Bloom. 1981. Gut hormone changes after jejunoileal(JIB) or biliopancreatic (BPB) bypass surgey for morbid obesity. Int. J. Obes. Relat. Metab. Disord. 5: 471–480.

Sausville, E. A., A.-M. Lebacq-Verheyden, E. R. Spindel, et al. 1986. Expression of the gastrin-releasing peptide in human small cell lung cancer. Evidence for alternative processing resulting in three distinct RNAs. J.Biol. Chem. 261: 2451–2457.

Scherubl, H., S. Faiss, T. Zimmer, et al. 1996. Neuroendocrine tumors of the gastroenteropancreatic system. 1. Diagnostic advances. Oncologie 19: 119–124.

Schiffmann, S. N., and J. J. Vanderhaeghen. 1991. Distribution of cells containing mRNA encoding cholecystokinin in the rat central nervous system. J. Comp. Neurol. 304: 219–233.

Schojldager, B., X. Molero, and L. J. Miller. 1989. Functional and biochemical characterization of the human gallbladder muscularis cholcystokinin receptor. Gastroenterology 96: 1119–1126.

Schubert, M. L., and J. Hightower. 1989. Inhibition of acid secretion by bombesin is partly mediated by release of fundic somatostatin. Gastroenterology 97: 561–567.

Schubert, M. L., B. Saffouri, J. H. Walsh, et al. 1985. Inhibition of neurally mediated gastrin secretion by bombesin. Am. J. Physiol. 248: G456–G462.

Schwartz, M. W., R. J. Seeley, L. A. Campfield, et al. 1996. Identification of targets of leptin action in the rat hypothalamus. J. Clin. Invest. 98: 1101–1106.

Segre, G., and S. Goldring. 1993. Receptors for secretin, calcitonin, parathyroid hormone (PTH)/PTH-related peptide, vasoactive intestinal peptide, glucagon-like peptide 1, growth hormone releasing hormone, and glucagon belong to a newly discovered G-protein–linked receptor family. Trends Endocrinol. Metab. 4: 309–314.

Singh, L., M. J. Field, J. C. Hunter, et al. 1996. Modulation of the in vivo actions of morphine by the mixed CCKA/B receptor antagonist PD 142898. Eur. J. Pharmacol. 307: 283–289.

Singh, P., B. Rae Venter, C. M. Townsend, Jr., et al. 1985. Gastrin receptors in normal and malignant gastrointestinal mucosa: Age-associated changes. Am. J. Physiol. 249: G761–G769.

Sjoqvist, A., and J. Fahrenkrug. 1986. Sympathetic nerve activation decreases the release of vasoactive intestinal polypeptide from the feline intestine. Acta Physiol. Scand. 127: 419–423.

Smith, G. P., and J. Gibbs. 1985. The satiety effect of cholecystokinin: Recent progress and current problems. Ann. N.Y. Acad. Sci. 448: 417–423.

Smith, J. P., J. G. Wood, and T. E. Solomon. 1989. Elevated gastrin levels in patients with colon cancer or adenomatous polyps. Dig. Dis. Sci. 34: 171–174.

Stanley, B. G., D. R. Daniel, A. S. Chin, et al. 1985. Paraventricular nucleus injections of peptide YY and neuropeptide Y preferably enhance carbohydrate ingestion. Peptides 6: 1205–1211.

Stephens, T. W., P. W. Bristow, S. G. Burgett, et al. 1995. The role of neuropeptide Y in the antiobesity action of the obese gene product. Nature 377: 530–532.

Taché, Y., T. Ishikawa, M. Gunion, et al. 1988. Central nervous system action of bombesin to influence gastric secretion and ulceration. Ann. N.Y. Acad. Sci. 547: 183–193.

Takahashi, Y., S. Fukushige, T. Murotsu, et al. 1986. Structure of human cholecystokinin gene and its chromosomal location. Gene 50: 353–360.

Takeda, J., Y. Seino, K. Tanaka, et al. 1987. Sequence of an intestinal cDNA encoding human gastric inhibitory polypeptide precursor. Proc. Natl. Acad. Sci. U.S.A. 84: 7005–7008.

Tangchristensen, M., P. J. Larsen, R. Goke, et al. 1996. Central administration of GLP-1 (7–36) amide inhibits food and water intake in rats. Am. J. Physiol. 40: R848–R856.

Tatemoto, K., M. Carlquist, and V. Mutt. 1981. Neuropeptide Y—a novel brain peptide with structural similarities to peptide YY and pancreatic polypeptide. Nature 296: 659–660.

Tatemoto, K., and V. Mutt. 1981. Isolation and characterization of the intestinal peptide porcine PHI (PHI-27), a new member of the glucagon/secretin family. Proc. Natl. Acad. Sci. U.S.A. 78: 6603–6607.

Taylor, I. L. 1985. Distribution and release of peptide YY in dog measured by specific radioimmunoassay. Gastroenterology 89: 1070–1077.

Uemura, S., S. Pompolo, and B. Furness. 1995. Colocalization of neuropeptide Y with other neurochemical markers in the guinea pig small intestine. Archi. Histol. Cytol. 58: 523–536.

Unger, R. H., and L. Orci. 1990. Glucagon. J. Clin. Invest. 74: 2296–2299.

Varndell, I. M., A. Harris, F. J. Tapia, et al. 1983. Intracellular topography of immunoreactive gastrin demonstrated using electron microscopy. Experientia 39: 713–717.

Wada, E., J. Way, A. M. Lebacq-Verheyden, et al. 1990. Neuromedin B and gastrin-releasing peptide mRNAs are differentially distributed in the rat nervous system. J. Neurosci. 10: 2917–2930.

Walsh, J. H. 1988. Peptides as regulators of gastric acid secretion. Annu. Rev. Physiol. 50: 41–63.

Walsh, J. H., H. C. Wong, and G. J. Dockray. 1979. Bombesin-like peptides in mammals. Fed. Proc. 38: 219–225.

Wank, S. A., 1995. Cholecystokin receptors. Editorial review. Am. J. Physiol. 269: G628–G646.

Wank, S. A., R. Harkins, R. T. Jensen, et al. 1992. Purification, molecular cloning and functional expression of the cholecystokinin receptor from rat pancreas. Proc. Natl. Acad. Sci. U.S.A. 89: 3125–3129.

Wank, S. A., J. R. Pisegna, and A. de Weerth. 1994. Cholecystokinin receptor family: Molecular cloning, gene structure, and functional expression in rat, guinea pig, and human. Ann. N.Y. Acad. Sci. 713: 49–66.

Whitcomb, D. C., I. L. Taylor, and S. R. Vigna. 1990. Characterization of saturable binding sites for circulating pancreatic polypeptide in brain. Am. J. Physiol. 259: G687–G691.

Wiesenfeld-Hallin, Z., and X.-J. Xu. 1996. The role of cholecystokinin in nociception, neuropathic pain and opiate tolerance. Regul. Peptides 65: 23–38.

Wolkowitz, O. M., B. Gertz, H. Weingartner, et al. 1990. Hunger in humans induced by MK-329, a specific peripheral type cholecystokinin receptor antagonist. Biol. Psychol. 28: 169–173.

Wood, S. M., M. E. Kraenzlin, T. E. Adrian, et al. 1985. Treatment of patients with endocrine tumours using a new long-acting somatostatin analogue: Symptomatic and peptide responses. Gut 26: 438–444.

Wu, J. Y., K. A. Henins, P. Gressens, et al. 1997. Neurobehavioral development of neonatal mice following blockade of VIP during the early embryonic period. Peptides 18: 1131–1137.

Yamagami, T., K. Ohsawa, M. Nishizawa, et al. 1988. Complete nucleotide sequence of human vasoactive intestinal peptide/PHM-27 gene and its inducible promoter. Ann. N.Y. Acad. Sci. 527: 87–102.

Yamaguchi, K., K. Abe, and T. Kameya. 1983. Production and molecular size heterogeneity of immunoreactive gastrin-releasing peptide in fetal and adult lungs and primary lung tumors. Cancer Res. 43: 3932–3939.

Chapter 17

Books and Literature Reviews

Bedecs, K., M. Berthold, and T. Bartfai. 1995. Galanin—10 years with a neuroendocrine peptide. Int. J. Biochem. Cell Biol. 27: 337–349.

De Pablo, F., L. A. Scott, and J. Roth. 1990. Insulin and insulin-like growth factor I in early development: Peptides, receptors and biological events. Endocr. Rev. 11: 558–577.

Hökfelt, T, T. Bartfai, D. Jacobowitz, et al., Eds. 1991. Galanin: A New Multifunctional Peptide in the Neuroendocrine System. New York, Macmillan.

Holzer, P. 1988. Local effector functions of capsaicin-sensitive endings: Involvement of tachykinins, calcitonin gene–related peptide and other neuropeptides. Neuroscience 24: 739–768.

Ishida-Yamamoto, A., and M. Tohyama. 1989. Calcitonin gene–related peptide in the nervous tissue. Prog. Neurobiol. 33: 335–386.

Johnson, L. R., Ed. 1986. Physiology of the Gastrointestinal Tract. New York, Raven Press.

Kahn, C. R., and G. C. Weir, Eds. 1994. Joslin's Diabetes Mellitus, 13th Ed. Philadelphia, Lea & Febiger.

Philippe, J. 1991. Structure and pancreatic expression of the insulin and glucagon genes. Endocr. Rev. 12: 252–271.

Samols, E., Ed. 1991. The Endocrine Pancreas. New York, Raven Press.

Taché, Y., P. Holzer, and M. G. Rosenfeld, Eds. 1992. Calcitonin gene–related peptide: The first decade of a pleiotropic peptide. Ann. N.Y. Acad. Sci. 657.

Walsh, J. H., and G. J. Dockray, Eds. 1994. Gut Peptides: Biochemistry and Physiology. New York, Raven Press.

Wimalawansa, U. J. 1996. Calcitonin gene–related peptide and its receptors: Molecular genetics, physiology, pathophysiology and therapeutic potentials. Endocr. Rev. 17: 533–585.

References

Aiyar, N., K. Rand, N. A. Elshourbagy, et al. 1996. A cDNA encoding the calcitonin gene–related peptide type 1 receptor. J. Biol. Chem. 271: 11325–11329.

Amara, S. G., V. Jonas, M. G. Rosenfeld, et al. 1982. Alternative RNA processing in calcitonin gene expression generates mRNAs encoding different polypeptide products. Nature 298: 240–244.

Backer, J. M., C. R. Kahn, and M. F. White. 1989. Tyrosine phosphorylation of the insulin receptor is not required for receptor internalization: Studies in 2,4-dinitrophenol-treated rats. Proc. Natl. Acad. Sci. U.S.A. 86: 3209–3213.

Banting, F. G., and C. H. Best. 1922. The internal secretion of the pancreas. J. Lab. Clin. Med. 7: 251–266.

Bauer, F. E., A. Zintel, M. J. Kenny, et al. 1989. Inhibitory effect of galanin on postprandial gastrointestinal motility and gut hormone release in humans. Gastroenterology 97: 260–264.

Bauerfeind, P. R., R. Hof, A. Hof, et al. 1989. Effects of hCGRP I and II on gastric blood flow and acid secretion in anesthetized rabbits. Am. J. Physiol. 256: G145–G149.

Bedecs K., M. Berthold, and T. Bartfai. 1995. Galanin—10 years with a neuroendocrine peptide. Int. J. Biochem. Cell. Biol. 27: 337–349.

Benmoussa, M., A. Chait, G. Loric, et al. 1996. Low doses of neurotensin in the preoptic area produce hyperthermia: Comparison with other brain sites and with neurotensin-induced analgesia. Brain Res. Bull. 39: 275–279.

Berthoud, H. R. 1996. Morphological analysis of vagal input to gastrin-releasing peptide and vasoactive intestinal polypeptide-containing neurons in the rat glandular stomach. J. Comp. Neurol. 370: 61070.

Blundell, T. L., J. F. Cutfield, S. M. Cutfield, et al. 1972. Three-dimensional atomic structure of insulin and its relationship to activity. Diabetes 21 (Suppl. 2): 492–505.

Boudin, H., D. Pelaprat, W. Rostene, et al. 1996. Cellular distribution of neurotensin receptors in rat brain—Immunohistochemical study using an antipeptide antibody against the cloned high-affinity receptors. J. Comp. Neurol. 373: 76–89

Bravenboer, B., P. H. Hendrikse, P. L. Oey, et al. 1994. Randomized double-blind placebo controlled trial to evaluate the effect of the ACTH 4–9 analog ORG 2766 in IDDM patients with neuropathy. Diabeticologia 37: 408–413.

Bretherton-Watt, D., M. A. Ghatei, H. Jamal, et al. 1992. The physiology of calcitonin gene–related peptide in the islet compared with that of islet amyloid polypeptide (amylin). Ann. N.Y. Acad. Sci. 657: 299–312.

Brown, J. C., M. A. Cook, and J. R. Dryburgh. 1973. Motilin, a gastric motor activity stimulating polypeptide: The complete amino acid sequence. Can. J. Biochem. 51: 533–537.

Carraway, R. E., and S. E. Leeman. 1973. The isolation of a new hypotensive peptide, neurotensin, from bovine hypothalami. J.Biol. Chem. 248: 6854–6861.

Carraway, R. E., S. P. Mitra, and G. Spaulding. 1992. Posttranslational processing of the neurotensin/neuromedin-N precursor. Ann. N.Y. Acad. Sci. 668: 1–6.

Changeux, J. P., A. Duclert, and S. Sekine. 1992. Calcitonin gene-related peptide and neuromuscular interactions. Ann. N.Y. Acad. Sci. 657: 361–375.

Chan-Palay, V., M. Ito, P. Tongroach, et al. 1982. Inhibitory effects of motilin, somatostatin, [Leu]enkephalin, [Met]enkephalin and taurine on neurons of the lateral vestibular nucleus. Proc. Natl. Acad. Sci. U.S.A. 79: 3355–3359.

Chakder, S., and S. Rattan. 1990. [Tyr^{o}]-calcitonin gene–related peptide 28–37 (rat) as a putative antagonist of calcitonin gene–related peptide responses on opossum internal anal sphincter smooth muscle. J. Pharmacol. Exp. Ther. 253: 200–206.

Cohen, B., D. Novick, and M. Rubinstein. 1996. Modulation of insulin activities by leptin. Science 274: 1185–1188.

Costa, M., J. B. Furness, and I. L. Gibbins. 1986. Chemical coding of enteric neurons. Prog. Brain Res. 68: 217–239.

Daikh, D. I., J. O. Douglass, and J. P. Adelman. 1989. Structure and expression of the human motilin gene. DNA 8: 615–621.

Dennis, T., A. Fourier, A. Cadieux, et al. 1990. $hCGRP_{8-37}$, a calcitonin gene–related peptide antagonist revealing calcitonin gene–related peptide receptor heterogeneity in brain and periphery. J. Pharmacol. Exp. Ther. 251: 718–725.

Depoorte, I., T. L. Peeters, and G. Vantrappen. 1991. Motilin receptors of the rabbit colon. Peptides 12: 89–94.

Dobner, P. R., D. L. Barber, L. Villa-Komaroff, et al. 1987. Cloning and sequence analysis of cDNA for the canine neurotensin/neuromedin N precursor. Proc. Natl. Acad. Sci. U.S.A. 84: 3516–3520.

Dumoulin, F. L., G. Ravich, C. A. Haas, et al. 1992. Calcitonin gene-related peptide and peripheral nerve regeneration. Ann. N.Y. Acad. Sci. 657: 351–360.

Dunne, M. J., C. Kane, R. M. Shepherd, et al. 1997. Familial persistent hyperinsulinemic hypoglycemia of infancy and mutations in the sulfanylurea receptor. N. Engl. J. Med. 336: 703–706.

DuVal, J. W., B. Saffouri, G. C. Weir, et al. 1981. Regulation of gastrin and somatostatin secretion by cholinergic and non-cholinergic intramural neurons. Am. J. Physiol. 243: G442–G447.

Edmondson, S., N. Khan, J. Shriver, et al. 1990. The solution structure of motilin from NMR distance constraints, distance geometry, molecular dynamics and iterative full relaxation matrix refinement. Biochemistry 30: 11271–11279.

Enriques, E., and L. Hallion. 1903. Reflexe acide de Pavloff et sécretine: Méchanisme humoral commune. C.R. Soc. Biol. (Paris) 55: 233–234.

Evers, B. M., Z. H. Zhou, V. Dohlen, et al. 1996. Fetal and neoplastic expression of the neurotensin gene in the human colon. Ann. Surg. 223: 464–470.

Eysselein, V. E., M. Reinshagen, A. Patel, et al. 1992. Calcitonin gene–related peptide in inflammatory bowel disease and experimentally induced colitis. Ann. N.Y. Acad. Sci. 657: 319–327.

Forster, E. R., and G. J. Dockray. 1991. The role of calcitonin gene–related peptide in gastric mucosal protection in the rat. Exp. Physiol. 76: 623–626.

Gabriel, S. M., L. M. Kaplan, J. B. Martin, et al. 1989. Tissue-specific sex differences in galanin-like immunoreactivity and galanin mRNA during development in the rat. Peptides 10: 369–374.

Gates, T. S., R. P. Zimmerman, C. R. Mantyh, et al. 1989. Calcitonin gene–related peptide-α receptor binding sites in the gastrointestinal tract. Neuroscience 31: 757–770.

Geddes, B. J., L. J. Parry, and A. J. S. Summerlee. 1994. Brain angiotensin II partially mediates the effects of relaxin on vasopressin and oxytocin release in anesthetized rats. Endocrinology 134: 118–1192.

Geppetti, P., M. Tramontana, S. Evangelista, et al. 1991. Differential effect on neuropeptide release of different concentrations of hydrogen ions on afferent and intrinsic neurons of the rat stomach. Gastroenterology 101: 1505–1511.

Graves, C. B., R. R. Goewert, and J. M. McDonald. 1986. The insulin receptor contains a calmodulin-binding domain. Science 230: 827–829.

Grønbach, J. E., and E. R. Lacy. 1995. Role of gastric blood flow in impaired defense and repair of aged rat stomachs. Am. J. Physiol. 269: G737–744.

Havrankova, J., J. Roth, and M. J. Brownstein. 1979. Concentrations of insulin and insulin receptors are independent of peripheral insulin levels. J. Clin. Invest. 54: 636–642.

Hellstrom, P. M. 1986. Vagotomy inhibits the effect of neurotensin on gastrointestinal transit in the rat. Acta Physiol. Scand. 128: 47–55.

Henquin, J.-C. 1994. Cell biology of insulin secretion. In: Joslin's Diabetes Mellitus, 13th Ed. Eds. C. R. Kahn and G. C. Weir. Philadelphia, Lea & Febiger, pp. 56–80.

Henry, J. L. 1982. Electrophysiological studies on the neuroactive properties of neurotensin. Ann. N.Y. Acad. Sci. 440: 216–227.

Hermansen, K., N. Yanaihara, and B. Ahrén. 1989. On the nature of the galanin action on the endocrine pancreas: Studies with six galanin fragments in the perfused dog pancreas. Acta Endocrinol. 121: 545–550.

Hoebel, B. G., P. Rada, G. P. Mark, et al. 1994. The power of integrative peptides to reinforce behavior by releasing dopamine. Ann. N.Y. Acad. Sci. 739: 36–41.

Hökfelt, T., Z. Wiesenfeld-Hallin, M. J. Villar, et al. 1987. Increase in galanin-like immunoreactivity in rat dorsal root ganglia after peripheral axotomy. Neurosci. Lett. 83: 217–220.

Hökfelt, T., X. Zhang, and Z. Wiesenfeld-Hallin. 1994. Messenger plasticity in primary sensory neurons following axotomy and its functional implictions. Trends Neurosci. 17: 22–30.

Holzer, P., Ch. Wachter, M. Jocič, et al. 1994. Vascular bed–dependent roles of the peptide CGRP and nitric oxide in acid-evoked hyperaemia of the rat stomach. J. Physiol. 480: 575–585.

Ido, Y., A. Vindigni, K. Chang, et al. 1997. Prevention of vascular and neural dysfunction in diabetic rats by C-peptide. Science 277: 563–566.

Ishida-Yamamoto, A., and M. Tohyama. 1989. Calcitonin gene–related peptide in the nervous tissue. Prog. Neurobiol. 33: 335–386.

Itoh, Z. 1990. Effect of motilin on gastrointestinal motor activity in the dog. In: Motilin. Ed. Z. Itoh. New York, Academic Press, pp. 133–153.

Kapas, S., K. J. Catt, and A. J. L. Clark. 1995. Cloning and expression of cDNA encoding a rat adrenomedullin receptor, J. Biol. Chem. 270: 25344–25347.

Kaplan, L. M., S. C. Hooi, D. R. Abraczinskas, et al. 1991. Neuroendocrine regulation of galanin gene expression. In: Galanin: A New Multifunctional Peptide in the Neuroendocrine System. Eds. T. Hökfelt, T. Bartfai, D. Jacobowitz, et al. New York, Macmillan, pp. 43–65.

Kappelle, A. C., G. Biessels, T. Vanburen, et al. 1994. The effect of diabetes mellitus on development of autonomic neuropathy in the rat—Beneficial effects of ACTH (4–9) analog ORG 2766 on existing diabetic neuropathy. Diabetes Nutr. Metab. 7: 63–70.

Kinsley, B. T., and D. C. Simonson. 1996. Evidence for a hypothalamic-pituitary versus adrenal-cortical effect of glycemic control on counterregulatory hormone responses to hypoglycemia in insulin-dependent diabetes mellitus. J. Clin. Endocrinol. Metab. 81: 684–691.

Kislauskis, E., B. Bullock, S. McNeil, et al. 1988. The rat gene encoding neurotensin and neuromedin N. J. Biol. Chem. 263: 4963–4968.

Kitamura, K., K. Kangawa, H. Matsuo, et al. 1995. Adrenomedullin: Implication for hypertension research. Drugs 49: 485–495.

Kurose, T., Y. Seino, S. Nishi, et al. 1990. Mechanism of sympathetic neural regulation of insulin, somatostatin and glucagon secretion. Am. J. Physiol. 258: E220–E227.

Lagny-Pourmire, I., A. M. Lorinet, N. Yanaihara, et al. 1989. Structural requirements for galanin ineraction with receptors from pancreatic beta cells and from brain tissue of the rat. Peptides 10: 757–761.

Lambert, P. D., R. Gross, C. B. Nemeroff, et al. 1995. Anatomy and mechanisms of neurotensin-dopamine interactions in the central nervous system. Ann. N.Y. Acad. Sci. 757: 377–389.

Lee, Y., Y. Shiotani, N. Hayashi, et al. 1987. Distribution and origin of calcitonin gene–related peptide in the rat stomach and duodenum: An immunohistochemical study. J. Neural. Transm. Gen. Sect. 68: 1–14.

Leibowitz, S. F. 1994. Specificity of hypothalamic peptides in the control of behavioral and physiological processes. Ann. N.Y. Acad. Sci. 739: 12–35.

Leibowitz, S. F., and R. D. Myers. 1987. The neurochemistry of ingestion. Chemical stimulation of the brain and in vivo measurement of transmitter release. In: Feeding and Drinking. Eds. F. M. Toates and N. E. Rowlands. Amsterdam, Elsevier, pp. 271–315.

LeRoith, D., S. A. Hendricks, M. A. Lesniak, et al. 1983. Insulin in brain and other extrapancreatic tissues of vertebrates and non-vertebrates. Adv. Metab. Dis. 10: 303–340.

Li, X.-M., L. Ferraro, S. Tanganelli, et al. 1995. Neurotensin peptides antagonistically regulate postsynaptic dopamine D_2 receptors in rat nucleus accumbens—a receptor-binding and microdialysis study. J. Neural Transmiss. Gen. Sect. 102: 125–137.

López, F. J., I. Merchenthaler, M. Ching, et al. 1991. Galanin: A hypothalamic-hypophysiotropic hormone modulating reproductive functions. Proc. Natl. Acad. Sci. U.S.A. 88: 4508–4510.

Maggi, C. A., S. Giuliani, and V. Zagorodnyuk. 1996. Calcitonin gene–related peptide (CGRP) in the circular muscle of guinea pig colon—role as inhibitory transmitter and mechanisms of relaxation. Regul. Peptides 61: 27–36.

Marshall, I. 1992. Mechanism of vascular relaxation by the calcitonin gene–related peptide. Ann. N.Y. Acad. Sci. 657: 204–215.

Mazella, J., J. M. Botto, E. Guillemare, et al. 1996. Structure, functional expression, and cerebral localization of the levocabastine-sensitive neurotensin/neuromedin N receptor from mouse brain. J. Neurosci. 16: 5613–5620.

Merchenthaler, I., F. J. López, D. E. Lennard, et al. 1991. Sexual differences in the distribution of neurons coexpressing galanin and luteinizing hormone–releasing hormone in the rat brain. Endocrinology 129: 1977–1986.

Merchenthaler, I., F. J. López, and A. Negro-Vilar. 1993. Anatomy and physiology of central galanin-containing neurons. Prog. Neurobiol. 40: 771–769.

Messell, T., H. Harling, G. Böttcher, et al. 1990 Galanin in the porcine pancreas. Regul. Peptides 28: 161–176.

Morley, J. E., S. A. Farr, and J. F. Flood. 1996. Peripherally administered calcitonin gene–related peptide decreases food intake in mice. Peptides 17: 511–516.

Mule, F., R. Serio, A. Postorino, T. Vetri, et al. 1996. Antagonism by Sr-48692 of mechanical responses to neurotensin in rat intestine. Br. J. Pharmacol. 117: 488–492.

Nemeroff, C. B., D. E. Hernandez, R. C. Orlando, et al. 1983. Cytoprotective effect of centrally administered neurotensin on stress induced gastric ulcers. Am. J. Physiol. 242: G342–G346.

Northam, E., P. Anderson, G. Werther, et al. 1995. Neuropsychological complications of insulin-dependent diabetes in children. Child Neuropsychol. 1: 74–87.

Nussdorfer, G. G., G. P. Rossi, and G. Mazzocchi. 1997. Role of adrenomedullin and related peptides in the regulation of the hypothalamo-pituitary-adrenal axis. Peptides 18: 1079–1089.

Olsen, R. D., A. J. Kastin, T. K. von Almen, et al. 1980. Systemic injections of gastro-intestinal peptides alter behavior in rats. Peptides 1: 383–385.

O'Meara, N., and K. S. Polonsky. 1994. Insulin secretion in vivo. In: Joslin's Diabetes Mellitus, 13th Ed. Eds. C. R. Kahn and G. C. Weir. Philadelphia, Lea & Febiger, pp. 81–96.

Orci, L., J. D. Vassalli and A. Perrelet. 1988. The insulin factory. Sci. Am. 259: 85–94.

Osheroff, P. L., and H. S. Phillips. 1991. Autoradiographic localization of relaxin binding sites in rat brain. Proc. Nat. Acad. Sci. U.S.A. 88: 6413–6417.

Peeters, T. L., M. J. Macielag, I. Depoortere, et al. 1992. D-amino acid and alanine scans of the bioactive portion of porcine motilin. Peptides 13: 1103–1107.

Phillis, J. W., and J. R. Kirkpatrick. 1980. The actions of motilin, luteinizing releasing hormone, cholecystokinin, somatostatin, vasoactive intestinal peptide, and other peptides on rat cerebral cortical neurons. Can. J. Physiol. Pharmacol. 58: 612–623.

Plata-Salaman, C. R. 1991. Insulin in the cerebrospinal-fluid. Neurosci. Biobehav. Rev. 15: 243–258.

Poitras, P. 1994. Motilin. In: Gut Peptides: Biochemistry and Physiology. Eds. J. H. Walsh and G. J. Dockray. New York, Raven Press.

Poitras, P., L. Trudel, R. G. Lahaie, et al. 1990. Stimulation of duodenal muscle contraction by porcine or canine motilin in the dog in vivo. Clin. Invest. Med. 13: 11–16.

Poitras, P., D. Gagnon, and S. St-Pierre. 1992. N-terminal portion of motilin determines its biological activity. Biochem. Biophys. Res. Commun. 183: 36–40.

Rattan, S., P. Gonnella, and P. K. Royal. 1988. Inhibitory effect of calcitonin-gene–related peptide and calcitonin on opossum esophageal smooth muscle. Gastroenterology 94: 284–293.

Rökaeus, A. 1994. Galanin. In: Gut Peptides: Biochemistry and Physiology. Eds. J. H. Walsh and G. J. Dockray. New York, Raven Press, pp. 525–552.

Rosasarellano, M. P., L. P. Solanoflores, and J. Ciriello. 1996. Neurotensin projections to the subfornical organ from arcuate nucleus. Brain Res. 706: 323–327.

Rossmanith, W. G., D. K. Clifton, and R. A. Steiner. 1996. Galanin gene expression in GnRH neurons of the rat: A model for autocrine regulation. Horm. Metab. Res. 28: 257–266.

Sabol, S. L., and H. Higuchi. 1990. Transcriptional regulation of the neuropeptide Y gene by nerve growth factor: Antagonism by glucocorticoids and potentiation by adenosine 3′5′-monophosphate and phorbol ester. Mol. Endocrinol. 4: 384–392.

Samson, W. K., and T. C. Murphy. 1997. Adrenomedullin inhibits salt appetite. Endocrinology 138: 613–616.

Schoelson, S., and P. A. Halban. 1994. Insulin biosynthesis and chemistry. In: Joslin's Diabetes Mellitus, 13th Ed. Eds. C. R. Kahn and G. C. Weir. Philadelphia, Lea & Febiger, pp. 29–55.

Schubert, M. L. 1991. The effect of vasoactive intestinal polypeptide on gastric acid secretion is predominantly mediated by somatostatin. Gastroenterology 100: 1195–1200.

Schubert, M. L., and J. Hightower. 1989. Inhibition of acid secretion by bombesin is partly mediated by release of fundic somatostatin. Gastroenterology 97: 561–567.

Schwartz, M. W., D. P. Figlewitcz, D. N. Baskin, et al. 1992. Insulin in the brain: A hormonal regulator of energy balance. Endocr. Rev. 13: 387.

Seino, S., and G. I. Bell. 1989. Alternative splicing of human insulin receptor mRNA. Biochem. Biophys. Res. Commun. 159: 312–316.

Sone, M., K. Takahashi, F. Satoh, et al. 1997. Specific adrenomedullin binding sites in the human brain. Peptides 18: 1125–1129.

Sternini, C., and K. Anderson. 1992. Calcitonin gene–related peptide–containing neurons supplying the rat digestive system: Differential distribution and expression patterns. Somatosens. Mo. Res. 9: 45–59.

Strauss, R. M., and L. M. Kaplan. 1991. Molecular analysis of human galanin: Peptide structure and species specific regulation of gene expression. Gastroenterology 100: A669–671.

Summerlee, A. J. S., and B. C. Wilson. 1994. Role of the subfornical organ in the relaxin-induced prolongation of gestation in the rat. Endocrinology 134: 2115–2120.

Sundler, F., R. Håkanson, S. Leander, et al. 1982. Light and electron microscopic localization of neurotensin in the gastrointestinal tract. Ann. N.Y. Acad. Sci. 400: 94–104.

Taché, Y. 1992. Inhibition of gastric acid secretion and ulcers by calcitonin gene–related peptide. Ann. N.Y. Acad. Sci. 657: 240–247.

Tanaka, K., M. Masu, and S. Nakanishi. 1990. Structure and functional expression of the cloned rat neurotensin receptor. Neuron 4: 847–854.

Tatemoto, K., A. Rokaeus, H. Jörnvall, et al. 1983. Galanin—A novel biologically active peptide from porcine intestine. FEBS Lett. 164: 124–128.

Tojo, C., T. Takao, T. Nishioka, et al. 1996. Hypothalamic-pituitary-adrenal axis in Wbn/Kob rats with non-insulin dependent diabetes mellitus. Endocr. J. 43: 233–239.

Tomlinson, D. R., P. Fernyhough, and L. T. Dienel. 1996. Neurotrophins and peripheral neuropathy. Philos. Trans. R. Soc. London (B. Biol. Sci.) 351: 455–462.

Varndell, I. M., and J. M. Polak. 1984. The use of double immunogold-staining procedures at the ultrastructural level for demonstrating neurochemical coexistence. In: Coexistence of Neuroactive Substances in Neurons. Eds. V. Chan-Palay and S. L. Palay. New York, Wiley, pp. 279–303.

Vincent, J. P. 1995. Neurotensin receptors—Binding properties, transduction pathways, and structure. Cell. Mol. Neurobiol. 15: 501–502.

Wagstaff, J. D., J. W. Gibb, and G. R. Hanson, 1996. Dopamine D-2 receptors regulate neurotensin release from the nucleus accumbens and striatum as measured by in vivo microdialysis. Brain Res. 721: 196–203.

Way, S. A., and G. Leng. 1992. Relaxin increases the firing rate of supraoptic neurons and increases oxytocin secretion in the rat. J. Endocrinol. 132: 149–158.

White, M. F., and C. R. Kahn. 1994. Molecular aspects of insulin action. In: Joslin's Diabetes Mellitus, 13th Ed. Eds. C. R. Kahn and G. C. Weir. Philadelphia, Lea & Febiger, pp. 139–162.

Wimalawansa, U. J. 1992. Isolation, purification and biochemical characterization of calcitonin gene–related peptide receptors. Ann. N.Y. Acad. Sci. 657: 70–87.

Wimalawansa, U. J. 1996. Calcitonin gene–related peptide and its receptors: Molecular genetics, physiology, pathophysiology, and therapeutic potentials. Endocr. Rev. 17: 533–585.

Wilden, P. A., C. R. Kahn, K. Siddle, et al. 1992. Insulin receptor kinase domain autophosphorylation regulates receptor enzymatic function. J. Biol. Chem. 267: 16660–16668.

Woods, S. C., and D. Porte Jr. 1983. The role of insulin as a satiety factor in the central nervous system. In: Advances in Metabolic Disorders: CNS Regulation of Carbohydrate Metabolism, Vol. 10. Ed. A. J. Szabo. New York, Academic Press, pp. 457–482.

Yano, H. Y. Seino, and J. Fujita. 1989. Exon-intron organization, expression and chromosomal localization of the human motilin gene. FEBS Lett. 2: 248–252.

Zhang, L., P. C. Colony, J. H. Washington, et al. 1989. Central neurotensin affects rat gastric integrity, prostaglandin E_2, and blood flow. Am. J. Physiol. 256: G226–G232.

Zhuang, H.-X., C. K. Snyder, S. F. Pu, et al. 1996. Insulin-like growth factors reverse or arrest diabetic neuropathy—effects on hyperalgesia and impaired nerve regeneration in rats. Exp. Neurol. 140: 198–205.

Chapter 18

Books and Literature Reviews

Azria, M. 1989. The Calcitonins. Physiology and Pharmacology. Basel, Karger.

Braverman, L. E., and R. D. Utiger, Eds. 1996. Werner and Ingbar's The Thyroid: A Fundamental and Clinical Text, 7th Ed. Philadelphia, Lippincott-Raven.

Davidson, N. C., and A. D. Struthers. 1994. Brain natriuretic peptide. Editorial Review. J. Hypertens. 12: 329–336.

Harvey, S., and R. A. Fraser. 1993. Parathyroid hormone: Neural and endocrine perspectives. J. Endocrinol. 139: 353–361.

Jacobs, J. W., and G. P. Vlasuk. 1987. Atrial natriuretic factor receptors. Endocrinol. Metab. Clini North Am. 16: 63–77.

Mallette, L. E. 1991. The parathyroid polyhormones: New concepts in the spectrum of peptide hormone action. Endocr. Rev. 12: 110–117.

Mallette, L. E. 1994. Parathyroid hormone and parathyroid hormone-related protein as polyhormones. In: The Parathyroids. Eds. J. P. Bilezikian, M. A. Levine, and R. Marcus. New York, Raven Press.

Martin, T. J., J. M. Moseley, and M. T Gillespie. 1991. Parathyroid hormone–related protein: biochemistry and molecular biology. Crit. Rev. Biochem. Mol. Biol. 26: 377–395.

Mulrow, P. J., and R. Schrier. 1987. Atrial Hormones and Other Natriuretic Factors. Bethesda, Md., American Physiological Society.

Rosenblatt, M., H. M. Kronenberg, and J T. Potts Jr. 1989. Parathyroid hormone physiology, chemistry, biosynthesis, secretion, metabolism and mode of action. In: Endocrinology. L. J. DeGroot, Ed. Philadelphia, W. B. Saunders.

Ruffolo, R. R. Jr., Ed. 1994. Angiotensin II Receptors. Vol. 1, Molecular Biology, Biochemistry, Pharmacology and Clinical Perspectives. Boca Raton, Fla., CRC Press.

Saavedra, J. M., and P. B. M. W. M. Timmermans, Eds. 1994. Angiotensin Receptors. New York, Plenum Press.

References

Adams, S. P. 1987. Structure and biologic properties of the atrial natriuretic peptides. Endocrinol. Metab. Clini. North Am. 16: 1–18.

Alderman, M. H., S. Madhavan, W. L. Ooi, et al. 1991. Association of the renin-sodium profile with the risk of myocardial infarction in patients with hypertension. N. Engl. J. Med. 324: 1098–1104.

Antunes-Rodrigues, J., S. M. McCann, L. C. Rogers, et al. 1985. Atrial natriuretic factor inhibits dehydration and angiotensin II–induced water intake in the conscious, unrestrained rat. Proc. Natl. Acad. Sci. U.S.A. 82: 8720–8723.

Antunes-Rodrigues, J., M. J. Ramalho, L. C. Reis, et al. 1993. Possible role of endothelin acting within the hypothalamus to induce the release of atrial natriuretic peptide and natriuresis. Neuroendocrinology 58: 701–708.

Barr, C. S., P. Rhodes, and A. D. Struthers. 1996. C-type natriuretic peptide. Peptides 17: 1243–1251.

Bartalena, L. 1990. Recent achievements in studies on thyroid hormone-biding proteins. Endocr. Rev. 11: 47–64.

Bergsma, D. J. 1994. Molecular biology of angiotensin II receptors. In: Angiotensin II Receptors. Vol. 1, Molecular Biology, Biochemistry, Pharmacology and Clinical Perspectives. Ed. Ruffolo, R. R. Jr. Boca Raton, Fla., CRC Press, pp. 33–51.

Blind, E., D. Flentje, and S. Fischer. 1990. Clinical application of intact parathyroid determination. In: Calcium Regulating Hormones, Vitamin D Metabolites, and Cyclic AMP: Assays and Their Clinical Application. Eds. H. Schmidt-Gayk, F. P. Armbruster, and R. Bouillon. Berlin, Springer-Verlag, pp. 3–23.

Brooks, D. T., and R. R. Ruffolo, Jr. 1994. Introduction: Angiotensin II receptors. In: Angiotensin II Receptors. Vol. 1, Molecular Biology, Biochemistry, Pharmacology and Clinical Perspectives. Ed. R. R. Ruffolo, Jr. Boca Raton, Fla., CRC Press, pp. 1–10.

Chambers, T. J., and A. Moore. 1983. The sensitivity of isolated osteoclasts to morphological transformation by calcitonin. J. Clin. Endocrinol. Metab. 57: 819–824.

Chan, Y. S., and T. M. Wong. 1995. Relationship of rostral ventrolateral medullary neurons and angiotensin in the central control of blood pressure. Biol. Signals 4: 133–141.

Christensen, G. 1995. Electrical activity and secretion of atrial natriuretic factor from atrial heart cells. In: The Electrophysiology of Neuroendocrine Cells. Eds. H. Schrübl and J. Hescheler. Boca Raton, Fla., CRC Press, pp. 189–203.

Clemo, H. F., C. M. Baumgarten, K. A. Ellenbogen, et al. 1996. Atrial natriuretic peptide and cardiac electrophysiology—Autonomic and direct effects. J. Cardiac Electrophysiol. 7: 149–162.

Copp, D. H., and E. C. Cameron. 1961. Demonstration of a hypocalcemic factor (calcitonin) in commercial parathyroid extract. Science 134: 2038–2039.

Craig, S. P., V. J. Buckle, A. Lamouroux, et al. 1986. Localization of the human tyrosine hydroxylase gene to 11p15: Gene duplication and evolution of metabolic pathways. Cytogenet. Cell Genet. 42: 29–32.

Czelusniak, J. M. Goodman, N. D. Moncrief, et al. 1990. Maximum parsimony approach to construction of evolutionary trees from aligned homologous sequences. Methods Enzymol. 183: 601–615.

De, A., S. Das, S. Chaudhury, and P. K. Sarkar. 1994. Thyroidal stimulation of tubulin and actin in rat brain cytoskeleton. Int. J. Dev. Neurosci. 12: 49–46.

De Bold, A. J. 1979. Heart atrial granularity. Effects of changes in water and electrolyte balance. Proc. Soc. Exp. Biol. Med. 161: 508–511.

De Bold, A. J., H. B. Borenstein, A. T. Veress, et al. 1981. A rapid and potent natriuretic response to intravenous injection of atrial myocardial extract in rats. Life Sci. 28: 89–94.

DeLong, G. R. 1996. The neuromuscular system and brain in thyrotoxicosis. In: Werner and Ingbar's The Thyroid; A Fundamental and Clinical Text, 7th Ed., Eds. L. E. Braverman and R. D. Utiger. Philadelphia, Lippencott-Raven, pp. 645–652.

Dewey, C. W., G. D. Shelton, C. S. Bailey, et al. 1995. Neuromuscular dysfunction in 5 dogs with acquired myasthenia gravis and presumptive hypothyroiditis. Prog. Vet. Med. 6: 117–123.

Dickson, P. W., A. R. Aldred, J. G. T. Menting, et al. 1987. Thyroxine transport in the choroid plexus. J. Biol. Chem. 262: 13907–13916.

Edwards, R. M., and R. R. Ruffolo, Jr. 1994. Angiotensin II receptor subclassification. In: Angiotensin II Receptors, Vol. 1, Molecular Biology, Biochemistry, Pharmacology and Clinical Perspectives. Ed. Ruffolo, R. R. Jr. Boca Raton, Fla., CRC Press, pp. 11–31.

Eggenberger, M., B. Fluhman, R. Muff, et al. 1996. Structure of a parathyroid hormone, parathyroid hormone–related peptide receptor of the human cerebellum and functional expression in human neuroblastoma SK-N-MC cells. Mol. Brain Res. 36: 127–136.

Ekins, R. P., A. K. Sinha, M. R. Pickard, et al. 1994. Transport of thyroid hormones to target tissues. Acta Med. Austriaca 21: 26–34.

Fitzsimons, J. T. 1969. The role of a renal thirst factor in drinking induced by extracellular stimuli. J. Physiol. (Lond.) 201: 349–368.

Fluharty, S. J., and A. N. Epstein. 1983. Sodium appetite elicited by intracerebroventricular infusion of angiotensin II in the rat. II Synergistic interaction with systemic mineralocorticoids. Behav. Neurosci. 97: 746–758.

Foster, G. V., A. Baghdiantz, M. A. Kumar, et al. 1964. Thyroid origin of calcitonin. Nature 202: 1303–1305.

Franci, C. R., J. A. Anselmo-Franci and S. M. McCann. 1997. Angiotensinergic neurons physiologically inhibit prolactin, growth hormone, and thyroid-stimulating hormone, but not adrenocorticotropic hormone, release in ovariectomized rats. Peptides 18: 971–976.

Fraser, R. A., H. M. Kronenberg, P. K. T. Pang, et al. 1990. Parathyroid messenger ribonucleic acid in the rat hypothalamus. Endocrinology 127: 2517–2522.

Freed, M. I., B. E. Ilson, N. H. Shusterman, et al. 1994. Therapeutic applications of angiotensin antagonists. In: Angiotensin II Receptors. Vol. 1, Molecular Biology, Biochemistry, Pharmacology and Clinical Perspectives. Ed. R. R. Ruffulo, Jr. Boca Raton, Fla., CRC Press, pp. 121–154.

Fukada, Y., Y. Hirata, H. Yoshimi. 1988. Endothelin is a potent secretogogue for atrial natriuretic peptide in cultured rat atrial myocytes. Biochem. Biophys. Res. Commun. 155: 167–172.

Fukayama, S., A. H. Tashjian, J. N. Davis, et al. 1995. Signaling by N-terminal and C-terminal sequences of parathyroid hormone–related protein in hippocampal neurons. Proc. Nat. Acad. Sci. U.S.A. 92: 10182–10186.

Galli, S. M., and M. I. Phillips. 1996. Interactions of angiotensin II and atrial natriuretic peptide in the brain—Fish to rodent. Proc. Soc. Exp. Biol. Med. 213: 128–137

Gardner, D. G., M. C. LaPointe, and J. Wu. 1988. Expression and regulation of the gene for atrial natriuretic factor. In: Fronti. Neuroendocrinol. 10: 45–61.

Geller, D. M., M. G. Currie, K. Wakitani, et al. 1984. Atriopeptins: A family of potent biologically active peptides derived from mammalian atria. Biochem. Biophys. Res. Commun. 120: 333–338.

Gower, W. R., Jr., S. Chiou, K. Skolnick, et al. 1994. Molecular forms of circulating atrial natriuretic peptides in human plasma and their metabolites. Peptides 15: 861–867.

Hilton, J. M., S. Y. Chai, and P. M. Sexton. 1995. In vitro autoradiographical localization of the calcitonin isoforms C_{1a} and C_{1b} in rat brain. Neuroscience 69: 1223–1237.

Hodin, R. A., M. A. Lazar, and W. W. Chin. 1990. Differential and tissue-specific regulation of multiple rat c-*erb*A messenger RNA species by thyroid hormone. J. Clin. Invest. 85: 101–105.

Hongo, T., J. Kupfer, H. Enomoto, et al. 1991. Abundant expression of parathyroid hormone–related protein in primary rat aortic smooth muscle cells accompanies serum induced proliferation. J. Clin. Invest. 88: 1841–1848.

Horne, W. C., J. F. Shyu, M. Chakraborty, et al. 1994. Signal transduction by calcitonin—Multiple ligands, receptors and signaling pathways. Trends Endocrinol. Metab. 5: 395–401.

Ichikawa, I., and R. C. Harris. 1991. Angiotensin actions in the kidney: Renewed insight into the old hormone. Kidney Int. 40: 583–596.

Inagami, T., K. Mizuno, M. Nakamaru, et al. 1988. The renin-angiotensin system: an overview of its intracellular function. Cardiovasc. Drugs Ther. 2: 453–458.

Ismael-Beigi, F. 1988. Thyroid thermogenesis: Regulation of (Na^+ and K^+)-adenosine triphosphatase and active Na, K transport. Am. Zool. 28: 363–371.

Jackson, I. M. D. 1996. Does thyroid hormone have a role as adjunctive therapy in depression? Thyroid 6: 63–67.

Jacobs, J. W. and G. P. Vlasuk. 1987. Atrial natriuretic factor receptors. Endocrinol. Metab. Clin. North Am. 16: 63–77.

Kangawa, K., and H. Matsuo. 1984. Purification and complete amino acid sequence of alpha–human atrial natriuretic polypeptide (alpha-hANP). Biochem. Biophys. Res. Commun. 118: 131–139.

Kemp, B. E., J. M. Moseley, C. P. Rodda, et al. 1987. Parathyroid hormone–related protein of malignancy: Active synthetic fragments. Science 238: 1568–1570.

Kisch, B. 1956. Electron microscopy of the atrium of the heart. I. Guinea pig. Exp. Med. Surg. 14: 99–112.

Koller, K. J., and D. V. Goeddel, 1992. Molecular biology of the natriuretic peptides and their receptors. Circulation 86: 1081–1088.

Koller, M., H. P. Krause, F. Hofmeister, et al. 1975. Endogenous brain angiotensin II disrupts passive avoidance behavior in rats. Neurosci. Lett. 14: 71–75.

Krenning, E. P., R. Docter, T. J. Visser, et al. 1983. Plasma membrane transport of thyroid hormone: Its possible pathological significance. J. Endocrinol. Invest. 6: 59–63.

Ku, Y.-H., and T. Zhang. 1994. Brain atriopeptin mediates AV3V depressor response. Peptides 15: 1053–1056.

Kuno, T., J. W. Andresen, Y. Kamisaki, et al. 1986. Co-purification of an atrial natriuretic factor receptor and particulate guanylate cyclase from rat lung. J. Biol. Chem. 261: 5817–5823.

Langub, M. C., C. M. Dolgas, R. E. Watson, et al. 1995. The C-type natriuretic peptide receptor is the predominant natriuretic peptide receptor messenger RNA expressed in rat hypothalamus. J. Neuroendocrinol. 7: 305–309.

Lappe, R. W., J. L. Dinish, F. Bex, et al. 1986. Regulatory role of atrial natriuretic factor on drinking responses to central angiotensin II. Pharmacol. Biochem. Behav. 24: 1573–1576.

Laurent, V., P. Bulet, and M. Salzet. 1995. A comparision of the leech *Theromyzon tessulatum* angiotensin I–like molecule with forms of vertebrate angiotensinogens—a hormonal system conserved in the course of evolution. Neurosci. Lett. 190: 175–178.

Lazar, M. 1993. Thyroid hormone receptors: Multiple forms, multiple possibilities. Endocr. Rev. 14: 184–193.

Lenkei, Z., M. Palkovits, P. Corvol, et al. 1996. Distribution of angiotensin-II type-2 receptor (AT_2) messenger RNA expression in the adult rat brain. J. Comp. Neurol. 373: 322–339.

Lewis, E. J., G. Hunsicker, R. P. Bain, et al. 1993. The effect of angiotensin-converting enzyme inhibition on diabetic neuropathy. N. Engl. J. Med. 329: 1456–1462.

Lim. A. T., R. C. Dow, Z. Yang, et al. 1994. ANP (5–28) is the major molecular species in hypophyseal portal blood of the rat. Peptides 15: 1557–1559.

Maack, T., D. N. Marion, M. J. F. Camargo, et al. 1984. Effects of auriculin (atrial natriuretic factor) on blood pressure, renal function and the renin-aldosterone system in dogs. Am. J. Med. 77: 1069–1075.

Makino, Y., N. Minamino, E. Kakishita, et al. 1996. Natriuretic peptides in water-deprived and salt-loaded rats. Peptides 17: 1031–1039.

Mallette, L. E. 1991. The parathyroid hormones: New concepts in the spectrum of peptide hormone action. Endocr. Rev. 12: 110–117.

Mallette, L. E. 1994. Parathyroid hormone and parathyroid hormone–related protein as polyhormones. In: The Parathyroids. Eds. J. P. Bilezitian, M. A. Levine, and R. Marcus. New York, Raven Press.

Mallette, L., J. Thornby, and H. T. Pretorius. 1986. Internal homology in preproparathyroid hormone. Four copies of a primitive gene. J. Bone Miner. Res. 1: 58–63.

Mangin, M., K. Ikeda, B. E. Dreyer, et al. 1988. Two distinct tumor-derived parathyroid hormone–like peptides arise from alternative ribonucleic acid splicing. Mol. Endocrinol. 2: 1049–1055.

Martin, T. J., J. M. Moseley, and M. Y. Gillespie. 1991. Parathyroid hormone–related protein: Biochemistry and molecular biology. Crit. Rev. Biochem. Mol. Biol. 26: 377–395.

Mattingly, M. T., R. R. Brandt, D. M. Heublein, et al. 1994. Presence of C-type natriuretic peptide in human kidney and urine. Kidney Int. 46: 744–747.

McKenzie, J. M. 1974. Long-acting thyroid stimulator in Graves' disease, In: Handbook of Physiology, Endocrinology III. Eds. M. A. Greer, and D. H. Solomon. Washington D.C., Amer. Physiol. Soc., pp. 285–301.

Medeiros-Neto, G., H. M. Targovnik, and G. Vassart. 1993. Defective thyroglobulin synthesis and secretion causing goiter and hypothyroidism. Endocr. Rev. 14: 165–183.

Motté, P., P. Ghillani, F. Troalen, et al. 1990. Design of new methods for measuring calcitonin and related peptides using monoclonal antipeptide antibodies. In: Calcium Regulating Hormones, Vitamin D Metabolites, and Cyclic AMP. Assays and Their Clinical Application. Eds. H. Schmidt-Gayk, F. P. Armbruster, and R. Bouillon. Berlin, Springer-Verlag, pp. 351–364.

Mukoyama, M., M. Nakajima, M. Horiuchi, et al. 1993. Expression cloning of type 2 angiotensin II receptor reveals a unique class of seven-transmembrane receptors. J. Biol. Chem. 268: 24539–24542.

Nakao, K., Y. Ogawa, S. Suga, and H. Imura. 1992. Molecular biology and biochemistry of the natriuretic peptide receptors J. Hypertens. 10: 1111–1114.

Nutley, M. T., S. A. Parimi, and S. Harvey. 1995. Sequence analysis of hypothalamic parathyroid hormone messenger ribonucleic acid. Endocrinology 136: 5600–5607.

Nuzzenzeig, D. R., J. A. Lewicki, and T. Maack. 1990. Cellular mechanisms of type C receptors of atrial natriuretic factor. J. Biol. Chem. 265: 20952–20958.

Ogawa, Y., H. Itoh, N. Tamura, et al. 1994. Molecular cloning of the complementary-DNA and gene that encode mouse brain natriuretic peptide and generation of transgenic mice that overexpress the brain natriuretic peptide gene. J. Clin. Invest. 93: 1911–1921.

Oikawa, S., M. Imai, C. Inuzuka, et al. 1985. Structure of dog and rabbit precursors of atrial natriuretic polypeptides deduced from nuecleotide sequence of cloned cDNA. Biochem. Biophys. Res. Commun. 132: 892–899.

Oppenheimer, J. H. 1985. Thyroid hormone action at the nuclear level. Ann. Intern. Med. 102: 374–384.

Oppenheimer, J. H., and H. L. Schwartz. 1985. Stereospecific transport of triiodothyronine from plasma to cytosol and from cytosol to nucleus in the rat liver, kidney and brain. J. Clin. Invest. 75: 147–154.

Overton, R. M., and D. L. Vesely, 1996. Processing of long-acting natriuretic peptide and vessel dilator in human plasma and serum. Peptides 17: 1155–1162.

Palkowits, M., U. Bahner, and H. Geiger. 1995. Preoptic neuronal circuit–atrial natriuretic peptide–containing neurons are sensitive to acute and chronic alterations in body fluid volume. Miner. Electrolyte Metab. 21: 423–427.

Porter, J. G., R. M. Scarborough, Y. Wang, et al. 1989. Recombinant expression of a secreted form of the atrial natriuretic peptide clearance receptor. J. Biol. Chem. 264: 14179–14184.

Porterfield, S. P. 1994. Vulnerability of the developing brain to thyroid abnormalities—Environmental insults to the thyroid system. Environ. Health Perspect. 102: 125–130.

Quiron, R., M. Dalpé, and T.-V. Dam. 1986. Characterization and distribution of receptors for the atrial natriuretic peptides in mammalian brain. Proc. Natl. Acad. Sci. U.S.A. 83: 174–178.

Rafferty, B., J. M. Zanelli, M. Rosenblatt, et al. 1983. Corticosteroidogenesis and adenosine 3′,5′-monophosphate production by the amino-terminal (1–34) fragment of human parathyroid hormone in rat adrenocortical cells. Endocrinology 113: 1036–1042.

Reid, I. A. 1992. Interactions between ANG III, sympathetic nervous system, and baroreceptor reflexes in regulation of blood pressure. Am. J. Physiol. 262: E763–778.

Reis, L. C., M. J. Ramalho, A. L. V. Favaretto, et al. 1994. Participation of the ascending serotoninergic system in the stimulation of atrial natriuretic peptide release. Proc. Soc. Natl. Acad. Sci. U.S.A. 91: 12022–12026.

Rodda, D. P., M. Kubota, J. A. Heath, et al. 1988. Evidence for a novel parathyroid hormone–related protein in fetal lamb parathyroid glands and sheep placenta: Comparisons with a similar protein implicated in humoral hypercalcemia of malignancy. J. Endocrinol. 117: 261–271.

Ryan, M. C., and A. L. Gundlach. 1995. Anatomical localization of a preproatrial natriuretic peptide messenger RNA in the rat brain by in situ hybridization histochemistry—Novel identification in olfactory regions. J. Comp. Neurol. 356: 168–182.

Saavedra, J. M. 1992. Brain and pituitary angiotensin. Endocr. Rev. 13: 329–380.

Samson, W. K. 1987. Atrial natriuretic factor and the central nervous system. Endocrinol. Metab. Clini. North Am. 16: 145–161.

Samson, W. K., F. L. Huang, and R. J. Fulton. 1993. C-type natriuretic peptide mediates the hypothalamic actions of the natriuretic peptides to inhibit luteinizing hormone secretion. Endocrinology 132: 504–509.

Schenk, D. B., L. K. Johnson, K. Schwartz, et al. 1985. Distinct atrial natriuretic factor receptor sites on cultured bovine aortic smooth muscle and endothelial cells. Biochem. Biophys. Res. Commun. 127: 433–442.

Shichiri, M. Hirata, Y., K. Kanno, et al. 1989. Effect of endothelin-1 on release of arginine-vasopressin from perfused rat hypothalamus. Biochem. Biophys. Res. Commun. 163: 1332–1337.

Silva, L. C. S., M. A. P. Fontes, M. J. Campagnole-Santos, et al. 1993. Cardiovascular effects produced by microinjection of angiotensin (1–7) on vasopressor and vasodepressor sites of the ventrolateral medulla. Brain Res. 613: 321–325.

Silva, O. L., and K. L. Becker. 1981. Immunoreactive calcitonin in extra-thyroid tissues. In: Calcitonin 1980. Proceedings of International Symposium, Milan. Ed. A. Pecile. Int. Congress Ser. 540. Amsterdam, Exerpta Medica pp. 144–153.

Simpson, J. B. 1981. The circumventricular organs and the central actions of angiotensin. Neuroendocrinology 32: 248–256.

Sinha, A. K., M. R. Pickard, J. D. Kim, et al. 1994. Perturbation of thyroid hormone homeostasis in the adult and brain function. Acta Med. Austriaca 21: 35–43.

Slatopolsky, E., K. Martin, J. Morrissey, et al. 1982. Current concepts of the metabolism and radioimmunoassay of parathyroid hormone. J. Lab. Clin. Med. 99: 309–316.

Standaert, D. G., P. Needleman, and C. B. Saper. 1988. Atriopeptin: Neuromediator in the central regulation of cardiovascular function. In: Fronti. Neuroendocrinol. 10: 63–78.

Stephenson, K. N., and M. K. Steele. 1992. Brain angiotensin receptor subtypes and the control of luteinizing hormone and prolactin secretion in female rats. J. Neuroendocrinol. 4: 441–447.

Strait, K. A., H. L. Schwartz, A. Perez-Castillo, et al. 1990. Relationship of *c-erb*A mRNA content to tissue triiodothyronine nuclear binding capacity in developing and adult rats. J. Biol. Chem. 265: 10514–10521.

Struckhoff, G., and A. Turzynski. 1995. Demonstration of parathyroid hormone–related protein in meninges and its receptor in astrocytes—Evidence for a paracrine meningo-astrocytic loop. Brain Res. 676: 1–9.

Sudoh, T., N. Minamino, K. Kangawa, et al. 1990. A new member of natriuretic peptide family identified in porcine brain. Biochem. Biophys. Res. Commun. 168: 863–870.

Suga, S., H. Itoh, Y. Komatsu, et al. 1993. Cytokine-induced C-type natriuretic peptide (CNP) secretion from vascular endothelial cells—Evidence for CNP as a novel autocrine/paracrine regulator from endothelial cells. Endocrinology 133: 3038–3041.

Suga, S., K. Nakao, K. Hosoda, et al. 1992. Receptor sensitivity of natriuretic peptide family, atrial natriuretic peptide, brain natriuretic peptide and C type natriuretic peptide. Endocrinology 130: 229–239.

Suva, L. J., K. A. Mather, M. T. Gillespie, et al. 1989. Structure of the 5′ flanking region of the gene encoding human parathyroid hormone–related protein (PTH-rP). Gene 77: 95–105.

Throsby, M., Z. Yang, D. L. Copolov, et al. 1994. Colocalization of atrial natriuretic factor and β-endorphin in rat thymic macrophages. Peptides 15: 291–296.

Tigerstedt, R., and P. G. Bergman. 1898. Niere und Kreislauf. Scand. Arch. Physiol. 8: 223–230.

Tsutsui, M., N. Yanagihara, M. Kouichiro, et al. 1994. C-type natriuretic peptide stimulates catecholamine synthesis through the accumulation of cGMP in cultured bovine adrenal medullary cells. J. Pharmacol. Exp. Ther. 268: 584–589.

Urena, P., X.-F. Kong, A.-B. Juppner, et al. 1993. Parathyroid hormone (PTH)/PTH–related peptide receptor messenger ribonucleic acids are widely distributed in rat tissues. Endocrinology 133: 617–623.

Verspohl, E. J., and I. K. Bernemann. 1996, Atrial natriuretic peptide (ANP)–induced inhibition of glucagon secretion: Mechanism of action in isolated rat pancreatic islets. Peptides 17: 1023–1029.

Vesely, D. L., M. A. Douglass, J. R. Dietz, et al. 1994. Negative feedback of atrial natriuretic peptides. J. Clin. Endocrinol. Metab. 78: 1128–1134.

Weaver, D. R., J. D. Deeds. K. C. Lee, et al. 1995. Localization of parathyroid hormone–related protein (PTH-rP) and PTH/PTH-rP receptor messenger RNAs in rat brain. Mol. Brain Res. 28: 296–310.

Whybrow, P. C. 1996a. Behavioral and psychiatric aspects of hypothyroidism. In: Werner and Ingbar's The Thyroid, A Fundamental and Clinical Text, 7th Ed., Eds. L. E. Braverman and R. D. Utiger. Philadelphia, Lippincott-Raven, pp. 866–870.

Whybrow, P. C. 1996b. Behavioral and psychiatric aspects of thyrotoxicosis. In: Werner and Ingbar's The Thyroid, A Fundamental and Clinical Text, 7th Ed., Eds. L. E. Braverman and R. D. Utiger. Philadelphia, Lippincott-Raven, pp. 696–700.

Wilcox, J. N., A. Augustine, D. V. Goeddel, et al. 1991. Differential regional expression of three natriuretic peptide receptor genes within primate tissues. Mol. Cell. Biol. 11: 3454–3462.

Winaver, J., A. Hoffman, Z. Abassi, et al. 1995. Does the heart's hormone, ANP, help in congestive heart failure? Trends Physiol. Sci. 10: 247–253.

Wright, J. W., A. J. Bechtholt, S. L. Chambers, et al. 1996. Angiotensin II and IV activation of brain AT_1 receptor subtype in cardiovascular function. Peptides 17: 1365–1371.

Wright, J. W., and J. W. Harding. 1994. Brain angiotensin receptor subtypes in the control of physiological and behavioral responses. Neurosci. Biobehav. Rev. 18: 21–53.

Yongue, B. G., J. A. Angulo, B. S. McEwen, et al. 1991. Brain and liver angiotensinogen messenger RNA in genetic hypertensive and normotensive rats. Hypertension 17: 485–491.

Zini, S, M. C. Fourniezaluski, E. Chauvel, et al. 1996. Identification of metabolic pathways of brain angiotensin II and angiotensin III using specific aminopeptidase inhibitors—Predominant role of angiotensin-III in the control of vasopressin release. Proc. Nat. Acad. Sci. U.S.A. 93: 11968–11973.

Chapter 19

Books and Literature Reviews

Breidbach, O., and W. Kutsch. 1995. The Nervous Systems of Invertebrates: An Evolutionary and Comparative Approach. Basel, Birkhäuser.

Harrison, L. M., A. J. Kastin, J. T. Weber, et al. 1994. The opiate system in invertebrates. Peptides 15: 1309–1329.

Holman, G. M., R. J. Nachman, and M. S. Wright. 1990. Insect neuropeptides. Annu. Rev. Entomol. 35: 201–217.

Holman, G. M., M. S. Wright, and R. J. Nachman. 1988. Insect neuropeptides: Coming of age. ISI Atlas of Science 1: 129–136.

Keller, R. 1992. Crustacean neuropeptides—Structures, functions and comparative aspects. Experientia 48: 439–448.

Kelly, T. J., E. P. Masler, and J. J. Menn. 1994. Insect neuropeptides. In: Natural and Engineered Pest Management Agents. Eds. P. A. Hedin, J. J. Menn, and R. M. Hollingsworth. ACS Symposium Series, Vol. 551. Washington, D.C., American Chemical Society, pp. 292–318.

Martini, L., and W. F. Ganong. 1967. Neuroendocrinology, Vol. 2. New York, Academic Press.

Menn, J. J., T. J. Kelly, and E. P. Masler, Eds. 1991. Insect Neuropeptides: Chemistry, Biology and Action. Washington, D.C., American Chemical Society.

Nässel, D. R. 1993. Neuropeptides in the insect brain: A review. Cell Tissue Res. 273: 1–29.

Raabe, M. 1992. Recent Developments in Insect Neurohormones. New York, Plenum Press.

Scharrer, E., and B. Scharrer. 1963. Neuroendocrinology. New York, Columbia University Press.

Schoofs, L., G. M. Holman, R. J. Nachman, et al. 1994. Structure, function, and distribution of insect neuropeptides. In: Perspectives in Comparative Endocrinology. Eds. K. Davey, R. E. Peter, and S. S. Tobe. Ottawa, National Research Council of Canada, pp. 155–165.

Schoofs, L., D. Veelaert, J. Vanden Broek, et al. 1997. Peptides in the locusts, *Locusta migratoria* and *Schistocerca gregaria*. Peptides 18: 145–156.

Thorndyke, M. C., and G. J. Goldsworthy, Eds.. 1988. Neurohormones in Invertebrates. Cambridge, U.K., Cambridge University Press.

References

Abernathy, R. L., R. J. Nachman, P. E. A. Teal, et al. 1995. Pheromonotropic activity of naturally occurring pyrokinin insect neuropeptides (FXPRLamide) in *Helicoverpa zea*. Peptides 16: 215–219.

Abernathy, R. L., P. E. A. Teal, J. A. Meredith, et al. 1996. Induction of pheromone production in a moth by application of a pseudopeptide mimic of a pheromonotropic neuropeptide. Proc. Natl. Acad. Sci. U.S.A. 93: 12621–12625.

Agricola, H.-J., and P. Bräunig. 1995. Comparative aspects of peptidergic signaling pathways in the nervous system of arthropods. In: The Nervous Systems of Invertebrates: An Evolutionary and Comparative Approach. Eds. O. Breidbach and W. Kutsch. Basel, Birkhäuser, pp. 303–327.

Araki, Y., G. J. Liu, W. Zhang, et al. 1995. Further mapping of the *Achatina* giant neuron types sensitive to the neuroactive peptides isolated from invertebrates. Gen. Pharmacol. 26: 1701–1708.

Belkin, K. J., and T. W. Abrams. 1993. FMRFamide produces biphasic modulation of the LFS motor neurons in the neural circuit of the siphon withdrawal reflex of *Aplysia* by activating Na^+ and K^+ currents. J. Neurosci. 13: 5139–5152.

Boer, H. H., and C. Montagne-Wajer, 1994. Functional morphology of the neuropeptidergic light yellow cell system in pulmonate snails. Cell Tissue Res. 277: 531–538.

Březina, V., B. Bank, E. C. Cropper, et al. 1995. Nine members of the myomodulin family of peptide cotransmitters at the B16 ARC neuromuscular junction of *Aplysia*. J. Neurophysiol. 74: 54–72.

Březina, V., C. G. Evans, and K. R. Weiss. 1994. Activation of K^+ current in the accessory radula closer muscle of *Aplysia californica* by neuromodulators that depress its contractions. J. Neurosci. 14: 4412–4432.

Brown, B. E., and A. N. Starratt. 1975. Isolation of proctolin, a myotropic peptide from *Periplaneta americana*. J. Insect Physiol. 21: 1879–1881.

Bungart, D., H. Dircksen, and R. Keller. 1994. Quantitative determination and distribution of the myotropic neuropeptide orcokinin in the nervous system of astacidean crustaceans. Peptides 15: 393–400.

Bylemans, D., Y.-J. Hua, S.-J. Chiou, et al. 1995. Pleitropic effects of trypsin modulating oostatic factor (Neb-TMOF) of the fleshfly *Neobellieria bullata* (Diptera Calliphoridae). Eur. J. Entomol. 92: 143–149.

Candelariomartinez, A., D. M. Reed, S. J. Pritchard, et al. 1993. SCP-related peptides from bivalve molluscs—Identification, tissue distribution and actions. Biol. Bull. 185: 428–439.

Coast, G. M. 1996. Neuropeptides implicated in the control of diuresis in insects. Peptides 17: 327–336.

Coast, G. M., G. M. Holman, and R. J. Nachman. 1990. The diuretic activity of a series of cephalomyotropic neuropeptides: The achetakinins on isolated malpighian tubules of the house cricket *Acheta domesticus*. J. Insect Physiol. 36: 481–488.

Coast, G. M., and I. Kay. 1994. The effect of *Acheta* diuretic peptide on isolated malpighian tubules from the house cricket *Acheta domesticus*. J. Exp. Biol. 187: 225–243.

Coast, G. M., R. C. Rayne, T. K. Hayes, et al. 1993. A comparison of the effects of two putative diuretic hormones from *Locusta migratoria* on isolated locust Malpighian tubules. J. Exp. Biol. 175: 1–14.

Coleman, M. J., P. H. Konstant, B. S. Rothman, et al. 1994. Neuropeptide degradation produces functional inactivation in the crustacean nervous system. J. Neurosci. 14: 6205–6216.

Cropper, E. C., V. Březina, F. S. Vilim, et al. 1994. FRF peptides in the ARC neromuscular system of *Aplysia*—purification and physiological actions. J. Neurophysiol. 72 (5): 2181–2195.

Davis, M.-T. B., V. N. Vakharia, J. Henry, et al. 1992. Molecular cloning of the pheromone biosynthesis–activating neuropeptide in *Helicoverpa zea*. Proc. Natl. Acad. Sci. U.S.A. 89: 142–146.

De Loof, A. 1987. The impact of the discovery of vertebrate-type steroids and peptide hormone–like substances in insects. Entomol. Exp. Appl. 45: 105–113.

Dickinson, P. S., C. Mecsas, and E. Marder. 1990. Neuropeptide fusion of two motor-pattern generator circuits. Nature 344: 155–158.

Ding, Q., B. S. Donly, S. S. Tobe, et al. 1995. Comparison of allatostatin neuropeptide precursors in the distantly related cockroaches *Periplana americana* and *Diploptera punctata*. Eur. J. Biochem 234: 737–746.

Dircksen, H., J. Stangier, and R. Keller. 1987. Proctolin-like, Famide-like and leu-enkephalin–like immunoreactivity in the thoracic ganglion–pericardial organs system of brachyuran *Callinectus*. Gen. Comp. Endocrinol. 66: 42–46.

Ewer, J., S. C. Gammie, and J. W. Truman. 1997. Control of insect ecdysis by a positive feedback endocrine system: Roles of eclosion hormone and ecdysis triggering hormone. J. Exp. Biol. 200: 869–881.

Fernlund, P., and L. Josefsson. 1972. Crustacean color-change hormone: Amino acid sequence and chemical synthesis. Science 177: 173–174.

Gade, G., A. Lopate, R. Kellner, et al. 1992. Primary structures of neuropeptides isolated from the corpora cardiaca of various *Cetonoid* beetle species determined by pulsed liquid phase sequencing and tandem fast atom bombardment mass spectometry. Biol. Chem. Hoppe Seyler. 373: 133–142.

Gammi, S. C., and J. W. Truman. 1997. Neuropeptide hierarchies and the activation of sequential motor behaviors in the hawkmoth, *Manduca sexta*. J. Neurosci. 17: 4389–4397.

Geraerts, W. P. M., A. B. Smit, K. W. Li, et al. 1992. The light green cells of *Lymnaea*: A neuroendocrine model for stimulus-induced expression of multiple peptide genes in a single cell type. Experientia 48: 464–473.

Grimmelikhuijzen, C. J. P., and D. Graff. 1986. Isolation of Glu-Gly-Arg-Phe-NH_2 (anthoRFamide), a neuropeptide from sea anenomes. Proc. Natl. Acad. Sci. U.S.A. 83: 9817–9821.

Grimmelikhuijzen, C. J. P., and J. A. Westfall. 1995. The nervous system of cnidarians. In: The Nervous Systems of Invertebrates: An Evolutionary and Comparative Approach. Eds. O. Breidbach and W. Kutsch. Basel, Birkhäuser, pp. 7–24.

Halton, D. W., C. Shaw, A. G. Maule, et al. 1992. Peptidergic messengers: A new perspective of the nervous system of parasitic platyhelminths. J. Parisitol. 78: 179–193.

Harrison, L. M., A. J. Kastin, J. T. Weber, et al. 1994. The opiate system in invertebrates. Peptides 15: 1359–1329.

Hasson, A., K. J. Shon, B. M. Olivera, et al. 1995. Alterations of voltage-activated sodium current by a novel conotoxin from the venom of *Conus gloriamaris*. J. Neurophysiol. 73: 1295–1302.

Holman, G. M., R. J. Nachman, and M. S. Wright. 1990. Insect neuropeptides. Annu. Rev. Entomol. 35: 201–217.

Holman, G. M., M. S. Wright, and R. J. Nachman. 1988. Insect neuropeptides: Coming of age. In: ISI Atlas of Science, Vol. 1, pp. 129–136.

Hooper, S. L., W. C. Probst, E. C. Cropper, et al. 1994. Myomodulin application increases cAMP-dependent protein kinase in the accessory radula closer muscle of *Aplysia*. Neurosci. Lett. 179: 167–170.

Horodyski, F. M., J. Ewer, L. M. Riddiford, et al. 1993. Isolation, characterization and expression of the eclosion hormone gene. Eur. J. Biochem. 215: 221–228.

Hua, Y.-J, R.-J. Jiang, and J. Koolman. 1997. Multiple control of ecdysone biosynthesis in blowfly larvae: Interaction of ecdysiotropins and ecdysiostatins. Arch. Insect Biochem. Physiol. 35: 125–134.

Ichikawa, T. 1992. Growth of axon collaterals of eclosion hormone neurons into a new release site during metamorphosis of *Bombyx mori*. Neurosci. Lett. 138: 14–18.

Jonas, E. A., R. J. Knox, L. K. Kaczmarek, et al. 1996. Insulin receptor in *Aplysia* neurons—Characterization, molecular cloning and modulation of ion currents. J. Neurosci. 16: 1645–1658.

Kandel, E. R. 1976. Behavioral biology of *Aplysia*. San Francisco, Freeman, p. 137.

Karlson, P., and M. Luscher. 1959. "Pheromones" a new term for a class of biologically active substances. Nature 183: 55–56.

Karagogeos, D., and G. C. Papadopoulos. 1994. Localization of molluscan R15 alpha 2 peptide immunoreactivity in the mammalian brain. Brain Res. 650: 275–282.

Keller, R. 1992. Crustacean neuropeptides: Structures, functions and comparative aspects. Experientia 48: 439–448.

Kellett, E., S. J. Perry, N. Santama, et al. 1996. Myomodulin gene of *Lymnaea*—Structure, expression and analysis of neuropeptides. J. Neurosci. 16: 4949–4957.

Kellett, E., S. E. Saunders, K. W. Li, et al. 1994. Genomic organization of the FMRFamide gene in *Lymnaea*—Multiple exons encoding novel neuropeptides. J. Neurosci. 14: 6564–6570.

Kelly, T. J., E. P. Masler, and J. V. Menn. 1994. Insect neuropeptides. In: Natural and Engineered Pest Manngement. Eds. P. A. Hedin, J. J. Menn, and R. M. Hollingsworth. ACS Symposium Series. Vol. 551. Washington, D.C., American Chemical Society, pp. 292–318.

Kopeč, S. 1922. Studies on the necessity of the brain for the inception of insect metamorphosis. Biol. Bull. 42: 323–342.

Kreiner, T., M. Schaefer, and R. H. Scheller. 1986. *Aplysia* neuroendocrine system. Front. Neuroendocrinol. 9: 1–29.

Kuramato, T., and A. Ebara. 1989. Contraction of flap muscles in the cardioarterial valve of *Panuliris japonicus*. Comp. Biochem. Physiol. 93A: 419–422.

Lange, A. B., I. Orchard, Z. Wang, et al. 1995. A non-peptide agonist of the invertebrate receptor for SchistoFLRFamide (PDVDHVFLRFamide), a member of a subfamily of insect FMRFamide-related peptides. Proc. Nat. Acad. Sci. U.S.A. 92: 9250–9253.

Laurent, V., P. Bulet, and M. Salzet. 1995. A comparison of the leech *Theromyzon tessulatum* angiotensin I–like molecule with forms of vertebrate angioteninogens—a hormonal system conserved in the course of evolution. Neurosci. Lett. 190: 175–178.

Leung, P. S., C. Shaw, C. F. Johnston, et al. 1994. Immunocytochemical distribution of neuropeptide F (NPF) in the gastropod mollusc, *Helix aspersa* and in several other invertebrates. Cell Tissue Res. 275: 383–393.

Li, K. W., R. M. Hoek, F. Smith, et al. 1994a. Direct peptide profiling by mass spectometry of single identified neurons reveals complex neuropeptide processing pattern. J. Biol. Chem. 269: 30288–30292.

Li, K. W., F. A. Vangolen, J. Vanminnen, et al. 1994b. Structural identification, neuronal synthesis, and role in male copulation of myomodulin-A of *Lymnaea*—A study involving direct peptide profiling of nervous tissue by mass spectrometry. Mol. Brain Res. 25: 355–358.

Lingueglia, E., G. Champigny, M. Lazdunski, et al. 1995. Cloning of the amiloride-sensitive FMRFamide peptide gated sodium channel. Nature 378: 730–733.

Loechner, K. J., and L. K. Kaczmarek. 1994. Autoactive peptides act at 3 distinct receptors to depolarize the bag cell neurons of *Aplysia*. J. Neurophysiol. 71: 195–203.

Madrid, K. P., D. A. Price, M. J. Greenberg, et al. 1994. FMRFamide-related peptides from the kidney of the snail, *Helisoma trivolvis*. Peptides 15: 31–36.

Martin, R., and K. H. Voigt. 1987. The neurosecretory system of the octopus vena cava. Experientia 43: 537–543.

Masler, E. P. 1997. Neurally derived factors that affect in vitro ecdysteroid production by prothoracic glands of the gypsy moth *Lymantria dispar*: Possible developmental regulators. Ann. N.Y. Acad. Sci. 814: 145–161.

Maule, A. G., D. W. Halton, and C. Shaw. 1995. Neuropeptide F—a ubiquitous invertebrate neuromediator. Hydrobiologia 305(1–3): 297–303.

Menn, J. J., T. J. Kelly, and E. P. Masler, Eds. 1991. Insect Neuropeptides: Chemistry, Biology and Action. Washington, D.C., American Chemical Society.

Mercier, A. J., M. Schiebe, and H. L. Atwood. 1990. Pericardial peptides enhance synaptic transmission and tension in phasic extensor muscles of crayfish. Neurosci. Lett. 111: 401–408.

Meredith, J., M. Ring, A. Macins et al., 1996. Locust ion transport peptide: Primary structure, cDNA and expression in a baculovirus system. J. Exp. Biol. 199: 1053–1059.

Muneoka, Y., and M. Kobayashi. 1992. Comparative aspects of structure and action of molluscan neuropeptides. Experientia 48: 448–456.

Muren, J. E., and D. R. Nässel 1996. Isolation of 5 tachykinin-related peptides from the midgut of the cockroach *Leucophaea maderae*—Existence of N-terminally extended isoforms. Regul. Peptides 65: 185–196.

Muren, J. E., and D. R. Nässel. 1997. Novel tachykinin-related peptides in the cockroach nervous system and intestine: Structure, distribution and actions. Ann. N.Y. Acad. Sci. 814: 312–314.

Nachman, R. J., G. M. Holman, and G. M. Coast. 1998. Mimetic analogs of the myotropic/diuretic insect kinin family. In: Arthropod Endocrinology: Perspectives and Recent Advances. Eds. G. M. Coast and S. G. Webster. Cambridge, Cambridge University Press. pp. 379–391.

Nachman, R. J., R. E. Isaac, G. M. Coast et al. 1997a. Aib-containing analogues of the insect kinin neuropeptide family demonstrate resistance to an insect angiotensin-converting enzyme and potent diuretic activity. Peptides 18: 53–57.

Nachman, R. J., E. H. Olender, V. A. Roberts, et al. 1996. A nonpeptidal peptidomimetic agonist of the insect FLRFamide myosuppressin family. Peptides 17: 313–320.

Nachman, R. J., V. A. Roberts, A. B. Lange, et al. 1997b. Active conformation and mimetic analog development for the pyrokinin/PBAN/diapause pupariation and myosuppressin insect neuropeptide families. In: Natural Pest Control Agents. Eds. P. Hedin, J. J. Menn, and R. M. Hollingworth. Washington, D.C. American Chemical Society. pp. 277–291.

Nässel. D. R. 1993. Neuropeptides in the insect brain: A review. Cell Tissue Res. 273: 1–29.

Norekian, T. P., and R. A. Satterlie. 1994. Small cardioactive peptide B increases the responsiveness of the neural system underlying prey capture reactions in the pteropod mollusc *Clione limacina*. J. Exp. Zool. 270: 136–147.

O'Shea, M., and M. Adams. 1986. Proctolin: From "gut factor" to model neuropeptide. In: Advances in Insect Physiology, Vol. 19. Eds. P. D. Evans and V. B. Wigglesworth. London, Academic Press, pp. 1–28.

Petri, B., M. Stengl, S. Wurden, et al. 1995. Immunocytochemical characterization of the accessory medulla in the cockroach *Leucophaea maderae*. Cell Tissue Res. 282: 3–19.

Phares, G. A., and P. E. Lloyd. 1996. Purification, primary structure, and neuronal localization of cerebral peptide 1. Peptides 17: 753–761.

Rachinsky, A., and S. S. Tobe. 1996. Role of 2nd messengers in the regulation of juvenile hormone production in insects, with particular emphasis on calcium and phosphoinositide signaling. Arch. Insect Biochem. Physiol. 33: 259–282.

Rao, K. R., and J. P. Riehm. 1989. The pigment-dispersing hormone family: Chemistry, structure-activity relations, and distribution. Biol. Bull. 177: 225–229.

Reich, G. 1992. A new peptide of the oxytocin-vasopressin family isolated from nerves of the cephalopod *Octopus vulgaris*. Neurosci. Lett. 134: 191–194.

Riddiford, L. M., and J. W. Truman. 1978. Biochemistry of insect hormones and insect growth regulators. In Biochemistry of Insects. Ed. M. Rockstein. New York, Academic Press, pp. 309–357.

Saito, H., Y. Takeuchi, R. Takeda, et al. 1994. The core and complementary sequence responsible for biological activity of the diapause hormone of the silkworm, *Bombyx mori*. Peptides 15: 1173–1178.

Salzet, M., P. Bulet, W. M. Weber, et al. 1996a. Structural characterization of a novel neuropeptide from the central nervous system of the leech *Erpobdella octoculata*—the leech osmoregulatory factor. J. Biol. Chem. 271: 7237–7243.

Salzet, M., P., M. Vergerbocquet, P. Bulet, et al. 1996b. Purification, sequence analysis and cellular localization of a prodynorphin-derived peptide related to the alpha-neoendorphin in the rhynchobdellid leech *Theromyzon tessulatum*. J. Biol. Chem. 271: 13191–13196.

Salzet, M., P. Bulet, C. Wattez, et al. 1994. FMRFamide-related peptides in the sex segmental ganglia of the pharyngobdellid leech *Erpobdella octoculata*—Identification and involvement in the control of hydric balance. Eur. J. Biochem. 221: 269–275.

Santama, N., K. W. Li, W. P. M. Geraerts, et al. 1996. Posttranslational processing of the alternative neuropeptide precursor encoded by the FMRFamide gene in the pulmonate snail *Lymnaea stagnalis*. Eur. J. Neurosci. 8: 968–977.

Santama, N., C. H. Wheeler, D. R. Skingsley, et al. 1995. Identification, distribution and physiological activity of 3 novel neuropeptides of *Lymnaea*—EFLRIamide and QFYRIamide encoded by the FMRFamide gene, and a related peptide. Eur. J. Neurosci. 7: 234–246.

Scharrer, B. 1975. The role of neurons in endocrine regulation: a comparative overview. In: Trends in Comparative Endocrinology. Ed. E. J. W. Barrington. Utica, N.Y., Thomas Griffiths, pp. 7–11.

Scharrer, B. 1987. Neurosecretion: Beginnings and new directions in peptide research. Annu. Rev. Neurosci. 10: 1–16.

Scharrer, B., and E. Scharrer. 1944. Neurosecretion. II: A comparison between the pars intercerebralis-cardiacum-allatum system in invertebrates and the hypothalamo-hypophyseal system of vertebrates. Biol. Bull. 87: 242–251.

Scharrer, E., and B. Scharrer. 1963. Neuroendocrinology. New York, Columbia University Press.

Schoofs, L., J. Van den Broeck, and A. De Loof. 1993. The myotropic peptides of *Locusta migratoria*: Structures, distribution, functions and receptors. Insect Biochem. Mol. Biol. 23: 859–881.

Schoofs, L., D. Veelaert, G. M. Holman, et al. 1994. Partial identification, synthesis and immunolocalization of locustamyoinhibin, the 3rd myoinhibiting neuropeptide isolated from *Locusta migratoria*. Regul. Peptides 52: 139–156.

Soyez, D. 1997. Occurrence and diversity of neuropeptides from the crustacean hyperglycemic family in arthropods: A short review. Ann. N.Y. Acad. Sci. 814: 509–512.

Spring, J. H. 1990. Endocrine regulation of diuresis in insects. J. Insect Physiol. 36: 13–22.

Stone, J. V., W. Mordue, K. E. Batley, et al. 1976. Structure of locust adipokinetic hormone, a neurohormone that regulates lipid utilization during flight. Nature 263: 207–211.

Swales, L. S., and P. D. Evans. 1995. Distribution of myomodulin-like immunoreactivity in the brain and retrocerebral complex of the locust *Schistocerca gregaria*. J. Comp. Neurol. 353: 407–414.

Teal, P. E. A., J. H. Tumlinson, and H. Oberlander. 1990. Endogenous suppression of pheromone production in virgin female moths. Experientia 46: 1047–1050.

Thompson, K. S. J., R. C. Rayne, C. R. Gibbon, et al. 1995. Cellular co-localization of diuretic peptides in locusts: A potent control mechanism. Peptides 16: 95–104.

Turner, C. W. D. 1966. General Endocrinology, 4th Ed. Philadelphia, W. B. Saunders, p. 70.

Van Kesteren, R. E., F. A. Vangolen, K. W. Li, et al., 1995. A novel method to study diversity and functions of peptides in neuronal networks—peptides of the network underlying male copulation behavior in the mollusk *Lymnaea stagnalis*. Neth. J. Zool. 45: (1–2): 57–63.

Wainwright, G., S. G. Webster, M. C. Wilkinson, et al. 1996. Structure and significance of mandibular organ-inhibiting hormone in the crab, *Cancer pagurus*. J. Biol. Chem. 271: 12749–12754.

Wells, M. J. 1968. Lower Animals. World University Library. New York, McGraw-Hill p. 179.

Wells, M. J., and J. Wells. 1959. The mechanism of hormonal control of gonad maturation in *Octopus*. J. Exp. Biol. 36: 1–33.

Wenning, A., and R. L. Calabrese. 1995. Endogenous peptide modulates the activity of a sensory neuron in the leech *Hirudo medicinalis*. J. Exp. Biol. 198: 1405–1415.

Wiens, B. L., and P. H. Brownell. 1994. Neuroendocrine control of egg-laying behavior in the nudibranch, *Archidoris montereyensis*. J. Comp. Neurol. 344: 619–625.

Appendix A: Abbreviations for Neuropeptides (synonyms in parentheses)

ACTH	adrenocorticotropic hormone (corticotropin)
ADH	antidiuretic horomne (vasopressin)
AKH	adipokinetic hormone
ANH	atrionatriuretic hormone
AT	angiotensin
AVP	arginine vasopressin
BCP	bag cell peptide
bGH	bovine growth hormone
BNP	brain natriuretic peptide
CCAP	calcitonin carboxyl-adjacent peptide (katacalcin); crustacean cardioactive peptide
CCK	cholecystokinin
CG	chorionic gonadotropin
CGRP	calcitonin gene–related peptide
CHH	crustacean hyperglycemic hormone
CLIP	corticotropin-like intermediate lobe peptide
C peptide	connecting peptide
CNP	C-type natriuretic peptide
CRH	corticotropin-releasing hormone
CT	calcitonin
DSIP	delta sleep–inducing peptide
EDNH	egg development neurosecretory hormone
EGF	epidermal growth factor
EH	eclosion hormone
ELH	egg-laying hormone
ETH	ecdysis-triggering hormone
FaRP	FMRFamide-related peptide
FMRFamide	Phe-Met-Arg-Phe-NH_2
FSH	follicle-stimulating hormone
GAP	GnRH-associated peptide
GH	growth hormone
GHIH	GH release–inhibiting hormone (somatostatin)
GHRH	growth hormone–releasing hormone
GHRP	growth hormone–releasing peptide
GIH	gonad-inhibiting hormone
GIP	gastric inhibitory peptide
GLP	glucagon-like peptide
GLU	glucagon
GnRH	gonadotropin-releasing hormone
GRF	gonadotropin-releasing factor
GRP	gastrin-releasing peptide
GRPP	glucagon-related pancreatic peptide
hCG	human chorionic gonadotropin
IGF	insulin-like growth factor
IP	intervening peptide
ITP	ion transport peptide
JP	joining peptide
LANP	long-acting natriuretic peptide
LDCV	large dense-core vesicle
LH	luteinizing hormone
LHRH	luteinizing hormone–releasing hormone
LHRH-lp	LHRH-like peptide
LVP	lysine vasopressin
LYCP	light yellow cell peptide
MCH	melanin-concentrating hormone
MIF	melanocyte-stimulating hormone release inhibiting factor
MIH	molt-inhibiting hormone

MIP	molluscan insulin–related peptide
MOIH	mandibular organ–inhibiting hormone
MPGF	major proglucagon fragment
MSH	melanocyte-stimulating hormone
NGF	nerve growth factor
NKA	neurokinin A (substance K)
NKB	neurokinin B (neuromedin K)
NmB	neuromedin B
NmN	neuromedin N
NPR	natriuretic peptide receptor
NPF	neuropeptide F
NP-γ	neuropeptide-γ
NPY	neuropeptide Y
OT	oxytocin
PACAP	pituitary adenylate cyclase–activating peptide
PBAN	pheromone biosynthesis–activating neuropeptide
PHI	peptide histidine isoleucine
PIF	prolactin release-inhibiting factor
PL	placental lactogen (choriomammotropin)
POMC	pro-opiomelanocortin
PP	pancreatic polypeptide
PPT	preprotachykinin
PRF	prolactin-releasing factor
PRL	prolactin
PTH	parathyroid hormone (parathormone)
PTH-rP	parathyroid hormone–related protein
PTTH	prothoracicotropic hormone (prothoracicotropin)
PY	peptide Y
PYY	peptide YY
RPCH	red pigment–concentrating hormone
SCP	small cardioactive peptide
SRIF	somatotropin release–inhibiting factor (somatostatin)
SP	substance P
T_3	triiodothyronine
T_4	tetraiodotyrosin thyroxine
TMOF	trypsin-modulating oostatic factor
TRH	thyrotropin-releasing hormone
TSH	thyroid-stimulating hormone
Tyr-MIF-1	Tyr-Pro-Leu-Gly-NH_2
Tyr-W-MIF-1	Tyr-Pro-Trp-Gly-NH_2
VIH	vitellogenesis-inhibiting hormone (gonad-inhibiting hormone)
VIP	vasoactive intestinal polypeptide
VP	vasopressin (antidiuretic hormone)

Appendix B: Miscellaneous Abbreviations

ACh	acetylcholine
ACE	angiotensin-converting enzyme
AMP	adenosine monophosphate
AP	action potential
ARC	accessory radula closer
ATP	adenosine triphosphate
BBB	blood-brain barrier
BNST	bed nucleus of stria terminalis
BUI	brain uptake index
CAL	calmodulin
cAMP	cyclic adenosine monophosphate
cDNA	complementary DNA
cGMP	cyclic guanosine monophosphate
CNS	central nervous system
CSF	cerebrospinal fluid
CVO	circumventricular organ
DA	dopamine
DIT	diiodotyrosine
DNA	deoxyribonucleic acid
DOPA	dihydroxyphenylalanine
DRG	dorsal root ganglion
ECF	extracellular fluid
EEG	electroencephalogram
EGTA	ethyleneglycoltetraacetic acid
EPSP	excitatory postsynptic potential
ER	endoplasmic reticulum
ERP	electroretinogram
GABA	γ-aminobutyric acid
GDP	guanosine diphosphate
GTP	guanosine triphosphate
GMP	guanosine monophosphate
GPCR	G protein-couple receptor
HPA	hypothalamic-pituitary-adrenal
HPG	hypothalamic-pituitary-gonadal
HPLC	high-performance liquid chromatography
HPT	hypothalamic-pituitary-thyroid
5-HT	5-hydroxytryptamine (serotonin)
ICF	intracellular fluid
i.c.v.	intracerebroventricular
IDDM	insulin-dependent diabetes mellitus
IL	interleukin
IP_3	inositol 1,4,5-triphosphate
IPSP	inhibitory postsynaptic potential
i.v.	intravenous
JH	juvenile hormone
LATS	long-acting thyroid stimulator
LPS	lipopolysaccharide
MAP	microtubule-associated protein
MBH	medial basal hypothalamus
MCR	melanocortin receptor
ME	median eminence
MEPP	miniature endplate potential
MIT	monoiodotyrosine
MMC	migrating motor complex
MPOA	medial preoptic area
mRNA	messenger ribonucleic acid
NA	noradrenalin
NE	norepinephrine
NGF	nerve growth factor
NIDDM	non–insulin-dependent diabetes mellitus
NMDA	*N*-methyl-D-aspartate
NO	nitric oxide
NOS	nitric oxide synthase
NPR	natriuretic peptide receptor
OVLT	organum vasculosum of the lamina terminalis

PAM	peptidylglycine α-amidating monoxygenase
PC	prohormone convertase
PCE	pro-opiomelanocortin–converting enzyme
PCR	polymerase chain reaction
PI	phosphatidylinositol
PCR	polymerase chain reaction
PIP_2	phosphatidylinositol 4,5-biphosphate
POA	preoptic area
PVN	paraventricular nucleus
REM	rapid eye movement
RER	rough endoplasmic reticulum
RIA	radioimmunoassay
rpHPCL	reversed phase high-performance liquid chromatography
RRA	radioreceptor assay
rRNA	ribosomal RNA
SAM	sympathoadrenal medullary
SCN	suprachiasmatic nucleus
SF	steroidogenic factor
SON	supraoptic nucleus
Tg	thyroglobulin
TNF	tumor necrosis factor
TTR	transthyretin
VM	ventral midline
VMN	ventromedial nucleus

Appendix C: Code Letters for Amino Acids

Alanine	Ala	A
Arginine	Arg	R
Asparagine	Asn	N
Aspartic acid	Asp	D
Cysteine	Cys	C
Glutamic acid	Glu	E
Glutamine	Gln	Q
Glycine	Gly	G
Histidine	His	H
Isoleucine	Ile	I
Leucine	Leu	L
Lysine	Lys	K
Methionine	Met	M
Phenylalanine	Phe	F
Proline	Pro	P
Serine	Ser	S
Threonine	Thr	T
Tryptophan	Trp	W
Tyrosine	Tyr	Y
Valine	Val	V

Index